Manual of Rheumatology and Outpatient Orthopedic Disorders

Diagnosis and Therapy

Fourth Edition

Manual of Rheumatology and Outpatient Orthopedic Disorders

Diagnosis and Therapy

Fourth Edition

Editors

Stephen A. Paget, M.D.
Joseph P. Routh Professor of Medicine
Weill Medical College of Cornell University;
Physician-in-Chief
Attending Rheumatologist and Chair
Division of Rheumatology
Hospital for Special Surgery;
New York Presbyterian Hospital
New York, New York

Allan Gibofsky, M.D., J.D.
Professor of Medicine and Public Health
Weill Medical College of Cornell University;
Professor of Law, Fordham University;
Attending Rheumatologist
Division of Rheumatology
Hospital for Special Surgery;
New York Presbyterian Hospital
New York, New York

John F. Beary, III, M.D.
Clinical Professor of Medicine
University of Cincinnati;
Attending Physician
Rheumatology Division
Veterans Administration Medical Center
Cincinnati, Ohio

Associate Editor
Paul Pellicci, M.D.
Associate Professor of Surgery (Orthopedic)
Weill Medical College of Cornell University;
Associate Attending Surgeon
Hospital for Special Surgery
New York, New York

Forewords by
John L. Decker, M.D.
National Institutes of Health
Bethesda, Maryland

Charles L. Christian, M.D.
Physician-in-Chief Emeritus
Hospital for Special Surgery
New York, New York

LIPPINCOTT WILLIAMS & WILKINS
A **Wolters Kluwer** Company
Philadelphia • Baltimore • New York • London
Buenos Aires • Hong Kong • Sydney • Tokyo

Acquisitions Editor: Richard Winters
Developmental Editor: Michelle LaPlante
Production Editor: Emily Lerman
Manufacturing Manager: Colin J. Warnock
Cover Illustrator: Patricia Gast
Compositor: Circle Graphics
Printer: R.R. Donnelley, Crawfordsville

530 Walnut Street
Philadelphia, PA 19106 USA
LWW.com

Printed in the USA

Library of Congress Cataloging-in-Publication Data

Manual of rheumatology and outpatient orthopedic disorders : diagnosis and therapy / editors, Stephen A. Paget, Allan Gibofsky, John F. Beary, III ; associate editor, Paul Pellicci ; forewords by John L. Decker, Charles L. Christian.—4th ed.
p. ; cm.
Includes bibliographical references and index.
ISBN 0-7817-1576-8 (alk. paper)
1. Rheumatology—Handbooks, manuals, etc. 2. Orthopedics—Handbooks, manuals, etc. I. Paget, Stephen A. II. Gibofsky, Allan. III. Beary, John F.
[DNLM: 1. Rheumatic Diseases—diagnosis—Handbooks. 2. Rheumatic Diseases—therapy—Handbooks. 3. Ambulatory Care—Handbooks. 4. Bone Diseases—Handbooks. WE 39 M294 2000]
RC927.M346 2000
616.7'23—dc21

99-045307

---

10 9 8 7 6 5 4 3 2 1

With love, we dedicate this book of knowledge to our families:
Sandra Paget, Daniel, Matthew, and Lauren
Karen Gibofsky, Lewis, Esther, and Laura
Bianca Beary, John Daniel, Vanessa, Webster, and Nina

CONTENTS

III. DIAGNOSIS AND THERAPY
A. CONNECTIVE TISSUE DISORDERS

E. OSTEOARTHRITIS, METABOLIC BONE, AND ENDOCRINE DISORDERS

F. OTHER RHEUMATIC DISORDERS

IV. ORTHOPEDIC SURGERY AND REHABILITATION: PRINCIPLES AND PRACTICE

APPENDICES

CONTRIBUTING AUTHORS

John P. Allegrante, M.D.
Senior Scientist, Research Division, Hospital for Special Surgery; Adjunct Associate Professor of Behavioral Science, Weill Medical College and Graduate School of Medical Sciences; Professor of Health Education, Teachers College, Columbia University, 525 West 120th Street, New York, New York 10027

John F. Beary, III, M.D.
Clinical Professor of Medicine, University of Cincinnati; Attending Physician, Rheumatology Division, Veterans Administration Medical Center, 3200 Vine Street, Cincinnati, Ohio 45220

Stephen E. Bloomfield, M.D.
Formerly Attending Physician, Department of Ophthalmology, Mt. Sinai Medical Center, 5 East 98th Street, New York, New York 10029

Stefano Bombardieri, M.D.
Associate Professor and Chief, Division of Clinical Immunology, Department of Internal Medicine, University of Pisa, Via Roma 67, 56126 Pisa, Italy

Barry D. Brause, M.D.
Associate Professor of Clinical Medicine, Weill Medical College of Cornell University; Attending Physician, Hospital for Special Surgery, 535 East 70th Street, New York, New York 10021

Gordon A. Brody, M.D.
Clinical Associate Professor, Division of Orthopedic Surgery, Department of Functional Restoration, Stanford University School of Medicine, 900 Blake Wilbur Drive, Stanford, California 94305

Lisa R. Callahan, M.D.
Assistant Professor of Orthopedic Surgery, Weill Medical College of Cornell University; Assistant Attending Physician, Hospital for Special Surgery, 525 East 70th Street, New York, New York 10021

Giovanna Cirigliano, M.D.
Fellow, Clinical Immunology Unit, University of Pisa, Via Roma 67, 56126 Pisa, Italy

Daniel J. Clauw, M.D.
Professor of Medicine and Chief, Division of Rheumatology, Department of Medicine, Georgetown University School of Medicine, 3800 Reservoir Road NW, Washington, D.C. 20007

Theresa Colosi, M.D.
Private Practice, San Jose, California 95113

Charles N. Cornell, M.D.
Associate Professor of Orthopedic Surgery, Weill Medical College of Cornell University, 1300 York Avenue, New York, New York 10021

Mary Kuntz Crow, M.D.
Professor of Medicine, Weill Medical College of Cornell University; Senior Scientist, Hospital for Special Surgery, 535 East 70th Street, New York, New York 10021

Keith B. Elkon, M.D.
Professor of Medicine, Weill Medical College of Cornell University; Senior Scientist and Director, Rheumatology Research Program, Hospital for Special Surgery, 535 East 70th Street, New York, New York 10021

Theodore R. Fields, M.D.
Associate Professor of Clinical Medicine, Weill Medical College of Cornell University; Associate Attending Physician, Hospital for Special Surgery-New York Presbyterian Hospital, 535 East 70th Street, New York, New York 10021

Harry E. Figgie, III, M.D.
Retired

Sandy B. Ganz, M.D.
Director of Rehabilitation, Amsterdam Nursing Home; Associate in Research, Hospital for Special Surgery, 535 East 70th Street, New York, New York 10021

Allan Gibofsky, M.D., J.D.
Professor of Medicine and Public Health, Weill Medical College of Cornell University Professor of Law, Fordham University; Attending Rheumatologist, Hospital for Special Surgery, 535 East 70th Street, New York, New York 10021

Toni Golin, P.T.
Senior Occupational Therapist, Hospital for Special Surgery, 535 East 70th Street, New York, New York 10021

James Halper, M.D.
Assistant Professor of Psychiatry, Weill Medical College of Cornell University; Director, Psychiatric Disorders Program, Payne Whitney Clinic, 425 East 61st Street, New York, New York 10021

Jo A. Hannafin, M.D., Ph.D.
Assistant Professor of Orthopedic Surgery, Weill Medical College of Cornell University; Assistant Attending Orthopedic Surgeon, Hospital for Special Surgery, 535 East 70th Street, New York, New York 10021

Louis L. Harris, M.D.
Senior Administrator and Director, Network Development and Planning, Burke Rehabilitation Hospital, 785 Mamaroneck Avenue, White Plains, New York 10605

John H. Healey, M.D.
Associate Professor of Orthopedic Surgery, Weill Medical College of Cornell University; Chief, Orthopedic Service, Memorial Sloan-Kettering Cancer Center, 1275 York Avenue, New York, New York 10021

Robert N. Hotchkiss, M.D.
Associate Professor of Clinical Orthopedic Surgery, Weill Medical College of Cornell University; Hospital for Special Surgery, 535 East 70th Street, New York, New York 10021

Robert D. Inman, M.D.
Professor of Medicine and Immunology and Director, Rheumatology Division, The Toronto Hospital, 339 Bathurst Street, Toronto, Ontario M5T 2S8, Canada

Michael I. Jacobs, M.D.
Clinical Assistant Professor of Dermatology, Hospital for Special Surgery; New York Hospital-Cornell University Medical Center, 407 East 70th Street, New York, New York 10021

Norman A. Johanson, M.D.
Associate Professor of Orthopedic Surgery Hospital for Special Surgery; Temple University School of Medicine; Medical Director, Temple Arthritis and Joint Center; Department of Orthopedics, Temple University Hospital, Broad and Ontario Streets, Philadelphia, Pennsylvania 19140

Alan T. Kaell, M.D.
Professor of Medicine, State University of New York, Stony Brook; Chief, Division of Rheumatology, St. Charles Health System, 7 Medical Drive, Port Jefferson, New York 11776

Lawrence J. Kagan, M.D.
Professor of Medicine, Weill Medical College of Cornell University; Attending Physician, New York Presbyterian Hospital; Attending Physician, Hospital for Special Surgery, 535 East 70th Street, New York, New York 10021

Stuart S. Kassan, M.D.
Clinical Professor of Medicine, University of Colorado Health Sciences Center; Colorado Arthritis Associates, 4200 West Conejos Place, Denver, Colorado 80204

Robert P. Kimberly, M.D.
Howard L. Holley Professor of Medicine and Director, Division of Clinical Immunology and Rheumatology, University of Alabama at Birmingham School of Medicine; Director, University of Alabama Arthritis and Musculoskeletal Center, Tinsley Harrison Tower, 1900 University Boulevard, Birmingham, Alabama 35294

Kyriakos A. Kirou, M.D.
Instructor in Medicine, Weill Medical College of Cornell University; Assistant Scientist, Hospital for Special Surgery, 535 East 70th Street, New York, New York 10021

Joseph M. Lane, M.D.
Professor of Orthopedic Surgery, Weill Medical College of Cornell University; Hospital for Special Surgery, 535 East 70th Street, New York, New York 10021

Thomas J. A. Lehman, M.D.
Professor of Clinical Pediatrics, Weill Medical College of Cornell University; Chief, Division of Pediatric Rheumatology, Hospital for Special Surgery, 535 East 70th Street, New York, New York 10021

David S. Levine, M.D.
Instructor in Orthopedic Surgery, Weill Medical College of Cornell University; Hospital for Special Surgery, 535 East 70th Street, New York, New York 10021

Michael D. Lockshin, M.D.
Professor of Medicine, Weill Medical College of Cornell University; Director, Barbara Volcker Center for Women and Rheumatic Disease, Hospital for Special Surgery, 535 East 70th Street, New York, New York 10021

Paul Lombardi, M.D.
Senior Clinical Associate in Orthopedic Surgery, Weill Medical College of Cornell University; Hospital for Special Surgery, 535 East 70th Street, New York, New York 10021

Michael E. Luggen, M.D.
Associate Professor of Medicine, University of Cincinnati Medical Center, Division of Immunology, 231 Bethesda Avenue, Cincinnati, Ohio 45267

C. Ronald MacKenzie, M.D.
Associate Professor of Clinical Medicine, Weill Medical College of Cornell University; Associate Attending Physician, Hospital for Special Surgery, 535 East 70th Street, New York, New York 10021

Steven K. Magid, M.D.
Associate Professor of Clinical Medicine, Weill Medical College of Cornell University; Associate Attending Physician, Hospital for Special Surgery, 535 East 70th Street, New York, New York 10021

Joseph A. Markenson, M.D.
Consultant, Memorial Sloan-Kettering Cancer Center; Professor of Clinical Medicine, Weill Medical College of Cornell University; Attending Physician, Hospital for Special Surgery, 535 East 70th Street, New York, New York 10021

Richard R. McCormack, M.D.
Associate Attending Orthopedic Surgeon, Hospital for Special Surgery; Associate Clinical Professor of Clinical Orthopedic Surgery, Weill Medical College of Cornell University, 1300 York Avenue, New York, New York 10021

Robert L. Merkow, M.D.
Deceased

Dror Mevorach, M.D.
Assistant Professor of Medicine, Tel-Aviv Sourasky Medical Center, 6 Weizman Street, Tel Aviv 64239, Israel

Alexander Miric, M.D.
Senior Clinical Associate Professor of Orthopedic Surgery, Weill Medical College of Cornell University; Hospital for Special Surgery, 535 East 70th Street, New York, New York 10021

Stephen Ray Mitchell, M.D.
Director, Residency Program, Department of Medicine, Georgetown University, 5PHC, 3800 Reservoir Road, Washington, D.C. 20007

Stephen A. Paget, M.D.
Joseph P. Routh Professor of Medicine, Weill Medical College of Cornell University; Physician-in-Chief, Attending Rheumatologist, and Chair, Division of Rheumatology, Hospital of Special Surgery, 535 East 70th Street, New York, New York 10021; New York Presbyterian Hospital

Edward J. Parrish, M.S., M.D.
Associate Professor of Clinical Medicine, Weill Medical College of Cornell University; Attending Physician, Hospital for Special Surgery, 535 East 70th Street, New York, New York 10021

Paul Pellicci, M.D.
Associate Professor of Surgery (Orthopedic), Weill Medical College of Cornell University; Associate Attending Surgeon, Hospital for Special Surgery, 535 East 70th Street, New York, New York 10021

Theodore Pincus, M.D.
Professor of Medicine, Division of Rheumatology, Vanderbilt University Medical Center, 203 Oxford House, Nashville, Tennessee 37232

J. Robert Polk, M.D.
Vice President of Clinical Services, St. Alphonsus Regional Medical Center, 1055 North Curtis Road, Boise, Idaho 83706

Tracey A. Revenson, PH.D.
Associate Professor of Psychology, City University of New York Graduate School and University Center, 33 West 42nd Street, New York, New York 10036

Michael Rubin, M.D.
Associate Professor of Clinical Neurology, Weill Medical College of Cornell University; Associate Attending Physician, Hospital for Special Surgery and New York Presbyterian Hospital, 535 East 70th Street, New York, New York 10021

Jane E. Salmon, M.D.
Professor of Medicine, Weill Medical College of Cornell University; Attending Physician, Hospital for Special Surgery and New York Presbyterian Hospital, 535 East 70th Street, New York, New York 10021

Lisa R. Sammaritano, M.D.
Assistant Professor of Medicine, Weill Medical College of Cornell University; Assistant Attending Physician, Hospital for Special Surgery and New York Presbyterian Hospital, 535 East 70th Street, New York, New York 10021

Nicholas P. Scarpa, M.D.
Clinical Assistant Professor, Department of Medicine and Rheumatology, New Jersey Medical School, 185 South Orange Avenue, Newark, New Jersey 07103

Eric S. Schned, M.D.
Medical Director, Park Nicollete Clinic, 3800 Park Nicollete Boulevard, Minneapolis, Minnesota 55416

Robert Schneider, M.D.
Associate Professor of Radiology, Weill Medical College of Cornell University; Attending Radiologist, Hospital for Special Surgery, 535 East 70th Street, New York, New York 10021

Thomas P. Sculco, M.D.
Professor of Clinical Orthopedic Surgery, Weill Medical College of Cornell University; Hospital for Special Surgery, 535 East 70th Street, New York, New York 10021

Nigel Sharrock, M.D.
Professor of Anesthesiology, Weill Medical College of Cornell University, 1300 York Avenue, New York, New York 10021

Robert F. Spiera, M.D.
Assistant Professor of Medicine, Weill Medical College of Cornell University; Assistant Attending Physician, Hospital for Special Surgery, 535 East 70th Street, New York, New York 10021

Richard Stern, M.D.
Clinical Associate Professor of Medicine, Weill Medical College of Cornell University; Attending Physician, Hospital for Special Surgery, 535 East 70th Street, New York, New York 10021

Russell F. Warren, M.D.
Professor of Orthopedic Surgery, Weill Medical College of Cornell University; Surgeon-in-Chief, Department of Orthopedics, Hospital for Special Surgery, 535 East 70th Street, New York, New York 10021

Scott S. Weissman, M.D.
Attending Physician, Columbia University College of Physicians and Surgeons; Attending Physician, Manhattan Eye and Ear Hospital; Attending Physician and Director, Uveitis Service, New York Eye and Ear Infirmary, 310 East 14th Street, New York, New York 10003

Thomas L. Wickiewicz, M.D.
Associate Professor of Clinical Orthopedic Surgery, Weill Medical College of Cornell University; Associate Attending Surgeon, Hospital for Special Surgery, 535 East 70th Street, New York, New York 10021

Riley J. Williams, M.D.
Instructor in Orthopedic Surgery, Weill Medical College of Cornell University, 1300 York Avenue, New York, New York 10021

Yusuf Yazici, M.D.
Postdoctoral Fellow in Rheumatology, Hospital for Special Surgery, 535 East 70th Street, New York, New York 10021

Arthur M. F. Yee, M.D.
Assistant Professor of Medicine, Weill Medical College of Cornell University; Assistant Attending Physician, Hospital for Special Surgery, 535 East 70th Street, New York, New York 10021

John B. Zabriskie, M.D.
Associate Professor of Clinical Microbiology and Immunology, Rockefeller University, 1230 York Avenue, New York, New York 10021

FOREWORD TO THE FIRST EDITION

Making and acting upon a decision are the critical events in any patient–physician encounter, although it is uncommon for either the patient or the physician to recognize the significance of this sequence. As the physician's experience with the problem at hand increases, the decisions and consequent actions often become more and more instinctual. In the early days of aviation, pilots, distrusting their primitive and frequently failing instruments, were said to have flown "by the seat of the pants"; so, too, may the physician go with the "feel" of the situation. This manual is built on facts. It describes the acquisition of needed facts from the physician–patient encounter in rheumatic disease, the integration of those data into a decision, and the action that logically results from that decision. It constitutes not only a reasonable substitute for experience for the younger physician but also an excellent yardstick against which the older can measure performance.

There was a time not long ago when the patient with rheumatoid arthritis was viewed as a collection of inflamed joints. The very concept of the disease as a systemic affliction, developed by clinicians of yesteryear such as Bauer, Ragan, Copeman, and Hench, was critical to the development of rheumatology as a discipline of internal medicine, while placing perhaps undue emphasis on systemic features. These pages help to restore the concepts that all that hurts is not systemic disease, that articular symptoms are the major feature of rheumatoid arthritis, and that those who would deal with disease manifesting as musculoskeletal pain must also be aware of local afflictions such as march fracture, tennis elbow, and slipped capital femoral epiphysis. These pages represent the happy juxtaposition of the medical and orthopedic surgical expertise of the Hospital for Special Surgery, a hospital with an enviable tradition of cooperation and of excellence in both disciplines.

The pearls are numerous and genuine, and yet no one will consider this manual all-encompassing. It would not be easy to compress a more practical and useful clinical introduction into fewer pages. The reader will use it as such: a personal introduction to the complex and fascinating pathophysiology of human locomotor disease.

John L. Decker, M.D.
National Institutes of Health
Bethesda, Maryland

FOREWORD

The composition and authorship of the *Manual of Rheumatology and Outpatient Orthopedic Disorders* continue to reflect the fact that rheumatology and orthopedic surgery have a seamless interface in pursuit of education and patient care goals relative to musculoskeletal disease. The interrelationship of these two disciplines is a special and unique feature of the Hospital for Special Surgery, where many of the authors have served.

The primary goal of this manual has been to serve the needs of students and physicians-in-training. Yet professionals of all ages (perhaps especially senior colleagues) find it useful for reviewing miscellaneous things not successfully committed to memory. These include: American College of Rheumatology Criteria for Diagnosis and Classification of Rheumatic Disease, neurologic dermatomes, molecular targets of autoantibodies, normal laboratory values, details in the formulary, etc. Between the third and fourth editions, there has been an explosion of the rheumatologic formulary; new antiinflammatories and other drugs in the DMARD category; some based on new insights relative to the pathogenesis of rheumatoid arthritis.

Over the span of four editions, several new chapters have been added: antiphospholipid syndrome, rheumatic associations with HIV infection, diagnostic imaging, patient education, perioperative management, measuring functional status, etc. The emphasis remains the discussion of practical aspects of management of musculoskeletal disorders.

Charles L. Christian, M.D.
Physician-in-Chief Emeritus
Hospital for Special Surgery
New York, New York

PREFACE

It is currently estimated that approximately 41 million people in the United States have a musculoskeletal condition. Of these, more than 50% have some limitation of functional activity and many have to stop work entirely. Musculoskeletal and rheumatic symptoms account for about 15% of physician visits. The purpose of this manual is to concentrate the knowledge explosion in musculoskeletal disease to a succinct and easily retrievable form in order to improve the lives of our patients.

Extraordinary advances have occurred in the field of rheumatology since the third edition of this manual was published in 1993, and they are featured in the body of our manual as well as in the Appendix on Therapeutics. These include the use of tumor necrosis factor alpha antagonists for the treatment of refractory rheumatoid arthritis, the ascendancy of the use and effectiveness of combination disease-modifying regimens in the treatment in inflammatory arthropathies, and the availability of Cox-2-specific nonsteroidal antiinflammatory drugs that are safer for the gastrointestinal tract. Disease modification is a reality today in rheumatology, not only in rheumatoid arthritis and systemic lupus erythematosus, but also in our treatment of Lyme disease, septic arthritis, gout, vasculitides such as Wegener's granulomatosis, polyarteritis nodosa, Kawasaki's disease, and the antiphospholipid syndrome.

Nearly all chapters are authored or coauthored by present and/or past members of the Division of Rheumatic Disease or the Department of Orthopedic Surgery at Hospital for Special Surgery in New York City. As is often the case in clinical medicine, some problems have more than one potential solution; in these instances, for the sake of clarity and brevity, we identify the areas of controversy, then detail the approach employed at our Hospital. In all instances, our physicians have tried to carefully balance their years of experience with an evidence-based approach to their diagnostic and therapeutic choices.

Although medical information is ever expanding and increasingly complex, the time to absorb it is limited. Given the increasing clinical, academic, social, and family pressures, the physician needs to have a "reliable, old friend" to enable him or her to rapidly make accurate, state-of-the-art clinical decisions. This fourth edition of the *Manual of Rheumatology and Outpatient Disorders* is designed to distill a massive body of knowledge to a user-friendly form for the busy clinician. Our aim is to bring the "laboratory bench" to the office and bedside so as to meet the needs of internists, family physicians, rheumatology trainees, house officers, and students.

Stephen A. Paget, M.D.
Allan Gibofsky, M.D.
John F. Beary, III, M.D.

ACKNOWLEDGMENTS

The authors gratefully acknowledge the assistance of their support staff, in particular Venus Te Eng Fo, Cookie Reyes, and Mary Kehoe, for all they have done to assist in the preparation of the manuscript. We are also grateful to so many of our colleagues who have offered helpful suggestions. Finally, our thanks to the excellent staff of Lippincott Williams & Wilkins, especially Michelle LaPlante, for their assistance in the preparation of this volume.

I. MUSCULOSKELETAL DATA BASE

1. MUSCULOSKELETAL HISTORY AND PHYSICAL EXAMINATION

Stephen A. Paget, Charles N. Cornell, and John F. Beary, III

The musculoskeletal or locomotor system, like other body systems, can be defined anatomically and assessed functionally. **Lower** extremities support the weight of the body and allow ambulation. They require proper alignment and stability. **Upper** extremities reach, grasp, and hold, thus allowing self-care, feeding, and work. They require mobility and strength. Diseases and disorders of the musculoskeletal system disturb anatomy and interfere with function.

Musculoskeletal History

A careful history is the most important and powerful of the information-gathering procedures used to define a patient's problems. In most musculoskeletal disorders, 80% of the diagnosis comes from this part of the clinical evaluation. The history of patients with rheumatic complaints should include the following: (a) reason for consultation and duration of complaints; (b) present medical care and medications; (c) chronologic review of present illness with emphasis on the locomotor system, consequences of time and disease, and present functional assessment; (d) past history of medical, surgical, and trauma; (e) social history, emotional and work impact of the disorder, and environmental and work site factors; (f) family history, especially as it relates to the musculoskeletal system; and (g) review of systems. These queries cover the spectrum of rheumatic complaints: pain, stiffness, joint swelling, lack of mobility, physical handicap, and fear of future disability and handicap. The interviewer should be flexible and tactful. Avoid interrupting the patient with too many questions; the interviewer should merely guide the flow of information. The objective is to define the patient's complaints and goals and to identify patterns of disease and areas of musculoskeletal involvement that can be further scrutinized on physical examination.

I. **Chief complaint.** Note duration.

II. **Primary physician.** Note name, telephone number, fax number, and e-mail address to assist in locating important data. A discussion with that physician may add greatly to your assessment, may avoid the need to repeat expensive tests already performed, and will better define the course and tempo of the disorder.

III. **History of rheumatic diseases**

- A. Determine the mode of onset, inciting events, duration, and pattern and progression of the musculoskeletal complaints.
    1. **Acute onset** is consistent with infectious, crystal-induced, or traumatic origin. It can also occur in the setting of a connective tissue disorder. Chronic complaints are seen with rheumatoid arthritis (RA), seronegative spondyloarthropathies, and osteoarthritis or the chronic sequelae of traumatic or degenerative back problems.
    2. The **pattern of joint involvement** is very important in defining the type of joint disorder. Symmetric polyarthritis of the small joints of the hands and feet is characteristic of RA, whereas asymmetric involvement of the large joints of the lower extremities is most typical of the seronegative spondyloarthropathies. A migratory pattern of joint inflammation is seen in rheumatic fever and disseminated gonococcemia. A monarticular arthritis is consistent with osteoarthritis, infectious arthritis, crystal-induced synovitis, or one of the seronegative spondyloarthropathies (e.g., psoriatic arthritis, Reiter's syndrome). An intermittent joint inflammation of the knee with remissions and exacerbations is typical of the tertiary phase of Lyme disease.
    3. **Location, pain characteristics, and associated findings** may all be important keys to the diagnosis. First, metatarsophalangeal joint inflam-

mation of an acute and severe type is quite characteristic of gouty arthritis. Sudden onset of low back pain in the setting of lifting or bending with associated pain radiating down the lateral leg is a common presentation for a disk herniation with sciatica.

Pain in the superolateral shoulder or upper arm occurring in the setting of tennis playing or painting a ceiling is typical of a supraspinatus tendinitis, or impingement syndrome.

B. Record the **severity of disease,** as revealed by a chronologic review of the following:

1. Ability to **work** during months or years.
2. Need for hospitalization or home confinement.
3. When applicable, ability to do household chores.
4. Activities of daily living and **personal care.**
5. Landmarks or significant **functional change,** such as retirement from work, need for household help, assistance for personal care, and use of cane, crutches, or wheelchair.

C. Assess **current functional ability.** This can be done in a question-and-answer format and quantified with the use of functional instruments such as the Health Assessment Questionnaire (HAQ) or the Arthritis Impact Measurement Scale (AIMS2), or functional ability can be measured with the use of a visual analog scale (0 representing no impact on function and 10 being the worst possible limitation in function).

1. At home: independence or reliance on help from family members and others.
2. At work: transportation and job requirements and limitations. Have the patient collect an hour-by-hour log of work activities, with an attempt to define actions that may cause or exacerbate musculoskeletal problems.
3. At recreational and social activities: limitations and extent to which patient is house-bound.
4. Review of a typical 24-hour period, with focus on abilities to transfer, ambulate, and perform personal care.

D. Obtain an overview of **management** for rheumatic disease.

1. Medications used in the past, with emphasis on dosages, duration of treatments, efficacy response, and possible adverse reactions. Record the present drug regimen and how well the patient complies with it, and also the patient's understanding of the reasons for and potential complications of the medication.
2. Instruction in and compliance with a **therapeutic exercise** program.
3. Surgical procedures on joints, including benefits and liabilities. Record the name of the surgeon, date of the surgery, and the hospital. Operative pathology reports may be helpful.

E. Determine the patient's understanding of the disease, therapeutic goals, and expectations.

F. Record **psychosocial** consequences of disease.

1. Anxiety, depression, insomnia. Obtain information about psychological/psychiatric intervention and a listing of psychotropic medications.
2. Economic impact of handicap and present means of support.
3. Family interrelationships.
4. Use of community resources.

IV. Past history. Follow traditional lines of questioning, with attention to trauma and joint operations. Also question the patient about those specific medical disorders that could have a significant impact on or association with the joint disorder.

Specific associations include psoriasis with psoriatic arthritis or gout; ulcerative colitis or Crohn's disease with inflammatory disease of the spine or peripheral or sacroiliac joints; diabetes with neuropathic, septic joints, or osteomyelitis; hemochromatosis with severe osteoarthritis; endocrinopathies such as hypothyroidism (carpal tunnel syndrome, myopathy), hyperparathyroidism (pseudogout), and acromegaly (severe osteoarthritis). A complete medication list is essential, as well as an inquiry into prior medications. Important in this context is drug-induced lupus associated with the use of hydralazine and procainamide, Raynaud's phenomenon associated with the use of beta blockers, eosinophilia-myalgia syndrome associated with L-tryptophan, or myositis associated with the use of "statin" drugs for hypercholesterolemia.

V. **Social history.** The physician must consider the following associations between the social history and types of musculoskeletal disorders:

A. **Work activities,** including the possibility of joint or back trauma, exposure to toxins, or overuse syndromes. Specific examples include low-back syndromes, exposure to vinyl chloride leading to scleroderma-type skin changes, and carpal tunnel syndrome resulting from typing at a computer terminal.

B. **Sexual history,** including sexual preference, sexual promiscuity, and the most recent sexual experience. Musculoskeletal disorders related to acquired immunodeficiency syndrome (AIDS) and venereal disorders such as gonococcal disease should be considered.

C. **Living site and conditions,** including overcrowding (e.g., rheumatic fever), living in an area where Lyme disease is endemic, or a recent or distant history of tick bite.

D. **Emotional or physical stress,** which could have an impact on the development or exacerbation of musculoskeletal disorders.

E. The presence of **medical problems within the family,** including infectious disorders in children (e.g., fifth disease caused by parvovirus B19, rubella) and adults (e.g., hepatitis B and C, Lyme disease, tuberculosis).

F. **Recent travel,** with specific emphasis on the development of dysentery caused by *Salmonella* or *Shigella* (e.g., reactive arthritis or Reiter's syndrome) or travel to an area where Lyme disease is endemic.

VI. **Family history.** Inquiry about arthritis and rheumatic disease in parents and siblings may elicit vague and unreliable statements, but they are nonetheless important. The presence of severely handicapped relatives with RA or other severe rheumatic disease might result in a significant psychological impact on the patient and should be brought out in the interview. Such information may also be important in relation to the genetic background of arthritis in the family. The physician should inquire about the following musculoskeletal disorders, which clearly have a tendency to run in families: gout and uric acid kidney stones; RA and other connective tissue disorders; ankylosing spondylitis and other seronegative spondyloarthropathies; osteoarthritis, especially nodal disease in the fingers; and "true" connective tissue disorders, such as Marfan syndrome.

VII. **Review of systems.** Emphasize diseases and system disorders related to rheumatic complaints and diseases of connective tissue. Especially inquire about eye disease (iritis, uveitis, conjunctivitis, dryness), mouth disorders (dryness, mouth sores, tightness), gastrointestinal problems (problems with swallowing, reflux symptoms, abdominal pain, diarrhea with or without blood, constipation), genitourinary complaints (including dysuria, urethral discharge, hematuria), and skin disorders (rash with or without sun sensitivity, nodules, ulcers, Raynaud's phenomenon, ischemic changes). The presence of constitutional symptoms is also important, including complaints of weight loss, fatigue, fever, chills, night sweats, and weakness.

Physical Examination with Emphasis on Rheumatic Disease

Five aspects of the physical examination that should be recorded are (a) **gait,** (b) **spine,** (c) **muscles,** (d) **upper extremities,** and (e) **lower extremities.** The patient should be properly attired in a short gown, open at the back to allow examination of the entire spine. Examination should be methodic and start with observation of the patient's attitude, comfort, apparent state of nutrition, ease of undressing, and method of rising from a chair and sitting down. The patient is examined while standing, sitting, and supine. The examiner should rely mainly on inspection. When using palpation and manipulation, the examiner should be gentle and forewarn the patient of potentially painful maneuvers.

I. Gait. Describe the gait, and note a limp or use of cane or crutches. The normal gait is divided into the phases of stance (60%) and swing (40%). Clinically important gaits include the following:

A. Antalgic gait, characterized by a short stance phase on the painful side.

B. Short-leg gait, with signs of pelvic obliquity and flexion deformity of the opposite knee.

C. Coxalgic gait, an antalgic gait with a lurch toward the painful hip.

D. Metatarsalgic gait, in which the patient tries to avoid weight bearing on the forefoot.

II. Standing position

A. Examining front and back, note **posture** (cervical lordosis, scoliosis, dorsal kyphosis, lumbar lordosis). Check if the pelvis is level by putting one finger on each iliac crest and noting asymmetry. Pelvic obliquity suggests unequal leg lengths. Note also if a tilt of the trunk to one side is present.

B. Examine **alignment of the lower extremities** for flexion deformity of the knees, genu varum (bowlegs), or genu valgum (knock-knees).

C. Observe **position of the ankles and feet** (varus or valgus heels, flat feet, inversion or eversion of feet).

D. Check **back motion** on forward bending (with rounding of the normal thoracolumbar spine), lateral flexion to each side, and hyperextension (see also section **IV.C**). The extent of **spinal flexion** can be assessed with a metal tape measure. One end of the tape is placed at the C-7 spinous process, and the other end is placed at S-1 with the patient standing erect. The patient is then asked to bend forward, flexing the spine maximally. The measuring tape will reveal an increase of 10 cm with normal spine flexion; 7.5 cm of the total increase results from lumbar spine (measured from spinous process T12-S1) mobility in normal adults. These measurements are useful for the serial evaluation of patients with spondyloarthropathy.

III. Seated position

A. Observe **head and neck motion** in all planes (Fig. 1-1).

B. Examine **thoracolumbar spine motion** with the pelvis fixed. Observe rounding and straightening of back, lateral flexion to each side, and rotation to right and left.

C. Check **temporomandibular joints.** Palpate, examine lower jaw motion, and measure the aperture between upper and lower teeth with the mouth fully open.

D. Proceed with the rest of the routine examination of the head and neck; describe eye, ear, nose, and throat findings.

E. Upper extremities

1. Shoulders

a. Note normal **contour** or "squaring" caused by deltoid atrophy. Palpate anteriorly for soft-tissue swelling and laterally under the acromion for tendon insertion tenderness.

b. Function of the entire shoulder complex is evaluated by elevating both arms from 0 degrees along the sides of body to 180 degrees straight above the head. Quantify **internal** rotation by having the patient reach with the dorsum of the hands the highest possible level of the back (Fig. 1-2); quantify **external** rotation by noting the position behind the neck or head that the hands can reach.

c. Isolate the **glenohumeral joint motion** from the scapulothoracic motion by **fixing the scapula**. Holding both hands, assist the patient in abducting arms to the normal maximum of 90 degrees, and note restriction of motion on either side. To determine internal and external rotation of the glenohumeral joint on each side, the examiner **places one hand on the shoulder to prevent scapular motion** and, with the other hand, assists each arm to full external rotation of 90 degrees and full internal rotation of 80 degrees (Fig. 1-3).

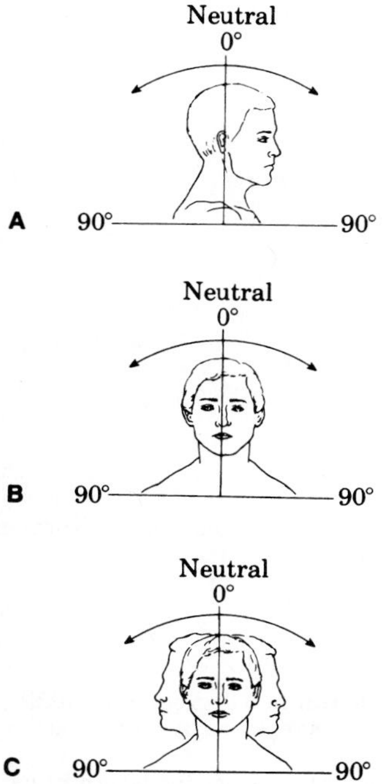

FIG. 1-1. Neck motion. **A:** Flexion and extension. **B:** Lateral bending. **C:** Rotation.

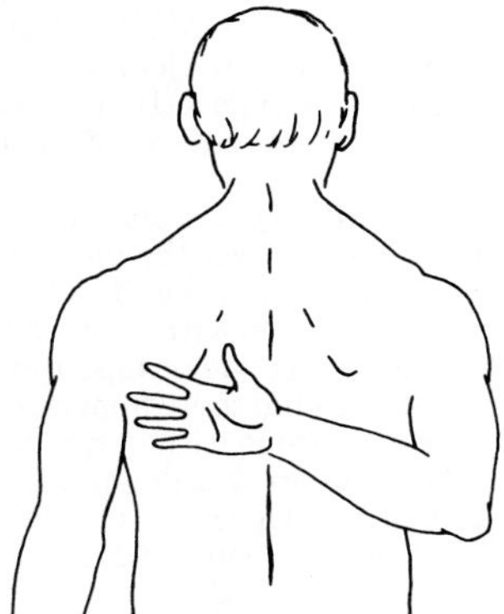

FIG. 1-2. Internal rotation of shoulder, posterior view. Record range of reach: Dorsum of hand to specific vertebral bodies.

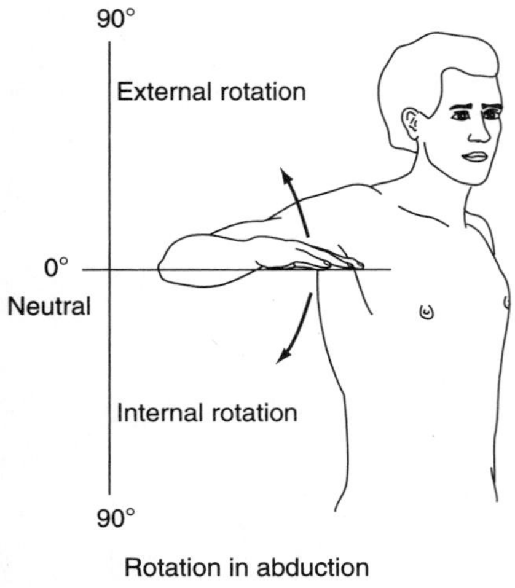

FIG. 1-3. Shoulder rotation (with arm in abduction).

2. Elbows

a. Inspect each elbow for **maximum extension** to 0 degrees and full flexion to 150 degrees. Less than full extension is reported in degrees as flexion deformity or lack of extension.

b. Inspection and palpation may reveal the presence of **olecranon bursitis** at the elbow tip or the soft-tissue swelling of **synovitis**, which is felt in the fossae between the olecranon and lateral epicondyle or between the olecranon and medial epicondyle.

c. Subcutaneous nodules and tophi should be sought in the olecranon bursa and over the extensor surface of the elbow and forearm.

3. Wrist and hands

a. Inspect and palpate wrists; metacarpophalangeal (MCP), proximal interphalangeal (PIP), and distal interphalangeal (DIP) joints of fingers; and carpometacarpal (CMC), MCP, and interphalangeal (IP) joints of thumbs (Fig. 1-4). Note shape and deformities: boutonniere, swan neck, and ulnar deviation.

b. Soft-tissue swelling has a spongy consistency and should be sought on the dorsum of the wrist distal to the ulna and over the radiocarpal joint. On the volar surface, the normal step-down from hand to forearm may be obliterated by soft-tissue swelling. Volar synovitis may be associated with carpal tunnel syndrome. Tapping on the volar aspect of the wrist may elicit paresthesias radiating into the radial three fingers, or even the forearm. This positive Tinel's sign is consistent with carpal tunnel syndrome. Thenar atrophy would further support this diagnosis.

c. All **finger joints** should be examined by inspection and palpation for soft-tissue swelling, capsular thickening, and bony enlargement.

d. Average wrist motion is dorsiflexion to 75 degrees, palmar flexion to 70 degrees, ulnar deviation of 45 degrees, and radial deviation of 20 degrees (Table 1-1).

e. The **fist** is described as 100% when all fingers reach the palm of the hand and the thumb closes over the fingers. Halfway fist closing is recorded as 50%; less than 50% and 75% are other possible intermediate measurements. The distance from fingertips to palm can also be recorded.

f. Grip is quantified by noting the patient's maximum strength in grasping two fingers of the examiner. **Pinch** is assessed by the force necessary to break the patient's pinch between index finger and thumb.

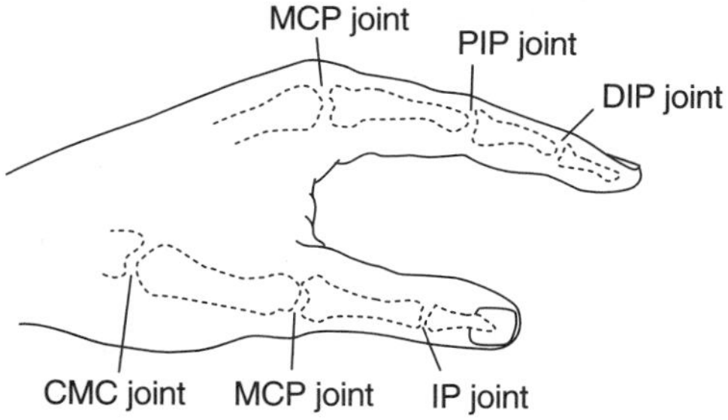

FIG. 1-4. Finger and thumb joints. *MCP,* metacarpophalangeal; *PIP,* proximal interphalangeal; *DIP,* distal interphalangeal; *CMC,* carpometacarpal; *IP,* interphalangeal.

g. **Pronation and supination** are combined functions of the elbow and wrist and are determined by having the patient hold the forearm horizontal and the thumb up. Pronation and supination are measured in degrees from the neutral position with the hand turning palm up and palm down (Fig. 1-5).

F. While the patient is sitting, customary physical examination of the **neck and chest** should be performed; it should include examination of sternoclavicular joints and measurement of **chest expansion,** which should be greater than 5 cm in the nipple line.

IV. **Supine position**

A. Start with the standard physical examination of the **abdomen,** and then proceed to the examination of the **lower extremities.**

B. Alignment of the **knees** is compared with the alignment noted on weight bearing (see section **II.B**). Palpate pedal pulses.

C. **Low back**

1. Inspection, palpation, and assessment of range of motion (see section **II.D**).
2. **Neurologic examination.** Look for radicular signs and root signatures (see section **I**).
3. **Traction maneuvers**

a. Straight leg-raising test to screen for lumbosacral nerve root symptoms; note angle of elevation that induces back or buttock pain.

b. **Gaenslen maneuver** to detect sacroiliac joint inflammation. Instruct the patient to lie supine on the examining table with knees flexed and one buttock over the edge. Ask the patient to drop the unsupported leg off the table. This maneuver will elicit pain in the sacroiliac joint ipsilateral to the extended hip. The maneuver exerts a traction force on the sacroiliac joint, which opens it up.

D. **Hips**

1. Hip function is screened by gently log-rolling each lower extremity and noting the freedom of motion of the **ball-and-socket joint.** Rolling also allows measurement of the **internal and external rotation** of the hip joint in extension.
2. With one hand fixing the pelvis, the other hand moves each hip to the normal 60 degrees of full **abduction** and to the normal 30 degrees of **adduction** while the hip is held in extension.
3. Each hip joint is then examined in **flexion;** both lower extremities are flexed at knees and hips and carried toward the chest, which gives the maximum angle (120 degrees) of flexion of each hip.
4. Normal hip **extension** is to minus 10 degrees. To avoid overlooking a hip flexion deformity for which accentuation of lumbar lordosis may compensate, the examiner keeps one lower extremity flexed over the chest, thus flatten-

Table 1-1. Average joint motion

Joint motion	Normal value
SPINE	
Cervical	
Forward flexion	40°
Lateral bending	30°
Extension	30°
Rotation	60°
Thoracic	
Rotation with pelvis fixed	45°
Chest expansion	>6 cm
Lumbar	
Forward flexion	90°
Lateral bending	30°
Extension	30°
UPPER EXTREMITIES	
Shoulder	
Abduction (arm at side and elevation above head)	180°
Rotation (arm in abduction to 90°)	
Internal	80°
External	90°
Elbow	
Flexion	150°
Extension	0°
Forearm	
Pronation	90°
Supination	85°
Wrist	
Extension	75°
Flexion	70°
Ulnar deviation	45°
Radial deviation	20°
Fist (in percentage)	
Full fist	100°
LOWER EXTREMITIES	
Hip	
Flexion	120°
Extension	-10°
In flexion	
Internal rotation	25°
External rotation	35°
Abduction	45°
Adduction	25°
In extension	
Abduction	60°
Adduction	30°
Knee	
Flexion	130°
Extension	0°
Ankle	
Flexion	15°
Extension	35°
Hind foot	
Inversion-eversion (subtalar) (in percentage)	
Full motion	100°

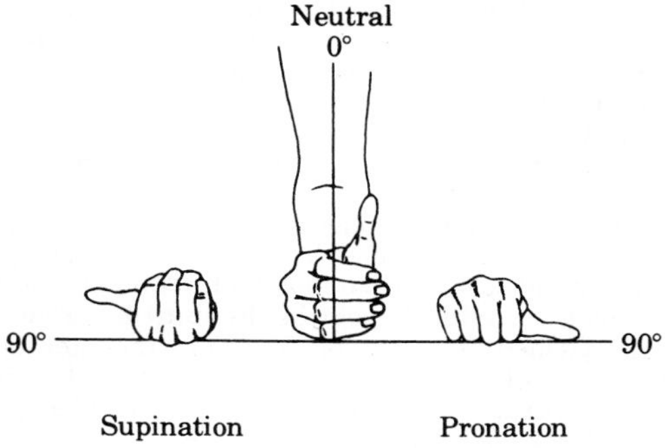

FIG. 1-5. Forearm pronation and supination.

ing the lumbar spine, while instructing the patient to extend fully the opposite leg.

5. With the hip in 90 degrees of flexion, the joint is evaluated for internal rotation (25 degrees), external rotation (35 degrees), abduction (45 degrees), and adduction (25 degrees) (Fig. 1-6).

E. Measurement of leg length (see Chapter 19).

F. Knees

1. By inspection and palpation, note position and mobility of **patellae.** Knee extension-flexion range is 0 to 130 degrees. Also palpate for the presence of osteophytes at tibiofemoral joint margin, which may also be tender.

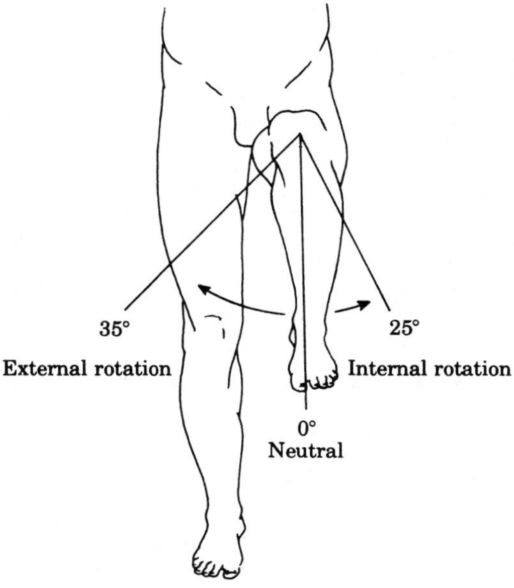

FIG. 1-6. Hip rotation in flexion.

2. **Soft-tissue swelling** is elicited by bimanual examination.
   a. Demonstrate intraarticular fluid by the **patellar click sign**. While compressing the suprapatellar pouch with one hand, push the patella against underlying fluid and the femoral condyle with the index finger of the other hand to elicit a click.
   b. For detection of a small amount of effusion, use the bulge sign. This maneuver is best executed by placing both hands on the knee so that the index fingers meet on the medial joint margin and the thumbs meet on the lateral aspect of the joint. Through a firm stroking motion of the fingers above and below the patella, fluid is "milked" into the interior of the joint, and the **medial aspect of the joint becomes flat**. The thumbs are then pushed suddenly and firmly into the lateral joint margin, thus producing a bulge of fluid on the medial side of the joint.
3. The **popliteal area** is examined for the presence of a synovial cyst. Standing makes the cyst more prominent.
4. **Knee stability** is evaluated by stressing medial and lateral **collateral ligaments.** Anteroposterior stability is assessed by holding the knee flexed with the foot firmly anchored on the bed and using both hands to pull and push the leg (drawer sign) to test the **cruciate ligaments.**

G. **Ankles and feet**
1. **Synovial soft-tissue swelling** of the ankles at both malleoli should be distinguished from periarticular edema and fat pads.
2. **Normal ankle motion** is 15 degrees flexion and 35 degrees extension.
3. **Subtalar motion,** which allows inversion and eversion of the foot, is best reported as a percentage of normal, with 100% meaning full mediolateral motion.

H. **Toes.** By inspection and palpation, note the following:
1. **Alignment** and deformity: hammertoes, claw toes, and hallux valgus.
2. **Soft-tissue swelling** and presence of inflammation, which are best documented by mediolateral squeezing across the metatarsal joints; pain may be elicited.

I. **Muscle examination.** Proximally and distally, note the following:
1. On inspection, muscle **wasting** and muscle **atrophy.**
2. On palpation, muscle **tenderness.**
3. On testing motion, muscle **strength** (Table 1-2).

J. **Neurologic examination**
1. Standard evaluation of **tendon reflexes.**
2. **Impairment of nerve root function** must be sought with care, and motor and sensory deficits recorded (see Chapters 14 and 18).
3. Look for **nerve entrapment** secondary to joint pathology (e.g., carpal tunnel syndrome).

V. **Systematic examination and joint chart**

A. Inspection, palpation, and movement of joints may reveal swelling, tenderness, temperature and color changes over the joint, crepitation, and deformity.
1. **Tenderness** on direct pressure over the joint and **stress pain** produced when the joint, at the limit of its range of motion, is nudged a little farther are important findings of inflammation. The number of tender and swollen

Table 1-2. Gradations of muscle weakness

Grade	Muscle involvement
0	No muscle contraction
1	Flicker or trace of contraction
2	Active movement possible with gravity eliminated
3	Active movement possible against gravity
4	Active movement possible against gravity and resistance
5	Normal muscle power

joints can be recorded and compared with future joint counts after the institution of therapy.

2. **Crepitation** is a palpable or audible sensation with joint motion caused by roughened articular or extraarticular surfaces rubbing each other. "Popping" sounds can also be heard and felt when tendons travel over bony prominences.
3. **Bony enlargement, subluxation, and ankylosis in abnormal positions cause deformity.**

B. **Quantification of findings**

1. **Range of motion** is reported in degrees and, when practical, in percentage of normal (i.e., fist and subtalar motions). See Table 1-1 for average values.
2. **Swelling and tenderness** are arbitrarily reported in grades 1, 2, and 3, which indicate size and severity ranging from minimal to severe. Numbers of swollen and tender joints can be recorded (called a joint count) for future comparison after treatment has been instituted, and for use in controlled clinical trials.
3. Other physical signs of joint abnormality include **warmth and erythema over the joint** and should be expressed as grades 1, 2, or 3 (mild, moderate, or severe).

VI. **Extraarticular features.** Examination is completed by recording specific findings important in rheumatic diseases, such as subcutaneous nodules, nail changes, rash, abnormal eye findings, sicca (dryness) signs of the eyes and mouth, lymphadenopathy, leg ulcers, and visceral involvement such as splenomegaly, pleural or pericardial signs, and neurologic abnormalities.

Assessment of Joint Structure and Function

The rheumatic disease history and systematic examination allow assessment of the following:

I. **Degree of joint inflammation.** Number of acute joints (tender and swollen) and their location and degree of involvement.

II. **Structural damage and deformity** (malalignment, subluxation, and instability). Findings are reported by a count of joints deformed or limited in their motion.

III. **Function.** Assessment is based on the following:

A. **Joint range of motion.**

B. **Muscle strength** (grip strength, abduction of shoulders, straight leg raising, rising from squatting and sitting positions, and walking on toes). See Table 1-2.

C. **Activities of daily living.** Mobility, personal care, special hand functions, and work and play activities.

D. Function can be reported in **four classes** based on the American College of Rheumatology classification:

Class 1 **Normal function without or despite symptoms**
Class 2 **Some disability but adequate for normal activity without special devices or assistance**
Class 3 **Activities restricted; special devices or assistance required**
Class 4 **Totally dependent**

Other, more quantitative instruments are available for the evaluation and prospective assessment of function, performance of social activities, and emotional status. Specialized pain and function instruments are also available for clinical trials.

In conclusion, a comprehensive clinical evaluation (history plus physical examination) focused on the musculoskeletal system and psychosocial consequences of disease, followed by a complete physical examination with a detailed musculoskeletal and joint evaluation, is the clinical basis for the diagnosis and individualized management of rheumatic disease. Such an approach allows the professional to distill large amounts of information rapidly to reach a specific diagnosis and formulate an appropriate, focused, and effective therapeutic plan.

Bibliography

Hoppenfeld S. *Physical examination of the spine and extremities.* New York: Appleton-Century-Crofts, 1976.

2. RHEUMATOLOGIC LABORATORY TESTS

Keith B. Elkon

The laboratory studies outlined in this chapter are helpful in the diagnosis and treatment of rheumatic diseases. They should be interpreted in the context of a careful history and physical examination. This chapter discusses erythrocyte sedimentation rate, C-reactive protein, auto-antibodies, complement, and other tests helpful in the serologic evaluation of rheumatic diseases. Synovial fluid analysis is discussed in Chapter 5, and uric acid metabolism in Chapter 37.

I. Acute-phase reactants

A. Erythrocyte sedimentation rate (ESR). The rate of fall in millimeters per hour of red blood cells (RBCs) in a standard tube (Westergren method) is a time-honored measurement of inflammation. Methods other than Westergren have been found to be less reliable. RBCs in inflammatory disorders tend to form stacks (*rouleaux*) that partly result from increased levels of fibrinogen and thus form sediment more rapidly. Falsely low ESRs are found in sickle cell disease, anisocytosis, spherocytosis, polycythemia, and heart failure. Prolonged storage of blood to be tested or tilting of the calibrated tube will increase the ESR.

Normal Westergren ESR values are 0 to 15 mm/h for male subjects and 0 to 20 mm/h for female subjects. A normal ESR value tends to exclude active inflammatory disorders such as acute rheumatic fever, systemic lupus erythematosus (SLE), rheumatoid arthritis (RA), and temporal arteritis-polymyalgia rheumatica (TA-PMR). The ESR is of some use in following the course (including therapeutic responses) of chronic inflammatory disorders.

B. C-reactive protein (CRP) is an acute-phase reactant serum protein that is present in low concentration in normal serum and was originally identified by its precipitin reaction with pneumococcal C polysaccharide. It is now commonly measured by a latex agglutination test or rocket electrophoresis. CRP levels rise rapidly under an inflammatory stimulus and then fall when inflammation subsides. In SLE and scleroderma, CRP levels are inappropriately low, unless infection is present. CRP testing may be performed on freeze-stored serum, which is its major advantage in comparison with ESR testing.

II. Rheumatoid factor (RF) is primarily associated with RA but is also found in other disorders (Table 2-1). RFs are immunoglobulins with specificity for the Fc portion of immunoglobulin G (IgG). Multiple immunoglobulin classes have RF activity, but conventional serologic systems (agglutination) detect primarily polymeric (IgM and IgA) RF.

A. Method. Agglutination of IgG-coated latex particles is the method used in most laboratories for measuring polymeric RF. RF activity is measured by using serial dilutions of the test sera. There are many other serologic systems for detection of RF, including bentonite flocculation, hemagglutination, nephelometry, and radioimmunoassay.

B. Interpretation. About 75% of RA patients have IgM RF, and patients with extraarticular disease are invariably RF-positive. Because IgM RFs are not specific for RA and only 75% of patients with RA have IgM RFs, the test is helpful only when combined with clinical information (see Table 2-1). High-titer RF activity is also found in the sicca (primary Sjögren') syndrome and mixed cryoglobulinemia, whereas in the other diseases listed, RF titers are usually low.

III. Antinuclear antibodies (ANAs). A wide array of antibodies to nuclear and cytoplasmic cellular antigens is found in lupus and other rheumatic diseases by immunofluorescence, immunoassay, and immunodiffusion. Different profiles of ANAs in rheumatic diseases have been described and have been correlated with

Table 2-1. Frequency of rheumatoid factor as measured by latex agglutination in rheumatic and nonrheumatic diseases

Disease	Approximate frequency (%)
Sicca syndrome	90
Mixed cryoglobulinemia	90
Rheumatoid arthritis	75
Systemic lupus erythematosus	30
Mixed connective tissue disease	25
Polymyositis	20
Systemic sclerosis (scleroderma)	20
Juvenile rheumatoid arthritis	10
Subacute bacterial endocarditis	40
Chronic interstitial pulmonary fibrosis	35
Pulmonary silicosis	30
Waldenström's disease (macroglobulinemia)	28
Cirrhosis	25
Infectious hepatitis	25
Leprosy	25
Elderly (>60 years)	15
Tuberculosis	15
Trypanosomiasis	15
Sarcoidosis	10
Syphilis	10

clinical features. The LE cell test is obsolete as a result of its poor sensitivity compared with ANA assay. (Some aspects of the clinical application of ANA data are discussed in Chapter 30.)

A. Indirect immunofluorescence for ANA testing

1. Immunofluorescence technique employs a cellular substrate, traditionally a thin section of frozen rat liver or kidney, placed on a glass slide. A cytocentrifuge preparation of white blood cells or cells from tissue culture can also be used. Sensitivity and pattern discrimination are optimal on tissue culture cell substrates (e.g., Hep-2). Test sera diluted to titers of 1:20 or greater are added to the cells, incubated, and then washed off. Fluorescein-labeled antibodies reactive with all immunoglobulins or specific for human IgG, IgM, or IgA are then layered over the sections, incubated, and washed off. Immunofluorescence microscopy detects the presence of antibodies in the test sera bound to cell membrane and intracellular components. Through indirect immunofluorescence, a variety of patterns representing antibodies to different cellular antigens can be detected. Percentages of ANA positivity and patterns of immunofluorescence observed are shown in Table 2-2.
2. ANA studies are usually reported by pattern, intensity of fluorescence (1 to 4+), or titer. Values of 2 to 4+ or titers greater than 1:40 are usually considered significant. Once positive ANA activity has been documented in a patient's serum, there is seldom need to repeat the test unless major changes in the patient's therapy or condition have taken place. Steroid or immunosuppressive therapy may change the ANA titer, but most physicians do not rely on serial changes in ANA to monitor disease activity. The usefulness of an ANA study is not its specificity but rather its sensitivity and technical simplicity. The ANA study should therefore be performed as an initial screening test for auto-antibodies. Greater diagnostic specificity is obtained by determining the reactivity of ANA-positive sera with nuclear constituents such as deoxyribonucleic acid (DNA), Smith antigen (Sm), or nuclear ribonuclear protein (nRNP) (see section **III. A. 3;B;C**).

Table 2-2. Patterns of immunofluorescence ("ANA")[a]

Disease	Diffuse (homogeneous)	Peripheral (rim)	Speckled	Nucleolar	ANA positivity (%)
SLE	++	++	+	0	≥90
MCTD	0	0	++	0	≥90
RA	+	0	0	0	30
Sicca syndrome	0	0	++	+	70
Scleroderma	+	0	+	++	≥70
Drug-induced SLE	+	+	0	0	≥90
Polymyositis	0	0	+0	0	≥70
WG[b]	+	0	0	0	30
PAN[b]	+	0	0	0	30
Elderly (>60 years)	+0	+0	+0	+0	20
Chronic liver disease	+0	+0	+0	+0	20
Idiopathic pulmonary fibrosis	+0	+0	+0	+0	10

[a] ANA patterns may vary considerably, and different tissue or cellular substrates may give different patterns and degrees of staining.
[b] With conventional substrates, approximately 30% of WG and PAN is ANA-positive. With neutrophils as substrate, approximately 80% of WG is positive for finely granular cytoplasmic staining, and approximately 60% of PAN is positive for a perinuclear cytoplasmic staining.
+, common; + +, most common; 0, less common; +0, variable pattern.
ANA, antinuclear antibody; SLE, systemic lupus erythematosus; MCTD, mixed connective tissue disease; RA, rheumatoid arthritis; WG, Wegener's granulomatosis; PAN, polyarteritis nodosa.

3. A special case of "ANA" are auto-antibodies that bind relatively selectively to cytoplasmic proteins within neutrophils (antineutrophil cytoplasmic antibody, or ANCA). The screening test for these auto-antibodies is similar to that described above except that human neutrophils are used as the cell substrate. Two patterns of IIF are obtained: **speckled** cytoplasmic, called c-ANCA, which is highly specific for Wegener's granulomatosis (present in approximately 80% of cases), and perinuclear (p-ANCA), which is present in polyarteritis nodosa and crescentic-glomerulonephritis.

B. Anti-DNA antibodies

1. Antibodies to DNA are measured by the **Farr method** (percent DNA binding). Equal volumes of complement-inactivated test serum and *Escherichia coli* double-stranded DNA (ds-DNA) radiolabeled with carbon 14 are incubated at 37°C for 1 hour and refrigerated overnight. Saturated ammonium sulfate is then added to the mixture; this step precipitates out all antibodies and any bound DNA. The mixture is then centrifuged, and the top half is counted as supernatant (S). The remaining precipitate is redissolved in saline solution and counted as precipitate (P). Percent DNA binding is calculated by the following formula:

$$\text{Percent DNA Binding} = [(P - S)/(P + S)] \times 100$$

2. Other methods for measuring ds-DNA antibodies are outlined and reviewed by Chubick (*Ann Intern Med* 1978;89:186). The most frequently used are millipore binding, *Crithidia* kinetoplast immunofluorescence, and solid-phase immunoassay. Because even highly purified ds-DNA may have single-stranded (ss) regions or nicks exposing single-stranded antigenic determinants, the conventional Farr assay probably measures a small amount of binding to ss-DNA. A positive Farr assay (>30%) is generally found only in SLE or mixed connective tissue disease (MCTD). The level of anti–ds-DNA antibodies is also of some value in assessing activity of SLE. Antibodies to ss-DNA are found in SLE and a variety of other autoimmune conditions, including drug-induced SLE and liver diseases.

C. **Antibodies to other intracellular constituents.** The heterogeneity of anti-"nuclear" antibodies, evident from varied patterns of ANAs, has been verified by immunodiffusion and counterimmunoelectrophoresis studies in which soluble components derived from cells as "extractable" antigens (ENAs) are used. In addition to nucleic acid antigens, several protein antigens from both the nuclei and cytoplasm have been identified. Table 2-3 summarizes the current knowledge regarding the cellular location of the antigens, immunofluorescence patterns, methods of detection, and primary disease associations. In many cases, the protein antigens have been molecularly cloned and have been expressed as fusion proteins. Solid-phase immunoassays utilizing these recombinant antigens are replacing many of the older assays for detection of specific protein antigens. Several of the antinuclear specificities are associated with "speckled" ANA pattern [Sm, nRNP, Ro (SS-A), La (SS-B), RANA]. Most of them are observed with multiple nuclear substrates, but at least one antigen, rheumatoid arthritis nuclear antigen (RANA), is present only in human B-lymphocyte lines. The two antinuclear specificities most characteristic of SLE are anti–ds-DNA and anti-Sm. High titers of anti-nRNP are usually associated with a mixed or undifferentiated pattern of MCTD; however, none of these reactivities can be considered diagnostic and must be interpreted in the context of the clinical presentation.

IV. **Complement.** The complement system, composed of at least 18 different plasma proteins, is a major effector of the humoral immune system. Activation of the system by immune complexes or polysaccharides can occur through either of two pathways, the classic or the alternative. Both pathways eventually cleave C3 with subsequent activation of the terminal components (C5b through C9), leading to lysis of target cells and the generation of multiple mediators of inflammation and anaphylaxis (Fig. 2-1). Serial measurements of complement levels may be helpful in assessing disease activity in SLE patients (see Chapter 30).

A. **Measurement** of complement or its components can be performed by functional (e.g., hemolytic) assays or by concentration with the use of antisera specific for individual components.

1. **Total hemolytic complement (CH50),** measured in hemolytic units, assays the ability of the test serum to lyse 50% of a standardized suspension of sheep RBCs coated with rabbit antibody.
2. By using stable intermediate complexes of complement components or sera known to be deficient in various components, **functional assays of individual components** have been developed.
3. **C3, C4, properdin, and factor B** are usually measured by radial immunodiffusion.

B. **Complement deficiency states.** Deficiencies of early classic pathway components C1 through C4 (of which C2 and C4 are the most common) are associated with SLE-like syndromes and an increased incidence of infection. Deficiencies of terminal components C5 through C9 have also been associated with rheumatic syndromes and in increased incidence of infection, particularly with *Neisseria.* Deficiency of the inhibitor of C1 esterase is associated with hereditary angioedema, and deficiency of C3b inactivator is associated with increased incidence of infection.

C. **Associations and interpretation.** CH50 measurements are often low in SLE and cryoglobulinemia as a result of decreased production or consumption by circulating or fixed immune complexes. Because numerous complement components are heat-labile, all test sera must be kept frozen at –20°C and assayed within 2 weeks or, preferably, frozen at –70°C and assayed within 2 years.

Table 2-3. Antibodies to nuclear and cytoplasmic antigens

Antigen	Cellular location	Immunofluorescence pattern	Method of detection	Disease association	Positivity (%)	Comments
Native ds-DNA	N	P, D	IA, IF, HA	SLE	≥65	Relatively specific for SLE
Denatured ss-DNA	N	P, D	IA, HA	SLE	80	Much lower specificity for SLE than anti–ds-DNA
				Drug-induced SLE	60	
				RA	50	
				Hepatitis	30	
				SS	10	
				Biliary cirrhosis	<10	
nRNP (U_1 RNP)	N	SP	ID, HA, CIE	MCTD or overlap	100	
Sm	N	SP	ID, HA, CIE	SLE	30	High specificity for SLE but less sensitive than ds-DNA
La (SS-B)	N	SP	ID, CIE	SS	40	Primary SS; also in about 30% SLE
Ro (SS-A)	N, ? C	SP	ID, CIE	SS	60	Same as above
SC1-70	N	D	ID	Scleroderma	20	Topoisomerase 1
Centromere	N	SP, coarse	IF	CREST variant	80	Definitive identification by IF on cycled cells or chromosome spread

RANA	N, B-lymphocyte lines	SP	ID	RA	65	EB virus-induced antigen similar to EBNA
DNA-histone (DNP)	N	P, D	LE cell test ID	SLE	50	Antigen responsible for LE phenomenon
Cytoplasmic ribosomes	C	Cytoplasmic, granular	ID, CIE IA	SLE	10	High specificity for SLE
PM-I	N	SP	ID	Polymyositis	50	Frequency increased when both diseases overlap
				Dermatomyositis	20	
Histone	N	D	IF, IA	Drug-induced SLE	30–50	Test not uniformly available
Jo-1	C	D	ID, CIE	Polymyositis	30	
Proteinase 3	C	D	IF, IA	WG	30–80	
Myeloperoxidase	C	PN	IF, IA	PAN, WG	50	
Elastase	C	?	IF		?	

For tests employing IA or HA, it is implied that the antigen used is pure. Relatively pure recombinant protein antigens are under evaluation and will replace CIE and ID. Specificity of CIE and ID is ensured by use of reference sera.

ds-DNA, double-stranded DNA; ss-DNA, single-stranded DNA; nRNP, nuclear ribonucleoprotein; Sm, Smith antigen; PM-I, polymyositis type I; RANA, rheumatoid arthritis nuclear antigen; N, nucleus; C, cytoplasm; P, peripheral; D, diffuse (homogeneous); SP, speckled; PN, perinuclear; IA, immunoassay [radio immunoassay (RIA) or enzyme-linked (ELISA)]; ID, immunodiffusion; HA, hemagglutination; CIE, counterimmunoelectrophoresis; IF, immunofluorescence; SLE, systemic lupus erythematosus; RA, rheumatoid arthritis; SS, sicca syndrome; MCTD, mixed connective tissue disease; WG, Wegener's granulomatosis; PAN, polyarteritis nodosa.

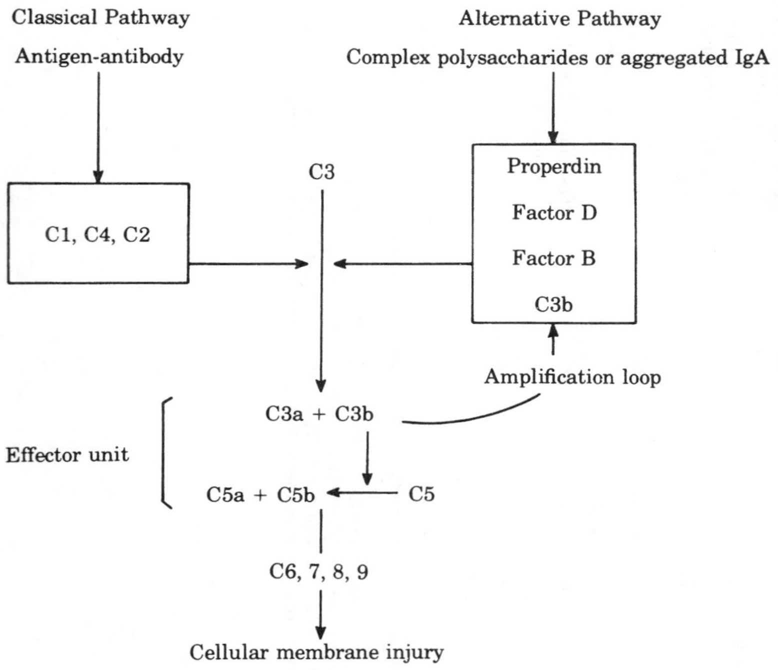

FIG. 2-1. Complement pathways.

Table 2-4 summarizes the serum and synovial fluid CH50 determinations in various rheumatic diseases.

V. Other serologic tests

A. Lupus anticoagulant. Lupus antibodies that inhibit the activation of thrombin can be identified by a **prolonged partial thromboplastin time** and a normal or slightly prolonged thromboplastin time in the absence of anticoagulant therapy. Antibodies in SLE sera that inactivate factors VII, XI, and XII have also been identified. Clinically significant bleeding is rare, whereas an association with vascular thrombosis is well documented.

B. False-positive serologic tests for syphilis and cardiolipin antibodies. False-positive serologic tests for syphilis are present in as many as 25% of SLE patients. The test is frequently positive in patients with the lupus anticoagulant; antibodies against phospholipid antigens are most likely responsible for both phenomena. Antibodies against cardiolipin are determined by immunoassays. High titers of IgG anticardiolipin antibodies in SLE are associated with thrombosis.

C. Hepatitis B (HB) and hepatitis C serologic tests (see Chapter 32). Syndromes associated with chronic HB surface (HBs) antigen include polyarteritis (approximately 30% of cases), essential mixed cryoglobulinemia (variable reported associations, up to 30%), and membranoproliferative glomerulonephritis. Patients with HBs-positive polyarteritis usually express HB early (HBe) antigen, have antibodies to HB core (HBc) antigen, and have immune complexes containing HBs reactants. Recently, an association between essential mixed cryoglobulinemia and hepatitis C virus infection has been reported.

Table 2-4. Complement activity (CH50) in serum and synovial fluid

Diagnosis	Serum	Synovial fluid
Normal	→	50% of serum level
Rheumatoid arthritis	↑ →	↓ →
RA vasculitis	↓ →	↓ →
SLE	↓ →	↓ →
Drug-induced SLE	→	→
Polymyositis	→	→
Scleroderma	→	→
Sicca syndrome	↑ →	→
Vasculitis	↔	↔
Rheumatic fever	↑ →	→
Gout	↑ →	↔
Pseudogout	↑ →	↔
Septic arthritis	↔	↔
HLA-B27–associated arthropathies	↑ →	↑ →
Cryoglobulinemia	↓ →	↓ →

↑, elevated; ↓, decreased; →, normal; ↔, variable.
RA, rheumatoid arthritis; SLE, systemic lupus erythematosis.

D. Immune complex assays. Several procedures have been developed for the detection and quantification of immune complexes in sera and other biologic fluids. Principles employed include size and solubility of complexes (vs. monomeric immunoglobulins), reactivity of complexes with complement (or its components), and affinity of complexes for receptors on cell membranes. Among these procedures, the two that have been most extensively applied are the following:

1. The **Raji cell assay,** which is based on the attachment of complexes to human lymphoblastoid cells through surface Fc and complement receptors.
2. The **C1q-binding assay** (as well as related techniques that depend on the affinity of purified C1q for IgG aggregates).

E. Cryoglobulins. The simplest test for immune complexes, based on their diminished solubility in the cold, is cryoprecipitation of sera at 0° to 5°C. Although it lacks sensitivity and is not readily quantified, cryoprotein screening is the basis for identification of the immune complex syndrome called mixed, or essential, cryoglobulinemia. Cryoglobulinemia is also a common feature of SLE. Blood to be studied for cryoproteins should not be processed by routine laboratory procedures; after clotting takes place in a 37°C bath, serum should be separated by a brief centrifugation at room temperature and an aliquot examined for precipitation after 2 days at 0° to 5°C. Turbidity caused by lipid can be distinguished by centrifugation in the cold (the lipid does not precipitate). Small amounts of cryoprotein (<30 μg/mL) may be seen in a wide variety of pathologic sera and are of questionable significance. Sera with very large quantities of cryoprotein may contain monoclonal immunoglobulins; the sera can be subjected to "cryocrit" measurements in calibrated hematocrit tubes.

Bibliography

Carson DA, et al. Physiology and pathology of rheumatoid factors. Springer Seminar. *Immunopathology* 1981;4(2):161.

Christian CL, Elkon KB. Autoantibodies to intracellular proteins: clinical and biological implications. *Am J Med* 1986;80(1):53.

Chubick A. An appraisal of tests for native DNA antibodies in connective tissue diseases. *Ann Intern Med* 1978;89(2):186.

Cooper NR. The complement system. In: Fudenberg HH, ed. *Basic and clinical immunology,* 5th ed. Los Angeles: Lange, 1984.

Harris EN, et al. Anticardiolipin antibodies: detection by radioimmunoassay and association with thrombosis in systemic lupus erythematosus. *Lancet* 1983;2(8361):1211.
Pepys MB, Baltz ML. Acute phase proteins with special reference to C-reactive protein and related proteins (pentaxins) and serum amyloid A protein. *Adv Immunol* 1983;34:141.
Plotz PH. Studies on immune complexes. *Arthritis Rheum* 1982;25(10):1151.
Tan EM. Antinuclear antibodies: diagnostic markers for autoimmune diseases and probes for cell biology. *Adv Immunol* 1989;44:93.

3. DIAGNOSTIC IMAGING TECHNIQUES

Robert Schneider

Numerous diagnostic imaging techniques may be used to supplement history, physical examination, and laboratory tests in the evaluation of bone and joint disease. Figure 3-1 illustrates some of these techniques as they were used in the workup of a patient with hip pain who was found to have septic arthritis. The decision regarding which imaging technique to use and in what sequence depends on the sensitivity and specificity of the technique for a particular problem and on the availability, cost, and risk of the technique and experience in its use. Providing clinical information when ordering an imaging examination will help the radiologist or technologist to tailor the examination to the problem under investigation. The goal is to make a confident diagnosis in the shortest time at the least cost and risk to the patient. For example, magnetic resonance imaging (MRI) has been shown to be the best method of detecting or ruling out hip fractures when radiographic findings are negative.

I. Imaging techniques

A. Plain roentgenography is usually the initial diagnostic imaging method in the evaluation of bone and joint pain. It provides excellent detail of bony anatomy and abnormalities. Structures other than bone, including cartilage, muscle, ligaments, tendons, and synovial fluid, all appear to have the same soft-tissue density on roentgenography, which makes evaluation of abnormalities of these tissues difficult unless fat or calcification is present. Cartilage destruction can be diagnosed if joint space narrowing is present (see Fig. 3-1). Synovitis may be detected in the knee, elbow, and ankle because of the displacement of adjacent fat pads, but it cannot be reliably detected in the hip and shoulder. Plain roentgenography is readily available and of relatively low cost. It is specific for the diagnosis of bony lesions, such as fractures, neoplasms, and osteomyelitis, but it is not as sensitive as other imaging techniques, such as radionuclide bone scanning and MRI, for the early diagnosis of these abnormalities.

B. Fluoroscopy may be used to determine position during surgical procedures (e.g., internal fixation of fractures and osteotomies); invasive radiologic procedures (e.g., myelography); injections of nerve root, facet, and epidural spine; percutaneous needle biopsy; diskography; and arthrography. Fluoroscopy can also be used for the evaluation of motion.

Care must be taken to limit fluoroscopic time to avoid excessive radiation exposure. Video disk and videotape recording may help reduce fluoroscopic radiation exposure.

C. Tomography supplements plain roentgenograms and provides better detail by blurring out areas above and below the plane of interest. Tomography has been replaced in most instances by computed tomography (CT) and MRI. Tomography is still occasionally used for detecting subtle fractures and evaluating spine fusions for pseudoarthrosis.

D. Radionuclide scanning

1. Bone scanning with use of technetium 99m phosphate complexes has been used most frequently in the evaluation of metastatic disease to the skeleton and has largely replaced routine roentgenographic skeletal surveys for this purpose. It is also used for the evaluation of benign bone disease, as abnormalities may be detected that are not visible on roentgenograms. Bone scanning detects physiologic changes in the bone, in comparison with the anatomic changes seen on roentgenograms. An *increased uptake of radionuclide* reflects increased blood flow to bone and increased osteoblastic activity associated with new bone formation. This can result from numerous causes, including infection, tumor, fractures, or synovitis. Thus, although bone scanning is sensitive in detecting abnormalities of the bones and joints, it is not specific. Bone scanning is indicated when bone or joint pain is present and roentgenographic findings are negative or inconclusive. It is useful in diagnosing early osteomyelitis, stress fractures, nondisplaced traumatic fractures, avascular necrosis, and metastatic disease as a cause of undiagnosed pain. Single-photon emission computed tomography (SPECT) may provide increased detail and can be helpful in diagnosing stress or traumatic spondylolysis and in detecting photopenic areas in avascular necrosis. Three-phase bone scanning, which includes blood flow and blood pool scans, as well as static images 2 to 4 hours or more after injection, should be ordered for the evaluation of localized bone or joint pain (see Fig. 3-1 B, C, D). The early phases show increased vascularity, which may be helpful in diagnosing synovitis, infection, and soft-tissue abnormalities. The

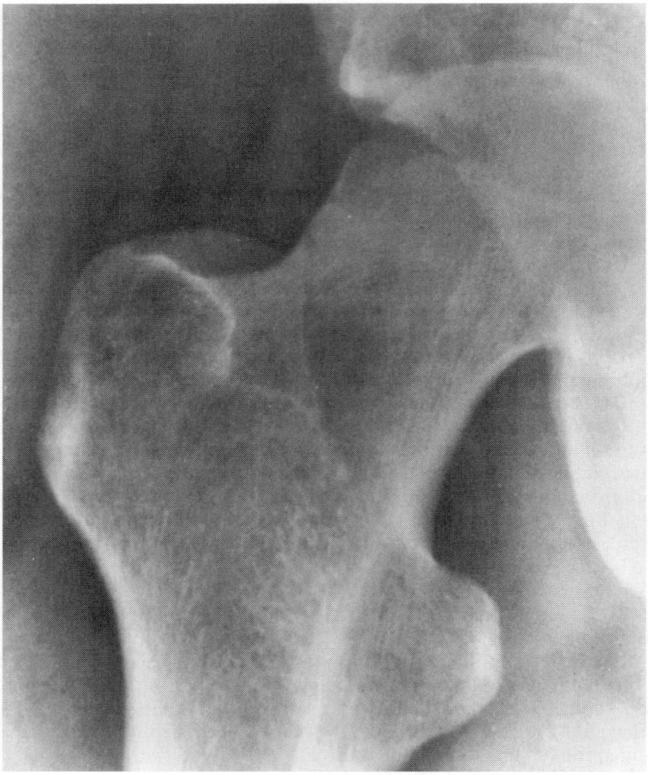

A

FIG. 3-1. Septic arthritis of the hip. **A:** Anteroposterior radiograph of the right hip shows marked narrowing of the joint space, indicating destruction of the articular cartilage. **B:** Dynamic flow scan shows increased vascularity in the right hip. **C:** Blood-pool scan shows increasing vascularity in the right hip. **D:** Delayed static image shows increased uptake in the right hip. **E:** Coronal T_1-weighted (TR/TE MSC 500/12) image shows a decreased signal in the right femoral head and neck and acetabulum. **F:** Coronal T_2-weighted (TR/TE MSCE 2000/80) image with fat suppression by chemical shift technique shows increased signal in the femoral head and neck and acetabulum caused by bone marrow edema, in the joint capsule caused by synovial effusion, and in the soft tissues caused by inflammation and edema. **G:** Hip arthrogram shows contrast material in the joint with irregularity of the joint capsule, indicating synovitis.

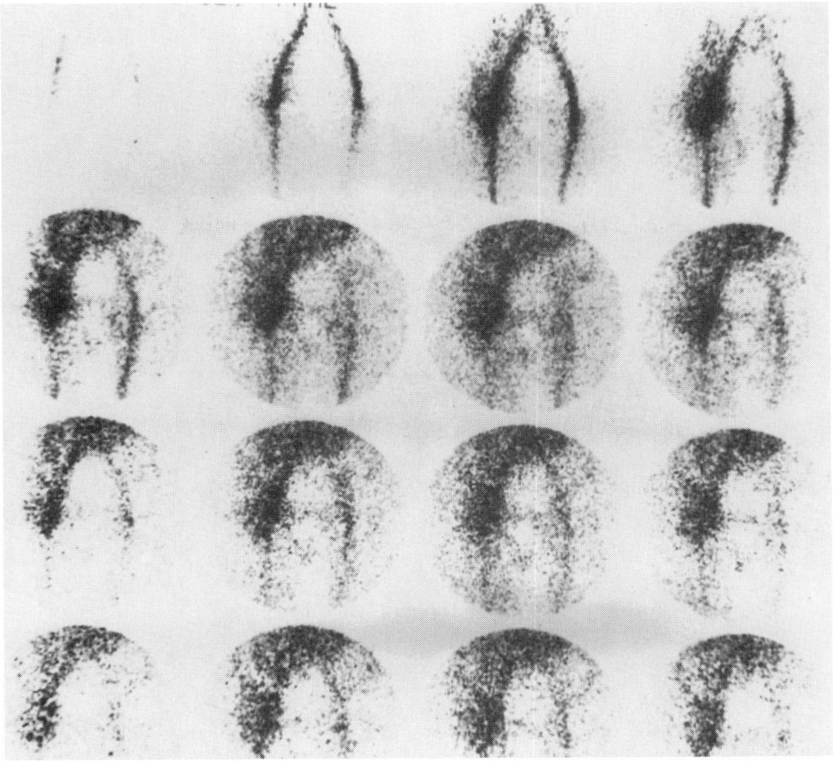

B

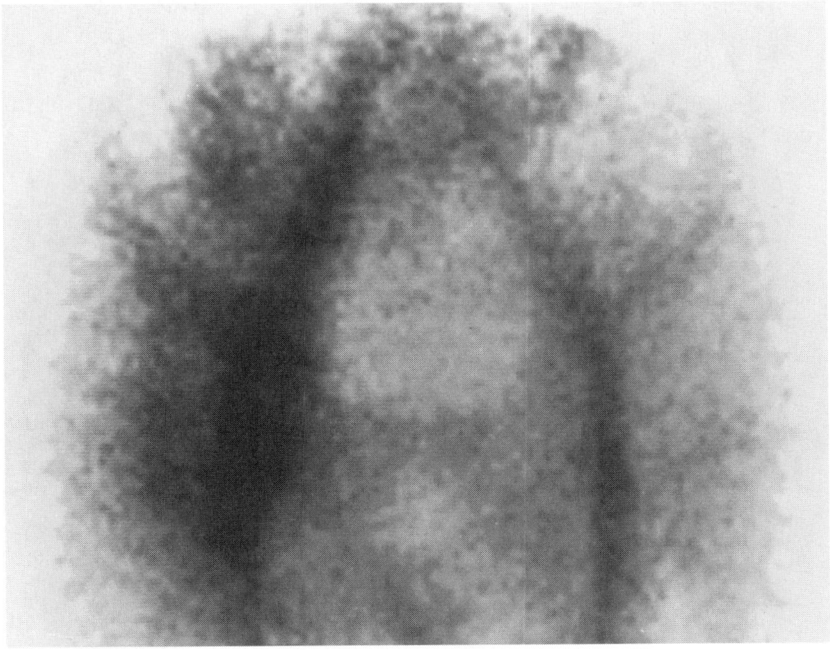

C

FIG. 3-1. *Continued.*

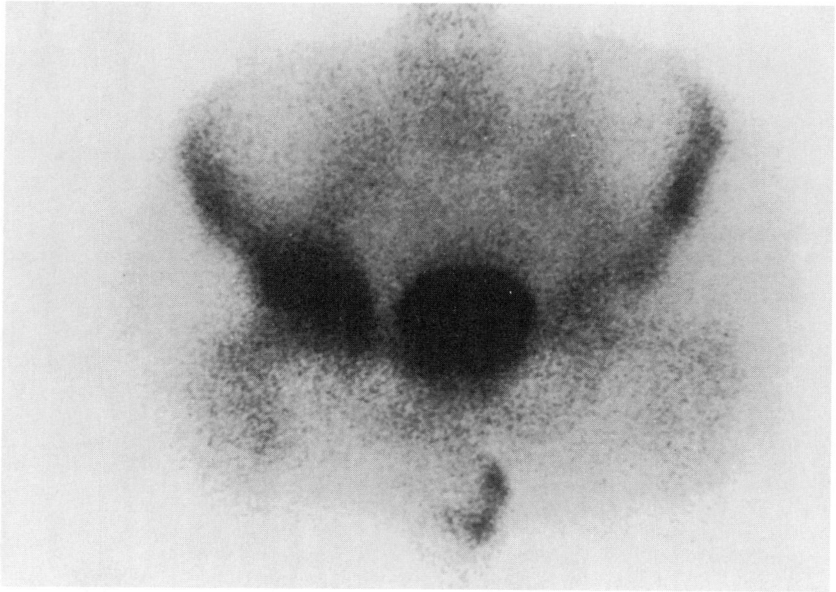

D

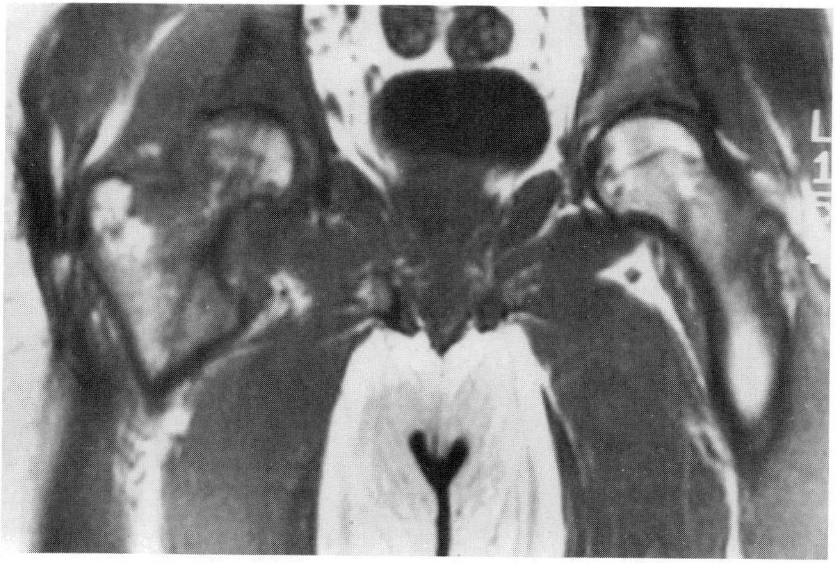

E

FIG. 3-1. *Continued.*

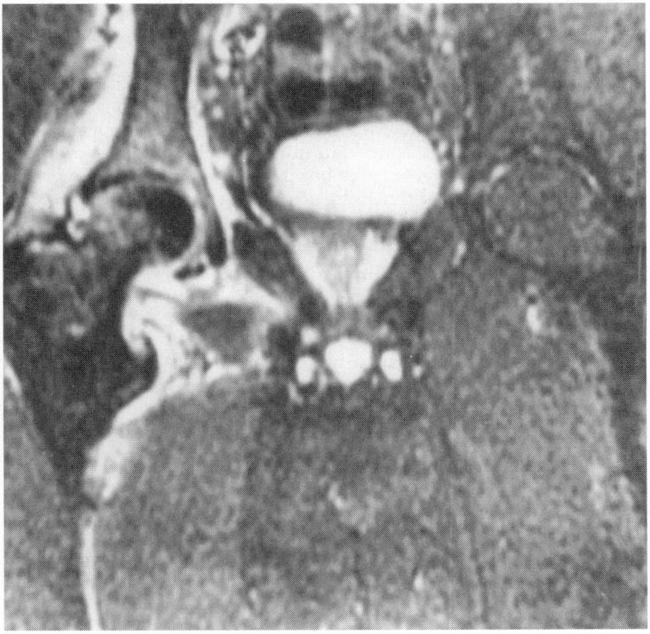

F

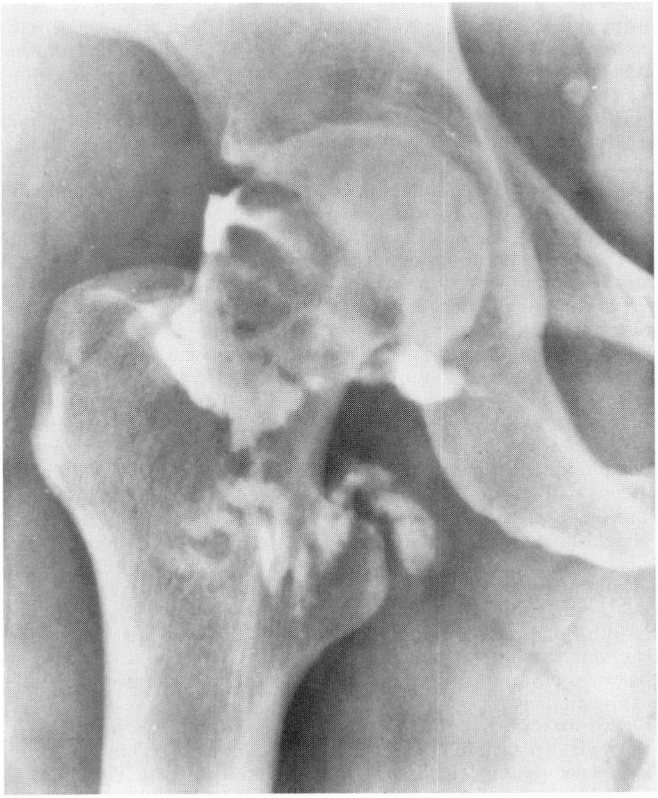

G

FIG. 3-1. *Continued.*

radiation exposure from a bone scan is similar to that from a roentgenographic series of the lumbar spine. MRI has a similar and in some cases better sensitivity than radionuclide bone scanning for early diagnosis of many bony and joint problems and in most cases has a better specificity. However, bone scanning is less expensive and has the advantage of *being able to survey the entire skeleton* during one examination.

2. **Radionuclide infection scanning**
   a. **Scanning with gallium citrate 67** shows increased uptake at sites of infection in the bones or soft tissues. It has a high sensitivity for infection but is nonspecific, as it may show increased uptake associated with other causes of increased bone turnover, including fractures or tumors, and also shows increased uptake in noninfectious inflammatory conditions, such as inflammatory arthritis. The specificity of a gallium scan for infection may be increased if it is compared with a bone scan. If the gallium scan shows more intense uptake than the bone scan at the affected site or if the uptake of gallium is not congruent with the uptake on the bone scan, then infection is likely. However, only one-third or fewer of bone infections meet these criteria. False-negative gallium scans may be seen in chronic infection or if the patient is treated with antibiotics before the scan is performed.
   b. **Scanning with indium 111- or technetium 99m-labeled leukocytes** can detect bone or joint infection and is more specific than bone scanning or gallium scanning. However, uptake may also be seen in noninfectious conditions. Comparison with bone scans or scans performed with radiolabeled colloids can increase the specificity for infection.

E. **Computed tomography (CT)** provides better soft-tissue contrast than does roentgenography, allowing the evaluation of soft-tissue abnormalities that cannot be visualized on roentgenograms. CT provides axial sections for visualization of cross-sectional anatomy, which often facilitates the evaluation of abnormalities in the pelvis and spine. This is especially valuable in evaluating pelvic fractures and localizing osteoid osteomas. Sagittal and coronal images can be obtained by reformatting thin axial sections or images obtained by helical scanning. CT is useful in evaluating the extent of bony and soft-tissue tumors. It can be used to diagnose intervertebral disk herniation and spinal stenosis. CT performed after the injection of contrast material (e.g., after myelography, diskography, or arthrography) provides additional information in these studies.

F. **Magnetic resonance imaging (MRI)** has the advantage of not using ionizing radiation. It provides multiplanar imaging capabilities without sacrificing image resolution.

1. **Spin echo technique.** The most commonly utilized imaging sequence is a multislice, multiecho spin echo technique, used with both T_1-weighted [short echo time (TE), short repetition time (TR)] and T_2-weighted (long TR/TE) images (see Fig. 3-1 E, F). Superior soft-tissue contrast is achieved by virtue of differential tissue relaxation times. Normal fatty bone marrow exhibits a bright signal intensity on T_1-weighted sequences, with a slightly less bright signal on T_2-weighted sequences. Conversely, pathologic processes (infiltrative disease, infection, bone marrow edema) will exhibit a low signal on T_1-weighted sequences (see Fig. 3-1E). Both cortical bone and fibrous tissue (including normal ligaments and tendons) maintain a low signal intensity on all pulse sequences. Fluid (synovial fluid, edema, cysts) exhibits a low signal intensity on T_1-weighted sequences, and a markedly bright signal intensity on T_2-weighted images (see Fig. 3-1 E, F). Intermediate-weighted or proton density images (long TR/short TE) reduce the differences in contrast between different tissues but provide a higher resolution for the evaluation of morphology.
2. **Gradient echo techniques.** Additional soft-tissue contrast is achieved through variation in pulse sequences. Gradient echo imaging provides rapid image acquisition with improved soft-tissue contrast. This is extremely useful in the evaluation of articular cartilage. Gradient echo techniques are also

advantageous in spine imaging; volumetrically acquired techniques allow for thin (>3 mm) slice acquisition within a relatively short time period. Such thin slices are essential in diagnosing subtle cervical disk disease.

3. **Fat-suppressed techniques.** Although visualized on spin echo images, bone marrow edema may be seen better with fat-suppressed techniques, such as short tau inversion recovery (STIR) and chemical shift techniques.
4. **Indications for MRI** include the following:
   a. Evaluation of internal derangement of the knee (meniscal tears; cruciate, collateral, and quadriceps mechanism tears; bone contusion).
   b. Osteonecrosis.
   c. Rotator cuff tears and glenohumeral instability.
   d. Tendon, ligament, and muscle tears and other abnormalities.
   e. Back pain.
   f. Evaluation of brain and spinal cord.
   g. Evaluation of bone and soft-tissue tumors.
   h. Assessment of occult fracture.

   In many cases, MRI obviates the need for the more invasive arthrogram or myelogram.
5. **Contraindications to MRI** include the presence of pacemakers, aneurysm clips, some prosthetic otologic and ocular implants, and some bullet fragments. Clinical concern is increased when the metallic object is anatomically close to a vital vascular or neural structure. Most prosthetic heart valves are felt to be safe for MRI. In addition, most orthopedic materials and devices are considered safe, including stainless steel screws and wires. However, ferromagnetic metallic implants will cause image artifact, with large areas of signal void and adjacent high signal ("flare" response), which may interfere with accurate image interpretation. Prior knowledge of the specific type (manufacturer, material) of metallic implant is essential before the patient is exposed to a strong magnetic field.
6. **Gadolinium diethylenetriamine pentaacetic acid (GD-DTPA)** is an MRI contrast agent that, when used in typical doses (0.1 mmol/kg of body weight), acts primarily to shorten T_1 relaxation times. Thus, regions that readily enhance with contrast will appear bright on T_1-weighted images. In the evaluation of the postoperative spine, contrast may help to distinguish scar from recurrent disk herniation (Fig. 3-2). Postoperative scar is felt to enhance with contrast by virtue of the rich vascularity of epidural granulation tissue. Conversely, the avascular adult disk will not demonstrate similar signal enhancement. A contrast-enhanced MRI examination performed long after surgery may not prove as reliable, as scar tissue may become progressively fibrotic, with less discernible contrast enhancement. Relative contraindications to GD-DTPA administration include hemolytic anemia, as the agent may promote extravascular hemolysis. Because GD-DTPA is cleared via glomerular filtration, caution should be utilized in patients with impaired renal function. The most common reported adverse reaction is mild headache (<10% of patients).

G. **Ultrasonography** may be used to evaluate soft-tissue masses and characterize them as either cystic or solid. Popliteal cysts can easily be detected. Tendons are more echogenic than muscle and can be evaluated for continuity and inflammation. Tenosynovitis can be detected as fluid in the tendon sheath. Ultrasonography has been used in the shoulder for evaluation of the rotator cuff tendons. Complete and partial tears and tendinopathy can be diagnosed. Tendons in most other parts of the body can be evaluated in a similar manner. Plantar fasciitis can be diagnosed by evaluating the thickness and appearance of the plantar fascia. Calcific tendinitis can be detected as focal areas of high echogenicity. Aspiration and injection of soft-tissue ganglia, calcific deposits, and tendon sheaths can be performed under ultrasound guidance. Foreign bodies in the soft tissue can be localized. Ultrasound is used for the evaluation of developmental dysplasia of the hip in infants to determine the position of the nonossified femoral head with respect to the acetabulum.

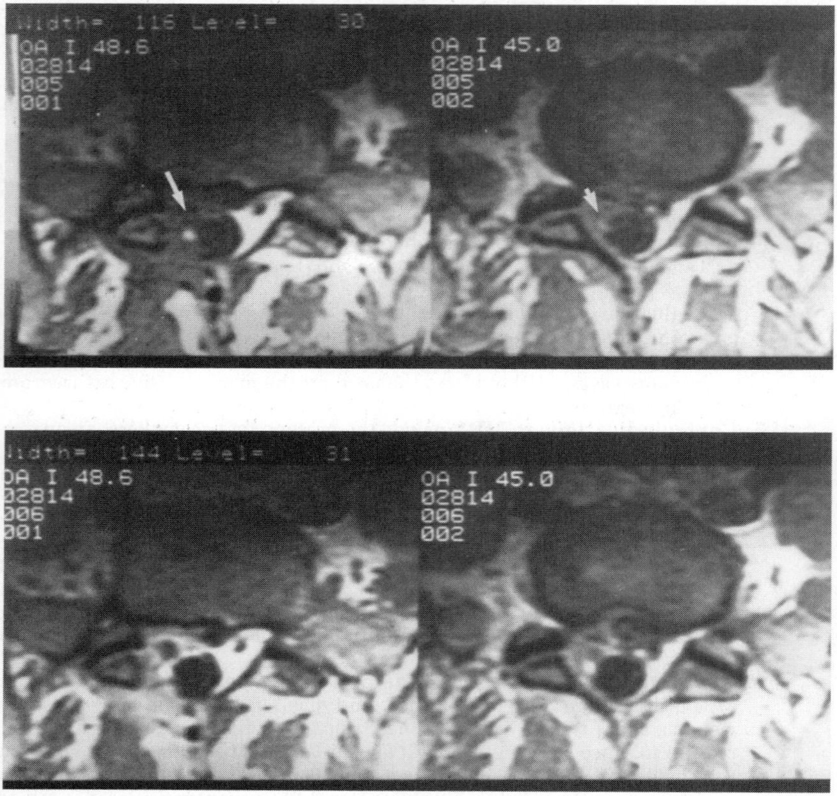

A

B

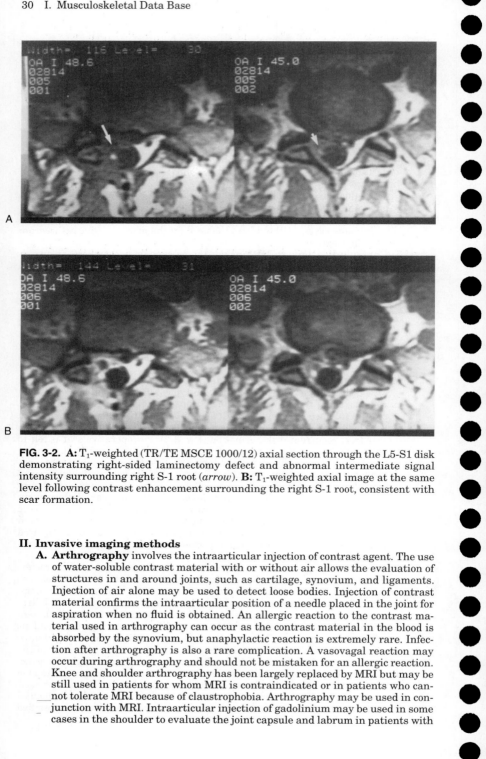

FIG. 3-2. A: T_1-weighted (TR/TE MSCE 1000/12) axial section through the L5-S1 disk demonstrating right-sided laminectomy defect and abnormal intermediate signal intensity surrounding right S-1 root (*arrow*). **B:** T_1-weighted axial image at the same level following contrast enhancement surrounding the right S-1 root, consistent with scar formation.

II. Invasive imaging methods

A. Arthrography involves the intraarticular injection of contrast agent. The use of water-soluble contrast material with or without air allows the evaluation of structures in and around joints, such as cartilage, synovium, and ligaments. Injection of air alone may be used to detect loose bodies. Injection of contrast material confirms the intraarticular position of a needle placed in the joint for aspiration when no fluid is obtained. An allergic reaction to the contrast material used in arthrography can occur as the contrast material in the blood is absorbed by the synovium, but anaphylactic reaction is extremely rare. Infection after arthrography is also a rare complication. A vasovagal reaction may occur during arthrography and should not be mistaken for an allergic reaction. Knee and shoulder arthrography has been largely replaced by MRI but may be still used in patients for whom MRI is contraindicated or in patients who cannot tolerate MRI because of claustrophobia. Arthrography may be used in conjunction with MRI. Intraarticular injection of gadolinium may be used in some cases in the shoulder to evaluate the joint capsule and labrum in patients with instability, in the hip to detect labral tears, and in the wrist to detect ligament tears.

1. **Hip arthrography** is used in children to evaluate the position of the cartilaginous femoral head with respect to the acetabulum in Legg-Perthes disease, developmental dysplasia of the hip, and coxa vara deformities. In adults, it is used to evaluate painful hip prostheses and the joint capsule after aspiration.

Bibliography

Berquist TH, ed. *MRI of the musculoskeletal system,* 3rd ed. New York: Raven Press, 1996.

Chan TW, Listerud J, Kressel HY. Combined chemical shift and phase selective imaging for fat suppression: theory and initial clinical experience. *Radiology* 1991;181(1):41.

Collier DB, Fogelman I, Rosenthall L, eds. *Skeletal nuclear medicine.* St. Louis: Mosby, 1996.

Formage B, ed. *Musculoskeletal ultrasound.* New York: Churchill Livingstone, 1995.

Glickstein MF, Sussman SK. Time-dependent scan enhancement in magnetic resonance imaging of the post-operative lumbar spine. *Skeletal Radiol* 1991;20(5):333.

Resnick D, ed. *Diagnosis of bone and joint disorders,* 3rd ed. Philadelphia: WB Saunders, 1995.

Shellock FG, Curtis JS. MR imaging and biomedical implants, materials, and devices: an updated review. *Radiology* 1991;180(2):541.

4. ARTHROCENTESIS AND INTRAARTICULAR INJECTION

Richard Stern

I. **Arthrocentesis** is a safe and relatively easy procedure that plays both diagnostic and therapeutic roles in the management of arthritis patients. It should be included in the initial evaluation of every patient with a joint effusion, especially those with monarthritis. Subsequent synovial fluid analysis can lead to a specific diagnosis in infectious and crystal-induced arthritis and can be of help in differentiating an inflammatory process such as rheumatoid arthritis from a noninflammatory state such as osteoarthritis.

A. **Diagnostic indications**

1. As part of an initial evaluation.
2. To rule out superimposed infection in an already diseased joint.

B. **Therapeutic indications**

1. Drainage of an effusion to relieve pain.
2. Instillation of medication.
3. Drainage of a septic joint.
4. Drainage of hemarthrosis (correct any coagulation disorder first).

C. **Contraindications**

1. Infection in overlying skin or soft tissue.
2. Severe coagulation disorder.

II. **Intraarticular injection.** Joint injection is primarily used to deliver intraarticular corticosteroids to treat inflamed joints, bursae, or tendons. Contraindications are the same as for arthrocentesis. Corticosteroid should not be injected into a joint until infection (including that caused by mycobacteria or fungi) has been excluded. There is some evidence that repeated injection into the small joints of the hand may lead to deformity. Similarly, injections into tendon insertions may result in rupture. Large joints should not be injected more than three or four times per year or 10 times cumulatively. Small joints should be injected less often, not more than two or three times per year or four times cumulatively.

III. **Supplies**

A. **Materials for aseptic skin preparation**

1. Sterile gloves.
2. Iodine solution.
3. Alcohol solution.
4. Sterile gauze pads.

B. **Materials for local anesthesia**

1. One percent lidocaine for skin, subcutaneous tissues, and joint structures.
2. Ethyl chloride spray for skin.

C. **Sterile 18- to 25-gauge needles,** depending on the size of the joint. Inflamed joint fluids may be thick and require a large-bore needle for removal.

D. **Syringes,** 3 to 50 mL in size, depending on the joint and amount of effusion.

E. **Tubes for synovial fluid analysis**

1. Chemistry tube for glucose.
2. Hematology tube [with ethylenediaminetetraacetic acid (EDTA)] for cell count and differential.
3. Sterile tube for cultures and smears.
4. Heparinized tube for crystal analysis. Ascertain that a powdered anticoagulant, which may interfere with crystal indentification, is not used.
5. Cytology bottle (if neoplasm is suspected).

IV. **Technique.** The most important maneuver before aspirating a joint is to locate the appropriate landmark and mark it with an indelible felt pen. Generous local anesthesia of the overlying skin and subcutaneous tissues is recommended. Long-acting intraarticular steroid preparations may induce a crystal synovitis 24 hours after the injection, which soon abates spontaneously or with application of ice and pain medications. Further, the needle itself may traumatize the joint, especially if the joint is small; for this reason, the patient should be warned of possible short-term aggravation of symptoms in the injected joint and receive appropriate instructions regarding analgesia.

A. Shoulder. The shoulder can be entered either anteriorly or posteriorly.

1. **Anterior approach** (Fig. 4-1). With the patient's hand in the lap and the shoulder muscles relaxed, the glenohumeral joint can be palpated by placing the fingers between the **coracoid process** and the humeral head. As the shoulder is internally rotated, the humeral head can be felt turning inward and the joint space can be felt as a groove just lateral to the coracoid. When the skin over this area is anesthetized, a 20- or 22-gauge needle can be inserted lateral to the coracoid. (Avoid the thoracoacromial artery, which runs on the medial aspect of the coracoid.) The needle is directed dorsally and medially into the joint space. The needle should be directed slightly superiorly to avoid the neurovascular bundle.
2. **Posterior approach** (Fig. 4-2). The posterior aspect of the shoulder joint is identified with the patient's arm internally rotated maximally. This position is achieved by placing the patient's ipsilateral hand on the opposite shoulder. The humeral head can then be palpated by placing a finger posteriorly along the **acromion** while the shoulder is rotated. The needle is inserted about 1 cm inferior to the **posterior tip of the acromion** and directed anteriorly and medially.

B. Elbow (Fig. 4-3). The **elbow joint** can be identified by placing the patient's relaxed arm in the lap. With the palm facing the patient, flex the elbow to a 45-degree angle. Place your finger on the **lateral epicondyle** and note the shallow depression distal to it, which represents the elbow joint. A 22-gauge needle is introduced perpendicular to the joint.

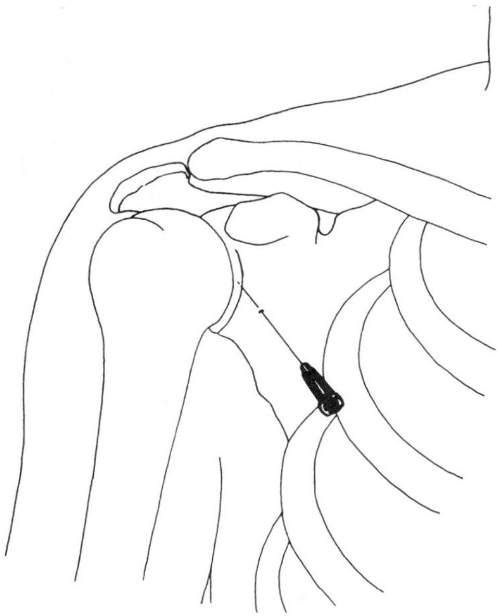

FIG. 4-1. Arthrocentesis of the shoulder, anterior approach.

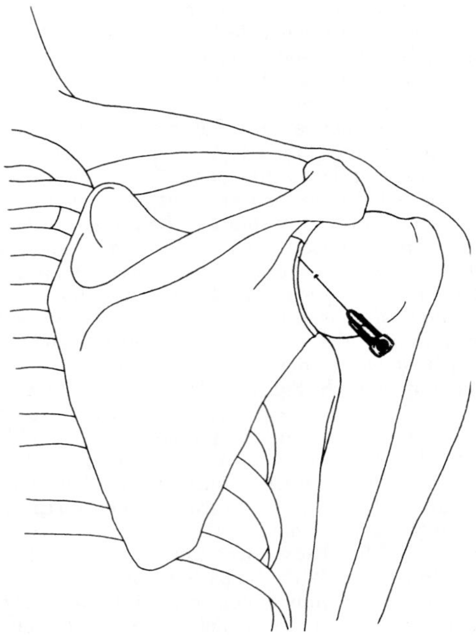

FIG. 4-2. Arthrocentesis of the shoulder, posterior approach.

C. **Wrist** (Fig. 4-4). Wrist aspiration is performed on the dorsal aspect just distal to the radius or ulna as indicated by clinical examination.
   1. **Radial entry.** The hand and wrist are relaxed in a slightly flexed position. The joint space can be located by palpating the edge of the distal radius just medial to the **thumb extensor tendon.** A 22-gauge needle should be directed into the joint from the dorsal aspect.
   2. **Ulnar entry.** Keep the wrist in the same relaxed position. The joint space can be identified by palpating just distal to the **distal ulna.** The 22-gauge needle is directed in a volar and radial direction.

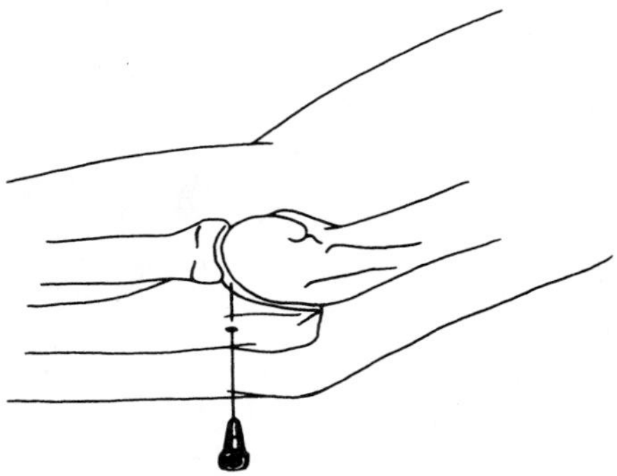

FIG. 4-3. Arthrocentesis of the elbow.

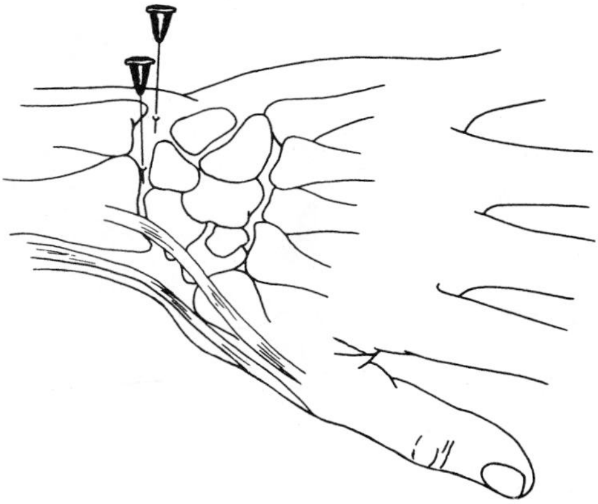

FIG. 4-4. Arthrocentesis of the wrist, medial and lateral approaches.

D. Ankle (Fig. 4-5). The ankle may be difficult to enter. For both approaches, the foot is first placed at about a 45-degree angle of plantar flexion.

1. **Medial approach.** A 22-gauge needle is placed about 1 in. proximal and lateral to the distal end of the **medial malleolus.** The flexor hallucis longus tendon is just lateral to this point. The needle is directed 45 degrees posteriorly, slightly upward, and laterally.
2. **Lateral approach.** A 22-gauge needle is placed about 1/2 in. proximal and medial to the distal end of the **lateral malleolus.** The needle should be directed 45 degrees posteriorly, slightly upward, and medially.

E. Knee (Fig. 4-6). The knee is the largest and easiest joint to enter. It may be entered either medially or laterally. The patient should be supine with the knee

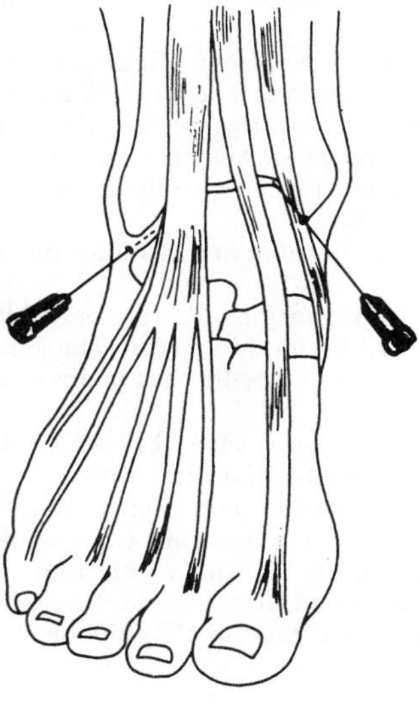

FIG. 4-5. Arthrocentesis of the ankle, medial and lateral approaches.

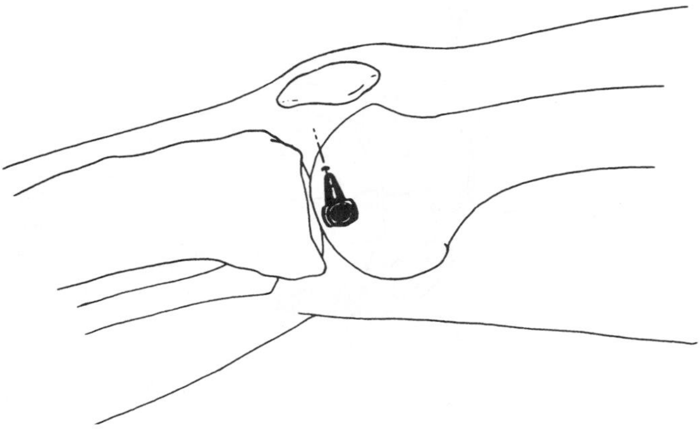

FIG. 4-6. Arthrocentesis of the knee, medial approach.

comfortably extended to relax the quadriceps muscle. If one can gently rock the patella medially and laterally, relaxation is adequate. By grasping the medial and lateral margins of the patella, a skin mark can be made that corresponds to the inferior plane of the patella. It is generally easier to aspirate at the medial aspect of the joint. After the skin and subcutaneous tissue are anesthetized, a 19-gauge needle is introduced in a direction parallel to the plane of the posterior surface of the patella. With thick exudative effusions, a larger-bore needle may be required. Drainage of the knee bursa can be facilitated by compressing the suprapatellar pouch during aspiration. With large knee effusions, the distended suprapatellar pouch can be aspirated directly from either the medial or lateral aspect of the quadriceps muscle mass.

F. Small joints of the hands and feet may be difficult to enter. Occasionally, the effusion bulges and facilitates aspiration. Often, a corticosteroid injection can be performed just adjacent to the joint rather than within; this results in an equivalent clinical response.

1. **The metacarpophalangeal (MCP) joint** can be easily palpated on its dorsal, lateral aspect with the finger slightly flexed and relaxed. The joint is entered on the dorsal-lateral aspect with a 22-gauge needle. Because this is a ball (distal metacarpal) and cup (first phalanx) joint, the needle should not be directed at a 90-degree angle but rather distally at about a 60-degree angle.
2. **The metatarsophalangeal (MTP) joint** is aspirated in a fashion similar to that for the MCP joint.
3. **The proximal interphalangeal (PIP) joint** margin is barely palpable but may be felt on its dorsal aspect just distal to the skin crease. The joint is entered from the dorsal aspect with a 25-gauge needle that is directed slightly distally.
4. **The distal interphalangeal (DIP) joint** is extremely small and difficult to enter. The technique is the same as for aspirating the PIP joint.

G. Other joints. There are external landmarks that can direct aspiration and injection of the hip joint, but success in this venture requires some experience. When the goal of aspiration is to secure synovial fluid for diagnostic studies, arthrocentesis should be performed under fluoroscopic or ultrasound control. The spinal and sacroiliac joints often demand fluoroscopic or CT guidance.

Table 4-1. Intraarticular therapy regimens

Joint	Needle gauge	Dose of methylprednisolone acetate (mg)
Knee, shoulder	16–24	40–80
Wrist, ankle, elbow	20–22	10–40
Interphalangeal	25–27	5–10

V. Intraarticular medications. At our institution, we use methylprednisolone acetate, a long-acting, insoluble corticosteroid preparation. The dose varies with the size of the joint. Doses and appropriate needle sizes are summarized in Table 4-1.

5. SYNOVIAL FLUID ANALYSIS

Richard Stern

Synovial fluid analysis is an extremely useful diagnostic tool in the evaluation of rheumatic diseases. It should be included in the initial evaluation of most arthritic conditions. It can yield a specific diagnosis in infectious and crystal-induced arthritis and can be helpful in the diagnosis of other arthritic diseases.

I. Synovial fluid studies

A. Gross examination alone can be quite helpful in establishing the nature of a joint fluid. After air bubbles are allowed to clear, a heparinized specimen is examined for the following:

1. **Color.** Normal synovial fluid is straw-colored. Inflammatory fluids range from yellow to greenish yellow. Hemarthrosis occurs in patients with coagulation disorders, trauma, neoplasms, and tuberculous arthritis and in patients receiving anticoagulant therapy.
2. **Clarity.** Normal synovial fluids are clear enough that print can be read through them. As inflammation increases from mild to marked, the fluid becomes first translucent and then opalescent.
3. **Viscosity.** Synovial fluid viscosity is tested by allowing a drop of fluid to fall from the needle tip. Normal synovial fluids are quite viscous, and a "string" of fluid will form. Because viscosity is decreased in inflammatory synovial fluids, no string sign is seen.
4. **Mucin clot.** If 1 mL of synovial fluid is added to 3 mL of 2% acetic acid, a firm mucin clot will form. When acetic acid is added to an inflammatory fluid, a poor clot results. This test is rarely used today.

B. Cell count. This is performed on a counting chamber. However, because often only few cells are present, the initial count can be taken with the specimen undiluted. If there are too many cells to count, appropriate dilution can be achieved with normal saline solution. (Diluents for white blood cells precipitate mucin.) Often, both red and white blood cells can be counted on the same chamber. Remember the ratio of RBCs/WBCs is ~750/1. This can be important in hemorrhagic fluids that are inflammatory or infected.

C. Polarizing microscopy of a specimen of heparinized fluid is used to perform a **crystal examination** (see Chapter 37). A useful mnemonic for differentiating urate crystals from calcium pyrophosphate is "U-Pay-Peb"; urate crystals parallel to the polarizer axis appear yellow, and urate crystals perpendicular to the polarizer axis appear blue. The opposite is true for the calcium pyrophosphate crystals of pseudogout. Urate crystals are needle-shaped and calcium pyrophosphate crystals are rhomboid. Remember that the finding of crystals does not rule out the possibility of an infection.

D. Microbiologic studies

1. **Stains** should include both Gram and acid-fast methods.
2. **Cultures** should include routine bacterial studies. Fungal and mycobacterial cultures are ordered as clinically necessary. Synovial fluids and extraarticular sites suspected of harboring gonococci should also be plated on Thayer-Martin material at the bedside, as gonococci are fastidious and difficult to grow.

E. Biochemical studies

1. **Glucose.** Determination of synovial fluid glucose, when interpreted with a simultaneous serum value, is helpful in diagnosing infectious arthritis. In bacterial infection or tuberculosis, the synovial fluid glucose will be less than half the serum value. Occasionally, low values may be seen in rheumatoid arthritis (RA).

Table 5-1. Synovial fluid analysis

Classification	Condition	Color	Clarity	Viscosity	WBC/µL	NTP (%)	Crystals	Glucose (% serum)	Complement	Culture/smear
Normal	Normal	Yellow	Translucent	High	<200	<25	0	Same	Normal	0
Group 1 (non-inflammatory)	Osteoarthritis	Yellow	Transparent	High	<2,000	<25	0	Same	Normal	0
Group 2 (non-inflammatory)	Trauma	Pink or red	Transparent	High	<2,000	<25	0	Same	Normal	0
	SLE	Yellow	Translucent	Slightly decreased	0–9,000	<25	0	Same	Normal	0
	Acute rheumatic fever	Yellow	Translucent	Slightly decreased	0–60,000	25–50	0	Same	Normal	0
	Pseudogout	Yellow or white	Translucent or opaque	Low	50–75,000	90	+	Same	Normal	0
	Gout	Yellow or white	Translucent of opaque	Low	100–160,000	90	+	Same	Normal	0
	Rheumatoid arthritis	Yellow or purulent	Translucent or opaque	Low	3,000–50,000	50–75	0	75–100	Normal or low	0
Group 3 (purulent)	Tuberculosis	Purulent	Opaque	Low	2,500–100,000	50	0	50–75	Normal or low	+
	Bacterial arthritis	Purulent	Opaque	Low	50,000–300,000	>90	0	<50	Normal or low	+[a]

WBC, white blood cells; NTP, neutrophils; SLE, systematic lupus erythematosus.
[a] Often negative in gonococcol arthritis.

2. **Protein** determination does not provide additional useful information and should not be routinely ordered.
3. **Complement** may be decreased in RA, but the test is rarely helpful for diagnosis because synovial fluid complement is usually normal in early RA.

II. Diagnosis by fluid group (Table 5-1). Synovial fluid can be divided into three groups based on the degree of inflammation.

A. Group 1 fluids are clear and transparent and have few white cells on cell count. They include normal, osteoarthritic, and systemic lupus erythematosus (SLE) joint fluids.

B. Group 2 fluids generally have a higher white cell count and are not as clear as group 1 fluids; they appear translucent. This group includes fluids from most noninfectious, inflammatory arthritic conditions such as gout, pseudogout, psoriatic arthritis, Reiter's syndrome, and RA. Leukemia or lymphoma occasionally presents in this category, but the differential count reveals more than 90% mononuclear cells.

C. Group 3 fluids are opalescent or purulent. Group 3 fluids include those from bacterial infections and tuberculosis (although joint fluid from gonococcal arthritis can be either group 2 or group 3). Group 3 fluids typically have 50,000 to 300,000 white blood cells per milliliter; these are mostly neutrophils. Occasionally, the synovial fluid from a patient with an inflammatory arthritic condition such as RA may have as many as 50,000 to 75,000 white cells per milliliter and appears opalescent or even purulent. As Table 5-1 shows, there is considerable overlap between the various arthritic diseases; this table is meant to serve as a guideline rather than provide a rigid set of criteria.

6. IMMUNOGENETIC ASPECTS OF RHEUMATIC DISEASES

Allan Gibofsky

The efforts of numerous investigators during the past three decades have resulted in the recognition of a major histocompatibility complex in humans consisting of the alleles of at least seven closely linked loci on the short arm of autosomal chromosome 6. The antigens that the genes of this region code for were first detected on white blood cells and were therefore originally referred to as human leukocyte antigens (HLA). Initially, these antigens interested primarily transplantation physicians, as similarity between donor and recipient seemed to influence allograft survival; soon, however, the hypothesis was advanced that certain clinical conditions might be associated with one or more antigens of this system. A large number of diseases have been studied, and individual or combinations of antigens have appeared with greater frequency than would be expected in the normal population. This increase is particularly true for rheumatic diseases and related syndromes with features of altered immunoreactivity, where, as will be discussed, the strongest and most significant associations have been demonstrated. This chapter reviews the basic concepts of immunogenetics, emphasizing the potential significance of the HLA system antigens in clinical rheumatology.

I. Immunogenetic nomenclature

A. Gene. Segment of DNA that directs the synthesis of a polypeptide chain or protein.

B. Allele. Alternative form of the same gene, resulting from mutation or duplication.

C. Locus. The position of a gene on any given chromosome.

D. Genotype. The genetic composition of an individual.

E. Phenotype. The observed expression of the genotype.

F. Haplotype. Closely linked loci, transmitted as a unit from each parent; two haplotypes constitute the genotype.

G. Allo-antigen. Product of the A, B, C, or DR, DP, or DQ loci; recognized on the cell surface by specific antibody.

H. Determinant. Product of the HLA-D locus; recognized by cell-cell interaction in the mixed lymphocyte culture technique.

II. Immunogenetic nomenclature

A. Loci definition. Seven closely linked loci, A, B, C, D, DR, DP, and DQ, were defined at the Ninth International Histocompatibility Workshop in 1984; the alleles of each are shown in Table 6-1. The products of the A, B, and C series are defined by using serologic reagents, most often with a lymphocytotoxicity assay.

The determinants of the D locus are defined by cell-cell interaction in the mixed lymphocyte culture.

Initial studies directed toward the development of serologic methods for the detection of HLA-D antigens have resulted in the recognition of several additional gene products, preferentially expressed on the surface of B lymphocytes. These B-cell antigens have extensive biologic and chemical homologies with the I-region antigens of the murine histocompatibility system and are therefore also referred to as Ia antigens. These Ia allo-antigens were primarily recognized with allo-antibodies that developed as a result of immunization with paternal antigens during pregnancy or in the sera of renal transplant recipients who became immunized against nonmatching antigens present on the homograft (see Table 6-1). These human Ia antigens are highly polymorphic and have certain allo-antigenic specificities related closely to HLA alleles. The studies from the Tenth International Histocompatibility Workshop indicate that the gene products of the HLA-D region appear to be highly complex, polymorphic, and not yet fully defined. Each product consists of a noncovalently

Table 6-1. Complete listing of recognized serologic and cellular HLA specificities

A	B	C	D	DR	DQ	DP
A1	B5	Cw1	Dw1	DR1	DQ1	DPw1
A2	B7	Cw2	Dw2	DR103	DQ2	DPw2
A203	B703	Cw3	Dw3	DR2	DQ3	DPw3
A210	B8	Cw4	Dw4	DR3	DQ4	DPw4
A3	B12	Cw5	Dw5	DR4	DQ5(1)	DPw5
A9	B13	Cw6	Dw6	DR5	DQ6(1)	DPw6
A10	B14	Cw7	Dw7	DR6	DQ7(3)	
A11	B15	Cw8	Dw8	DR7	DQ8(3)	
A19	B16	Cw9(w3)	Dw9	DR8	DQ9(3)	
A23(9)	B17	Cw10(w3)	Dw10	DR9		
A24(9)	B18		Dw11(w7)	DR10		
A2403	B21		Dw12	DR11(5)		
A25(10)	B22		Dw13	DR12(5)		
A26(10)	B27		Dw14	DR13(6)		
A28	B2708		Dw15	DR14(6)		
A29(19)	B35		Dw16	DR1403		
A30(19)	B37		Dw17(w7)	DR1404		
A31(19)	B38(16)		Dw18(w6)	DR15(2)		
A32(19)	B39(16)		Dw19(w6)	DR16(2)		
A33(19)	B3901		Dw20	DR17(3)		
A34(10)	B3902		Dw21	DR18(3)		
A36	B40		Dw22	DR51		
A43	B4005		Dw23	DR52		
A66(10)	B41		Dw24	DR53		
A68(28)	B42		Dw25			
A69(28)	B44(12)		Dw26			
A74(19)	B45(12)					
A80	B46					
	B47					
	B48					
	B49(21)					
	B50(21)					
	B51(5)					
	B5102					
	B5103					
	B52(5)					
	B53					
	B54(22)					
	B55(22)					
	B56(22)					
	B57(17)					
	B58(17)					
	B59					
	B60(40)					
	B61(40)					
	B62(15)					
	B63(15)					
	B64(14)					
	B65(14)					
	B67					
	B70					
	B71(70)					
	B72(70)					
	B73					

Table 6-1. (*continued*)

A	B	C	D	DR	DQ	DP
	B75(15)					
	B76(15)					
	B77(15)					
	B78					
	B81					
	Bw4					
	Bw6					

HLA, human leukocyte antigen.

associated combination of an alpha and a beta chain. The alpha and beta chains are substantially different from each other, and there is evidence for at least six alpha-chain genes and seven beta-chain genes, all in the HLA region. These genes appear to be arranged in subsets corresponding to three distinct products, all of which are class II molecules: (a) DR molecules, with homology to murine I-E antigens (one alpha and two or three beta chains); (b) DQ molecules, with homology to murine I-A antigens (two alpha and two beta chains); and (c) DP molecules, intermediate in structure between I-A and I-E (two alpha and two beta chains), which appear not to be serologically defined. The alpha- and beta-chain genes of each series' products are significantly more similar to each other than to genes of one of the other allelic series.

B. Genetics of inheritance. The antigens of this system are inherited in classic mendelian fashion. Unlike those phenotypic characteristics that exhibit dominant and recessive forms (e.g., eye color and ABO type), the HLA antigens are co-dominant; if a gene has been inherited from a parent, the corresponding HLA antigen will be expressed on the cell surface. Given the number of alleles at each locus, the number of possible phenotypic combinations is very large, indicating the enormous immunogenetic heterogeneity of an outbred population. Thus, the finding of an altered frequency of a particular antigen in a patient group is likely to prompt intense interest in the biologic role of this system in the regulation of the immune response and disease susceptibility.

III. Disease associations. Of the many conditions thus far investigated and shown to be associated with particular alleles of the HLA system, the rheumatic diseases have been the most important. Although the associations are high, they are neither absolute nor diagnostic; the presence of an antigen is not the sole factor in disease pathogenesis, for the antigen also occurs in disease-free persons.

Nevertheless, knowledge of the association may prove useful in permitting subdivisions of clinical groups within the larger population (e.g., pauciarticular juvenile rheumatoid arthritis). This knowledge could facilitate the search for possible etiologic agents and confirm or refute the following suggested mechanisms for HLA and disease associations:

1. The HLA antigen may be structurally similar to the antigenic component of an infectious agent.
2. The HLA antigen may be part of a neo-antigen, formed in combination with an infectious agent.
3. The HLA antigen may be a receptor for an infectious or environmental toxin.
4. There may be linkage disequilibrium with one or more immune response genes.

A. Ankylosing spondylitis. The most significant association of any HLA antigen occurs in this disease. Between 85% and 90% of white patients have HLA-B27, which seems to be a marker for seronegative axial arthropathy in this group.

Ethnic differences may be important as well, because the antigen occurs with different frequency in both patient and control nonwhite groups. The lower association in Pima Indians and American blacks, groups in which the disease itself is less frequent, would suggest that B27 is not involved directly in pathogenesis but rather may be linked to the predisposing gene. Thus far, no HLA-D or -DR association has been recognized, which suggests that susceptibility to ankylosing spondylitis may involve mechanisms different from those involved in the other rheumatic diseases.

B. Reiter's syndrome. Nearly 80% of white patients with the classic triad of symptoms have the antigen B27. This antigen is also seen in slightly lower frequency in incomplete forms of the syndrome. It has been suggested that the reactive arthritis seen following infection with *Yersinia* or *Salmonella* is comparable to the form of Reiter's syndrome following bacterial dysentery. In these conditions also, HLA-B27 is increased.

C. Rheumatoid arthritis (RA). The B lymphocyte allo-antigen HLA-DR4 has been reported in 60% to 80% of white patients with classic adult seropositive RA, in comparison with 24% to 28% of controls. In contrast, no significant HLA association has been detected in adult patients with clinically similar seronegative disease, which suggests that seronegative and seropositive RA may have a different immunogenetic basis.

D. Systemic lupus erythematosus (SLE). Both HLA-DR antigens DR2 and DR3 have been found to be increased in white patients with SLE. This immunogenetic diversity would support the clinical diversity seen in this disease. Some data have suggested that clinical subgroups of patients with SLE show an association with one or the other HLA-DR antigen (e.g., with DR3 in skin disease and with DR2 in vasculitis), but not necessarily with both.

E. Sicca syndrome. White patients with primary sicca syndrome show a strong association with HLA-DW3 and the related B-cell antigen HLA-DR3. Of interest was the report that HLA-DR4 is increased in frequency in patients with secondary sicca syndrome, which no doubt reflects the high incidence of RA seen in this population.

F. Psoriatic arthritis. The HLA antigens A26, B38, Cw6, DR4, and DR7 have been reported to be increased in patients with psoriatic arthritis. In addition, B2 has been reported to be increased in patients with axial skeletal disease. Different antigens have been associated with skin disease alone.

G. Inflammatory bowel disease (IBD). Patients with IBD and ankylosing spondylitis show an increased frequency of HLA-B27. No increase in the frequency of this antigen is seen in patients with enteropathic peripheral arthritis as a manifestation of IBD.

H. Behçet's disease. The HLA antigen Bw51 is increased in white patients with this condition. The association is even more significant in Oriental patients.

I. Lyme disease. HLA-DR2 and HLA-DR4 are increased in white patients with this disorder, which results from a Borrelia bergdorferi spirochete transmitted by an Ixodes scapularis.

J. C2 deficiency. The gene coding for the second component of complement is located on chromosome 6 and is part of the major histocompatibility complex. Fu and associates have reported several family studies of patients with C2 deficiency and an SLE-like illness in whom the deficient C2 gene segregated with the same haplotype (A10-B18).

K. Rheumatic fever. In several groups of patients with this disease, a B-cell allo-antigen not related to HLA-D has been detected in virtually all patients tested. The relationship of this allo-antigen to other genes located within the major histocompatibility complex remains to be determined.

L. Juvenile rheumatoid arthritis. HLA-B27 has been reported in 40% of patients with combined pauciarticular and axial disease. Associations with the B-cell allo-antigens HLA-DR5 and HLA-DRw8 have also been reported.

7. MEASURING FUNCTIONAL STATUS IN RHEUMATIC DISEASES

C. Ronald MacKenzie and Theodore Pincus

Functional status refers to a patient's level of performance in the activities of daily living. Although functional status is clearly of major importance to patients and health care professionals, it is not assessed with laboratory tests, radiographs, and other imaging procedures and therefore has not been formally measured in traditional medical care settings. During the last decade, several questionnaire instruments have been studied extensively to assess functional status in individual patients in clinical research, clinical trials, and clinical practice. The development of these questionnaires has been based on rigorous scientific methods and provides new insights into the long-term course of various rheumatic diseases. In this chapter, a brief review is presented of the methodologic requirements and clinical applications of functional status questionnaires, as well as a brief description of several of the most widely used questionnaires.

I. **Methodologic requirements.** Applications of functional status measures include **quantitative evaluation** of a patient's baseline level of function for comparison over time in clinical trials or clinical practice, **discrimination** between individuals (or groups) according to a given component or criterion of functional status, and **prediction** of a subsequent functional level in patients at risk for functional compromise in the future. Although the structural characteristics of the functional measures vary depending on the purpose for which the scale is to be used, several requirements pertain to all questionnaires.

A. **Quantification.** The questionnaire should provide a quantitative "score," preferably with an absolute zero or "normal" value, to allow for arithmetic and statistical comparisons.

B. **Standardized data collection.** The questionnaire should be collected according to an established methodology, analogous to a laboratory procedure, including rules for distribution, recording, and scoring of the data.

C. **Reliability.** Reliability or consistency includes both of the following:

1. **External consistency.** Similar results are seen when an index is applied by different users at the same time and by the same person (including the patient) at different times.
2. **Internal consistency.** Specific scale items measuring similar attributes elicit the same responses from the patients.

D. **Validity.** The questionnaire should measure what it purports to measure.

1. **Face validity** (i.e., what is noted on simple inspection of the questionnaire makes sense).
2. **Content validity** (i.e., the questionnaire represents a specified construct, in this case functional capacity).
3. **Criterion validity** (i.e., agreement of the index with another measure of the same phenomenon, the "gold standard").

E. **Responsiveness.** Responsiveness or **sensitivity to change** refers to the capacity of a questionnaire to detect a change in patient status when a clinical impression exists that a change has occurred (e.g., with the application of an effective therapy), and to indicate no change when no change in functional status is seen.

F. **Feasibility.** Although not generally emphasized, a most important consideration in the use of questionnaires in clinical settings involves feasibility—that is, the questionnaire should be brief, "patient-friendly," nonthreatening, and easily distributed and collected by the office staff.

II. **Demonstrated clinical applications.** Functional status questionnaires correlate well with traditional end points of evaluation in the rheumatic diseases, such as joint counts, radiographic findings, and results of various laboratory investigations. Moreover, questionnaires appear to provide useful information concerning a number of important clinical phenomena that have been difficult or impossible to quantify with traditional measures. These include the following:

A. Documentation and prediction of long-term functional declines and work disability associated with the rheumatic diseases.

B. Prediction of mortality in patients with rheumatoid arthritis, including identification of patients with projected 5-year survivals in the range of 50%, as in patients with cardiovascular and neoplastic diseases.

C. Identification of health service utilization by patients with rheumatic diseases.

D. Provision of measurable insights into psychosocial problems of patients with rheumatic diseases.

E. Detection of changes in clinical status in patients enrolled in clinical trials, as effective as physical or laboratory measures. Although the use of these questionnaires has been largely limited to clinical research, the demonstrated utility of self-reported questionnaires in patient assessment and monitoring has led to their more recent use in routine patient evaluation as adjuncts to patient evaluation.

III. Functional status questionnaires. Many questionnaires have been developed to measure various aspects of functional status in patients with the rheumatic diseases. Among the most widely used measures of overall functional capacity, all of which meet appropriate methodologic standards, are the following:

A. Health Assessment Questionnaire (HAQ). This questionnaire measures performance in activities of daily living, emphasizing difficulty and the need for equipment and physical assistance to complete common tasks. Scores on eight subscales derived from 20 questions are averaged to create a disability index with scores ranging from 0 to 3 on each scale. A visual analog subscale measures intensity of pain. The HAQ is self-administered and takes 8 to 10 minutes to complete.

B. Modified Health Assessment Questionnaire (MHAQ). This self-administered questionnaire includes a modification of the HAQ; the original 20 questions were reduced to eight, and supplemental questions concerning patients' perceived satisfaction with their health, global status, morning stiffness, pain, gastrointestinal symptoms, and fatigue were added.

C. Arthritis Impact Measurement Scale (AIMS). The AIMS questionnaire consists of 48 multiple-choice questions grouped into nine subscales measuring physical, social, and mental health. The questionnaire is comprehensive and evaluates a patient's performance across the entire spectrum of functional activity, including general physical activity, lower extremity function, household activities, activities of daily living, basic self-care techniques, interaction with friends and family, anxiety, depression, and pain. A revision of the questionnaire (AIMS2) has recently been published. In its new form, three scales have been added to evaluate arm function, work, and social support, as have sections to assess satisfaction with function, attribution of problems to arthritis, and self-designation of priority areas for improvement. The possible range of scores on each subscale is 0 to 10, with subscale results averaged to obtain an overall scale. The AIMS takes 20 to 30 minutes to complete.

D. MACTAR Patient Preference Disability Questionnaire. This questionnaire is designed to identify individual disabilities caused by arthritis and assess their relative importance to the patient. Although patients may report any activity of their choosing, they are prompted by an interviewer with a "menu" of activities, including mobility, self-care, work, and leisure. Activities are subsequently ranked by the patient according to their order of importance. The questionnaire requires about 10 minutes to administer, and standardized scores ranging from 0 (worst function) to 1.0 (optimal function) are calculated. This questionnaire differs from the others in that its design is patient-specific and that an interviewer is required to administer it.

Bibliography

Kirshner BK, Guyatt G. A methodologic framework for assessing health indices. *J Chron Dis* 1985;38:27.

Liang MH, Jette AM. Measuring functional ability in chronic arthritis: a critical review. *Arthritis Rheum* 1981;24(1):80.

Meenan RF, et al. AIMS2: the content and properties of a revised and expanded arthritis impact measurement scale's health status questionnaire. *Arthritis Rheum* 1992;35(1):1.

Pincus T, et al. Self-report questionnaire scores in rheumatoid arthritis reflect traditional physical, radiographic, and laboratory measures. *Ann Intern Med* 1989; 110(4):259.

Wolfe F, Pincus T. Standard self-report questionnaire in routine clinical and research practice: an opportunity for patients and rheumatologists. *J Rheumatol* 1991;18(5):643.

8. PATIENT EDUCATION

John P. Allegrante

Patient education is an integral part of the comprehensive clinical care of the patient with arthritis and musculoskeletal diseases. Most patients believe that education is very important to the management of their disease or condition. Planned educational interventions that specify measurable goals for knowledge, skills, and behavioral change, and that combine multiple educational and behavioral strategies, have been shown to have the greatest chance of producing potentially beneficial psychological, behavioral, and health outcomes in patients with arthritis and other chronic diseases. In addition to the impact on patient knowledge and attitude, there is substantial evidence demonstrating that patient education can enhance patient adherence to therapeutic regimens, produce physiologic and immunologic changes in response to behavioral change, and result in clinically significant improvements in health outcomes.

I. Definition. Patient education is defined as any combination of planned learning experiences designed to help people who are having or have had experience with illness or disease to make voluntary adaptations of behavior that will lead to better health. Education promotes understanding of the disease, a positive attitude toward recommended therapy, and the development of skills necessary to comply with therapy and cope with the illness experience. Patient education should be a process designed and tailored to help patients **adopt, maintain,** and **prevent relapse of** disease-relevant behavior.

II. Goals of patient education. The goals of patient education in the context of rheumatic and musculoskeletal diseases are to enable the patient to

- **A.** Understand the disease and treatment(s).
- **B.** Control or relieve pain and other symptoms.
- **C.** Enhance psychosocial well-being by decreasing anxiety and depression and improving morale and motivation.
- **D.** Control (if not alter) disease activity and its consequences.
- **E.** Prevent or minimize disability.
- **F.** Decrease inappropriate use of health services.
- **G.** Increase the opportunities for independent living and enhanced functional health status, including employment and social functioning.
- **H.** Improve skills to communicate with the clinician regarding symptom experience and treatment preferences.

III. Diagnostic approach to patient education. Several studies have shown that patients are often poorly informed about their disease and treatment and that large percentages of patients do not adhere to therapeutic regimens as prescribed. One approach to this problem is for the clinician to make an educational diagnosis and prescribe an educational plan. Educational diagnosis begins by assessing individual patient and family educational needs that are relevant to the disease and therapeutic goals.

A. Behavioral diagnosis. Determine what specific behaviors (e.g., keeping appointments, taking medications, exercising, changing diet, managing stress) are most likely to contribute to achieving the desired clinical outcome.

Prioritize these behaviors in terms of importance and potential for change, and focus on one or two behaviors that the patient is likely to adopt early and successfully.

B. Educational diagnosis. Once target behaviors have been specified, identify those predisposing, enabling, and reinforcing factors that are most likely to contribute to the performance of the behavior(s) of interest.

1. Predisposing factors. Patient beliefs about the disease and efficacy of treatment play an important role in determining patient compliance with medical regimens. Patients' beliefs about their ability to cope with and control the effects of their disease appear to be especially important in managing the symptomatic experience of chronic illness. The first step in an educational diagnosis is to assess the patient's knowledge and beliefs about the disease and disease process, including perceived susceptibility, severity, and seriousness of the disease or condition and perceived costs and benefits of treatment. Assessment of psychological factors such as patient motivation, self-esteem, perceived self-efficacy, and locus of control is also important. Several standardized measures are available to assess these and other patient beliefs.

2. **Enabling factors.** Research in health education has shown that although knowledge is necessary before behavioral change can occur, knowledge is not sufficient. Patients need to possess the skills and resources necessary to make behavioral changes. Communication skills and the skills to perform specific disease-related management tasks, such as exercising, taking medications, and monitoring and documenting progress accurately, permit patients to put into action what they know.
3. **Reinforcing factors.** Family members, members of the health care team (physician, nurse, physical therapist, occupational therapist, social worker), and even other patients can play an important role in reinforcing patient behavior through their attitudes, values, and behavior. When possible, assess the impact of these reinforcing factors and coordinate patient teaching and reinforcement of instructions to patients with other professionals, family members, and significant others.

IV. Measurable impact and outcomes of patient education

A. Patient knowledge, attitudes, and disease-management skills.

B. Informed consent.

C. Decision-making skills and coping behavior.

D. Communication skills.

E. Frequency, duration, and quality of behavior (e.g., complying with therapeutic regimens, keeping appointments, and other coping or disease-management behavior).

F. Health outcomes (e.g., measures of functional status).

G. Use of health services (e.g., reducing cost of episodic hospital care, rate of rehospitalization).

V. Types of patient education

A. Preoperative education prepares the patient for the experience of surgery and what can be expected, by teaching relaxation and other coping skills that can reduce patient anxiety, length of hospital stay, postsurgical complications, use of pain medications, and overall hospital costs.

B. Medication self-administration education programs educate patients and family members to take responsibility for administering medications in the context of home health care, often with medication error rates that are comparable with or below those of nurses and other health professionals.

C. Outpatient education programs include pre-admission education designed to orient the patient to diagnostic and therapeutic procedures in the hospital, community education designed to focus interest on population-wide disease risk factors and screening, and post-discharge education designed to foster social support for groups of patients.

D. Discharge planning education facilitates the transition from hospital care to home health care or nursing home care by educating the patient and family about the patient's post-hospital needs and how to access community resources to meet those needs.

E. Family education is typically incorporated into most types of patient education, but it is especially important in the treatment of patients with severely disabling diseases and conditions, elderly patients, and patients who experience complications during their hospital stay.

F. Peer education and social support programs enlist the cooperation of lay volunteers who have experienced an illness or condition in teaching patients and providing social support; these have been shown to be especially valuable in cases of chronic diseases and illnesses that stigmatize, limit social interaction, or result in severe functional impairments.

G. **Cooperative care** is inpatient hospital care that encourages the participation of a family member in providing patient care and uses education to improve family knowledge and satisfaction with care, adherence to treatment, and self-management.

H. **Early discharge education** has been developed in response to the cost-containment tool of "diagnosis-related groups." It is used with patients who meet strict eligibility criteria for early discharge from the hospital and is designed to facilitate the development of appropriate patient self-care skills before the patient leaves the hospital.

I. **Home health education programs** educate patients and family members to perform clinical procedures and use technologies that are typically confined to hospitals and require professional supervision.

J. **Mutual aid and self-help groups** can be hospital- or community-based and led by lay or professional people. They provide patients who have chronic illnesses and their families with an important source of education about the disease, emotional and instrumental social support, and advocacy.

VI. Educational and behavioral strategies for patient teaching

A. **Use direct instruction** during the clinical visit, and **repeat** and **reinforce** instructions to patients during subsequent visits.

B. **Encourage patients to take notes** during the clinical visit and to write down or record instructions.

C. **Have patients clarify instructions** by repeating them back to the instructor, and encourage questions during the clinical visit.

D. **Have patients set short-term goals** for behavior change that are challenging yet manageable and that are reinforced with predetermined rewards.

E. **Encourage patients to use self-monitoring strategies,** such as checklists, diaries, and other devices, that help them to measure progress and document achievement of goals.

F. **Have patients sign a written contract** that specifies the frequency, duration, and quality of behaviors that are expected to be performed; have a family member witness and co-sign the behavioral contract.

G. **Prepare written instructions and tip sheets** for patients about medication and other complex aspects of a therapeutic regimen in advance of the clinical visit; distribute these in clinic or office waiting areas.

H. **Telephone patients** a day or two following an office visit to follow up, clarify, and reinforce instructions.

I. **Include a family member** or significant other when presenting instructions to patients; have the family member take notes.

J. **Utilize a variety of audiovisual aids** when teaching patients, including printed materials such as diagrams, tip sheets, pamphlets, newsletters, and videotape cassette presentations.

K. **Provide language translations and large-type versions of instructions** to patients as appropriate.

VII. Selected sources of patient education materials and resources

A. **American Hospital Association, Chicago, IL,** promulgates guidelines and policy statements and sets standards for patient education as part of the hospital accreditation process.

B. **Arthritis Foundation, Atlanta, GA** (telephone: 1-800-283-7800) and local chapters produce a range of printed information pamphlets and educational audiovisual programs for patients, publish a patient newsletter, and will provide information about mutual aid and self-help groups for people with arthritis. These include the SLESH (systemic lupus erythematosus self-help) course, PACE (people with arthritis can exercise) course, and ASH (arthritis self-help) course.

C. **Arthritis Health Professions Association, Atlanta, GA,** publishes *Arthritis Care and Research,* which contains articles about research and evaluation studies of arthritis patient education.

D. **International Patient Education Council, Rockville, MD,** publishes *Patient Education and Counseling,* a leading journal devoted exclusively to issues, reports of research, and case studies of patient education.
E. **National Institute for Arthritis and Musculoskeletal and Skin Diseases, Bethesda, MD,** provides information about patient education research in arthritis and musculoskeletal diseases being conducted at multipurpose arthritis centers, through which technical assistance in developing patient education programs is usually available.
F. **National Project for Self-Help Groups, Fairfax, VA,** serves as a clearinghouse and provides access to hundreds of mutual aid and self-help groups for patients with chronic diseases throughout the nation.
G. **Society for Public Health Education, Washington, DC,** publishes *Health Education and Behavior,* a leading journal devoted to health education research and practice, including patient education.
H. **Ankylosing Spondylitis Association.** 14827 Ventura Blvd., Suite 119, Box 5872, Sherman Oaks, CA 91403.
I. **SLE Foundation.** 149 Madison Avenue, Suite 205, New York, NY 10016.
J. **Scleroderma Foundation.** 2320 Bath Street, Suite 315, Santa Barbara, CA 93105.
K. **Sjögren's Syndrome Foundation.** 333 North Broadway, Suite 2000, Jericho, NY 11753.
L. **Wegener's Granulomatosis Foundation.** 9000 Rockville Pike, Bldg. 31, Rm. 1B 30 W, Bethesda, MD 20892.
M. **Osteoporosis Foundation.** 1232 22nd Street NW, Washington, DC 20037-1292.

Bibliography

Allegrante JP. The role of physical activity and patient education in the management of osteoarthritis. In: Baker JR, Brandt K, eds. *Reappraisal of the management of patients with osteoarthritis.* Springfield, NJ: Scientific Therapeutics Information, 1993:31.

Allegrante JP, et al. A walking education program for patients with osteoarthritis of the knee: theory and intervention strategies. *Health Educ Q* 1993;20:63.

Bartlett EE. Which patient education strategies will pay off under prospective pricing? *Patient Educ Counsel* 1988;12:51.

Becker MH, Maiman L. Strategies for enhancing patient compliance. *J Community Health* 1980;6:113.

Belcon MC, Haynes RB, Tugwell P. A critical review of compliance studies in rheumatoid arthritis. *Arthritis Rheum* 1984;27:1227.

Buckley LM, Vacek P, Cooper SM. Educational and psychosocial needs of patients with chronic disease: a survey of preferences of patients with rheumatoid arthritis. *Arthritis Care Res* 1990;3:5.

Daltroy LH. Doctor-patient communication in rheumatological disorders. *Baillieres Clin Rheumatol* 1993;7:221.

Daltroy LH, Liang MH. Patient education in the rheumatic diseases: a research agenda. *Arthritis Care Res* 1988;1:161.

Daltroy LH, Liang MH. Advances in patient education in rheumatic disease. *Ann Rheum Dis* 1991;50:415.

Deyo RA. Compliance with therapeutic regimens in arthritis: issues, current status, and a future agenda. *Semin Arthritis Rheum* 1982;12:233.

DiMatteo MR, DiNicola DD. *Achieving patient compliance: the psychology of the medical practitioner's role.* New York: Pergamon, 1982.

Donovan J. Patient education and the consultation: the importance of lay beliefs. *Ann Rheum Dis* 1991;50:418.

Glanz K, Lewis FM, Rimer BK, eds. *Health behavior and health education: theory, research, and practice,* 2nd ed. San Francisco: Jossey Bass, 1997.

Green LW, Kreuter MW. *Health promotion planning: an educational and environmental approach.* Mountain View, CA: Mayfield, 1991.

Haynes RB, Taylor DW, Sackett DL, eds. *Compliance in health care.* Baltimore: Johns Hopkins University Press, 1979.

Janz NK, Becker MH. The health belief model: a decade later. *Health Educ Q* 1984;11:1.
Jette AM. Improving patient cooperation with arthritis treatment regimens. *Arthritis Rheum* 1982;25:447.
Liang MH. Compliance and quality of life: confessions of a difficult patient. *Arthritis Care Res* 1989;2:S71.
Lorig K, Holman H. Arthritis self-management studies: a twelve-year review. *Health Educ Q* 1993;20:17.
Lorig K, Konkol L, Gonzalez V. Arthritis patient education: a review of the literature. *Patient Educ Counsel* 1987;10:207.
Lorish C, et al. Rheumatoid arthritis patients' knowledge of their disease and treatment: a survey of hospitalized patients. *Arthritis Rheum* 1983;26[Suppl]:S82.
Lorish CD, Richards B, Brown S. Missed medication doses in rheumatic arthritis patients: intentional and unintentional reasons. *Arthritis Care Res* 1989;2:3.
Maycock JA. Role of health professionals in patient education. *Ann Rheum Dis* 1991;50:429.
Mazzuca SA. Does patient education in chronic disease have therapeutic value? *J Chron Dis* 1982;35:521.
McClellan W. The physician and patient education: a review. *Patient Educ Counsel* 1986;8:151.
Meichenbaum D, Turk DC. *Facilitating treatment adherence: a practitioner's guidebook.* New York: Plenum Publishing, 1987.
Mullen PD, et al. Efficacy of psychoeducational interventions on pain, depression, and disability in people with arthritis: a metaanalysis. *J Rheumatol* 1987;14[Suppl]:33.
Potts M, Weinberger M, Brandt KD. Views of patients and providers regarding the importance of various aspects of an arthritis treatment program. *J Rheumatol* 1984;11:71.
Robbins L. Patient education. In: Klippel J, Weyand C, Wortmann R, eds. *Primer on the rheumatic diseases,* 11th ed. Atlanta, GA: Arthritis Foundation, 1997:416.
Robbins L, Horton R, Engelhard E. The use of video and written curriculum in rheumatology health education intervention for patients and health professionals. *Arthritis Care Res* 1993;6:S27.
Silvers IJ, et al. Assessing physician/patient perceptions in rheumatoid arthritis. *Arthritis Rheum* 1985;28:300.
Squyres WD, ed. *Patient education: an inquiry into the state of the art.* New York: Springer-Verlag, 1980.
Steckler A, et al. Health education intervention strategies: recommendations for future research. *Health Educ Q* 1995;22:307.
Stewart M, Roter D, eds. *Communicating with medical patients.* Newbury Park, CA: Sage, 1989.
Strecher VJ. Improving physician-patient interactions: a review. *Patient Counsel Health Educ* 1982;4:129.
Svarstad BL. Physician-patient communication and patient conformity with medical advice. In: Mechanic D, ed. *The growth of bureaucratic medicine.* New York: John Wiley and Sons, 1976:220.
Tucker M, Kirwan JR. Does patient education in rheumatoid arthritis have therapeutic potential? *Ann Rheum Dis* 1991;50:422.
Wade KJ, Brown S, Wasner CK. Rheumatoid arthritis patient education: a consensus on main topics. *Arthritis Rheum* 1982;25[Suppl]:S86.
Weinberger M, et al. Can the provision of information to patients with osteoarthritis improve functional status? A randomized, controlled trial. *Arthritis Rheum* 1989;32:1577.
Winfield JB, and the ACR/AHPA/AF/NAAB Task Force on Arthritis Patient Education. Arthritis patient education. *Arthritis Rheum* 1989;32:1330.

II. CLINICAL PRESENTATIONS

9. MONARTHRITIS/POLYARTHRITIS: DIFFERENTIAL DIAGNOSIS

Stephen Ray Mitchell and John F. Beary, III

The *number of joints* and the *time course* during which a joint disorder develops guide the approach to differential diagnosis. Acute monarthritis may represent septic arthritis, which is a rheumatologic emergency. Prompt diagnosis and treatment of a potentially septic process are required. The single abnormal joint that persists beyond 2 months presents a different diagnostic challenge. In each case, one must view the overall clinical presentation, including factors such as associated extraarticular visceral involvement, constitutional signs and symptoms, severity of illness and limitation of function, potential foci of infection, skin lesions, hyperuricemia, and history of trauma or bleeding disorders. Usually, an aggressive initial approach is indicated, including joint aspiration with synovial fluid analysis and occasionally referral for synovial biopsy or arthroscopy. Therapy will vary significantly depending on the presumptive diagnosis. Specific therapy of each disease is discussed in later chapters. Tables 9-1 and 9-2 summarize the diagnostic approach to this group of disorders.

I. Acute monarthritis

A. Infectious arthritis generally develops with an abrupt onset and marked inflammatory response. Because prompt therapy is required to prevent joint damage or systemic sepsis, it is important to diagnose bacterial infection promptly.

One may be deceived, however, in a partially treated patient on oral antibiotics or in an immunosuppressed patient by the mild appearance of the joint. A prudent approach includes careful examination for associated infectious foci and clues (e.g., cutaneous pustules with neisserial infection), prompt joint aspiration, synovial fluid culture and Gram's stain, and empiric antibiotics (depending on age and epidemiology). A viral process is typically polyarticular (except transient synovitis of the hip in childhood, which is thought to be viral or postviral in origin). Lyme arthritis, caused by a Borrelia spirochete, can present acutely as recurring knee monarthritis, but more often it presents early in the course of the disease as migratory polyarthralgias (see Chapter 41).

B. Crystal-induced disease

1. **Gout** classically presents as "podagra" with abrupt, intense onset of pain in the first metatarsophalangeal joint; it often affects the midfoot and ankle but can involve any joint or bursa. Typically, a man in his thirties or a postmenopausal woman (often using thiazide diuretics, which cause hyperuricemia) presents with monarthritis of the lower extremity. However, 30% present with polyarticular synovitis. Between episodes, the joints return to normal unless chronic disease develops. Check carefully for tophi on the ears, elbows, or feet. At a younger age of onset, one must think of lymphoma or other disorders associated with rapid cell turnover. Joint aspiration is diagnostic for negatively birefringent, needle-shaped crystals within white blood cells. Note that gout can coexist with pseudogout, and both can coexist with infection (see Chapter 37).
2. **Calcium pyrophosphate dihydrate (CPPD) deposition disease (pseudogout)** is an acute or subacute process in the elderly with involvement of large or small joints (including the second and third metacarpophalangeal joints).

   Chondrocalcinosis can often be defined radiographically in the knee, symphysis pubis, or triangular cartilage of the wrist. Crystals found within white blood cells are rhomboid-shaped and positively birefringent. In those patients who present at a younger age, other diagnostically important, treatable medical conditions, such as hemochromatosis, hyperparathyroidism, or Wilson's disease, must be considered (see Chapter 38).

Table 9-1. Differential diagnosis of monarthritis by presentation

Monarthritis	Common	Less common
Acute	Bacterial arthritis Gout (CPPD) Spondyloarthropathies Reiter's disease Psoriatic arthritis Inflammatory bowel disease Juvenile RA Hemarthrosis Trauma Anticoagulant therapy	Leukemia Rheumatoid arthritis Sarcoid arthritis Hemarthrosis Coagulopathy Dialysis Osteochondromatosis PVNS
Chronic	Osteoarthritis Spondyloarthropathies Lyme disease (recurring)	Fungal arthritis Tuberculous arthritis Bacterial arthritis Monarticular RA CPPD Sarcoid arthritis PVNS Osteochondromatosis

RA, rheumatoid arthritis; CPPD, calcium pyrophosphate dihydrate deposition disease; PVNS, pigmented villonodular synovitis.

C. **Hemarthrosis** is defined as the aspiration of bloody joint fluid.

1. **Trauma** usually is associated with a relevant history of injury. A layer of fat (from the bone marrow) seen on top of bloody fluid implies intraarticular fracture even in the presence of negative radiographs.
2. **Internal derangement.** Meniscal tears involving avascular portions of knee fibrocartilage may not be bloody but can cause intermittent locking, giving way, and a positive Macmurray maneuver (a painful click produced by extending the knee when the foot is internally or externally rotated). Instability of the collateral and cruciate ligaments is also a clue to this condition (see Chapter 22).

Table 9-2. Differential diagnosis of polyarthritis by presentation

Polyarthritis	Common	Less common
Acute		
Migratory	*Neisseria* infection Acute rheumatic fever Lyme disease (early)	Viral
Nonmigratory	Rheumatoid arthritis Serum sickness Systemic lupus Polyarticular JRA	Hematologic disorders Polyarticular gout
Chronic		
	Rheumatoid arthritis Polyarticular JRA Systemic lupus Polyarticular gout	Sarcoid arthritis CTD and overlap syndromes Spondyloarthropathy

JRA, juvenile rheumatoid arthritis; CTD, connective tissue disease.

3. **Nontraumatic hemarthrosis** may be seen with anticoagulation, after dialysis, or with benign neoplasms such as pigmented villonodular synovitis, synovial osteochondromatosis, or hemangioma of the synovium. Diagnosis is confirmed with synovial biopsy, arthroscopy, or magnetic resonance imaging (MRI).

D. **Periarticular syndromes.** Any of the tissues surrounding the joint can be involved in an inflammatory or traumatic process. A careful musculoskeletal examination can distinguish between tendinitis, bursitis, overuse syndromes, and surrounding cellulitis. Erythema nodosum is often seen with drug reaction, inflammatory bowel disease, or acute sarcoidosis. It often causes a periarthritis about the ankles and can result in an associated joint effusion. Osteomyelitis or neoplasia should be considered with focal bone pain. Severe periarticular pain in a child, nocturnal in nature, is uncommon with juvenile arthritis and should always suggest leukemia.

E. **Noninfectious inflammatory conditions**

1. **Seronegative spondyloarthropathies.** Because of the highly inflammatory, monarticular nature of some episodes of joint inflammation associated with Reiter's syndrome or psoriatic arthritis, the clinical presentation may be indistinguishable from that of infection. The diagnosis may be supported by the presence of characteristic extraarticular features, such as a psoriasiform rash, eye inflammation, or urethritis. A history of low back symptoms or tenderness over the sacroiliac joints suggests the diagnosis of spondyloarthritis and is an indication for radiographic study of the sacroiliac joints (see Chapter 33).
2. **Juvenile rheumatoid arthritis (JRA).** The child who presents with monarthritis and a negative infection workup may well have *pauciarticular* (fewer than four joints) JRA (see section **II.B.3** and Chapter 25). **Transient synovitis of the hip** characteristically presents as a monarthritis of the hip in a child following a viral illness. The child is nontoxic in appearance and has a culture-negative joint effusion. This self-limited disorder is felt to be mediated by a virus or immune complexes and responds to bed rest and antiinflammatory medications.

F. **Monarticular presentation of a polyarticular disease.** Although rheumatoid arthritis (RA) characteristically evolves into a symmetric polyarthritis, some patients present, at the onset of the disorder, with a monarticular synovitis. Attacks of "palindromic rheumatism" resemble gout. These are intense inflammatory episodes that involve a single joint and periarticular tissues. They last days at a time, with a return to normal between episodes. Later, the more typical, polyarticular pattern of RA emerges (see Chapter 28).

II. **Chronic monarthritis.** A single involved joint that persists beyond 2 months represents a somewhat different group of diseases. Some conditions will resolve; others will progress to a polyarticular presentation. The finding of other involved joints alters the diagnosis significantly, in that the presence of oligoarthritis makes infection and neoplasia much less likely.

A. **Infectious conditions**

1. **Pyogenic bacterial infections.** Most untreated pyogenic bacterial infections present in an acute fashion because of their virulence. These processes rarely persist in a chronic fashion unless they are partially treated.
2. **Bacterial osteomyelitis.** There is the rare occurrence of an associated bacterial osteomyelitis or an organism that is a low-virulence bacterial pathogen.
3. **Fungal infection** in an immunocompromised host, or following penetration of a splinter or plant thorn, may develop subacutely and persist in a single joint.
4. **Lyme arthritis** commonly persists for months to years after the primary infection as a recurring, inflammatory monarthritis, most commonly in the knee. In children in endemic areas, it is equally as common for the child to have Lyme disease as to have JRA.
5. **Tuberculous arthritis** usually presents subacutely as an inflammatory process in a single joint. Often, but not always, there is evidence of prior mycobacterial disease in the lung, and the patient demonstrates a positive

skin test reaction to tuberculin. In contrast to a bacterial process, tuberculous arthritis may arise from a subchondral focus of osteomyelitis and often leads to bony erosions with the absence of joint space narrowing.

B. Noninfectious inflammatory disorders

1. **Seronegative spondyloarthropathies** may be the most common causes of chronic inflammatory monarthritis. Important clinical clues include the presence of low-back or buttock pains with morning stiffness reflecting spinal involvement or inflammation of the sacroiliac joints; extraarticular features, such as pitting of the nails or a scaling skin rash (psoriasis); characteristic skin lesions, such as keratoderma blennorrhagicum or circinate balanitis, associated with urethritis and conjunctivitis (Reiter's disease); a history consistent with inflammatory bowel disease (ulcerative colitis or Crohn's disease); or a history of uveitis.
2. **Rheumatoid arthritis** can present as chronic monarthritis and requires additional months of observation before the typical symmetric joint distribution develops.
3. **Pauciarticular JRA** is often monarticular. The joint involvement may be much less impressive than the potentially devastating, asymptomatic chronic iridocyclitis that can occur in patients with antinuclear antibodies.
4. **Sarcoid arthropathy** can be associated with monarthritis, and associated erythema nodosum and hilar adenopathy will often suggest the diagnosis. More typically, there will be oligoarthritic involvement, with a prominent periarthritis about the ankles.

C. Noninflammatory conditions

1. **Osteoarthritis** is called osteoarthrosis in Europe to emphasize the noninflammatory nature of the disease. Osteoarthritis usually is of an insidious onset in the hands and weight-bearing joints. It is less common, in the absence of trauma, in the wrist, ankle, elbow, or shoulder. Patients present with pain or brief morning stiffness in one or more hand joints or in a single weight-bearing joint. Symptoms may occur at the end of the day or following activity. Studies reveal normal laboratory data, a noninflammatory joint fluid, and a radiograph that may show asymmetric joint space narrowing, subchondral sclerosis, or osteophyte (spur) formation. The presence of chondrocalcinosis on radiographs may account for symptoms in joints uncommonly involved in osteoarthritis, such as the wrist or second or third metacarpophalangeal joints.
2. **Internal derangement of the knee** (see section **I.C.2**). If untreated, this problem can lead to recurrent effusion, pain, and premature osteoarthritis.
3. **Avascular necrosis of bone.** Avascular necrosis of bone (also called **osteonecrosis**) is associated with monarticular pain and decreased range of motion in hips, knees, or shoulders resulting from ischemic necrosis of bone and the underlying bone marrow. While half of patients have no obvious cause, this condition is associated with steroid use, systemic lupus erythematosus (with or without a history of corticosteroid therapy), alcoholism, hemoglobinopathies, and Gaucher's disease.

   Avascular necrosis of bone may involve multiple sites, and some of them remain asymptomatic and are defined only radiologically. Typical radiographic changes are subchondral crescent-shaped, lucent areas (the "crescent" sign) within the femoral head. This may be followed by bone remodeling and collapse if weight bearing is not interrupted. In the chronic phase, secondary degenerative changes may occur. If the findings on plain films are normal, an early diagnosis can be made by a nuclear bone scan or MRI (see Chapter 45).
4. **Neoplasia.** As noted above, the most common benign joint neoplasms are synovial chondromatosis and pigmented villonodular synovitis. The best preoperative diagnostic test is an MRI study, which will reveal radiolucent cartilaginous or synovial lesions.

III. Acute polyarthritis. The involvement of two to four joints (oligoarthritis) or more than four joints (polyarthritis) raises the possibility of several diseases listed in Table 9-2. The pattern in which the arthritis develops is often diagnostically helpful.

A. Infectious conditions. When an acutely painful, warm, swollen joint develops then returns to normal while synovitis occurs in another joint, the patient is categorized as having **migratory polyarthritis.** This group of disorders includes important, treatable diseases for which prompt diagnosis is crucial.

1. **Bacterial infection.** The young adult with migratory polyarthritis, often associated with tenosynovitis and cutaneous pustular lesions, may have a disseminated bacterial process such as **disseminated neisserial infection.** Most commonly seen with *Neisseria gonorrhoeae,* the same syndrome can occur with *Neisseria meningitidis.* Both require prompt treatment with parenteral antibiotics. Most pyogenic bacteria produce a monarthritis, as does the late presentation of gonococcal arthritis. Polyarticular bacterial arthritis is unusual except in the immunocompromised host (see Chapter 40).
2. **Reactive (or postinfectious) arthritis**
   a. **Acute rheumatic fever** should be strongly considered in the young patient with migratory polyarthritis. A search for serologic evidence of a recent streptococcal infection with a rising antistreptolysin O (ASO) titer will support this diagnosis. Although the Jones criteria are helpful in making the diagnosis, acute rheumatic fever may occur in the absence of carditis, rash, or chorea. The arthritis associated with acute rheumatic fever typically is exquisitely painful, sometimes out of proportion to any effusion or synovitis, and is usually abrupt in onset (see Chapter 43).
   b. **Reiter's syndrome** can also cause an acute, reactive polyarthritis following dysentery or urethral infection. The arthritis is often more explosive and usually more sustained than in acute rheumatic fever. Patients may or may not demonstrate the characteristic Reiter's triad of arthritis, urethritis, and conjunctivitis.
3. **Spirochetal infection.** *Borrelia burgdorferi* infection during the primary, early stage of **Lyme disease** can lead to a migratory polyarthralgias associated with low-grade fever and symptoms typical of viral infection. Late Lyme disease assumes a more oligoarthritic pattern that waxes and wanes. The diagnosis is supported by the clinical presentation, the presence of an erythema chronicum migrans rash, and serologic testing.
4. **Viral infection.** Classically, viral arthritis is polyarticular and may, at times, be migratory. The prodromal, preicteric phase of hepatitis B can present classically with rash and arthritis. Other viruses known to produce a polyarticular presentation are rubella virus (including after vaccination), mumps virus, Epstein-Barr virus (infectious mononucleosis), and parvovirus B19. Parvovirus causes fifth disease or erythema infectiosum, a febrile exanthem in children. It can mimic acute rheumatic fever with a migratory polyarthritis or can produce an RA-like, seronegative chronic polyarthritis in adults and some children.
5. **Miscellaneous infections.** Infections with *Rickettsia,* fungi, or parasites can lead to polyarticular disease but are less common.

B. Noninfectious inflammatory conditions

1. **Rheumatoid arthritis.** Although usually insidious in onset, RA can present with an acute polyarthritis. Early on, these patients may be seronegative for rheumatoid factor but may have fatigue, anemia, and thrombocytosis. Fever is not commonly seen in RA.
2. **Polyarticular JRA** may present differently in subsets of children.
   a. The younger child has a **seronegative oligoarthritis** that is often **insidious in onset.** Serum in approximately 25% will be positive for antinuclear antibodies. A potentially destructive iridocyclitis is seen in this group of children.
   b. Another group of children may present with **systemic-onset JRA,** with high spiking fevers, a transient rash, hepatosplenomegaly, lymphadenopathy, and polyarticular or oligoarticular joint complaints that develop later.
   c. **The preadolescent girl,** in contrast, may present with rheumatoid factor positivity, nodules, and an erosive polyarticular joint disease similar to adult RA (see Chapter 25).

3. **Systemic lupus erythematosus (SLE)** is a classic immune complex disorder that characteristically presents with an RA-like polyarthritis of the small joints of the hands and feet. Marked proliferative synovitis speaks against the diagnosis of SLE. Erosive disease is rare, but the presence of reversible deformity is not. Other clinical features, such as serositis, fever, skin rash, and renal disease, may provide clues to the diagnosis. Laboratory abnormalities can include the presence of serum antinuclear antibodies, anemia, and thrombocytopenia (see Chapter 30).
4. **Other connective tissue diseases** include a spectrum of disorders that produce inflammatory disease of muscles, soft tissues, small blood vessels, and viscera. The initial presentation may include polyarthritis, but more diagnostic features evolve, including Raynaud's phenomenon with digital infarcts, skin thickening, dysphagia, and pulmonary fibrosis suggestive of scleroderma; proximal myopathy and skin rash characteristic of polymyositis/dermatomyositis; and overlap features seen in mixed connective tissue disease.
5. **Seronegative spondyloarthropathies.** This group of diseases is characterized by presence of the class I histocompatibility antigen HLA-B27; axial arthritis, including spondylitis and sacroiliitis; and inflammatory disease of the eye, skin, and ligamentous insertions (enthesopathy). The joint pattern is usually oligoarthritic and asymmetric, and large joints of the lower extremity are involved. Rheumatoid factor and antinuclear antibodies are not usually found in the serum of these patients. The specific diagnosis is usually defined by the associated clinical features: psoriatic arthritis by the presence of psoriasis, Reiter's syndrome by the concomitant conjunctivitis and urethritis, and enteropathic arthritis by the presence of ulcerative colitis or Crohn's disease.
   a. **Ankylosing spondylitis** has perhaps the least association with peripheral joint involvement of the group; it usually presents insidiously with symptoms in the axial spine. However, inflammatory involvement of the peripheral joints may develop in 25% to 30% of patients at some point in the disease. This most often involves the hips and shoulders (see Chapter 33).
   b. **Reiter's syndrome** typically has a markedly acute presentation of polyarthritis. The triad of conjunctivitis, urethritis, and asymmetric oligoarthritis may not always occur simultaneously, and limited disease has been recognized. Disease onset often follows dysentery or urethritis caused by a number of pathogens. Enthesopathy (inflammation of ligamentous or tendon insertions) and joint inflammation cause the classic "sausage digit" or dactylitis that enlarges the joints and soft tissues of the toes or fingers.

      Extraarticular features that are most helpful in diagnosis include circinate balanitis (a psoriasiform rash encircling the glans penis) or a hyperkeratotic rash on the feet (keratoderma blennorrhagicum) (see Chapter 36).
   c. **Psoriatic arthritis** can present as asymmetric oligoarticular arthritis of large and small joints; it can also present as a symmetric polyarthritis indistinguishable from RA. Dactylitis, psoriasis, and nail dystrophy are clinical features used to distinguish psoriatic arthritis from RA. Nail involvement, often simple pitting, may be present in 60% of patients with arthritis and psoriasis and is found in only 5% of those with psoriasis alone (see Chapter 35).
   d. **Enteropathic arthritis** usually presents as an asymmetric polyarthritis of the lower extremities, which can predate known inflammatory bowel disease by months to years. It is typically nonerosive, and the peripheral joint inflammation usually responds to therapy of the underlying bowel disease. The axial arthritis may not respond as well. Clues to the diagnosis include abdominal pain, abnormal bowel movements, erythema nodosum, or pyoderma gangrenosum associated with a spondylitic presentation (see Chapter 34).

6. **Crystal-induced disease**
   a. **Gout** can present as polyarticular disease in the setting of long-established tophi. In men, there generally will be a history of previous, typical, acute oligoarticular attacks; however, in postmenopausal women on thiazides, there is a well-described presentation of diffuse tophaceous, polyarticular disease without previous episodic disease. Virtually every joint can be involved, and significant fever and leukocytosis can be present. Diagnostic clues include palpable tophi in the olecranon bursa or along the pinna of the ear and characteristic erosions on radiographs of the hands or feet. Characteristic negatively birefringent crystals in the synovial fluid white blood cells and polyarticular or tophaceous disease make a septic process much less likely, but gout and joint sepsis can coexist. Similarly, gout and pseudogout crystals can be found in the same inflamed joint (see Chapter 37).
   b. **Calcium pyrophosphate dihydrate deposition disease.** The presentations of CPPD deposition disease include (a) acute monarticular pseudogout, (b) atypical osteoarthritis, (c) Charcot-like knee disease, and (d) polyarticular disease in the hands and wrists that can mimic RA. Clues include radiographic evidence of chondrocalcinosis of the triangular cartilage of the wrist, the symphysis pubis, or the knees and the identification of typical, weakly positively birefringent rhomboid crystals in synovial fluid white blood cells. As previously discussed, it is important to exclude associated treatable medical illnesses such as hyperparathyroidism and hemochromatosis (see Chapter 38).
7. **Serum sickness** presents as an acute, sometimes migratory polyarthritis that develops 10 to 14 days after antigen exposure stimulates the formation of immune complexes. The antigen can be antibiotics or other drugs, or biologics such as horse or human antisera. The clinical response is fever, polyarthritis, pruritus, and a rash. The rash is often urticarial and sometimes petechial. Adenopathy and occasionally renal disease may occur. Laboratory assessment reveals mild leukocytosis, normal or mild elevation of the sedimentation rate, rare eosinophilia, and decreased serum complement. The heterophil reaction may be positive, and circulating immune complexes can be detected.
8. **Sarcoidosis** presents as a periarthritis or polyarthritis associated with hilar adenopathy, erythema nodosum, and fever (Löfgren syndrome). A similar disorder can occur without adenopathy and can be due to infections (streptococci, TB, coccy), inflammatory bowel disease, and drug reactions.
9. **Vasculitis**
   a. **Small-vessel involvement.** Polyarthritis may be seen in types of vasculitis in which **small vessels** are inflamed. This includes the leukocytoclastic angiitis **Henoch-Schönlein purpura.** Typically, dependent and at times confluent areas of nonthrombocytopenic purpura are present from the feet to the waistline in association with inflammatory arthritis of the ankles and knees.
   b. **Medium-sized vessel involvement.** An inflammatory arthritis may also be present when medium-sized vessel involvement leads to systemic necrotizing vasculitides, such as **Wegener's granulomatosis** or **polyarteritis nodosa.**
   c. In children, **Kawasaki disease** is characterized by a febrile exanthem associated with adenopathy, mucositis, ocular changes, and devastating coronary arteritis. This disorder, thought to be the most common vasculitis of childhood, causes an inflammatory polyarthritis in one-third of patients (see Chapter 25).
10. **Hematologic disorders.** Polyarthritis may be the presenting or an early manifestation of leukemia, lymphoma, or sickle cell disease. Diagnostic clues are periarticular pain, bone pain, and nocturnal pain, as well as an associated known hematologic disorder. In children who present with these

symptoms, a bone marrow aspirate is indicated, even in the presence of a normal peripheral blood smear.

IV. Chronic polyarthritis involves four or more joints and persists longer than 2 months. Oligoarthritis involves fewer than four joints, often in an asymmetric fashion.

A. Rheumatoid arthritis. The arthritis is usually an **additive** (joints do not return to normal between episodes), **symmetric polyarthritis** of the small joints of the hands and feet. Larger joints of the upper and lower extremities and neck are also commonly involved. Rheumatoid factor may not be present in the serum early in the disease. However, eventually 80% of patients are positive for rheumatoid factor. Extraarticular manifestations include constitutional features such as weight loss and fatigue, subcutaneous nodules, and anemia (see Chapter 28).

B. Systemic lupus erythematosus. Nearly 70% of patients will present with joint complaints. The arthropathy is usually an RA-like polyarthritis that is nonerosive. The diagnosis of SLE is based on the multisystem clinical presentation and is supported by the finding of serum antinuclear antibodies.

C. Other connective tissue diseases and overlap syndromes

1. **Scleroderma** (progressive systemic sclerosis) often produces arthralgias and morning stiffness, but signs of joint inflammation are uncommon. The diagnosis of scleroderma is based on a history of Raynaud's phenomenon, multisystem illness involving the lungs, kidneys, and gastrointestinal tract, and characteristic skin findings.
2. **Polymyositis.** Arthralgias may be reported in about one-third of patients with polymyositis, but joint problems are not a major aspect of this disease.
3. **Overlap syndrome** is a term that recognizes that connective tissue diseases such as RA, SLE, scleroderma, and polymyositis have overlapping clinical and serologic features.

D. Seronegative spondyloarthropathies (see section **III.B.5**). In patients with psoriatic arthritis, Reiter's syndrome, or ankylosing spondylitis, a chronic phase may develop. Characteristic features include sacroiliitis, asymmetric oligoarthritis or polyarthritis of the lower extremities, and spondylitis. Even **Reiter's disease,** with its typical episodic flares of activity, becomes chronic in nearly 75% of patients.

E. Crystalline disease (see section **III.B.6**). As acute gouty attacks become more frequent, the joints may no longer return to normal. Patients begin to experience constant symptoms, including morning stiffness. Radiographs of patients with untreated chronic tophaceous gout can sometimes demonstrate joint changes similar to those of RA; such abnormalities may also be seen with the symmetric, polyarticular variant of CPPD deposition disease.

F. Osteoarthritis. Despite the lack of systemic features, osteoarthritis in some people can be diffuse in distribution, mildly inflammatory, and associated with significant, if slowly progressive, deformity and disability. The joint distribution typically involves the first carpometacarpal joint of the thumb; first metatarsophalangeal joint; distal and proximal interphalangeal joints of the hands, hips, and knees; and the cervical and lumbar spine (see Chapter 44).

10. MUSCLE PAIN AND WEAKNESS

J. Robert Polk and Lawrence J. Kagen

Muscle pain and weakness are commonly encountered in clinical medicine. Evaluation of a patient with these symptoms and signs begins with a careful history and thorough physical examination. Family history and medication history are important and if possible should be verified personally by the primary physician. *Proximal weakness is the usual symptom and sign of myopathy.* Muscle pain and tenderness may also be present but are experienced less often than weakness. Syndromes of muscular pain and weakness can be divided into neurologic and myopathic categories.

Neurologic Causes

I. **Upper motor neuron disease** includes brain and brainstem hemorrhages, infarctions, and neoplasms. Some demyelinating diseases may present in this category. Spasticity, increased deep tendon reflexes, pathologic reflexes, sensory abnormalities, and impaired cerebral functions may be noted.

II. **Lower motor neuron disease.** Brainstem lesions such as progressive bulbar palsy and poliomyelitis may present with weakness but usually have other features, such as cranial nerve dysfunction, that lead to the correct diagnosis. Anterior horn cell lesions can cause muscle weakness. Segmental involvement of muscles, which are flaccid, fasciculations, and loss of deep tendon reflexes are seen. Sensory abnormalities do not occur. Muscle atrophy occurs early.

III. **Nerve root disease** presents with muscle weakness if the ventral root is involved. Loss of deep tendon reflexes and muscle atrophy also occur. Muscles are hypotonic. Atrophy is less pronounced than in anterior horn cell lesions. Pain and sensory loss may occur with dorsal root dysfunction.

IV. **Peripheral nerve disease** presents with loss of deep tendon reflexes and hypotonia. Sensory abnormalities may or may not occur. Characteristically, several peripheral nerves are involved simultaneously. Distal weakness occurs early. These diseases can easily be confused with primary myopathies, especially during later stages when a primary myopathy may have features of proximal and distal weakness, muscle atrophy, and loss of deep tendon reflexes.

V. **Myoneural junction disease.** Myasthenic syndromes resemble myopathies more than neuropathies. Muscle weakness is often more proximal than distal, without early reflex changes or sensory abnormalities. Myasthenia gravis is characterized by increased muscle fatigue with continued exertion. Improvement occurs with rest.

Ocular muscles are frequently involved. An edrophonium test along with electromyography (EMG) can be used to confirm the diagnosis. The Eaton-Lambert syndrome may present with similar features, but repetitive electrical stimulation on EMG causes augmented muscle response at higher frequencies. Drugs that induce a myasthenic syndrome include D-penicillamine and the aminoglycoside antibiotics.

Myopathic Causes

The major causes of myopathy are drugs, toxins, metabolic disturbances, inflammatory syndromes, endocrinopathies, infections, and muscle dystrophies.

I. **Toxin and drug-induced myopathy**

A. **Steroid myopathy.** The insidious onset of proximal muscle weakness in a patient on steroids should suggest steroid myopathy. Myopathy can occur while a patient is on low or high doses of steroids, frequently after a recent increase in dose.

The duration of steroid treatment does not correlate with the time of onset. Patients with steroid myopathy frequently have at least two other steroid side effects, such as osteoporosis, cushingoid facies, hyperglycemia, hypertension, or psychiatric disorders. Concomitant hypokalemia is usually not seen. Inflammation is not present.

1. **Laboratory studies.** Serum muscle enzymes—creatine kinase (CK), aldolase, and aspartate aminotransferase (AST, previously known as SGOT)—are not increased; urinary creatinine excretion, however, is increased.

   EMG studies generally are not helpful. Muscle biopsy in patients with Cushing's syndrome has shown predominantly type 2 fiber atrophy, but biopsy in steroid myopathy has yielded conflicting results and has not been helpful.

2. **Treatment** is to reduce the steroid dose as much as possible or to discontinue the drug.

B. Hypokalemic myopathy. Any drug or pathologic condition causing hypokalemia can cause muscle weakness. Several drugs have been implicated, some with better substantiation than others; those usually implicated are diuretics and cathartics. Hypokalemia can also exacerbate muscle weakness due to other types of myopathies.

1. An **acute** syndrome of muscle pain, tenderness, and weakness of proximal and axial muscles may be seen. More generalized weakness can also occur.

   Serum muscle enzymes are elevated, and muscle biopsy may show vacuolar myopathy, with or without fiber necrosis and regeneration. EMG may show myopathic changes. Reflexes may be depressed or absent.

2. **Chronic** hypokalemia can result in a painless proximal or generalized myopathy, also with depressed or absent reflexes. As in the acute syndrome, serum muscle enzymes are elevated, and muscle biopsy shows vacuolar myopathy. Diagnosis is based on demonstration of hypokalemia and identification of the offending drug.

3. **Treatment** is restoration of a normal serum potassium level.

C. Alcoholic myopathy. Alcohol has been shown to be a direct hepatotoxin; proof of its muscle toxicity still rests largely on clinical interpretations. Three types of myopathy are caused by alcohol.

1. **Acute.** This form presents with cramps and, at times, with fulminant rhabdomyolysis and myoglobinuria, which usually occur together with swelling and tenderness of proximal muscles. Muscle enzymes are markedly elevated. Muscle biopsy shows necrosis and phagocytosis with little regeneration. Recovery occurs with abstinence.

2. **Chronic.** This form is least common and may occur even in the absence of a history of the acute clinical variety, described in the preceding section. Proximal muscles are weak, atrophied, and mildly tender. Unless alcoholic neuropathy is also present, distal muscle strength remains intact. Muscle enzymes are moderately elevated, and EMG shows myopathic changes. The lower extremities are affected prominently, with both atrophy and tenderness. Histopathologic findings include fiber necrosis, a mild increase in fibrous tissue, focal fat infiltration, a large variability in muscle fiber size, and regeneration of fibers.

3. **Subclinical.** In this form, muscle enzyme elevation occurs without clinical weakness and may be common in confirmed alcoholics. Diagnosis of alcoholic myopathy is based on the standard tests mentioned previously (enzymes, EMG, and muscle biopsy), but it should be remembered that a coexistent peripheral neuropathy caused by nutritional deficiency or another toxin may be present.

D. Drug-induced rhabdomyolysis and myoglobinuria. Features include severe muscle pain with swelling and tenderness, markedly elevated serum muscle enzymes, and gross (dark red-brown) pigmenturia. The urine is positive by "dipstick" (benzidine or orthotolidine). If hemolysis is suspected, the urine is reddish, the serum is pink, and a low serum haptoglobin is present. Immunoassays and electrophoresis can definitely differentiate hemoglobin and myoglobin and, in doubtful instances, should be performed. Renal failure is the worst consequence of myoglobinemic states. Emphasis from the outset should be placed on maintaining urinary output with furosemide and mannitol, as needed. Other acute laboratory abnormalities are hypocalcemia and hyperkalemia. Several drugs and toxins can induce acute rhabdomyolysis, including cocaine, illicit heroin mixtures, amphetamines, alcohol, some antimalarial drugs, anesthetics, and other drugs that cause hypokalemia. Lipid-lowering agents (e.g., lovastatin and other "statins," gemfibrozil) can also produce this syndrome. Other causes of myoglobinuria include McArdle disease, phosphofructokinase (PFK) deficiency, exertion, crush injury, prolonged pressure, injury during surgery, immobilization resulting from neurologic disorders, ischemia, and malignant hyperthermia syndrome.

II. Metabolic myopathies

A. A group of closely related abnormalities are characterized by **inborn errors of glycogen metabolism.** Distinct enzyme abnormalities cause myopathic symptoms.

1. Acid maltase deficiency. The infantile form (Pompe's disease) presents a few months after birth with diffuse muscle weakness, severe hypotonia, and cardiomyopathy with congestive heart failure. Death caused by cardiorespiratory failure occurs within 2 years. The adult or late-onset form is caused by a partial deficiency of acid maltase activity. The late-onset form presents in childhood or adult life with gradually progressive limb-girdle weakness. The pelvic girdle muscles are more involved than the shoulder muscles. Clinical heart or liver involvement has not been seen. Respiratory muscle involvement, seen in 25% to 50% of cases, leads to chronic respiratory insufficiency. The late-onset form may be mistaken for polymyositis, limb-girdle dystrophy, or spinal muscular atrophy.

a. Laboratory studies. Serum CK is increased, and the EMG changes are similar to those of polymyositis. Muscle biopsy shows a vacuolar myopathy. Biochemical assay revealing decreased or absent enzyme activity in muscle confirms the diagnosis. Also useful in diagnosis is decreased urinary excretion of acid maltase.

b. Treatment. There is no proven effective therapy for either the infantile or late-onset form.

2. Deficiency of enzymes in the glycolytic pathway

a. Muscle phosphorylase deficiency (McArdle disease). This inherited deficiency of skeletal muscle phosphorylase is more common than acid maltase deficiency or PFK deficiency; 60 cases have been reported. The female-to-male ratio is 1 : 4. Childhood symptoms of fatigue are usually overlooked. A characteristic pattern of exercise-induced muscle pains, stiffness, and weakness, which resolves with rest, occurs after puberty. Prolonged exercise results in severe cramps of the exerted muscles. Myoglobinuria and muscle necrosis may occur if exercise is strenuous; however, exercise tolerance may improve after a nonstrenuous warm-up period ("second-wind" phenomenon). As the result of recurrent attacks of myoglobinuria, some patients have a persistent proximal myopathy. The muscle cramps are actually contractions, which may last several hours.

(1) Laboratory studies. Serum CK is increased. Venous lactic acid levels do not rise with the ischemic forearm exercise test (see final the section of this chapter, Laboratory Aids to Diagnosis). Muscle biopsy shows vacuoles that stain with periodic acid–Schiff (PAS) beneath the sarcolemma and scattered necrotic or regenerating muscle fibers.

(2) Treatment. There is no long-term effective treatment.

b. Muscle phosphofructokinase deficiency results in a syndrome similar to McArdle disease. Easy fatigability occurs during childhood. Later, exercise-induced muscle pain or cramps with myoglobinuria occur. However, unlike those of McArdle disease, exercise-induced symptoms here often include nausea and vomiting. This is an autosomal recessive disease.

(1) **Laboratory studies.** Serum CK is increased. Venous lactate levels do not rise after the ischemic forearm exercise test. A mild hemolytic anemia occurs when PFK is absent from erythrocytes, which may be helpful diagnostically. Diagnosis is confirmed by the absence of PFK activity on direct measurement in muscle biopsy by biochemical or histochemical methods.

(2) **Treatment.** No generally effective therapy is available.

c. **Deficiency of other enzymes in the glycolytic pathway** also may lead to myopathy with impaired generation of lactate from glucose. These include the following:

(1) Glycogen debrancher.

(2) Phosphoglycerate kinase.

(3) Phosphoglycerate mutase.

(4) Lactate dehydrogenase (M subunit).

B. **Disorders of lipid metabolism.** Glycogen provides energy for work of short duration, whereas fatty acids provide energy for periods of rest, prolonged low-intensity exercise, and fasting. This knowledge allows prediction of the symptoms of abnormal fatty acid metabolism in muscle.

1. **Carnitine palmityltransferase (CPT) deficiency** is inherited as an autosomal recessive disorder with a male preponderance. Patients with CPT deficiency tolerate short periods of exercise normally. However, after prolonged exercise or fasting, muscular pains and myoglobinuria develop. Muscle strength is normal between attacks. There is no second-wind phenomenon.

a. **Laboratory studies.** Serum CK is normal at rest but elevated during attacks. There is a normal rise in venous lactate with the ischemic forearm exercise test. Hypertriglyceridemia, which is probably related to the impaired fatty acid utilization of CPT deficiency, may be found. The muscle biopsy specimen may be normal or show intrafiber lipid droplets. A screening test is a 38-hour fast, which will cause an elevation in serum CK.

Diagnosis is confirmed by biochemical assay of CPT activity in muscle.

b. **Treatment.** Therapy consists of eating regular meals and avoiding prolonged exertion. A diet high in carbohydrates and low in fats is effective in reducing the incidence of acute attacks.

2. **Carnitine deficiency** occurs in two forms, an isolated myopathy or a systemic disorder.

a. **Isolated muscle carnitine deficiency** is characterized by childhood onset of a slowly progressive limb-girdle weakness. Facial and pharyngeal muscles may be involved. Deep tendon reflexes are decreased or absent.

(1) **Laboratory studies.** Serum CK is moderately increased. EMG reveals a myopathic pattern. Serum carnitine levels are normal or slightly decreased. Muscle biopsy shows prominent intrafiber lipid droplets, especially in type 1 fibers. Carnitine levels in muscle are reduced to one-tenth to one-fifth of normal.

(2) **Treatment.** Preferred long-term treatment is oral administration of carnitine with a medium-chain triglyceride diet. Prednisone is effective but not desirable as long-term treatment.

b. **Systemic carnitine deficiency** presents with myopathy and hepatic insufficiency. Hepatic encephalopathy and attacks of lactic acidosis occur. Death usually occurs by age 20.

(1) **Laboratory studies.** Patients uniformly have decreased levels of serum carnitine. Carnitine deficiency states are often associated with other primary metabolic defects.

(2) **Treatment** with oral carnitine has resulted in improved strength and normalization of hepatic function in some cases.

C. **Disorders associated with abnormal serum potassium.** These interrelated syndromes of muscular weakness are associated with either hypokalemia or hyperkalemia. The exact pathogenetic role of potassium in these disorders is largely unknown.

1. **Familial periodic paralysis.** An autosomal dominant disease, this disorder is characterized by attacks of intense weakness of limb muscles that progress to complete paralysis. Attacks begin in adolescence or early adulthood and occur less frequently with age. There is marked hypotonia and absent-to-decreased tendon reflexes during attacks. Strenuous exercise or a high intake of carbohydrates may precipitate attacks. Chronic myopathy may occur after repeated attacks.
   a. **Laboratory studies.** Serum CK is elevated and *serum potassium is low* during attacks. Muscle biopsy shows vacuolar changes.
   b. **Differential diagnosis.** Hyperaldosteronism and hyperthyroidism with periodic paralysis may mimic the syndrome. The use of diuretics or cathartics may also cause similar symptoms.
   c. **Treatment** is with oral potassium (2 to 8 g of potassium chloride until the attack resolves) or intravenous potassium (50 mEq over several hours).
2. **Adynamia episodica hereditaria (Gamstorp's disease).** This autosomal dominant disease is characterized by attacks of weakness or paralysis of skeletal muscle, similar to those of familial periodic paralysis. The onset is between ages 5 and 10 years. The disease is most active during the adolescent years, after which it subsides. Attacks are precipitated by prolonged exertion or by administration of 2 to 5 g of potassium chloride.
   a. **Laboratory studies.** During attacks, the serum potassium is elevated, although high normal values have been noted. Between attacks, the patient is asymptomatic and serum potassium is normal, although persistent weakness may last for several days after an attack. Serum CK is elevated.
   b. **Treatment** with potassium-lowering agents, such as 50 to 100 mg of hydrochlorothiazide PO daily, is effective in preventing attacks.

D. **Deficiency of myoadenylate deaminase.** Deficiency of this enzyme has been associated with post-exertional cramps and myalgia. It has been suggested that impairment in the function of adenylate deaminase may lead to reduced entry of adenine nucleotides into the purine nucleotide cycle during exercise and that this may be responsible for the observed abnormalities.

E. **Mitochondrial myopathies.** Abnormalities in mitochondrial genetics can produce a variety of myopathic disorders, from ophthalmologic states to myopathies associated with encephalopathy and lactic acidoses. In addition, mitochondrial dysfunction can be manifested in different phenotypes affecting skeletal and cardiac muscle, the nervous system, and the kidneys. Diagnosis can be approached by family history, which may demonstrate a pattern of maternal inheritance; microscopy of biopsied tissue demonstrating structural abnormalities of mitochondria (e.g., subsarcolemmal aggregates in myofibers, the so-called "ragged red" fibers); and biochemical studies demonstrating abnormalities in components of oxidative phosphorylation, such as cytochrome oxidase.

III. Endocrine myopathies

A. **Hypothyroid myopathy.** The most commonly recognized endocrine myopathy occurs as a feature of hypothyroidism; it may antedate the diagnosis of hypothyroidism by several months. Symptoms and signs of this entity range from mild aches and pains, muscle cramps, and proximal weakness to apparent muscle hypertrophy and the mounding phenomenon, or myoedema (a transient focal ridging of muscle in response to percussing or pinching the muscle). In the usual form, proximal weakness may be observed, although atrophy is rare.

Hypertrophic muscles may exhibit myotonia-like contractions that are electrically silent on EMG.

1. **Laboratory studies.** Serum CK is often markedly elevated. A variety of EMG changes have been noticed, most of which indicate a myopathic

process. Muscle biopsy may show focal necrosis, regeneration, and vacuolization of fibers, but findings are usually normal. Fiber size is quite variable. Sarcolemma nuclei are numerous, enlarged, and centrally placed. Mucoprotein deposits occur in one-third of patients. Histochemical staining has shown a decrease in type 2 fibers that is directly proportional to disease severity and serum CK levels. CK levels are not increased in hypopituitarism, and a myopathy has not been reported with hypopituitarism; nonetheless, in a patient with hypothyroidism, hypopituitarism should be considered.

2. **Treatment** of hypothyroidism is thyroid hormone replacement. With proper therapy, serum CK levels return to normal over several months.

B. **Thyrotoxic myopathy.** The manifestations of this disorder range from complaints of diffuse weakness, easy fatigability, and mild atrophy to severe proximal muscle weakness with pronounced atrophy. Laryngeal and pharyngeal muscles are not involved. Serum muscle enzymes are not elevated, even in the severe form; creatinuria, however, is present. EMG may show myopathic changes. Muscle biopsy may reveal only small fiber size or atrophy of fibers with replacement of fat and lymphocyte infiltrates. (Less common myopathies in association with hyperthyroidism are exophthalmic ophthalmoplegia, thyrotoxic periodic paralysis, and the association of Graves' disease in 5% of patients with myasthenia gravis).

C. **Acromegalic myopathy.** Proximal muscle weakness and easy fatigability occur in up to 50% of patients with acromegaly. Myalgia and cramps may occur in a few patients. Muscle mass, however, is increased. Serum CK and aldolase are usually normal but may be slightly elevated. EMG shows myopathic findings. Muscle biopsy shows no consistent pattern, but there is some evidence that type 2 fiber hypertrophy may occur. With treatment of the pituitary tumor, strength recovers gradually over months or years.

IV. **Muscular dystrophy.** This group of primary muscle diseases is characterized by degeneration of muscle fibers, which occurs on a genetic basis. Although there is no specific treatment for these disorders, it is important to distinguish them from treatable forms of myopathy. Genetic counseling is suggested for patients and their families.

A. **Duchenne's pseudohypertrophic muscular dystrophy.** The onset of this sex-linked disease is usually in early childhood. Pelvic-girdle involvement, manifested by frequent falls, difficulty in climbing stairs, difficulty in rising from the floor, and a peculiar gait, is characteristic. The onset is insidious, and progression is slow. Gradually, the trunk and shoulder muscles become involved, causing the patient to require a wheelchair by age 12. Patients usually die in their twenties of either pulmonary infection or the cardiomyopathy associated with the disease.

1. **Physical examination** early in the disease reveals enlarged, firm (pseudohypertrophic), but weak calves and sometimes quadriceps and deltoids. Facial and distal muscles usually retain normal strength.

2. **Laboratory studies.** Serum muscle enzymes are increased. Creatinuria is present. Muscle biopsy shows fiber size variation and fat infiltration, depending on the stage of the disease. Dystrophin, a normal muscle protein bound to the sacrolemma, is absent. EMG reveals low-amplitude potentials of short duration. Electrocardiographic abnormalities, such as a prolonged PR interval, slurred QRS complex, ST-segment depression or elevation, and usually right bundle-branch block, are seen late in the disease. Female carriers may have mild abnormalities of serum CK, muscle biopsy, and EMG but are clinically asymptomatic.

B. **Becker's muscular dystrophy** is similar to the Duchenne form but milder, with later manifestations of disability. It is also an X-linked dystrophinopathy, with reduced synthesis of dystrophin.

C. **Fascioscapulohumeral dystrophy** is an autosomal dominant disease that affects female and male subjects equally. The usual age of onset is between 9 and 20 years, although adult onset has been recognized. The symptoms vary in severity; thus, diagnosis may be difficult. Shoulder-girdle weakness and winged scapulae are usually the first findings. Facial muscles are involved and may be the first muscles affected in some patients. The face is flattened, and the mouth moves asymmetrically, unable to pucker or whistle. Axial and pelvic muscles may become involved late in the disease; however, distal muscles are usually spared. Cardiac disease is rare, and patients usually live a normal life span. Serum muscle enzymes may be elevated slightly, and elevated urinary creatine is common.

D. **Limb-girdle dystrophy** is inherited in an autosomal recessive form and affects female and male subjects equally. Its onset occurs during the second or third decades. Shoulder- or pelvic-girdle muscles are involved first, with gradual progression to other muscle sites over years, although facial muscles are spared. Cardiac disease resulting from limb-girdle dystrophy is rare.

1. **Laboratory studies.** Serum muscle enzymes are slightly elevated, and creatinuria is present. Muscle biopsy shows fibrous and fatty replacement with necrosis of single fibers. Sarcolemmal nuclei are increased in number, forming chains centrally in the fibers. These changes may also be seen in Duchenne's dystrophy and fascioscapulohumeral dystrophy.

   Some forms of this disorder are secondary to a genetic lack of production of dystrophin-associated glycoproteins.

E. **Myotonic dystrophy.** Myotonia is an inability to relax a muscle normally after contraction. It may be elicited by grasping with the hand or by directly percussing muscle groups, such as those of the forearm or tongue, or the thumb adductors.

Myotonic dystrophy is an inherited disease that begins early in adult life. It is manifested by distal muscle weakness and atrophy. Deep tendon reflexes are reduced. Ptosis may be present, and closure of the eyelids is also weak. Atrophy of the temporalis and sternocleidomastoid muscles is severe. Other clinical features include early frontal alopecia, cataracts, blepharitis, conjunctivitis, and testicular atrophy. Mental retardation may occur. Dystrophic cardiac disease occurs late. The disease can be quite variable, and some patients and affected family members may manifest only one or two features.

1. **Laboratory studies.** EMG reveals myopathic changes and characteristic afterpotentials of myotonia. Serum muscle enzymes are usually normal, and creatinuria is rare. Histopathologic features are similar to those of other dystrophies; however, there may be prominent rows of sarcolemmal nuclei, spirals of myofibrils, and areas of clear sarcoplasm, devoid of myofibrils. Type 1 fiber atrophy is present. Peripheral nerves and anterior horn cells are normal. This disease is associated with an expanded cytosine-thymine-guanine (CTG) repeating motif in the noncoding region of the myotonin protein kinase gene.
2. **Treatment.** Quinine in a dose of 300 to 600 mg PO q6h can relieve the myotonia; however, there is no known cure. Supportive therapy and physical therapy may prolong mobility and prevent contractures.

F. **Congenital myopathies** are rare inherited diseases that begin during infancy. Progression may be quite insidious. Diagnosis rests on muscle biopsy.

V. **Inflammatory myopathies.** This group of myopathies is characterized by inflammation of unknown etiology within the muscles.

A. For full discussions of idiopathic polymyositis, dermatomyositis, myositis of other rheumatic diseases, and myositis associated with carcinoma, see Chapter 27.

B. **Sarcoid myopathy.** Muscle biopsies in small numbers of sarcoid patients without symptoms of muscle pain or weakness have revealed noncaseating granulomas typical of the disease. The occurrence of asymptomatic muscle involvement has clouded the issue of whether a true sarcoid myopathy exists. Nonetheless, there are sarcoid patients with symptomatic muscle involvement. Muscle pain and tenderness are most often seen in acute sarcoidosis with erythema nodosum. Symmetric proximal muscle weakness can be seen in chronic sarcoid (see Chapter 51).

1. **Laboratory studies.** EMG shows a nonspecific myopathic pattern. Muscle biopsy shows noncaseating granulomas, surrounding lymphocytic infiltrates, muscle fiber necrosis, and fiber regeneration.
2. **Differential diagnosis.** Similar granulomatous reactions have been seen in various malignancies, leprosy, syphilis, tuberculosis, Crohn's disease, drug reactions, and several fungal infections.
3. **Treatment.** Administration of 20 to 40 mg of prednisone daily has been effective in about half of patients.

VI. Infectious myositis and myopathy. Several microorganisms have been implicated in the onset of myositis. Both diffuse and proximal myopathies have been reported. This group of myopathies is to be distinguished from the isolated muscle involvement seen in tropical pyomyositis, streptococcal myositis, and clostridial myonecrosis.

A. Trichinosis is caused by the nematode *Trichinella spiralis.* It is transmitted by ingestion of uncooked or poorly cooked pork or bear meat. Within 2 days of ingestion of the cysts, diarrhea, nausea, abdominal pain, and fever occur. By the end of the first week, patients may have fever, periorbital edema, conjunctivitis, muscle pain and tenderness, and an erythematous maculopapular rash. Muscle weakness may be mild but is often quite severe. Muscle invasion may last 6 weeks. Myocarditis and encephalitis may occur during this stage of illness. The most commonly invaded muscles are those of the diaphragm, eye, tongue, shoulder, and calf.

1. **Laboratory studies.** Biopsy of the deltoid or gastrocnemius muscle should be performed during the third or fourth week of illness. Pressing the tissue between glass slides will reveal the uncalcified larvae. Calcified cysts represent former infection. The muscle shows a severe myositis with neutrophilic, eosinophilic, and lymphocytic infiltrates. Fiber degeneration and necrosis are present. Serum muscle enzymes are characteristically elevated. By the end of the second week, a 15% to 50% eosinophilia is present. Serologic tests become positive by the end of the third week.
2. **Treatment** is with 25 mg of thiabendazole per kilogram twice daily for 7 days. Patients with myocarditis, encephalitis, or severe hypersensitivity manifestations should be treated with 40 mg of prednisone daily during thiabendazole administration.

B. Toxoplasmosis. *Toxoplasma gondii* has been proved to cause myositis in an occasional patient. A recent case report of a patient with polymyositis and cerebellar ataxia is an example of this problem. The patient had severe muscle cramps, coarse fasciculations, and no weakness or muscle tenderness. Serum CK was markedly elevated. EMG indicated a chronic peripheral neuropathy. Muscle biopsy showed chronic interstitial myositis, fiber necrosis, and encysted *T. gondii. Toxoplasma* organisms were grown in mice injected with a suspension of the muscle biopsy.

Serologic evidence of *Toxoplasma* infection in patients with polymyositis consists of elevated complement-fixation titers, positive findings on Sabin-Feldman dye tests, and specific immunoglobulin M antibodies in a subgroup of patients. Most rheumatologists do not routinely order these tests. However, some patients with positive serologies defined early in the disease course did respond to antibiotic therapy for toxoplasmosis.

C. Viral myositis. A number of different viruses may cause an illness similar to polymyositis. Often, a prodromal illness is caused by the virus. It is unclear whether the myositis is a post-infectious immune phenomenon or a true infection of muscle. Virus-like particles have been found in muscle in some cases. Biopsy shows myositis with fiber necrosis and regeneration. Myoglobinuria may occur, especially with influenza and herpes group myositis. Viruses implicated are hepatitis B and C virus, echovirus, coxsackie virus, herpes simplex virus, and influenza virus. Late atrophy of muscles may occur. In addition, muscle biopsy findings at times may be normal. Human immunodeficiency virus (HIV) and medications such as zidovudine (AZT) can be responsible for severe myopathy as well as a syndrome indistinguishable from polymyositis.

D. **Miscellaneous infections causing myopathy.** It should be noted that numerous other microorganisms have been implicated as etiologic agents in myositis. Some have occurred only in immunocompromised patients. Agents found include *Candida tropicalis, Mycoplasma pneumoniae, Trypanosoma cruzi,* and *Echinococcus alveolaris.*

VII. **Fibromyalgia** presents as variable muscle pain and multiple tender points with normal muscle strength. The sedimentation rate and muscle enzymes are normal. It is a diagnosis of exclusion. (See Chapter 49 for a full discussion.)

VIII. **Polymyalgia rheumatica** presents in patients over 50 with proximal soreness and stiffness and constitutional symptoms. It may be associated with temporal arteritis. The Westergren sedimentation rate is elevated to over 50 mm/h in most patients, and many are anemic. (See Chapter 26 for a full discussion.)

IX. **Miscellaneous disorders presenting as myopathy.** The following disorders may present with muscle pain:

A. Primary amyloidosis.
B. Stiff-man syndrome.
C. Cervical and lumbar spondylosis.
D. Parkinson's disease.

Laboratory Aids to Diagnosis

I. **Serum chemistries.** As a result of the association of hypokalemia, hyperkalemia, hypocalcemia, hypercalcemia, hypomagnesemia, and hypophosphatemia with muscle weakness, tetany, and sometimes cramps, it is prudent to obtain serum chemistry values if clinical suspicion so indicates.

Muscle enzymes commonly measured are CK, aldolase, lactic dehydrogenase (LDH), and AST. CK is probably the most reliable indicator of muscle damage because skeletal muscle, compared with other tissues, contains relatively more of it. However, heart, brain, and smooth muscle also contain CK. Strenuous physical exertion as well as intramuscular injections may increase CK and cause elevated values for a week. Serum myoglobin is elevated in polymyositis in essentially all patients with active disease. However, this test is only performed in the setting of red urine or renal compromise. An immunoassay should be performed to detect myoglobinemia. Plasma cortisol, growth hormone, thyroid-stimulating hormone (TSH), and thyroxine values are indicated if one of the endocrine myopathies is suspected. CK may also be elevated in amyotrophic lateral sclerosis.

II. **Hematologic studies.** The erythrocyte sedimentation rate (ESR) may be elevated in inflammatory myopathy. It is useful for following patients but is not a specific test for any myopathy. Atypical lymphocytosis may occur in viral illness or toxoplasmosis. Eosinophilia may occur in infections and polymyositis. Cold agglutinins may indicate *Mycoplasma* infection.

III. **Urinary studies.** Steroid myopathy and some muscular dystrophies may be associated with elevated creatine-creatinine urinary excretion ratios with normal muscle enzymes:

$$\% \text{ creatinuria} = \text{creatine (mg/24 hr)}/\text{creatine (mg/24 hr)} + \text{creatine (mg/24 hr)} \times 100$$

This ratio should be calculated on at least two 24-hour urine collections, as day-to-day variability may occur. A ratio above 6% in adults is elevated. Urinary studies for heavy metals may be useful if a peripheral neuropathy is suspected. Myoglobinuria occurs in several diseases of muscle. Both hemoglobin and myoglobin give positive reactions to orthotolidine and benzidine. Immunoassay and electrophoresis techniques can measure myoglobin. The ammonium sulfate test has often proved unreliable or difficult to interpret. Excretion of acid maltase is decreased in acid maltase deficiency.

IV. **Provocative studies**

The **ischemic forearm exercise test** is of value in detecting deficiencies of enzymes of glycolysis. The test is performed with the patient at rest and fasting. After a baseline venous lactate level has been obtained through an indwelling catheter, a blood pressure cuff on the upper arm is inflated above systolic pressure. The patient exercises this arm for 1 minute to produce lactic acid. Sufficient work can be generated by compressing another blood pressure cuff at a rate of one stroke per second; a rise in the mercury column can then be observed. After 1 minute of exercise, the cuff is deflated and serial lactate levels are obtained at 1, 2, 3, and 5 minutes after work. Patients with enzyme deficiency will not show the expected rise in venous lactate. However, decreased lactate production is also seen following alcohol ingestion. In addition to decreased lactate production, a progressive contracture of forearm muscle that is electrically silent on EMG may develop in patients with myophosphorylase deficiency. Assay of these samples for ammonia can be used as a screening test for myoadenylate deficiency.

V. Electromyography and electroneurography

A. Nerve conduction velocities are an informative way to detect peripheral neuropathies. Diseases such as infectious polyneuritis (Landry-Guillain-Barré syndrome), Charcot-Marie-Tooth disease, and several others characteristically are associated with a slowed nerve conduction velocity.

B. EMG abnormalities are helpful in the diagnosis of polymyositis, myasthenia gravis, myotonic dystrophy, Eaton-Lambert syndrome, and McArdle disease. Characteristic findings in polymyositis are mentioned in Chapter 27. Note, however, that trichinosis and several muscular dystrophies may cause a myopathic EMG pattern similar to that of polymyositis. In myasthenia gravis, repetitive stimulation gives a characteristic decremental response, which is opposite to the pattern seen in Eaton-Lambert syndrome. In myotonic dystrophy, electrical silence after a brief voluntary contraction does not occur; instead, there is a burst of electrical activity that subsides in minutes. In McArdle disease, the muscular cramping that occurs is electrically silent.

VI. Muscle biopsy is of major diagnostic value in inflammatory muscle disease, steroid myopathy, muscular dystrophy, and infectious myositis. It is also valuable in the diagnosis of myopathy associated with various connective tissue diseases, including vasculitis. The site for a muscle biopsy should be the deltoid or quadriceps in most cases. EMG abnormalities identify areas of pathology. A biopsy specimen of the muscle contralateral to that subjected to EMG should be taken to detect artifacts that may have been produced by EMG needles. The muscle chosen for biopsy should not be atrophied or severely weak.

VII. Other modalities of imaging or assessing muscle, such as magnetic resonance imaging and ultrasound, can also provide valuable information regarding extent and activity of disease.

Bibliography

Lane RJM, ed. *Handbook of muscle disease.* New York: Marcel Dekker, 1996.

Griggs RC, Mandell JR, Miller RG. *Evaluation and treatment of myopathies.* Philadelphia: FA Davis Co, 1995.

Engel AG, Francini-Armstrong C. *Myology: basic and clinical.* New York: McGraw-Hill, 1994.

Walton J, Karpati G, Hilton-Jones D. *Disorders of voluntary muscle.* New York: Churchill Livingstone, 1994.

11. RASH AND ARTHRITIS

Michael I. Jacobs

The differential diagnosis of rash and arthritis is complex. Knowledge of the plethora of cutaneous manifestations of the arthritic diseases is important in making a correct diagnosis. A complete examination of the body surface is essential, because it may reveal lesions of psoriasis or discoid lupus erythematosus (DLE) that are hidden in the scalp, psoriatic pitting of the nails, or infiltration of old scars secondary to sarcoidosis. The purpose of this chapter is to provide the physician with diagnostic information about specific cutaneous findings in each disorder. Where applicable, immunofluorescent techniques, which may help confirm the diagnosis, are described.

I. **Behçet's syndrome.** Originally described as the triad of iritis and recurrent oral and genital ulcerations, Behçet's syndrome is a multisystem disease involving the eyes, mucous membranes, skin, blood vessels, joints, bowel, kidneys, nervous system, lungs, and heart.

   A. The **oral lesions** resemble those of aphthous stomatitis. They begin as small areas of macular erythema that then develop into superficial gray ulcers. Larger, deeper ulcerations occasionally occur.

   B. **Genital ulcerations** are most frequently located on the scrotum and labia but may also be found on the penis or in the vagina.

   C. **Other cutaneous manifestations** of Behçet's syndrome are erythema nodosum-like lesions on the lower extremities, folliculitis-like lesions, pustules, furuncles, and superficial phlebitis. A positive pathergy test can be elicited at 24 or 48 hours (i.e., the development of a pustule at the site of skin trauma such as a needle stick).

II. **Dermatomyositis/polymyositis.** The cutaneous manifestations specific for dermatomyositis are heliotrope rash and Gottron's papules. Additional cutaneous findings common to other connective tissue diseases are seen.

   A. **Heliotrope rash** is a violaceous discoloration of the upper eyelids accompanied by edema. It develops early in the course of the disease and often coincides with a similar violaceous eruption on the butterfly area of the face, neck, anterior chest, and other sun-exposed regions. On the extremities, the rash characteristically involves the extensor surfaces of both large and small joints, in contrast to the rash of lupus erythematosus, which involves the skin between the joints on the dorsum of the hand.

   B. **Poikiloderma,** which consists of speckled hyperpigmentation and hypopigmentation, telangiectasis, and cutaneous atrophy, appears later in the course of the disease.

   C. **Gottron's papules,** which are violaceous and flat-topped and appear on the extensor aspect of the interphalangeal joints, are a late manifestation.

   D. **Calcification** of skin, fascia, and muscle occurs in those patients, especially children, with severe muscle involvement.

   E. **Other findings** seen in dermatomyositis are Raynaud's phenomenon, erythema, papules, and ulcerations or leukoplakia of the mucous membranes. There is generally no correlation between the extent of cutaneous involvement and the severity of the myositis. Correlation exists between the degree of nailfold capillary abnormality, as viewed with a wide-field microscope, and the number of organ systems involved by the disease process.

III. **Erythema nodosum (EN)** appears as crops of discrete, tender subcutaneous nodules that are erythematous and whose centers are slightly raised. Lesions are usually 2 cm or more in size and are characteristically located on the shins and ankles, but they may occur symmetrically on the extensor aspect of the extremities and, infrequently, on the face. Prodromal symptoms may include fever, chills, malaise, and polyarthralgia. Lesions heal without scarring or ulcerations and undergo color changes similar to those of bruises.

A. Etiology. EN is a hypersensitivity reaction involving the vasculature of the subcutaneous tissue and should alert the physician to search for an underlying disease process. Specific etiologies follow.

1. Infection

a. β-Hemolytic streptococci. EN may appear within 3 weeks of an upper respiratory infection.

b. Tuberculosis was once a common cause of EN. Skin lesions appear 3 to 8 weeks after the primary infection.

c. Deep fungal infection. Coccidioidomycosis, histoplasmosis, and North American blastomycosis can produce EN lesions.

d. Lepromatous leprosy. When accompanied by EN, iritis, orchitis, lymphadenopathy, and polyneuritis, the disease is referred to as erythema nodosum leprosum.

2. Sarcoidosis. Lofgren syndrome, consisting of bilateral hilar adenopathy and EN, is a benign form of sarcoidosis.

3. Drug allergy. Allergy to sulfonamides, bromides, iodides, oral contraceptives, and other drugs has been associated with EN.

4. Inflammatory bowel disease. Both ulcerative colitis and Crohn's disease produce EN in about 10% of cases.

5. Behçet's syndrome. EN is seen in association with other cutaneous manifestations of this disease.

B. Differential diagnosis. Diseases to be considered in the differential diagnosis of EN are erythema induratum, Weber-Christian disease, subcutaneous nodular fat necrosis in association with pancreatic disease, recurrent thrombophlebitis, cutaneous arteritis, and lupus profundus.

IV. Juvenile rheumatoid arthritis (JRA). The characteristic rash of JRA is seen in approximately 30% of patients, mostly those with systemic-onset disease. It is more common in patients under the age of 2 years. Lesions are erythematous and flat or very slightly raised; they vary in diameter from 3 to 10 mm and have diffuse borders. Lesions occur on the trunk, extremities, and face and may become confluent. The rash is evanescent, is often associated with fever spikes, and occurs most frequently in the early evening. It may be pruritic. Koebner's phenomenon is common (i.e., rash is triggered by skin trauma).

The cutaneous eruption does not correlate with presence of rheumatoid factor (RF) in the serum, although the rash is often present during periods of active systemic disease. Skin nodules are rarely found in younger patients.

Teens with RF may have subcutaneous nodules similar to those in patients with adult RA.

V. Lupus erythematosus

A. The lupus band test (LBT) demonstrates deposits of immunoglobulin and complement at the dermal-epidermal junction by direct immunofluorescent staining of the skin. Biopsy of cutaneous lesions in DLE or systemic lupus erythematosus (SLE) yields a positive LBT in about 90% of patients.

Clinically normal skin of patients with DLE demonstrates a negative LBT. The LBT in clinically normal skin of patients with SLE varies with sun exposure. Approximately 50% of patients with SLE have a positive LBT in clinically normal, sun-protected skin, whereas 80% have a positive LBT in clinically normal, sun-exposed areas.

B. Discoid lupus erythematosus. The characteristic lesion of DLE is a scaly plaque that ranges in color from red to violaceous, with sharply-defined borders, central atrophy, telangiectasia, and areas of hypopigmentation or hyperpigmentation. Keratinous plugging of the hair follicles can sometimes be detected as tiny rough projections across the lesion. Lesions may be multiple and asymmetric and are most commonly found on the head and neck, particularly in the malar areas, ears, and scalp. When the scalp is involved, hair loss with scarring at the site of the lesion results. Lesions on the oral and nasal mucosae may ulcerate. Lesions of DLE produce scarring; those that result in severe scarring may, infrequently, produce skin cancer.

When discoid lesions are present below the neck, the term generalized DLE is used. SLE develops in fewer than 10% of patients who present with lesions of DLE.

C. **Systemic lupus erythematosus.** Cutaneous manifestations of SLE comprise several of the criteria for the classification of SLE. These criteria are facial erythema, DLE lesions, photosensitivity, and oral or nasopharyngeal ulceration.

1. **Facial erythema.** The classic butterfly rash of SLE occurs in up to 40% of patients. It begins as a transient erythematous, edematous eruption across the bridge of the nose and malar areas. It is often exacerbated by sun exposure and may accompany a flare of systemic disease. If the rash is persistent, atrophy, telangiectasia, and scaling will develop.
2. **Discoid lesions** seen in SLE are identical to those of DLE and occur in approximately 20% to 30% of patients. Patients with DLE only above the neck are at less risk for development of SLE.
3. **Photosensitivity** will often precipitate butterfly-pattern erythema, the rash of subacute lupus erythematosus, and lesions of DLE. The active spectrum is ultraviolet light of 280 to 320 nm (ultraviolet B), which normally produces sunburn erythema. Ultraviolet A (320 to 400 nm) has been implicated in lesions of subacute cutaneous lupus erythematosus (SCLE). Sunlight may also cause a flare of systemic disease.
4. **Oral or nasopharyngeal ulcerations** are shallow and have gray bases with red borders. They are often painful and usually seen in patients with severe cutaneous disease.
5. **Raynaud's phenomenon** is seen in up to 30% of cases.
6. **Alopecia** can be of two types in SLE.
   a. **Scarring** alopecia is produced when discoid lesions affect the scalp; these lesions are easily recognized.
   b. More subtle is the **reversible** (diffuse or patchy) alopecia that may arise. Diffuse alopecia is more common than patchy alopecia. It may accompany a clinical flare of SLE and is sometimes elicited only by specifically questioning the patient about increased hair loss. The frontal hairline may consist of short, broken hairs, as in traction alopecia.
7. **Subacute cutaneous lupus erythematosus** is a nonscarring photosensitive eruption with papulosquamous and annular-polycyclic patterns. The distribution is over sun-exposed areas. Patients have a high frequency of anti-Ro auto-antibodies and generally have a milder systemic disease.
   a. The **papulosquamous** eruption is composed of confluent and discrete scaly erythematous papules and plaques.
   b. In the **annular-polycyclic** type, scaly erythematous borders surround central areas of subtle hypopigmentation and telangiectasia.
8. **Vasculitis**
   a. Arteritis may result in focal areas of gangrene on the fingers or toes.
   b. Livedo reticularis is a purple, netlike, deep vascular discoloration that is most common on the lower extremities.
   c. All manifestations of leukocytoclastic vasculitis (see section **XIV.A.2**) may be observed.
   d. Painful ulcers may develop over the forearms, hands, and fingers, and near the malleoli.
9. **Periungual telangiectasia** develops on the fingers. This disorder commonly occurs in scleroderma, dermatomyositis, and, less frequently, RA.
10. **Urticaria** may be the presenting cutaneous manifestation of SLE.
11. **Lupus profundus** is characterized by firm vasculitic nodules in the subcutaneous fat. Erythema of the overlying skin sometimes occurs. The nodules may be found on the forehead, cheeks, buttocks, and upper arms.

VI. **Lyme arthritis.** This multisystem inflammatory disorder is caused by the spirochete *Borrelia burgdorferi,* which is transmitted by the bite of an Ixodes tick.

Erythema migrans, present in up to 75% of patients, is a rapidly expanding annular erythematous lesion that begins at the site of the tick bite. The central portion may remain erythematous, clear, or rarely become necrotic. The rash appears within days to 4 weeks after the tick bite. Patients at this stage will often have fever, fatigue, headache, and arthralgias. A secondary rash consisting of multiple annular lesions resembling those of secondary syphilis may follow. The nervous system, heart, eyes, and joints can become involved weeks to years later. *Borrelia* has also been implicated in some cases of **acrodermatitits chronica atrophicans,** morphea, and progressive facial hemiatrophy of Parry-Romberg.

VII. Psoriasis. This chronic disease involves the skin and joints and may present at any age. There is a family history of the disease in approximately 30% of cases. Psoriasis has been estimated to affect about 2% of the population in the United States.

A. Characteristics. Psoriasis is characterized by increased epidermal proliferation. The typical skin lesion is a well-delineated, raised, erythematous plaque covered by a loosely adherent silvery scale. As the scale accumulates, the lesion may even appear white. Lesions vary in size from small papules to extensive plaques and occasionally assume an annular or gyrate configuration. Lesions of psoriasis heal without scarring.

B. Distribution

1. Although psoriasis usually has a **symmetric** distribution, a solitary lesion is sometimes seen.
2. **Sites of predilection** include the elbows, knees, scalp, and lumbosacral region.
3. Any clinical pattern of psoriasis may be associated with psoriatic arthritis. However, **nail involvement** is seen in 80% of patients with arthritis and in only 30% of patients without joint involvement.

C. Medications that may cause psoriasis to flare include chloroquine and lithium; withdrawal of systemic corticosteroids is also a possible cause.

D. Koebner's phenomenon is the appearance of new lesions at sites of trauma, such as scratching, sunburn, or physical injury. Bluntly scraping off the scale to reveal punctate areas of bleeding underneath produces the **Auspitz** sign.

E. The **chronic plaque type** is seen on the sites of predilection noted in **B** and on the trunk and extremities. Lesions may become confluent.

F. Inverse psoriasis is localized to intertriginous areas.

G. Guttate psoriasis is characterized by teardrop-shaped lesions on the trunk and proximal extremities; it is often precipitated by a β-hemolytic streptococcal infection.

H. Palmar psoriasis is characterized by scaly, erythematous patches on the palms and fingers. This form may be mistaken for a dermatophyte infection.

I. Pustular psoriasis may present as localized sterile pustules of the palms, soles, or paronychial skin or as severe generalized pustules accompanied by fever, arthralgia, and leukocytosis.

J. Exfoliative erythroderma, in which the skin of the entire body is thickened, erythematous, and scaly, may be precipitated by an infection, drug allergy, sunburn, or severe contact dermatitis.

K. Nail changes include surface pits, yellow discoloration of the nail plate, lifting of the nail bed, subungual keratotic accumulation, thickening, crumbling, grooving, and splitting.

VIII. Pyoderma gangrenosum is frequently associated with ulcerative colitis, Crohn's disease, RA, myeloproliferative disorders, and leukemia. Rarely, it is associated with chronic active hepatitis, myeloma, sarcoidosis, and diabetes mellitus. It begins as a tender pustule that rapidly expands to become a large ulcer many centimeters in diameter with a bluish, undermined border and a necrotic, purulent center. Lesions most frequently occur on the legs and trunk and heal with scar formation. Cutaneous trauma may exacerbate existing ulcers or cause the formation of new lesions.

Skin biopsy of pyoderma gangrenosum is not diagnostic. The diagnosis can be made only when other causes of cutaneous ulcerations, such as vasculitis, syphilis, tuberculosis, and bacterial, fungal, and protozoal infection, are excluded.

IX. **Reiter's syndrome** consists of the tetrad of arthritis, urethritis, conjunctivitis, and mucocutaneous lesions. The mucocutaneous lesions, present in about 80% of cases, may be divided into the following categories:

A. **Mucosal lesions.** The penis is commonly affected by superficial ulcerations around the urethral meatus. Eroded red papules involve the corona and glans and become confluent (**balanitis circinata**). Erosion, erythema, and purpura are seen frequently in the mouth and pharynx.

B. **Cutaneous lesions**

1. **Red macules** may develop on the palms and soles, then form pustules and progress to thick hyperkeratotic plaques (**keratoderma blennorrhagica**).
2. **Psoriasiform plaques,** which may form pustules, are sometimes found scattered on the scalp, trunk, extremities, and scrotum.
3. **Nail changes** include subungual hyperkeratosis and thickening of the nail plate.
4. **Generalized exfoliative erythroderma** may be seen in severely ill patients.

X. **Rheumatic fever.** Three type of skin lesions are observed in rheumatic fever. They are listed in decreasing order of frequency.

A. **Subcutaneous nodules** are usually less than 0.5 cm in diameter and are found over bony prominences of the elbows, knuckles, ankles, and occiput. Nodules may persist up to a month or recur over several months and are frequently associated with carditis.

B. **Erythema marginatum** is most commonly seen on the trunk, extremities, and the axillary vault. These flat or slightly raised polycyclic and annular lesions begin as small erythematous macules or papules that rapidly spread peripherally. The outlines of the lesions may become irregular. Usually associated with carditis, the lesions often erupt soon after the onset of arthritis and may recur for months.

C. **Erythema papulatum,** an extremely rare manifestation of rheumatic fever, is characterized by indolent papules that are found over the flexor and extensor surfaces of large joints.

XI. **Rheumatoid arthritis.** Rheumatoid nodules and manifestations of vasculitis are the major cutaneous findings in RA and are observed primarily in patients with RF.

A. **Rheumatoid nodules** are found in approximately 20% of patients. They are firm, up to several centimeters in diameter, and most frequently located subcutaneously, although they can involve tendon sheaths and periosteum. They are found in skin subjected to repeated minor trauma, such as the juxta-articular region of the elbows, Achilles tendons, ischial tuberosities, scapular areas, and hands and feet. If they occur on the sclera, scleromalacia with possible globe perforation may result. Rheumatoid nodules may rarely soften and ulcerate.

B. **Vasculitic lesions** are commonly found on the digits. They present as tiny nail infarcts or red or purpuric macules or papules that can progress to painful subcutaneous nodules or ulcers, 2 to 3 mm in diameter. In severe cases of digital arteritis, gangrene of the finger pulp can ensue. Vasculitis frequently affects the dependent lower extremities, manifesting as purpuric macules and papules, urticarial lesions, hemorrhagic bullae, painful ulcers, and livedo reticularis.

C. **Other rare cutaneous features** of RA are palmar erythema and skin atrophy of the hands.

XII. **Sarcoidosis.** All cutaneous manifestations of sarcoidosis, except EN and transient maculopapular eruptions, show histologic evidence of sarcoid granulomas on skin biopsy.

Circulating immune complexes may be responsible for both EN and transient maculopapular eruptions, either of which may be a presenting sign of the disease.

A. **Erythema nodosum** is a septal panniculitis that appears as painful, erythematous, slightly raised, rounded lesions symmetrically distributed on the extensor aspect of the extremities, often localized to the shins. Fever and polyarthralgias may occur. When healing, the lesions assume the color of a bruise. Recurrent lesions appear in crops. EN is not specific for sarcoidosis, but the condition is termed **Lofgren syndrome** when accompanied by bilateral hilar adenopathy.

B. Transient maculopapular eruptions occur on the trunk, face, or extremities and may be accompanied by acute uveitis, peripheral lymphadenopathy, and parotid enlargement.

C. Granulomatous cutaneous lesions of sarcoidosis include the following:

1. **Papules.** Translucent, reddish brown; they are found on the periorbital area, ala nasi, and upper torso.
2. **Annular lesions.** Formed from papules coalescing in rings.
3. **Nodules.** Rarely found on the extremities or trunk.
4. **Plaques.** Purple to reddish brown; they are symmetrically located on the extremities and buttocks. Plaques on the face, ears, fingers, or toes are referred to as lupus pernio.
5. **Ichthyosis-like lesions.** Large scales, usually located on the lower extremities.
6. **Generalized erythroderma.**
7. **Infiltration of old scars.** A phenomenon peculiar to sarcoidosis; scars become purple and raised.

XIII. Scleroderma and variants. Scleroderma may present as a disease localized to the skin or as a systemic process.

A. Localized scleroderma

1. **Morphea** is a discrete, well-defined plaque of scleroderma that is smooth, indurated, and yellowish white in color. It has a violaceous halo when the disease is active.
2. **Generalized morphea.** Numerous large plaques may involve almost the entire body, usually sparing the face. Underlying muscle atrophy is often prominent on the extremities.
3. **Guttate morphea** consists of small, white, sclerotic lesions usually located on the chest and shoulders.
4. **Linear scleroderma** generally begins during childhood, is unilateral, and may result in joint contractures secondary to involvement of muscle and bone.
   - a. **Facial hemiatrophy** may be associated with facial linear scleroderma.
   - b. ***Coup de sabre*** refers to linear scleroderma that involves the face and scalp.

B. Systemic scleroderma (progressive systemic sclerosis, or PSS). Skin involvement in PSS may be classified by type of onset and presence or absence of Raynaud's phenomenon.

1. **Acrosclerosis** is the predominant type, accounting for 90% of cases. It is characterized at an early stage by edema of the hands, fingers, feet, and legs and by Raynaud's phenomenon. Later, the skin of the hands and feet becomes indurated, thick, taut, smooth, and bound down. The process may extend onto the extremities. The face, neck, and trunk are commonly involved. Cutaneous manifestations include the following:
   - a. **Sclerodactyly.** Smooth, shiny, tapered fingers with taut, bound-down skin from the MCPs to the fingertips.
   - b. **Joint contractures** occur principally over small joints but may involve large joints as well. Hand contractures result in "claw hand" deformity.
   - c. **Ulcerations** usually develop over the fingers, toes, malleoli, and knuckles and may result in infection.
   - d. **Facial involvement** may result in either a waxy, expressionless facies or in a pinched facies with thin lips, radial furrows about the mouth, sunken cheeks, and a beaklike nose.
   - e. **Pigment alterations** appear as three types.
     - (1) The most common type is **post-inflammatory hyperpigmentation** or **hypopigmentation** in sclerotic areas.

(2) In areas of normal skin, **complete pigment loss,** dotted centrally by perifollicular pigment resembling vitiligo, may develop.
(3) Rarely, generalized **hyperpigmentation** similar to that seen in Addison's disease occurs.

f. **Matlike telangiectases** may occur on the face, lips, hands, oral mucosa, and upper trunk. There is a high correlation between the degree of nail fold capillary abnormality, as viewed with a wide-field microscope, and the extent of internal organ involvement in scleroderma.

g. **Bullae** may rarely occur in areas of sclerosis.

h. **Calcinosis cutis** generally occurs late in the course of scleroderma and is usually limited to the skin over joints. The **CREST syndrome** consists of **c**alcinosis, **R**aynaud's phenomenon, **e**sophageal dysfunction, **s**clerodactyly, and **t**elangiectasia. It identifies a group of PSS patients with a more favorable prognosis.

2. **Diffuse systemic sclerosis** often begins on the trunk and rapidly spreads to involve the extremities and face.

3. The **differential diagnosis** of fibrotic skin includes the following:
   a. Eosinophilic fasciitis.
   b. Tryptophan-induced eosinophilia myalgia syndrome.
   c. Borreliosis.
   d. Graft-versus-host disease.
   e. Porphyria cutanea tarda.
   f. Scleroderma.
   g. Carcinoid syndrome.
   h. Scleromyxedema.
   i. Lichen sclerosis et atrophicus.
   j. Bleomycin-induced sclerosis.
   k. Chlorinated hydrocarbon-induced sclerosis (polyvinyl chloride).
   l. Occupational trauma.
   m. Primary amyloidosis.
   n. Melorheostosis with linear scleroderma.
   o. Progeria.
   p. Werner syndrome.
   q. Phenylketonuria.
   r. Toxic oil syndrome (caused by adulterated rapeseed oil).

C. **Eosinophilic fasciitis** can usually be distinguished from systemic scleroderma by examination of the skin. On the trunk and proximal extremities, localized areas of induration develop that are firmly bound to underlying tissues. A cobblestone or puckered surface is formed secondary to involvement of the subcutaneous fibrous tissue and is most obvious during overhead extension of the upper extremities. Raynaud's phenomenon and internal organ involvement do not occur. A biopsy specimen that includes skin, fascia, and muscle is necessary for diagnosis. Fibrotic thickening and a cellular infiltrate, often including eosinophils, are found in the deep fascia and may also be present in the lower dermis, fat, and muscle. Laboratory abnormalities include blood eosinophilia in 30% of patients, an increased erythrocyte sedimentation rate, and hypergammaglobulinemia. A history of tryptophan ingestion should be elicited.

D. **Tryptophan-induced eosinophilia myalgia syndrome.** In 1989, a disease characterized by peripheral eosinophilia and myalgia with features of both eosinophilic fasciitis and systemic scleroderma was seen following tryptophan ingestion. Clinical features include fever, fatigue, weakness, muscle cramps, arthralgia, cutaneous edema, rashes, pruritus, and thickening of the skin. The degree of both eosinophilia and myalgia is variable. Scleroderma-like skin changes can involve the extremities as in eosinophilic fasciitis, or become more generalized as in PSS.

E. **Undifferentiated connective tissue syndrome,** also known as mixed connective tissue disease, denotes combined clinical features of SLE, scleroderma, and polymyositis. High titers of antibodies to U1RNP occur in many of these patients. Some authorities feel that undifferentiated connective tissue syndrome represents a prodrome of SLE or scleroderma in most patients (see Chapter 31). Raynaud's phenomenon and swollen hands are the most frequent skin manifestations.

Direct immunofluorescent studies of clinically normal skin in patients with undifferentiated connective tissue syndrome reveal subepidermal immunoglobulin deposits in approximately one-third of cases.

XIV. **Vasculitis, cutaneous** (See also Chapter 32.)

A. **Classification.** Cutaneous vasculitis includes septic and leukocytoclastic categories.

1. **Septic vasculitis.** Skin manifestations of the **gonococcal arthritis-dermatitis syndrome** occur during the initial bacteremic phase and are accompanied by fever, rigor, tenosynovitis, and migratory polyarthritis. The skin lesions are usually tender, few in number, and located on the distal extremities. They may present as petechiae, small ecchymoses, hemorrhagic papules, vesiculopustules on a hemorrhagic base, or hemorrhagic bullae. It is difficult to culture gonococci from skin lesions.
2. **Leukocytoclastic vasculitis.** Lesions of "palpable purpura" on the lower extremities may be easily recognized. The morphologic expression of the immune complex vasculitis that involves the postcapillary venules of the skin is manifold. Lesions are usually concentrated on the legs and distributed symmetrically. They may begin as erythematous macules or urticarial papules. These lesions then become purpuric. The vasculitis may rapidly progress to form hemorrhagic vesicles and bullae, nodules, or superficial ulcers covered by eschars. Such lesions are painful and may appear in recurrent crops that last for weeks. Three important syndromes manifested by leukocytoclastic vasculitis follow.

a. **Henoch-Schönlein purpura** occurs primarily in children and young adults following an upper respiratory tract infection. Purpuric lesions develop over the extensor surfaces and buttocks. Edema of the lower legs is common; edema of the hands, scalp, and periorbital areas occurs in young children. Arthritis, abdominal pain, gastrointestinal bleeding, and renal involvement presenting as proteinuria and hematuria are other features. Serum complement levels are usually normal. Immunofluorescent staining of skin biopsy specimens of early lesions reveals mainly immunoglobulin A and complement deposition in the walls of affected vessels.

b. **Hypocomplementemic vasculitis** is characterized by recurrent attacks of urticarial skin lesions accompanied by arthritis and hypocomplementemia. The urticarial lesions may last for days, and small purpuric lesions may occasionally be present. Abdominal pain, edema of the face and larynx, and mild renal disease may occur. Biopsy and immunofluorescent staining of early skin lesions reveal immunoglobulin and complement deposition in vessel walls.

c. **Mixed cryoglobulinemia** demonstrates the spectrum of cutaneous manifestations of leukocytoclastic vasculitis and is accompanied by immune complex renal disease (often severe), hepatosplenomegaly, and lymphadenopathy. The presence of mixed cryoglobulinemia, positive RF, and hypocomplementemia help to define this disease. A majority of patients have hepatitis C infection. Immunofluorescent staining of early skin lesions reveals immunoglobulins and complement in the walls of affected vessels.

B. **Differential diagnosis of cutaneous vasculitis**

1. **Infectious agents.** *Gonococcus, Meningococcus, Staphylococcus aureus,* β-hemolytic streptococci, hepatitis B virus, hepatitic C virus, human immunodeficiency virus, *Mycobacterium leprae,* endocarditis-producing bacteria.

2. **Drugs.** Penicillin, sulfonamides, thiazides, phenothiazines, aspirin, allopurinol.
3. **Rheumatic disease.** SLE, RA, sicca syndrome, Henoch-Schönlein syndrome, hypocomplementemic vasculitis, mixed cryoglobulinemia, hyperglobulinemic purpura, paraproteinemia, Wegener's granulomatosis, polyarteritis nodosa, polyangiitis syndrome.
4. **Malignancies.** Lymphoproliferative disorder, Hodgkin's disease, carcinoma.
5. **Systemic diseases.** Serum sickness, ulcerative colitis, chronic active hepatitis, primary biliary cirrhosis, bowel bypass syndrome, Goodpasture syndrome, retroperitoneal fibrosis.
6. **Genetic disorders.** C2 deficiency.

12. RAYNAUD'S PHENOMENON

Kyriakos A. Kirou and Mary Kuntz Crow

Raynaud's phenomenon (RP) is characterized by episodic ischemia of the digits. Typically, exposure to cold or emotional stress produces vasospasm and occlusion of the digital arteries, with well-demarcated ischemic blanching of the involved digits. This may be followed sequentially by cyanosis and rubor, although the classic triphasic color change is not common. Numbness and sometimes pain occur, especially during the reactive hyperemia phase (rubor). An attack may last from several minutes to hours (usually 10 to 30 minutes). Upper extremities are most frequently involved, but 40% of patients have symptoms in their lower extremities.

The phenomenon is named after Maurice Raynaud, who first described it in 1862. It can occur in otherwise healthy persons (primary RP) or in association with other disorders (secondary RP). In 1932, Allen and Brown defined the criteria for diagnosing primary RP: (a) appearance of symptoms with exposure to cold or emotional upset; (b) bilateral symmetric involvement of the hands; (c) presence of normal pulses; (d) absence of, or only superficial, digital gangrene; (e) absence of an underlying disorder commonly associated with the symptom complex; (f) presence of symptoms for at least 2 years without the appearance of an underlying cause.

These guidelines for diagnosis remain valid. However, a systemic disease may develop in patients with presumed primary RP many years after the onset of symptoms. LeRoy and Medsger have proposed a stricter definition of primary RP that would exclude all patients with evidence of digital pitting, ulcerations, or gangrene; abnormal nailfold capillaries; a positive antinuclear antibody (ANA) test; or an abnormal erythrocyte sedimentation rate (ESR) at presentation. According to a recent metaanalysis of ten studies, a connective tissue disease (CTD) developed in 80 of 639 patients with primary RP (12.5%) after a mean follow-up of 2.8 years. An abnormal nailfold capillary pattern was the best predictor of transition, with a positive predictive value of 47% (Spencer-Green). In another study (Landry et al.), a CTD developed after 10 years of follow-up in 19 of 80 patients (24%) who had what appeared to be primary RP. This value increased to 55% for seropositive patients [for antinuclear antibody (ANA) or rheumatoid factor (RF)] and to 81.8% for seropositive patients with evidence of fixed arterial obstructions (on vascular laboratory evaluation).

Population-based studies estimate a prevalence of RP of 5.8% to 20.2% among women and 4.1% to 12.7% among men, with the highest rates noted in the coldest geographic regions. Primary is much more common than secondary RP, and it usually affects young women (onset in teens is characteristic of primary RP).

I. Pathogenesis. Vasospasm of the digital arteries and cutaneous arterioles is the *sine qua non* of RP. Neural signals, including sympathetic, parasympathetic, and sensory-motor fibers (that release substance P and calcitonin gene-related peptide), and the endothelium are the major determinants of vascular reactivity. Circulating hormones and mediators released from circulating cells are also very important. Some of the neurotransmitters and mediators act directly. Notably, epinephrine (released by sympathetic nerves) acts directly on α_2-adrenoreceptors, abundantly present on smooth-muscle cells of small digital and cutaneous arteries, to cause vasoconstriction. Others act indirectly by activating endothelial cells to produce either vasodilators (i.e., nitric oxide) or vasoconstrictors (i.e., endothelin-1). Reduced digital blood flow can be triggered by either a whole-body exposure to cold (through a sympathetic reflex mechanism) or local digital cooling.

A. Vasospasm alone, without an underlying arterial structural abnormality, is responsible for **primary RP.** Residence in cold climates may predispose to it. Patients with primary RP have an increased α_2-adrenoreceptor sensitivity to cold. The underlying mechanism remains unknown.

B. **Secondary RP** is associated with many and diverse disorders. Vasospasm is important, but a structural arterial abnormality compromising even the resting digital blood flow is likely to exist also.

1. **Connective tissue disease**

   a. **Systemic sclerosis (SSc) or scleroderma.** There are two forms of SSc, a diffuse cutaneous form, associated with auto-antibodies to topoisomerase-1, and a limited cutaneous form, the CREST syndrome (calcinosis, RP, **e**sophageal dysmotility, **s**clerodactyly, and **t**elangiectasia), associated with anti-centromere antibodies. Most (90% to 95%) patients with SSc exhibit RP, which is frequently the presenting feature of the disease. RP is usually worse in limited SSc. On examination, sclerodactyly, evidence of ischemic tissue necrosis with digital pitting, digital ulcerations, and even gangrene may be present. Nailfold capillary microscopic abnormalities include enlargement of the capillary loops and the presence of intervening avascular areas. The latter predict transition to diffuse SSc. Endothelial cell damage or dysfunction is a prominent and early characteristic in the disease course, but the underlying mechanisms are unknown. Oxygen free radicals generated during reperfusion injury from repeated ischemic attacks may contribute. Histologically, intimal hypertrophy and thrombosis in small (including the digital) arteries occur. Adventitial fibrosis is common and has been implicated in digital ischemia, by virtue of external compression. Cold-induced vasospasm in the heart and other internal organs has been noted in SSc and is called systemic or visceral RP. Scleroderma-overlap CTD syndromes such as mixed connective tissue disease **(MCTD),** characterized by features of SSc, SLE, polymyositis, and anti-U1RNP antibodies, and tRNA synthetase-associated syndromes, characterized by antibodies to tRNA synthetases and features of myositis and fibrosing alveolitis, have a similarly high prevalence of RP.

   b. **Systemic lupus erythematosus (SLE).** RP occurs in 10% to 35% of cases of SLE. Nailfold capillaroscopy may show increased capillary tortuosity. It is usually benign without occurrence of tissue necrosis.

   c. **Sjögren's syndrome.**

   d. **Rheumatoid arthritis.**

   e. **Systemic vasculitis.** Inflammatory occlusion of the involved vessels frequently leads to severe digital ischemia and gangrene.

   f. **Polymyositis.**

2. **Traumatic vasospastic disease.** Persons who are exposed to repetitive trauma to the digits are at increased risk for the development of RP. It has been postulated that chronic stimulation of the pacinian corpuscles in the hands may result in digital artery vasospasm through a reflex that involves the sympathetic system. It most commonly occurs in workers who use vibratory tools such as pneumatic hammers and chain saws. The term **vibration-induced white finger** is used for this condition. Typists and pianists may also be affected. Interestingly, frostbite predisposes to the development of RP in the body parts involved.

3. **Occlusive arterial disease.** Atherosclerosis and thromboangiitis obliterans (Buerger's disease) may result in RP in the distribution of the narrowed blood vessels. Thrombotic or embolic occlusions of digital or larger proximal arteries are also in the working differential diagnosis.

4. **Nerve compression.** RP can result from a thoracic outlet syndrome. Compression (e.g., by a cervical rib or a pectoralis minor tendon) of brachial plexus sympathetic fibers and the subclavian artery have been implicated. RP may also be seen in patients with the carpal tunnel syndrome.

5. **Drugs and chemicals.** Ergot alkaloids have a direct vasoconstrictive action on blood vessels. Methysergide may cause intimal fibrosis. Exposure to vinyl chloride and bleomycin can cause a scleroderma-like illness with RP. Beta blockers, sympathomimetics, cocaine, cyclosporine, interferon-alfa, vinblastine, and cisplatin have been all implicated in the development of RP.

6. **Hematologic abnormalities.** RP has been reported in cryoglobulinemia, cold agglutinin disease, polycythemia, and macroglobulinemia. Blood hyperviscosity is the presumed underlying mechanism.
7. **Other disorders** associated with RP include malignancy, and hypothyroidism.

II. Diagnosis

A. History. The diagnosis of RP is based on a history of the classic triad of sequential digital pallor, cyanosis, and rubor in response to cold exposure or emotional stimuli. However, white alone, white and blue-purple, or white and red color changes are frequently seen. Male sex and age above 40 suggest secondary RP. A thorough history including exposure to drugs, trauma, and occupational hazards should be taken to differentiate primary from secondary RP.

B. Physical examination. Examination of patients with primary RP between attacks is unrevealing. Moreover, attempts to reproduce an attack during clinical evaluation are usually unsuccessful and not recommended. Nevertheless, the clinician should look for clues of an underlying disease. Asymmetric involvement and abnormal peripheral pulses should prompt vascular surgical evaluation and exclusion of thromboembolic disease (especially in an acute setting and history of trauma). Puffy hands, sclerodactyly, tendon friction rubs, and telangiectasia are features of SSc and scleroderma-overlap CTD syndromes. Similarly, **nailfold capillary microscopy,** performed with placement of grade B immersion oil on the nailfolds and a stereo-zoom microscope (or even an ophthalmoscope set at 40 diopters), may reveal important scleroderma-specific abnormalities (see above). The presence of digital trophic skin changes, ulcers, severe pain, and gangrene indicate a compromised resting blood flow, as would occur with a fixed arterial obstruction. Maneuvers to detect thoracic outlet compression or carpal tunnel syndrome should be undertaken.

C. Laboratory studies

1. A complete blood count with differential, urinalysis, and tests for ESR, ANA, and RF can help identify an underlying systemic disorder in the initial evaluation. Additional tests should be ordered accordingly. Evaluation for the presence of a hypercoagulable state, cryoglobulins, hypothyroidism, and anti-centromere and anti-topoisomerase antibodies may be necessary. Chest radiography might reveal a bony cervical rib or basal lung fibrosis. Echocardiography is useful for exclusion of thromboemboli or septic emboli, and nerve conduction studies for nerve compression syndromes.
2. **Vascular laboratory evaluation** may include a Doppler study of vessels to assess the patency of the superficial palmar arch and proximal larger arteries. Additionally, finger photoplethysmography and finger blood pressure determination (with a pneumatic cuff placed around the proximal phalanx and a photoplethysmograph placed over the distal phalanx), performed at a warm ambient temperature to avoid vasoconstriction, may prove very useful. Abnormal photoplethysmographic waveforms and brachial-finger pressure gradients of more than 20 mm Hg indicate fixed arterial obstruction somewhere in the vascular pathway supplying the terminal phalanx.
3. **Arteriography** (or magnetic resonance angiography) is necessary only when a proximal embolic source is suspected or microsurgical arterial reconstruction of the superficial palmar arch is contemplated. Sympathetic blockade is recommended prior to angiograpy in order to avoid reflex vasospasm due to vascular trauma.

D. Differential diagnosis. RP, which is an episodic disorder, must be differentiated from processes characterized by persistent vasospastic ischemia. In the disorders described below, vasoconstriction is probably limited to arterioles and does not involve the digital arteries.

1. **Acrocyanosis,** like RP, is exacerbated by low temperatures and emotional stress. However, cyanosis is not confined to the digits but extends diffusely to the hands or feet. Its idiopathic form is a benign disorder.

2. **Livedo reticularis,** characterized by a persistent purple or blue mottling of the skin, predominantly involves the extremities; it is usually a benign condition. However, it may be vasculitic in nature (livedo reticularis with ulceration or *atrophie blanche*) or secondary to a systemic disorder such as SLE or the antiphospholipid syndrome.

III. Treatment. Adequate reassurance and patient education on how to avoid cold exposure is often all that is needed for patients with mild primary RP. Temperature biofeedback, in combination with different relaxation techniques or conditioning treatment, has also been helpful for such patients. Severe primary RP compromising quality of life because of frequent uncomfortable attacks and the constant need to practice cold avoidance will usually respond to pharmacologic therapy with calcium channel blockers. Therapy of secondary RP should address both vasospasm and the underlying disorder. Notably, vasculitis will require corticosteroids or immunosuppressive therapy. Antiphospholipid syndrome, other thrombophilic disorders, and thromboembolic events require appropriate anticoagulation therapy. Severe involvement of large vessels (secondary to trauma, atherosclerosis, or vasculitis) will require vascular surgery. Microsurgical revascularization, if available, can be effectively employed for occlusive lesions affecting the wrist arteries and superficial palmar arch. Notably, these are frequently seen in SSc.

A. **General measures.** Avoidance of cold temperatures and the use of warm clothing, mittens, and even electrically heated gloves cannot be overemphasized. Tobacco smoking should be discontinued. Repetitive traumatic injury to the extremities should be avoided. Beta blockers, if used, should be appropriately substituted. For acute and severe ischemic pain, which may further augment sympathetically mediated vasospasm, adequate analgesia will be necessary. Extreme care should be undertaken to prevent or treat infection (usually with *Staphylococcus*) of ischemic ulcers.

B. **Drug therapy of vasospasm.** Vasodilators are more helpful in cases in which the vasospastic component is prominent. If a significant occlusive component is present, the benefit may be less significant.

1. **Calcium channel blockers** are the best-studied agents and the usual first choice. Some calcium channel blockers, in addition to causing vasodilation, may inhibit *in vivo* platelet activation and enhance the thrombolytic activity of blood. However, they can aggravate esophageal reflux or constipation. They should be avoided during pregnancy.

   a. **Nifedipine** can decrease the number and severity of episodes of RP. Side effects are common and include headache, tachycardia, flushing, lightheadedness, and edema. The initial dosage is 10 mg orally three times daily with upward titration to the maximum tolerated dose. The slow-release preparations (30 or 60 mg once daily) are thought to have fewer side effects. Because amlodipine is very closely related to nifedipine, it is also used (5 to 10 mg daily).

   b. **Diltiazem,** another calcium channel inhibitor, may be efficacious in patients with primary or vibration-induced RP. The dosage is 30 mg three to four times daily.

2. **Alpha blockers**

   a. **Prazosin,** an α_1-adrenoreceptor blocker, is beneficial in primary RP, yet the clinical improvement may not be sustained with prolonged treatment. Syncope may occur with the first dose but can be prevented by giving the drug at bedtime and limiting the dose to 1 mg. Subsequent doses are better tolerated. Most patients can be managed on 1 to 2 mg orally three times daily.

   b. **Phenoxybenzamine** is a potent alpha blocker. The weak evidence supporting its use in RP and the high incidence of side effects (postural hypotension, palpitations, diarrhea, impotence) limit its clinical usefulness.

3. **Presynaptic sympathetic inhibitors,** such as guanethidine and reserpine, have been largely replaced by other, better studied and tolerated agents.

4. **Nitrates.** Topical nitroglycerin ointment and sustained-release transdermal glyceryl trinitrate patches can reduce the number and severity of attacks in both primary and secondary RP, but their use is limited by the high incidence of headaches.
5. **Prostaglandins,** besides being **potent vasodilators** and platelet aggregation inhibitors, probably have additional biologic properties of longer-lasting benefit to microcirculation. Although they are effective when given intravenously, there is not yet sufficient evidence for the clinical usefulness of available oral prostaglandin preparations.
   a. **Iloprost** is a chemically stable prostacyclin analog. Recent controlled studies have shown that intravenous infusions of iloprost promote healing of digital ischemic ulcerations and may reduce the frequency and severity of RP attacks in patients with SSc. Improvement in microcirculation after 5-day iloprost infusion therapy (0.5 to 2 ng/kg per minute for 6 hours daily) can last for 2 to 4 weeks; thereafter, repeated monthly 1-day infusions may maintain these effects. Therapy is probably more effective in early ischemia, before extensive tissue damage has occurred. Side effects are common during infusion and include headaches, nausea, and jaw, thigh, or chest pains. Therapy should be avoided in pregnancy and in patients with coronary disease, stroke, or bleeding disorders. Iloprost is currently not available in the United States. **Prostacyclin (prostaglandin I_2)** itself has also been effective in RP secondary to SSc. It is approved for use in primary pulmonary hypertension where it is given continuously (via a portable infusion pump linked to a central vein) at a starting dose of 2 ng/kg per minute.
   b. **Prostaglandin E_1** is probably less effective but better tolerated than iloprost. It requires a central intravenous line and has been given in infusions of 6 to 10 ng/kg per minute over a 72-hour period. It is available in the United states for maintaining the patency of the ductus arteriosus.
6. **Serotonin receptor inhibitors.** Ketanserin, an antagonist of 5-hydroxytryptamine$_2$ receptors on vascular smooth muscle and platelets, may be effective in both primary RP and RP secondary to CTD. It is not available in the United States.
7. The role of **angiotensin-converting enzyme inhibitors** in RP needs further exploration.

C. **Other drugs.** Antiplatelet agents such as low-dose aspirin and pentoxifylline have been advocated by several experts, but there is little supporting evidence for their use in RP. Temporary improvement in skin blood flow has been observed with infusions of recombinant tissue plasminogen activator in SSc-associated RP.

D. **Sympathetic blocks and sympathectomy.** Sympathectomy is not recommended for upper-extremity RP, as it does not offer long-term benefits. However, peripheral or proximal sympathetic blocks have a place in the acute management of severe digital ischemia (digit at imminent risk for tissue loss) in CTD, and they will often sufficiently stabilize the condition to allow maintenance therapy with a calcium channel blocker. For cases refractory to such treatment and to maximum pharmacologic therapy (including vasodilators and sometimes aspirin and heparin), **digital sympathectomy** (adventitial stripping) can be digit-saving, often with immediate restoration of blood flow. The technique, in experienced hands, is a relatively safe procedure. Alternatively, in such critical conditions, prostaglandin infusions can be tried first. For lower-extremity RP, lumbar sympathectomy is usually effective.

E. **Exercises** to strengthen the shoulder muscles are highly recommended for thoracic outlet syndrome. Refractory cases will require surgical decompression.

IV. **Prognosis.** Primary RP has an excellent prognosis. However, as noted above, in a proportion of patients with apparent primary RP, especially those presenting with abnormalities on nailfold capillaroscopy or serology testing, a CTD will eventually develop. Careful clinical follow-up is warranted in such cases. The prognosis of secondary RP depends on the character of the underlying disease. The presence of fixed arterial obstructions on vascular laboratory evaluation not only increases the probability of transition to a CTD in a patient with RP and abnormal serology, but also strongly correlates with digital ulcerations (half of patients) and amputations (10% to 20% of patients).

Bibliography

Ceru S, et al. Effects of five-day versus one-day infusion of iloprost on the peripheral microcirculation in patients with systemic sclerosis. *Clin Exp Rheumatol* 1997;15:381.

Coffman JD. *Raynaud's phenomenon.* New York: Oxford University Press, 1989.

Landry GJ, et al. Long-term outcome of Raynaud's syndrome in a prospectively analyzed patient cohort. *J Vasc Surg* 1996;23:76.

LeRoy EC, Medsger TA Jr. Raynaud's phenomenon: a proposal for classification. *Clin Exp Rheumatol* 1992;10:485.

Maricq HR, et al. Geographic variation in the prevalence of Raynaud's phenomenon: a five-region comparison. *J Rheumatol* 1997;24:879.

Matucci Cerinic M, et al. New approaches to the treatment of Raynaud's phenomenon. *Curr Opin Rheumatol* 1997;9:544.

Spencer-Green G. Outcomes in primary Raynaud phenomenon. *Arch Intern Med* 1998;158:595.

Wigley FM, Flavahan NA. Raynaud's phenomenon. *Rheum Dis Clin North Am* 1996; 22:765.

Yee AMF, et al. Adventitial stripping: a digit-saving procedure in refractory Raynaud's phenomenon. *J Rheumatol* 1998;25:269.

13. OCULAR FINDINGS IN RHEUMATIC AND CONNECTIVE TISSUE DISORDERS

Scott S. Weissman and Stephen E. Bloomfield

The eye and its associated orbital structures may exhibit pathologic changes in patients afflicted with many connective tissue or collagen diseases. In certain inflammatory joint diseases, such as rheumatoid arthritis (RA), there is a similarity in the pathologic processes occurring in the joints and the eye. Inflammation in the conjunctiva and sclera seems to be somewhat analogous to that occurring in the synovium and cartilage, where uncontrolled and relentless immunologically-mediated inflammation in either organ results in its destruction. For the purposes of classifying the ocular manifestations of collagen disease, it is convenient to conceptualize the eye anatomically as a structure consisting of three concentric spheres or coats: an outer collagen coat, or scleral shell; a middle vascular coat, known as the uveal tract; and the inner, retinal layer. *Each of the various collagen diseases shows a characteristic pattern involving one or more of these structures.* For example:

1. The outer collagen or corneoscleral layer becomes involved with RA, and a scleritis results.
2. The middle or uveal coat is more often involved with the seronegative spondyloarthropathies, such as ankylosing spondylitis or juvenile arthritis, and iridocyclitis develops.
3. The inner, retinal layer is involved in systemic lupus erythematosus (SLE), so that a characteristic retinal vasculitis, retinopathy, or choroidopathy results. In the following sections, the ocular manifestations found in each of the rheumatic diseases is considered.

I. **Rheumatoid arthritis.** The most characteristic and potentially serious ocular manifestation of RA is inflammation of the sclera, cornea, or both. The most common manifestation of RA is keratoconjunctivitis sicca.

A. **Scleritis.** The clinical spectrum of scleritis may range from a mild, localized, superficial episcleritis to a dramatically painful, necrotizing scleritis with dire prognostic systemic implications.

The various types of scleritis are probably different manifestations of a single pathologic process, which appears similar to that operating in the joints. An immune complex vasculitis in the sclera appears to be responsible for the inflammatory process. The specific clinical entity produced depends on the site, depth, and extent of the pathologic process.

1. **The incidence of scleritis** in RA is about 5%; thus, scleritis will develop in one of every 20 patients in the rheumatology clinic during the evolution of their disease. Also of interest is the incidence of RA in patients who consult an ophthalmologist and are given a diagnosis of scleritis. The incidence of RA in patients with scleritis is approximately 33%. Therefore, every scleritis patient in an ophthalmology clinic should be evaluated for arthritis.
2. **Prognosis for life and sight.** The prognostic significance of rheumatoid scleritis is dramatically illustrated by a study in which 45% of patients with scleritis died within 5 years of being given the diagnosis, compared with 18% of a matched control sample of RA patients without scleritis. In mild forms of scleral inflammation, such as local or generalized episcleritis, the swelling and inflammatory process is superficial, although painful, and it is usually easy to control with topical medications and resolves without serious sequelae. Deep scleritis, however, is one of the few severely painful eye problems, has serious prognostic implications for sight and life, and requires systemic, often long-term treatment with one of several antiinflammatory agents. In **necrotizing scleritis,** the most dramatic and destructive form of scleritis, a scleral

vessel is suddenly occluded, causing an avascular patch (sequestrum) that eventually dissolves and exposes the underlying uveal tissue. Necrosis occurring slowly over time and without inflammation is called **necrotizing scleritis without inflammation;** it is referred to in the older classic literature as **scleromalacia perforans.** Necrotizing scleritis represents the eye changes of the malignant phase of a systemic tissue disorder and usually occurs in patients who have manifested the advanced stages of the disease. It is also seen in polyarteritis nodosa, Wegener's granulomatosis, and SLE. Scleritis itself has serious ocular complications other than the production of a scleral defect; it can result in keratitis, cataracts, uveitis, and glaucoma.

3. **Treatment.** Because of the depth and severity of the inflammatory process in scleritis, long-term (years) systemic antiinflammatory agents are required. Those that have been reported to be effective include indomethacin, diflunisal, corticosteroids, azathioprine, cyclophosphamide, and cyclosporin A. In the most severe and sight-threatening cases, cyclophosphamide along with intravenous corticosteroids must be used. With the latter two drugs, the clinician is in the unenviable position of balancing toxic treatments versus a destructive disease.

B. Corneal complications. Corneal manifestations associated with RA are serious problems whose importance and occurrence are not generally appreciated. Corneal involvement may accompany inflammation of the adjacent sclera or may occur in the absence of any other ocular complications. One form is the development of peripheral ulcers or furrows at or near the limbus (limbal guttering), frequently occurring in the absence of significant inflammation. These ulcers may be nonprogressive or go on to cause marked thinning and perforation of the cornea. Central corneal ulcers and perforations can be seen in clinically quiet eyes. These patients are usually in an advanced stage of their disease and are often on maintenance doses of systemic corticosteroid drugs.

C. Sicca syndrome (keratoconjunctivitis sicca) (see Chapter 29). Keratoconjunctivitis sicca is one of the most common ocular manifestations of RA. It also occurs with several of the other collagen diseases and as an isolated entity. The syndrome as originally described by Sjögren consists of dry eye, dry mouth, and arthritis. Today, the term has come to be used to describe patients with joint disease and a dry eye. The xerostomia may or may not be present.

1. **Signs and symptoms.** The symptoms that patients complain of are a foreign-body sensation or a feeling of "something" (sand or lashes) in their eyes. The clinical spectrum of a patient with keratoconjunctivitis sicca may vary from symptoms only, with very few signs seen by the ophthalmologist, to mild signs consisting of punctate erosions on the inferior half of the cornea, with or without filaments that consist of a mixture of surface cells and mucus. There is one particularly devastating variation in which corneal infiltration and necrosis sometimes develop, leading to possible corneal perforation. Fortunately, this is quite rare.
2. **Treatment** of a dry eye consists of keeping the eye moist and clean with a minimum number of drugs and devices, as these treatment methods have their own complications. The eye can be kept moist with tear replacements and by decreasing evaporation through the use of moist-chamber glasses or contact lenses.
   - **a.** The first line of defense is replacement of tear volume through the use of artificial tears. This works best when combined with nightly eyelash lavage with baby shampoo to clean off accumulated debris that the compromised tear film cannot handle. Variable success has been reported with artificial tear inserts, such as Lacriserts.
   - **b.** Another simple expedient is the use of moist-chamber glasses, which are an extension of the glasses frame. Clear plastic extends to the face, trapping any moisture produced and thereby decreasing evaporation.

c. More severe cases require more aggressive treatments, all of which have inherent risks. Occlusion of the punctum can reduce the drainage of tears but should only be used if less than 3 mm of wetting is noted on Schirmer's test. Therapeutic soft contact lenses are extremely useful when foreign-body symptoms are so extensive that patients cannot keep their eyes open. This is also the case when filaments develop in a dry eye.

The filaments, as mentioned, consist of mixtures of desiccated, loose, surface epithelial cells combined with mucus, which is produced in greater quantities in these patients. The problem with contact lenses in patients with dry eyes is the possible development of corneal infections.

D. **Differential diagnosis of "red eye."** These diagnostic possibilities hold for all the collagen diseases but are presented in this section because RA is the most common underlying entity and is associated with the greatest number of possible causes of a red eye.

1. **Scleritis,** either local or general. Pain is usually present.
2. **Keratitis sicca** results in the eyes becoming irritated from lack of a normal tear volume to lubricate and protect the surface.
3. **Conjunctivitis** occurs secondary to a tear volume deficit, which deprives the eye of its natural protection against infection.
4. **Iridocyclitis** usually occurs acutely in seronegative spondyloarthropathies, with light sensitivity, a miotic pupil on the affected side, and a peripupillary red ring (ciliary flush). A more chronic iridocyclitis, with a white and quiet external appearance, is more typical of children with juvenile rheumatoid arthritis (JRA).
5. **Glaucoma,** secondary either to scleritis and inflammation of the trabecular meshwork or to corticosteroid therapy.
6. **Herpetic keratitis,** complicating immunosuppressive drug regimens used to treat this group of patients.

II. **Juvenile rheumatoid arthritis (JRA)** is sufficiently different in its ocular manifestations to warrant consideration as a separate entity. Adult RA affects the outer collagenous coat of the eye, producing scleritis, whereas in JRA, inflammation of the middle coat or a uveitis is the classic ocular complication. The uveitis in JRA is an insidious inflammation of the anterior uveal tract (iridocyclitis). Scleral inflammation in JRA is rare.

A. The **incidence of uveitis** in JRA is approximately 10%, and uveitis is more common in patients with pauciarticular involvement than with polyarticular disease. The uveitis usually develops after the arthritis but may precede it by many years.

B. **Signs and symptoms.** Acute iridocyclitis usually manifests with redness, pain, photophobia, and tearing, but the low-grade, chronic iridocyclitis of JRA may be asymptomatic, which makes it a particularly dangerous problem because extensive ocular disease may occur before the condition is recognized or show no correlation with joint inflammation. The most common sequela of iridocyclitis is the deposition of calcium beneath the corneal epithelium, causing band keratopathy. Band keratopathy is a nonspecific condition that develops after any longstanding inflammation. Chronic iridocyclitis also produces cataracts and secondary glaucoma. This chronic form of iridocyclitis can be unrelenting and have a progressive downhill course that leads to visual loss. The treatment itself, which consists of topical or systemic corticosteroid therapy, can result in glaucoma and cataracts.

III. **Ankylosing spondylitis (AS).** Iridocyclitis is so common in AS that it might be regarded as a clinical feature rather than a complication of the disease. Iridocyclitis occurs at some point in the life of almost all these patients and may be the presenting feature, antedating the joint symptoms by as much as 12 years or occurring when the disease is entirely quiescent. The iridocyclitis tends to affect one eye at a time and is generally fulminant in onset. In 20% of patients, it is the most disabling feature of the disease, because of both its severity and the frequent recurrences.

In addition to anterior uveitis being found in a large number of patients with AS, spondylarthropathy is found in a significant percentage of patients presenting to an ophthalmologist with iritis. *Young men with iridocyclitis should be investigated* for signs and symptoms relating to AS. There is a striking association of this disease with the presence of the histocompatibility antigen HLA-B27, which is found in only 5% to 8% of controls but in approximately 90% of white patients with AS.

IV. **Reiter's syndrome.** The classic diagnostic triad of Reiter's syndrome includes non-gonococcal urethritis, arthritis, and conjunctivitis. The ocular findings may be the presenting feature of this disease, although they usually follow the other symptoms. Conjunctivitis, part of the classic triad, is the most common ocular manifestation of the disease. It is usually mild and presents with some burning and tearing. Among the connective tissue diseases, Reiter's syndrome and psoriatic arthropathy are the *only conditions in which conjunctivitis is a complication.* Anterior uveitis occurs in 8% to 40% of patients with this entity. It is more common with recurrent disease than in the initial stage of illness. Reiter's syndrome also shows an association with the HLA-B27 antigen.

V. **Enteropathic arthropathy** is the form of polyarthritis associated with inflammatory bowel disease, including ulcerative colitis and Crohn's disease. Ocular findings associated with these entities involve mainly the uveal tract and manifest as an iridocyclitis. Scleritis has also been reported. The incidence of ocular findings in enteropathic arthropathy, however, is less than in the more common arthritis syndromes.

VI. **Systemic lupus erythematosus,** unlike some of the other connective tissue disorders, can involve almost every structure in the eye. The inner eye is rarely involved in RA, and the outer eye is rarely involved in the seronegative arthritides.

These distinctions can be clinically important, because if a fundus lesion or an anterior uveitis is seen in a patient with scleritis, it is likely that the disease syndrome is related to SLE. The fundus changes involve the inner retinal layer through an immune complex-mediated occlusive vasculitis.

A. The most common **retinal findings** are cotton-wool spots, retinal hemorrhages, and edema of the disk and surrounding retina. Similar changes can result from the associated hypertension seen in SLE patients with nephritis. The findings associated with vasculitis are sometimes called lupus retinopathy.

B. **Anterior segment involvement** may take the form of conjunctivitis, sicca syndrome, or scleritis. Ptosis and proptosis have been reported secondary to myositis of the extraocular muscles. Drug-induced SLE can also be associated with ocular manifestations.

VII. **Temporal arteritis (TA) and polymyalgia rheumatica (PMR).** Temporal arteritis, also known as giant-cell or cranial arteritis, can result in sudden, dramatic, and disastrous loss of vision. Polymyalgia rheumatica is included in this section because a small percentage of PMR patients have occult TA and 50% of TA patients have PMR. The two disorders are parts of a single disease spectrum.

A. **Temporal arteritis.** Ocular manifestations may occur in 30% of patients and are among the most serious consequences of this illness. Ocular complications occur usually several weeks to months after the onset of systemic symptoms but may also occur years later or develop first in the absence of systemic signs, a situation referred to as occult temporal arteritis. Inflammation of the ophthalmic, central retinal, or posterior ciliary arteries is responsible for the various ocular problems.

1. The most frequent and disastrous problem is the sudden, irreversible **loss of vision** caused by inflammation either in the central retinal artery, which is the terminal branch of the ophthalmic artery, or in the posterior ciliary arteries, which supply the optic nerve; the latter situation can result in an ischemic optic neuritis. An altitudinal visual field deficit is characteristic of optic nerve inflammation in temporal arteritis.
2. **Diplopia** also occurs from involvement of the posterior ciliary arteries, which supply the extraocular muscles.

3. When several of the extraocular muscles are involved, the syndrome of **anterior segment necrosis** may occur, which essentially is ischemia of the front of the eye that results in uveitis, iris necrosis, and scleritis.
4. **Treatment,** which must be instituted rapidly, consists of systemic corticosteroids in doses sufficient to suppress the clinical and laboratory evidence (especially the erythrocyte sedimentation rate) of disease activity. Any visual symptoms must be treated aggressively, at times with prednisone doses over 100 mg/day or intravenously with 500–1000 mg of Solumedrol. In some cases, vision is lost despite massive doses of systemic antiinflammatory medication. Unfortunately, bilateral blindness may occur in up to 25% of patients with temporal arteritis. The purpose of treatment is really prevention. Improvement of visual acuity in an involved eye after steroid therapy has begun is only rarely noted.

B. **Polymyalgia rheumatica** is the descriptive term coined by Barber in 1957 for the syndrome consisting of pain and stiffness in the shoulder and pelvic girdles in elderly patients, an associated high erythrocyte sedimentation rate, and a prompt and dramatic clinical response to modest doses of systemic prednisone, in the range of 10 to 15 mg/d. The importance of recognizing this entity lies in the fact that, in some patients, it is an occult pattern of temporal arteritis.

VIII. **Polyarteritis nodosa**

A. **Ocular manifestations** involve almost every tissue of the eye in this inflammatory disease affecting small and medium-sized arteries. The most common and serious manifestation is scleral keratitis, which is similar to that seen in RA but usually more painful and sharply demarcated. Guttering of the peripheral cornea develops in the limbal region, which may spread circumferentially to form a ring. Bilateral involvement can be present, and the associated pain may be intense. The process may extend centrally to involve much of the cornea, producing extensive scarring, vascularization, and perforation.

B. **Clinical syndromes** have been described in which polyarteritis nodosa is associated with specific eye and ear findings.

1. In Cogan's syndrome, an interstitial keratitis (deep corneal haze and vascularization) is associated with audiovestibular disease, characterized by profound deafness, vertigo, and tinnitus.
2. Another variation is an association of polyarteritis, scleritis, and otitis media. Anterior uveal involvement is manifested as iridocyclitis. The retinopathy of polyarteritis includes retinal vasculitis and changes secondary to coexistent hypertension. A host of ocular signs and symptoms of polyarteritis reflect central nervous system complications.

IX. **Wegener's granulomatosis.** Ocular and orbital complications are fairly common in Wegener's granulomatosis, the reported incidence being as high as 60%. If the orbit is involved by direct spread of the granuloma from the paranasal sinuses, the patient can have proptosis, limitation of movement of the globe, and a rapid destruction in vision from either involvement of the optic nerve or an exudative retinal detachment secondary to a posterior scleritis. Nasolacrimal duct obstruction may also be the presenting sign.

A. **Proptosis,** which is a common clinical feature and can be severe, results from invasion of the orbit, and later the sclera, by granulomatous tissue. The sclera becomes infiltrated, and the underlying collagen is attacked by granulation tissue. The histologic picture differs from that usually seen in scleral inflammatory disease in that the invasion is from the outside rather than from foci within the sclera.

B. **Other types of scleritis** are also seen in which intrascleral inflammation develops first. A particularly painful peripheral ulcerative keratitis or necrotizing scleritis may occur and be the presenting feature of the disease.

X. **Polymyositis and dermatomyositis.** Polymyositis is an inflammatory disease of striated skeletal muscle. When a characteristic skin rash is present, the term dermatomyositis is used. The most common ocular finding, indeed one of the more characteristic findings of dermatomyositis, is lid discoloration. There is a lilac discoloration of the upper eyelids, often associated with periorbital edema. This violaceous discoloration, called heliotrope rash, is considered pathognomonic.

Other ocular findings have been reported, but none is specific. Extraocular muscle weakness is uncommon and may be caused by the myositis itself or by coexistent myasthenia gravis. In children with dermatomyositis, retinal vasculitis is a relatively common feature.

XI. Scleroderma. The most common ocular manifestation of this chronic disease of connective tissue is involvement of the skin of the lids, which may have secondary effects on the cornea and conjunctiva. The eyelids lose their freedom of movement and become thin, smooth, and shiny. Tightness of the lids may result in only minimally decreased mobility or marked restriction of lid movement. Lid restriction may in turn lead to a severe exposure keratitis, especially when it is combined with a hyposecretion of tears occasionally seen with this disease. Sicca syndrome is a significant feature of scleroderma, as it is with the other connective tissue syndromes.

Bibliography

Foster CS, Forstot SL, Wilson LA. Mortality rate in rheumatoid arthritis patients developing necrotizing scleritis or peripheral ulcerative keratitis: effects of systemic immunosuppression. *Ophthalmology* 1984;91:1253.

Foulks GN. Non-infective inflammation of the anterior segment. *Int Ophthalmol Clin* 1983;23(1):3.

Gold OH. Ocular manifestations of connective tissue diseases. In: Duane T, ed. *Clinical ophthalmology,* vol 5. Hagerstown, MD: Harper & Row, 1980:1B.

McGavin OOM, et al. Episcleritis and scleritis: a study of their clinical manifestations and association with rheumatoid arthritis. *Br J Ophthalmol* 1976;60:192.

Theodore FH, Bloomfield SE, Mondino BJ. *Clinical allergy and immunology of the eye.* Baltimore: Williams & Wilkins, 1983.

Watson PG, Hazleman BL. *The sclera and systemic disorders.* London: WB Saunders, 1976.

14. NECK PAIN

Thomas P. Sculco and Alexander Miric

I. Anatomic considerations. The cervical area is composed of an integrated complex of structures whose dysfunction singly or in combination can result in neck or radicular pain. These structures include the following:

- **A.** Vertebrae.
- **B.** Intervertebral disks.
- **C.** Apophyseal and uncovertebral joints.
- **D.** Vertebral arteries.
- **E.** Spinal cord and nerve roots.
- **F.** Ligamentous complex.
  - **1.** Anterior and posterior longitudinal ligaments.
  - **2.** Interspinous and supraspinous ligaments.
- **G.** Paracervical musculature.

II. History

A. Mode of onset

1. A history of neck trauma may allow one to localize the injured structures and increases the probability that cervical films will reveal the injury.
2. If unrelated to trauma, acute severe restriction of motion can indicate paracervical muscle spasm ("wry neck").
3. If symptoms are more chronic in nature and began after frequent neck rotation, neck pain can indicate cervical disk degeneration and osteoarthritis.

B. Duration and localization of pain

1. **Acute onset** of pain usually suggests muscle spasm or nerve root irritation; radiation to the occiput or interscapular area may suggest a nerve root lesion.
2. **Chronic neck pain** that occurs intermittently with or without radicular symptoms may be seen in cervical osteoarthritis.
3. **If radiculitis is severe,** pain radiation to the shoulder and arm indicates nerve root compression resulting from either a disk herniation or foraminal encroachment by the osteophytes associated with osteoarthritis.
4. **Shoulder pain** either may be a radicular symptom secondary to root compression or may represent primary pain with associated referred neck and trapezial pain.

C. Relief and aggravation of pain. Rest in the supine position usually relieves local neck pain produced by muscle spasm but may have little or no effect on processes primarily involving osseous or ligamentous structures.

D. Neurologic signs and symptoms

1. **Paresthesias** radiating from the neck to the arm are an important indicator of nerve root irritability as the origin of the pain.
2. **Numbness and weakness of the arm or hand** indicate more severe nerve root compromise; careful neurologic examination will often localize the cervical nerve root involved (see Appendix B).
3. Patients with **vertebral artery** compromise may complain of dizziness, visual dysfunction, and syncopal episodes.
4. **Cervical myelopathy** can be identified in cases of severe cervical osteoarthritis; patient complaints may range from mild to severe difficulty with ambulation or handling objects.

E. Past medical history should be thoroughly explored. A history of malignancy, previous neck problems, associated musculoskeletal disorders, metabolic bone diseases, and smoking habits should be pursued. Patients with a history of rheumatoid arthritis often exhibit signs and symptoms of C1–2 instability. Patients with a history of psoriatic arthritis, ankylosing spondylitis, severe rheumatoid arthritis, or juvenile rheumatoid arthritis also often have associated cervical pathology. A history of intravenous drug abuse or a compromised immune system increases the chance of an infectious process. Because myocardial ischemia and aortic disease can present as neck pain, a complete medical history is needed.

F. The **occupational history** may provide the inciting cause of pain. Patients who perform extensive overhead work, such as painting or hanging wallpaper, may have increased pain after work. Patients with work-related symptoms often require longer periods of therapy.

III. Physical examination. The patient should disrobe sufficiently to allow full visualization of the neck and thoracic spine.

A. Patient standing

1. Observe the position in which the neck is held. With severe **unilateral paracervical spasm,** the head may be flexed laterally to that side and rotated to the opposite side.
2. Severe **paracervical muscle spasm** can be visualized and palpated posteriorly.
3. Evaluate the presence of neck or paracervical **muscle atrophy.** Also compare trapezial and shoulder musculature symmetry.
4. Examine **shoulder strength and range of motion,** and palpate for localized shoulder tenderness in an effort to rule out shoulder pathology as the source of pain.

B. Patient sitting

1. Record active and passive **neck range of motion.**
   - **a.** Normal **flexion** ends with the chin against the chest.
   - **b.** Normal **extension** ends with the occiput near C-7.
   - **c.** Normal **rotation** approaches 70 degrees to each side.
   - **d.** Normal **lateral bending** approaches 50 to 60 degrees.
2. Examine for **supraclavicular lymphadenopathy** and **carotid artery pulses.**
3. Perform a **neurologic examination** of the upper extremities.
   - **a. Sensory examination** with pin and cotton ball as well as tuning fork.
   - **b. Motor testing,** particularly of deltoid, biceps, triceps, wrist flexors and extensors, finger flexors and extensors, and interossei.
   - **c. Reflex examination** should include biceps, triceps, and brachioradialis.

C. Patient prone, forehead on pillow

1. Palpate paracervical area and spinous process for specific areas of tenderness or trigger points.
2. Evaluate deep percussion sensitivity in interscapular area.

IV. Laboratory studies

A. Radiographs, when needed, should be taken in anteroposterior, oblique, and lateral views. These films may be supplemented with an open-mouth view of the odontoid or flexion-extension films when instability is suspected. In cases of mild neck pain, a therapeutic trial for osteoarthritis might be tried before radiography is ordered. As symptoms and signs worsen, radiographic procedures become more appropriate.

1. **Alignment of the spine** in the anteroposterior and lateral projections should be evaluated.
   - **a.** The anteroposterior film should reveal approximately the same distance between spinous processes.
   - **b.** The lateral film should reveal vertebral bodies forming a gentle curve that is concave posteriorly.
2. **Narrowing of the disk space** is best seen on the lateral view. Such narrowing is most commonly seen at the C5–6 level, followed by the C6–7 and C4–5 levels.
3. The oblique view should demonstrate **neural foramina** of relatively uniform size through which the cervical nerve roots traverse. Isolated narrowing or the presence of an osteophyte may sometimes be identified.
4. The **uncovertebral joints** (joints of Luschka) are best seen on the anteroposterior view; cervical osteoarthritis often leads to narrowing of these joints.
5. The presence of a **cervical rib** should be noted as well.

6. **Congenital fusions of cervical vertebrae** or other bony anomalies may be present.

B. Further diagnostic studies

1. **Magnetic resonance imaging** is an excellent way to visualize the spinal cord and soft tissues in relation to bony anatomy.
2. **Computed tomography** is useful in determining spinal stenosis and areas of nerve root compression by osteophytes.
3. **Myelography** is indicated in patients with intractable neck pain and radiculopathy to localize spinal cord or nerve root compromise by disk, osteophyte, neoplasm, or other space-occupying process. Originally used in conjunction with plane radiographs, myelography is now often performed along with computed tomography in an effort to visualize the canal better (see section **IV. B.2**).
4. **Bone scan** may demonstrate osseous involvement by neoplasm, vertebral compression fracture, or infection in the cervical spine.
5. **Electromyography** may be useful in demonstrating spinal stenosis and areas of nerve root compression by osteophytes.
6. **Standard blood work** may reveal abnormal values, such as an elevated white blood cell count, erythrocyte sedimentation rate, or serum glucose level (in diabetic patients), that suggest an infectious process.

V. Differential diagnosis

A. Neck pain without radiculopathy. Referral to the occiput and upper back may or may not be present.

1. **Vertebrae**
   - **a.** Fracture, traumatic or osteoporotic (rare).
   - **b.** Septic spondylitis.
   - **c.** Tumor.
     - **(1)** More likely to be **primary** if patient is young (<20 years).
     - **(2)** More likely to be **metastatic** if patient is older (>50 years).
2. **Intervertebral disk**
   - **a.** Herniated cervical disk.
   - **b.** Disk space infection is rare in the cervical area but may present with severe neck pain and torticollis.
   - **c.** Disk degeneration.
3. **Apophyseal and uncovertebral joints**
   - **a. Osteoarthritis.**
   - **b. Rheumatoid arthritis** may lead to destruction of these joints with resultant pain and instability, particularly at the C1–2 level.
4. **Soft tissues**
   - **a.** Ligamentous injury to the neck results in pain and cervical instability.
   - **b.** Acute muscular spasm can produce acute pain and torticollis ("wry neck"). Wry neck may arise after trauma (e.g., whiplash), prolonged exposure to cold, prolonged period in an awkward position, or other activities that strain and require considerable neck rotation or positioning.
   - **c. Polymyalgia rheumatica** may lead to neck and shoulder pain in an elderly patient with systemic complaints or headache.
   - **d.** Tension and anxiety can produce severe paracervical muscle spasm.
5. **Surrounding structures.** Neck pain may be referred from the shoulder or periscapular structures. Cervical lymphadenopathy, if painful, can produce severe restriction in neck motion. Occipital headaches may produce secondary neck pain and muscle spasm. In addition, trigeminal and glossopharyngeal neuralgias have been described to cause neck pain.

B. Neck pain with radiculopathy. Objective neurologic deficit may or may not be present.

1. **Vertebrae.** Tumors or infections may produce radicular signs and symptoms.
2. **Intervertebral disk.** Herniation or degeneration of an intervertebral disk may produce specific radicular patterns, depending on the level of involve-

ment. Considerable overlap exists among the patterns outlined below. C5–6 and C6–7 are far more commonly involved than C7-T1 or C4–5.

a. **C5–6 (C-6 nerve root).** Pain will radiate to the shoulder or lateral arm and dorsal forearm. Anesthesia and paresthesias may be present in the thumb and index finger. Weakness, if present, will involve the biceps and wrist extensors. The biceps reflex is often decreased or absent.

b. **C6–7 (C-7 nerve root).** The pain distribution is similar to that of a C-6 radiculopathy. Anesthesia and paresthesias, when present, involve the index and long fingers. Weakness, if present, is noted in the triceps, wrist flexors, and finger extensors. The triceps reflex is often decreased or absent.

c. **C7-T1 (C-8 nerve root).** Pain may occur along the medial aspect of the upper arm and forearm. Anesthesia and paresthesias involve the ring and small fingers. Weakness, if present, is noted in the finger flexors and intrinsic musculature of the hand. The triceps reflex may be reduced.

3. **Apophyseal and uncovertebral joints.** Degenerative arthritis affecting these joints in the cervical area can lead to secondary encroachment of the cervical intervertebral foramina with nerve root irritation.

4. **Surrounding structures**

a. **Thoracic outlet syndrome.** Radicular symptoms with or without neurologic deficit can occur with compression of the subclavian vessel by a cervical rib or tight scalenus anterior muscle.

b. **Brachial plexus injuries** can lead to marked neurologic deficits with retrograde pain to the cervical area.

c. **Pancoast tumors** of the lung apex may occasionally produce neck pain and neurologic deficits.

d. **Visceral disease with referred pain** can originate in the aorta, the heart, or the lung.

VI. Therapy

A. **Rest** is the cornerstone of therapy for patients with neck pain, whether or not radiculopathy is present.

1. The patient should be advised to avoid activities that are particularly stressful to the neck; examples are driving, overhead lifting, athletic activities such as golf and tennis, and sitting at a desk for prolonged periods reviewing written material or working at a computer.
2. The neck should be supported by a firm cervical collar, fitted so that cervical motion is limited 60% to 70% and the patient is comfortable. The collar should be worn full-time initially; as symptoms recede, the patient may be weaned from the collar. Soft foam collars provide little, if any, cervical immobilization but may be useful during sleep if the firm collar is uncomfortable.
3. Neck pain is usually worse at night because of the positioning during sleep. Avoidance of more than one small pillow or the use of a cervical pillow often helps to decrease pain and spasm.

B. **Moist heat** generally relaxes tight, spastic musculature. A moist, warm towel can be wrapped around the neck as a collar; as the towel cools, this action can be repeated. A hydroculator or a hot water bottle wrapped in a moist towel can also be used.

C. **Medications** may be useful depending on the origin of the neck pain.

1. If there is inflammation or cervical radiculitis, 650 to 975 mg of **aspirin** PO four times daily or other nonsteroidal antiinflammatory drugs may help decrease inflammation and relieve pain provided the patient is at low risk for gastrointestinal bleeding.
2. If pain is severe, 60 mg of **codeine** PO q4h is used as needed.
3. **Muscle relaxants,** such as Flexeril, may aid in relief of paracervical muscle spasm. Powerful medications such as codeine and muscle relaxants should be used to manage acute, severe pain and not to treat chronic pain syndromes.

D. **Physical therapy** is useful if an osseous spur is compromising the intervertebral foramina to cause nerve root entrapment.

1. Three to five sessions per week of **intermittent cervical traction,** each lasting 20 to 30 minutes and reaching a maximum of 20 to 35 lb, may be used.
2. Traction may be preceded by **ultrasound** or **diathermy** to the upper neck and upper back.
3. If pain is severe, travel to the therapy center should be minimized. For these patients, **home cervical traction** may be prescribed.
4. Patients who improve during supervised cervical traction should also obtain home traction units for use twice daily. The length of the sessions should be gradually decreased as symptoms resolve.

E. Exercises should be encouraged only if they do not exacerbate the pain. Active range of motion can easily be performed in a shower or sauna. As the patient improves, isometric exercises in various positions of neck rotation and lateral bending may be prescribed (see Chapter 56). If weakness remains after cervical pain has diminished, exercises performed while swimming in a pool may prove useful.

F. Surgery rarely is needed. However, in the setting of refractory pain or neurologic deficits unresponsive to a conservative regimen, it may be considered.

15. SHOULDER PAIN

Russell F. Warren

The diagnosis and treatment of problems of the shoulder region require an understanding of the anatomy and function of this joint.

I. **Anatomy and function.** The shoulder consists of three joints and two gliding planes, which allow an exceedingly large range of motion at the expense of glenohumeral stability. As a result, the glenohumeral joint is the most commonly dislocated joint in the body. The gliding planes consist of the scapulothoracic surface and the subacromial space. The three joints are the acromioclavicular, sternoclavicular, and glenohumeral articulations. Elevation of the arm is produced by the combined rotation between the scapula and chest wall as well as by the glenohumeral joint. The rotator cuff consists of four muscles: the supraspinatus, the infraspinatus, the teres minor, and the subscapularis. In addition to assisting in internal and external rotation, these muscles act as a depressor on the humeral head during shoulder elevation. In this manner, a fulcrum that allows the deltoid to elevate the arm is established. As long as some depressor action of the rotator cuff remains, surprisingly large tears of the rotator cuff may be compatible with full elevation of the arm.

II. **Types of pain.** Pain may be related to intrinsic lesions of the shoulder, or it may be referred from other sites.

A. **Cervical spondylosis** of C5–6 often results in a referred type of pain to the shoulder. If the radiculopathy includes weakness of shoulder abduction and external rotation, it may closely mimic a torn rotator cuff. Cervical types of shoulder pain are usually increased by neck motion, particularly extension with rotation to the involved side.

B. **More than one basis** for pain may be present; for example, in patients with cervical spondylosis and referred pain to the shoulder, limitation of shoulder motion secondary to adhesive capsulitis may also develop (see section **C.2**). Also, pain can be referred from diseases involving the heart, lung, or gall bladder.

C. **Intrinsic shoulder pain** is generally worse at night and is increased by lying on the shoulder. Shoulder motion will generally aggravate the pain, particularly full elevation in the forward flexed position or abduction to 90 degrees. Tears of the rotator cuff may also cause pain radiating into the forearm and, rarely, the hand. Specific problems of the shoulder region tend to occur at certain age intervals.

1. From ages **20 to 30 years,** the impingement syndrome and instability problems may present as a painful shoulder.
2. From ages **40 to 50 years,** the impingement syndrome, calcific tendinitis, and adhesive capsulitis become more common.
3. From ages **50 to 70 years,** the impingement syndrome may progress to a full-thickness rotator cuff tear. In addition, adhesive capsulitis is common. Degenerative lesions of the acromioclavicular, sternoclavicular, and occasionally the glenohumeral joints become more frequent. Pain from metastatic disease should be considered.

III. **Physical examination.** On examining the shoulder region, one should note that the musculature of the dominant extremity may be somewhat hypertrophied about the shoulder and arm, particularly in athletic persons.

A. **Observation**

1. The **position of the shoulder** relative to the contralateral side should be noted. Elevation or dependency of the shoulder may be related to scoliosis, Sprengel's deformity, or simply athletic activity.

2. **Swelling** about the shoulder may be secondary to inflammation of a bursa or associated with rotator cuff tears.
3. View the shoulder from both the **anterior and posterior aspects.** Observe the **range of motion** from behind as the arm is elevated to note the scapulohumeral rhythm.
4. **Specific muscle atrophy** may indicate either rotator cuff tears or neurologic involvement.

B. Palpation

1. The **supraclavicular fossa** should be carefully palpated for masses as well as for tenderness of the brachial plexus, which is seen in thoracic outlet syndrome.
2. **Local tender spots** indicative of trigger points should be sought along the interscapular region and overlying musculature of the shoulder. If pressure is applied to these spots, radiation of pain into the upper arm may be observed.
3. Specific sites of tenderness should be noted anteriorly over the biceps tendon and laterally over the subdeltoid bursa and rotator cuff.
4. The **acromioclavicular and sternoclavicular joints** should be carefully examined for tenderness.

C. Motion

1. In examining the shoulder, one should observe the full range of **active** and **passive** motion, noting any discrepancy such as that sometimes seen in a rotator cuff tear. Active elevation in the plane of the scapula may demonstrate altered scapular thoracic rhythm with a "shrug sign" if a rotator cuff tear is present.
2. Shoulder motion is recorded as **abduction** in degrees and forward flexion in degrees. **External rotation** of the humerus is noted with the arm at the side as well as in the abducted position of 90 degrees. **Internal rotation** is recorded by placing the hand behind the back and noting which spinous process the thumb will reach. It is also tested at 90 degrees of abduction.
3. The **impingement sign** is positive in patients with rotator cuff inflammation and is noted by flexing the arm forward to the full overhead position. Pain is present during the last 10 degrees of passive elevation. Passive abduction to the 90-degree position with internal rotation will similarly produce pain.
4. The **adduction test** consists of fully adducting the humerus across the chest. This test stresses the acromioclavicular joint and will cause pain if degeneration of the joint is present. Placing the arm in adduction and resisting elevation may be painful if a slap lesion is present (superior labral tear).
5. In cases in which **instability of the glenohumeral joint** is a possibility, the joint should be carefully stressed in the following manner: The patient is placed in the supine position, and after maximal muscle relaxation is achieved, the shoulder is adducted and internally rotated with pressure placed in the posterior direction. If **posterior instability** is present, a click or a clear subluxation may be noted during this maneuver. To evaluate **anterior instability,** the shoulder is placed in the abducted, externally rotated position with gentle pressure placed in an anterior direction behind the humeral head. In some patients, inferior instability is demonstrated by distracting the arms inferiorly to see if a sulcus forms (sulcus sign) distal to the acromion. This sign is frequently present in multidirectional instability.

D. Neurovascular examination

1. A complete **neurologic examination** should be performed. Weakness may be the result of intrinsic shoulder lesions, as in a cuff tear, or of nerve lesions of the brachial plexus or cervical roots. Strength testing at 0 degrees and 90 degrees of elevation is important. Weakness of external rotation with the arm at the side is present with large rotator cuff tears involving the infraspinatus or with C5–6 nerve root problems. The lift-off test for subscapularis tears is performed by placing the back of the hand over L-5 and pushing away from the back. Loss of strength is associated with subscapularis tears.
2. The pain of a **carpal tunnel syndrome** may be referred proximally to the shoulder region.

3. Because **thoracic outlet syndrome** may be present, the circulation of the arm and the hand must be carefully evaluated.
   a. **Adson's test,** which may be positive, consists of palpating the radial pulse while the patient's head is turned to the involved side and performing a Valsalva maneuver. A positive test result—a decrease in the pulse—is not diagnostic; it occurs in a significant percentage of asymptomatic subjects. A reduced radial pulse on testing should be compared with the pulse on the contralateral side. It is better to test with the arm abducted and externally rotated, noting any decrease in the pulse. In addition, the Roos test is useful. This test is performed with patients in a similar position, but they open and close their hands for 1 to 2 minutes in an attempt to reproduce their symptoms.
   b. In the arterial type of thoracic outlet syndrome, **auscultation** of the supraclavicular region may demonstrate a bruit with the arm in position. The blood pressure may also be significantly reduced in the abducted position.

IV. **Radiographs**

A. **Standard views** of the shoulder generally have included internal and external rotation. Although helpful in the diagnosis of calcific tendinitis, they provide little information regarding the anteroposterior alignment of the shoulder or the width of the glenohumeral joint. Because the scapula lies on the chest wall at approximately a 40-degree angle, radiographs should be taken at a right angle to the scapula and glenohumeral joint rather than to the chest.

B. **Lateral and axillary views** of the scapula are useful in identifying degenerative changes of the glenohumeral joint and calcification of the rotator cuff; they are particularly important in the evaluation of acute injuries to the shoulder.

V. **Common shoulder problems.** The most common shoulder problems are impingement syndrome with rotator cuff tears, calcific tendinitis, adhesive capsulitis, acromioclavicular joint pain, thoracic outlet syndrome, and shoulder instability.

A. **Impingement syndrome** generally develops during the fifth decade and may progress to a rotator cuff tear by age 55. The underlying pathology consists of degeneration of the tendons of the rotator cuff. As a result, the insufficient cuff fails to prevent superior migration of the humeral head during elevation. This results in pressure on the rotator cuff and increasing pressure on the bone. Spurs may develop within the coracoacromial ligament over time with cuff degeneration. In some patients, a hooked acromion will increase the pressure on the cuff.

1. In young patients, cuff injury secondary to a contusion may occur, with hemorrhage and edema decreasing cuff function. This can mimic a tear. In addition, secondary impingement may develop in the second and third decades in throwing athletes. This happens when an underlying instability is present.
   a. **Pain** is generally noted with overhead elevation at 90 degrees with rotation. The pain may increase during specific activities, such as throwing and swimming.
   b. The **impingement sign** may be positive and the impingement test will relieve pain. The radiographic findings of young patients are often negative, but magnetic resonance imaging (MRI) may show cuff degeneration with a partial tear of the articular side of the supraspinatus and labral injury in some.
   c. **Treatment** is based on activity modifications and temporary avoidance of the offending positions.
      (1) Any contractures about the shoulder region must be eliminated by a stretching program.
      (2) Oral antiinflammatory agents may be helpful, particularly 25 mg of indomethacin four times daily for 7 to 10 days.
      (3) A muscle-strengthening program of exercise must be established because shoulder pain often leads to weakness, particularly of the rotator cuff. In carrying out these exercises, the patient should avoid the pain-producing positions.
      (4) A subacromial injection of 40 mg of methylprednisolone acetate (Depo-Medrol) is administered if the previous methods have failed, but injections should be limited to one or two during a 3-month period.

(5) After 6 months, if there is no improvement, arthroscopy with cuff debridement, followed by physical therapy, may be of value. If instability is present, it needs to be addressed with capsular plication or arthroscopic heating of the capsule. This will shrink the ligaments about 15%. This technique is experimental but to date has been useful in a limited number of patients involved in throwing or swimming sports activities.

2. During the **fourth or fifth decade,** a similar picture is noted, particularly in middle-aged tennis players, who often complain of pain while serving or hitting an overhead shot.
   a. **Radiography** may show some sclerosis of the greater tuberosity or of the acromion. MRI may show a partial or complete cuff tear.
   b. **Treatment** is similar to that in the older age groups.
3. During the **sixth or seventh decade,** further rotator cuff degeneration develops as a result of decreased vascularity of the supraspinatus tendon.
   a. The rotator cuff becomes attenuated as well as degenerative, with subsequent partial tearing that may progress to full-thickness tearing in some patients.
   b. The findings are similar to those of the younger patient but increased in severity. Crepitation of the subacromial space from an inflamed, thickened subacromial bursa may be present. In this age group, **biceps tendinitis** and **subacromial bursitis** are rarely separate entities and form part of the impingement syndrome.
   c. **Atrophy of the infraspinatus and supraspinatus regions** will increase in severity, particularly if a cuff tear is developing.
   d. When a small tear of the rotator cuff is present, shoulder motion may initially be normal, but as the tear increases, elevation will gradually be replaced by a shoulder-shrugging movement.
   e. **Loss of external rotation** may develop; however, it is seen only in patients with large, extensive tears that involve both the supraspinatus and infraspinatus.
   f. In patients with large tears of the rotator cuff, a **drop sign** will be positive. This sign is elicited by having the patient elevate the arm either actively or passively into the full overhead position, then lowering it in the place of the scapula. At approximately the 90-degree position, marked weakness is noted, and the arm will drop 30 to 40 degrees, often with pain.
   g. **Shoulder radiographs** will demonstrate sclerosis of the acromion with a reversal of the normal convexity of the inferior surface of the acromion.
      (1) Occasionally, a large spur will develop at the anterior inferior edge of the acromion in the coracoacromial ligament. An outlet radiograph of the shoulder may demonstrate the spur, a curved acromion, or both.
      (2) If a cuff tear is suspected or if the patient does not respond to treatment, an MRI should be obtained, which will demonstrate cuff degeneration and a tear if present. Tear size can be noted in addition to the degree of retraction and muscle atrophy.
      (3) For older patients, surgical treatment consists of acromioplasty and, if a tear is present, rotator cuff repair.
   h. The **conservative treatment** of older patients is similar to that of younger patients unless a rotator cuff tear is obvious.
      (1) Stretching, strengthening, and antiinflammatory agents can often be beneficial.
      (2) Injection of the subacromial space on one or two occasions may be helpful in allowing the patient to restore shoulder function; a long, repeated course of injections, however, will lead to further degenerative changes of the rotator cuff.

B. **Calcific tendinitis** may be present in either an acute or chronic form.
1. In the **acute** process, the patient notes the sudden occurrence of severe shoulder pain and will present holding the arm carefully at the side to avoid all shoulder movement.

a. A distinct swelling may be seen overlying the humeral head, and gentle **palpation** reveals a well-localized area of extreme tenderness.

b. All movements of the shoulder are resisted by pain.

c. **Shoulder radiographs** will generally show a fluffy calcific deposit within the rotator cuff tendons, most commonly the supraspinatus.

d. **Treatment** of the acute situation consists of injecting the deposit with 2 to 3 mL of 1% lidocaine and 40 mg of methylprednisolone acetate. After some local anesthesia is achieved, the deposit should be needled in an attempt to break it up, thus allowing the deposit to migrate into subacromial bursae, where it will be absorbed. Occasionally, the calcific deposit will rupture spontaneously, with prompt resolution of the patient's pain.

(1) Because pain may be temporarily increased following injection of the calcium deposit, ice should be applied to the shoulder for 20 to 30 minutes on several occasions during the next 24 hours.

(2) In addition, indomethacin is given for 3 to 4 days at a dosage of 25 mg four times daily.

(3) When pain abates, full shoulder motion should be encouraged to avoid development of a contracture.

2. In the **chronic** situation, the calcific deposit becomes indurated within the rotator cuff.

a. There is a long history, often of multiple attacks of shoulder pain. Complaints will often mimic those of the impingement-type syndromes.

b. **Treatment** is similar to that of acute tendinitis. Oral antiinflammatory agents (75 mg of sustained-release indomethacin twice daily for 7 days) and exercises are prescribed. Injections of 40 mg of methylprednisolone acetate are administered if no improvement is seen following conservative management. If pain persists or repeated attacks occur, operative removal of the calcium may be required.

c. It should be noted that some patients 40 years of age or more have asymptomatic calcium deposits in the shoulder.

C. **Adhesive capsulitis (frozen shoulder),** frequently seen during the fifth and sixth decades, may develop as a result of intrinsic shoulder pathology or occur secondary to extrinsic causes, particularly cervical spondylosis. Often, no specific etiologic factor can be found.

1. Motion will generally be restricted to elevation of 90 degrees, external rotation of 0 degrees, and a loss of internal rotation. Pain is present, particularly at the extremes of motion and at night.

2. On occasion, a large **loss of shoulder motion** will develop so slowly that the patient is unaware of the magnitude of the problem. Conversely, the onset may be sudden and severe, with marked loss of glenohumeral motion and a restriction of abduction to the 90-degree range.

3. **Tenderness** is present but poorly localized.

4. A history of **diabetes** is frequently obtained.

5. **Radiographic findings** will often be negative in the early stage but with time will show osteoporosis.

6. The region of the cervical spine, as well as chest and diaphragmatic lesions, should be carefully considered. Complete radiographic evaluation, including cervical spine, chest, and shoulder views, may be required.

7. **Metastatic lesions** involving the shoulder, spine, or brachial plexus may present as an adhesive capsulitis.

8. **Therapy** is directed toward achieving an improved range of motion. Steroid injections in the joint and oral antiinflammatory agents may be useful, depending on the stage of disease. A vigorous program of physical therapy is instituted both actively and passively at home and with a therapist. Improvement in range of motion is variable, but 95% of patients show significant, but slow, improvement by 3 months. If improvement does not occur, arthroscopic capsular release has been useful in a number of patients.

D. **Acromioclavicular joint.** Pain secondary to pathology of the acromioclavicular joint is frequently overlooked. The joint lies directly over the rotator cuff, and thus any alterations of the inferior surface will result in inflammation of the supraspinatus tendon deep to this joint.

1. **Degenerative lesions** of this joint may result in thickening and swelling and create an impingement syndrome.
2. **Pain** will occur with overhead activity of the arm and be aggravated by adduction of the arm across the chest. Pain occurs at night and is often increased by lying on the shoulder.
3. **Tenderness** is well localized to the involved joint.
4. **Radiographs** demonstrate narrowing of the joint with sclerosis and marginal osteophytes. Specific views taken at a 15-degree cephalic tilt allow better visualization of the acromioclavicular joint.
5. **Therapy** of the chronic situation consists of antiinflammatory medication, lidocaine injected locally, and Depo-Medrol. The degree of relief obtained from these injections confirms the diagnosis.
   - **a.** In the posttraumatic condition, muscle-strengthening exercises, particularly for the deltoid and trapezius, will result in improvement if significant degenerative changes are not present.
   - **b.** In the chronic situation in which pain persists despite one or two injections, resection of the outer 2 cm of the clavicle may be warranted.

E. Subluxation of the shoulder is an important cause of pain in the younger population. Often, the patient will state that the shoulder "comes out," although some patients will complain only of shoulder pain, particularly in the posterior humeral region.

1. **Specific testing** for shoulder instability should be performed, and any positions associated with apprehension should be noted.
2. **Radiographic evaluation** may provide confirmatory evidence of shoulder instability.
3. In those patients who have subluxation of the shoulder without dislocation, **rotation exercises** may be helpful. If symptoms persist despite this approach, surgical stabilization may be required.

F. Additional shoulder conditions. Although the more common causes of shoulder pain have been discussed, a wide variety of conditions may affect the shoulder.

1. The **thoracic outlet syndrome** with vascular or brachial plexus involvement may be the basis for extremity pain or fatigue.
2. Any type of **arthropathy,** including rheumatoid arthritis, degenerative joint disease, and syndromes such as polymyalgia rheumatica, may be expressed as rheumatic shoulder pain; however, in contrast to the conditions reviewed in this chapter, such problems are part of more generalized rheumatic syndromes.
3. **Osteonecrosis (avascular necrosis)** commonly affects the humeral head and should be considered in the differential diagnosis of shoulder pain (see Chapter 45).
4. The **shoulder-hand syndrome (reflex sympathetic dystrophy),** a poorly understood and uncommon basis for shoulder pain, is associated with diffuse swelling, pain, and vasomotor changes in the distal upper extremity (see Chapter 53). The problem occurs in elderly subjects and is sometimes related to myocardial infarction or other cardiopulmonary conditions. Unless an exercise program is vigorously instituted, supported by the use of analgesics and antiinflammatory drugs, **adhesive capsulitis** may be the outcome. If agents such as indomethacin (100 to 150 mg/24 h) do not control pain sufficiently to permit exercise, a short course of prednisone (25 mg/24 h for 3 to 4 days) may be instituted.
5. A variety of **intrathoracic problems** (including coronary ischemia, pulmonary embolus, pleuritis, and pneumonitis) and **diaphragmatic irritation** from abdominal lesions should be considered in the differential diagnosis of pain referred to the shoulder region.

16. ELBOW PAIN

Robert N. Hotchkiss

I. Anatomy

A. Joint. The articular anatomy of the elbow is unique because it contains two independent axes of motion in the same synovial pouch. The ulnohumeral joint determines flexion and extension, and the radiocapitellar joint pronation and supination of the forearm. The axis of rotation moves very little throughout flexion and extension, making a nearly perfect hinge that is highly constrained. The normal range of motion is 0 to 140 degrees of flexion and extension, 80 degrees of pronation, and 90 degrees of supination.

The elbow naturally deviates away from the body, the "carrying angle," which varies from person to person.

B. Stability. The hemi-circumferential articulation of the humerus and ulna combined with tension in the biceps-brachialis and triceps makes the elbow extremely stable. The radial head also contributes to stability by providing a wider base of support.

1. **Ligaments**
   - **a.** Because of the natural valgus (away from the body) angulation, valgus stress develops when a load is thrown or borne load. The medial collateral ligament, specifically the anterior portion, is the most important stabilizer.
   - **b.** On the lateral side, the radial collateral ligament helps to stabilize the ulna and humerus. The annular ligament wraps around the radial head, securing the proximal radius to the proximal ulna while allowing rotation of the radius.

C. Muscles

1. **Flexors.** The biceps and brachialis combine to function as the most powerful muscles in the upper extremity. Because of the location of the long head of the biceps, proximal ruptures can occur. The distal biceps tendon can also rupture. Depending on the patient's needs, some of the ruptures should be surgically repaired.
2. **Extensors.** The triceps is less powerful than the combined flexors. Active extension is needed for throwing and is especially important for patients who use their arms in transferring from bed to wheelchair or while using crutches. The triceps is much less prone to injury or rupture than the biceps.

D. Nerves. The medial, ulnar, and radial nerves all cross the elbow. The ulnar nerve is subcutaneous along the medial side and is palpable posterior to the medial epicondyle in the cubital tunnel. The radial nerve courses along the lateral side and is not palpable. The median nerve lies next to the brachial artery in the cubital fossa.

II. Examination

A. Etiology. In the examination of a painful elbow, it is helpful to categorize patients according to the suspected etiology.

1. **Acute pain** after trauma will be most likely associated with fracture or dislocation. Muscle tears of the biceps in middle-aged men can also occur. Acute pain on the medial or lateral sides of the elbow may be associated with sports such as golf or tennis, as the result of an acute muscle tear. Without a history of trauma, inflammation from gout, infection, rheumatoid arthritis (RA), or other rheumatic conditions should be investigated.
2. **Chronic pain** that develops slowly may be related to repetitive use; it is sometimes seen in assembly line workers or tennis enthusiasts. RA can present as recurrent warm effusions in the elbow or progressive, indolent loss of motion.
3. **Episodic pain,** characterized as sudden twinges and locking of the elbow, may be caused by loose cartilaginous fragments, commonly referred to as loose bodies.

B. Localization of pain by the patient is the single most important part of the examination. If the patient can specifically identify a reproducible location for the pain, the chances of diagnosis are greatly enhanced. Once the pain has been localized, or at least regionalized, the most common causes of pain in the given region can be investigated.

C. Palpation

1. **Point of maximal tenderness.** Once the pain is localized by the patient, examine for tenderness at that same location. Does direct pressure (gently applied) reproduce the discomfort? If pressure causes pain, local inflammation, from any of the sources listed below, should be suspected.
2. **Synovitis and effusions.** Proliferative synovium is usually associated with RA. Unlike effusions in the the knee, effusions in the elbow are often difficult to notice. Effusions can sometimes be palpated just anterior or posterior to the radial head, where arthrocentesis is performed.
3. **Crepitus.** Grinding and popping in a joint as it moves through a range of motion can often indicate severe erosions of articular cartilage. Both flexion-extension and pronation-supination should be checked. By placing a thumb over the radiocapitellar joint during passive forearm rotation, the status of the radial head can be assessed.

D. Range of motion

1. **Flexion-extension.** Flexion and extension should be recorded both actively and passively. With mild inflammation or minor trauma, extension is lost first. It is helpful to compare active and passive extension in the affected joint with the range of motion on the other side.
2. **Pronation-supination.** Forearm rotation should also be measured and compared with that on the other side.

III. Imaging and other diagnostic techniques

A. Plain radiographs. Plain radiographs of the elbow should include a true lateral and an anteroposterior film. The lateral film is the most difficult to obtain. If a flexion contracture exists, an anteroposterior film of the distal humerus and of the proximal forearm can be helpful. A radiocapitellar view can sometimes be helpful in assessment of the radiocapitellar joint. In the normal elbow, the head of the radius always points toward the capitellum in all views. If an effusion is present, the lateral view may demonstrate displacement of the anterior or posterior fat pad.

B. Bone scans can be useful in an attempt to localize or diagnose pain of unknown origin. A single-phase, "bone static" image may show uptake in a particular region and lead to closer scrutiny.

C. Computed tomography (CT) of the elbow can be useful in fracture and reconstructive problems. It is important to review the clinical history with the radiologist and to describe the area of interest, so that proper angulation of the cuts can be made.

D. Magnetic resonance imaging (MRI). The effectiveness of MRI in detecting a variety of painful conditions is steadily improving. The detail and resolution of images obtained with specialized surface coils permit visualization of ligament, cartilage, nerve, and muscle.

E. Arthrocentesis. As in all conditions of the joints, analysis of joint fluid can be valuable. (Analysis and technique are reviewed in other chapters.) Tapping the elbow requires knowledge of the surface anatomy to visualize effective needle placement.

In addition to synovial fluid analysis, instillation of 1% lidocaine or 0.5% bupivacaine can be diagnostically helpful if the examiner is unsure whether the source of the pain is intraarticular.

IV. Specific problems

A. Lateral elbow pain

1. **Lateral epicondylitis**
   a. **Sports-related. "Tennis elbow"** or lateral epicondylitis associated with racquet sports is common in amateurs and professionals. Onset can be rather acute or build slowly over months.

(1) The **diagnosis** is made by palpating the area of the lateral epicondyle with the elbow in nearly full extension and asking the patient to extend the wrist against resistance. This usually reproduces pain.

(2) Proper racquet size and proper backhand technique can lessen the severity of pain. The **first line of treatment** is rest, a short course of antiinflammatory medicine, and a wrist splint. Specialized braces that increase pressure in the forearm have also been used with success.

(3) The **second line of treatment** is local steroid injection in the area of greatest pain and symptom. The patient should be warned of possible skin depigmentation. It is mandatory for the patient to reduce the load on the elbow for at least 2 weeks after the injection.

(4) **If these measures fail,** excision of the degenerative fascia (Nirschl procedure) can be helpful in decreasing pain and restoring function.

Surgery should be reserved for severe, recalcitrant cases. Consideration should also be given to a change in avocation (i.e., avoiding racquet sports).

b. Cumulative trauma from work. Lateral elbow pain from repetitive labor is typically more resistant to treatment than is sports-related "tennis elbow." The onset can be insidious or begin with a direct blow to the lateral elbow. The pain is usually more diffuse throughout the extensor muscle mass. The same conservative measures listed in section **IV.A.1.a** should be tried. Return to work is often difficult.

2. Radial tunnel syndrome

a. Diagnosis. Entrapment of the posterior interosseous nerve, a branch of the radial nerve at the elbow, is a diagnosis that can be difficult to make. These patients frequently are indistinguishable from those with lateral elbow pain caused by work trauma (see section **IV.A.1.b**). Exquisite but dull pain over the anterior lateral elbow, distinct from the lateral epicondyle, may be present. Direct pressure over this same area should reproduce the symptoms. Weakness and pain during active extension of the middle finger can be present but is not necessarily diagnostic of this condition. Nerve conduction studies and electromyography have not been helpful the way they are in carpal tunnel syndrome.

b. Treatment. Surgical release of the radial and posterior interosseous nerves has been advocated for this condition, but consistent and effective treatment remains elusive.

3. Radial head fracture. People who fall on an outstretched hand are at special risk for this fracture.

a. The **diagnosis** is frequently missed because of inadequate radiography and examination. The symptoms may be a vague discomfort of the elbow, with little swelling. An ipsilateral fracture of the distal radius (Colles' fracture) may draw attention away from the elbow, and the radial head fracture goes unrecognized. Palpation of the radial head during gentle passive pronation and supination can be diagnostic, revealing exquisite tenderness or crepitation. Anteroposterior and lateral radiographs usually are diagnostic.

b. Treatment depends on the degree of displacement and other features. Most nondisplaced fractures require no splinting and benefit from early active motion.

4. Bicipital tendinitis and distal biceps rupture. Distal bicipital tendinitis can occur and may presage a distal biceps rupture.

a. Diagnosis. A patient who describes a heavy lifting activity followed by tenderness and soreness along the distal biceps tendon should be warned and the arm put at rest. A bone scan at this time can show increased uptake along the tendon, down to the insertion at the proximal radius. The biceps tendon can rupture at either end, but it is the distal end that can present as elbow pain or weakness. The rupture is usually seen in men 40 to 50 years of age, but it can also occur in younger weight lifters.

Most patients feel a sudden snap or tearing in the elbow while lifting and notice a sudden bulge in the distal forearm with weakness of supination. Ecchymosis may or may not be evident. Given the appearance of the arm, the amount of discomfort can be surprisingly minimal.

b. Treatment. The decision to repair this rupture surgically must be individualized. If repair is contemplated, it is best accomplished within days of injury.

B. Medial elbow pain

1. Medial epicondylitis. Inflammation of the medial side of the elbow is less common than inflammation of the lateral side. Overuse at work or **throwing sports** can initiate the process. As in lateral epicondylitis, there may be some tearing of the fibers of the muscle that originate from the medial side of the elbow.

a. Diagnosis. Direct palpation over the medial epicondyle usually elicits pain. This tenderness can be accentuated by resisted active flexion of the wrist. The zone of tenderness in medial epicondylitis is usually less discrete than that on the lateral side. The cubital tunnel, through which the ulnar nerve passes, is posterior to the epicondyle, and the examiner should attempt to distinguish between medial epicondylitis and cubital tunnel syndrome. Entrapment of the ulnar nerve can occur in patients with medial epicondylitis (often in throwing athletes), but the two conditions are separable and should be distinguished.

b. The **treatment** of medial epicondylitis is the same as that for the lateral side, but success is less predictable.

2. Cubital tunnel syndrome. Entrapment of the ulnar nerve at the elbow can occasionally begin as pain in the elbow. Associated with the local pain are the symptoms of nerve entrapment, paresthesias, numbness, and weakness in the ulnar nerve distribution. If the ulnar nerve subluxates over the medial epicondyle during flexion and extension, the pain can have quite an "electric" quality. It is useful to try to palpate the nerve during flexion and extension if you suspect subluxation. Tapping the ulnar nerve (Tinel's sign) may elicit paresthesia or dysesthesia in the distribution of the ulnar nerve. A full assessment of ulnar nerve function by motor and sensory examination is essential. Nerve conduction studies can be helpful to detect slowing of conduction across the elbow.

3. Valgus strain. Falls on an outstretched hand can cause sudden valgus loading or near dislocations. Tenderness along the medial side of the elbow is usually present, with swelling. Look for fractures of the radial head or avulsions of the medial epicondyle. It is not uncommon to see the medial collateral ligaments calcify several months later. This usually causes no functional loss and does not require any treatment.

C. Stiffness and contracture

1. Posttraumatic. Stiffness of the elbow after trauma is quite common, and physical therapy is usually required to minimize it. The functional range of motion of the elbow is in an arc of approximately 30 to 130 degrees of flexion, and 50 to 150 degrees of pronation-supination range. Each patient must be examined individually to determine whether treatment should be tried and which specific modality is appropriate. Forced, sudden, passive motion can be deleterious.

2. Heterotopic bone formation. Loss of motion may also be caused by juxta-articular bone formation at the elbow. Patients who have experienced cranial trauma are especially prone to heterotopic bone formation and may require excision and contracture release.

D. Olecranon bursitis. Acute inflammation of the olecranon bursa is a common condition that can result from infection or an acute gouty attack. Distinguishing infection from nonseptic inflammatory conditions such as gout or RA is often impossible on clinical examination alone. It becomes especially difficult in the diabetic patient with a history of gout. Both demonstrate erythema, fluctuance, and generalized tenderness. Adenopathy may be more prominent in infection, but it is not always present. Traumatic bursitis can cause bursal swelling and even some warmth. Fluid analysis demonstrates bloody or xanthochromic fluid that is culture negative.

1. **Laboratory studies.** Aspirating the bursal fluid for Gram's stain, culture, crystal examination, and cell count is most helpful, and findings can be diagnostic. Unfortunately, some patients are placed on antibiotics before specimens are taken, and the diagnosis remains elusive. The simultaneous use of antiinflammatory agents and antibiotics, although not technically graceful, may be prudent in some of these patients until the final culture results are available. Because *Staphylococcus aureus* is most commonly cultured, dicloxacillin or a cephalosporin should be started pending the results of the culture. In those patients with infection who do not respond to a 1- to 2-day course of oral antibiotics, intravenous therapy is indicated. Daily aspiration of the bursa is also mandatory.
2. **Treatment.** Recurrent bouts of inflammatory olecranon bursitis can be treated with repeated aspirations. In noninfectious cases, treatment of the underlying systemic disorder or avoidance of local trauma are indicated. However, if the frequency and severity of the episodes do not abate, operative bursectomy should be considered.

E. **Osteoarthritis.** Primary symptomatic osteoarthritis is less common in the elbow than in the weight-bearing joints of the lower extremities and interphalangeal joints of the hands. Inflammatory arthritis of the elbow is more likely to be a crystal-based arthropathy than a primary degenerative joint disease.

F. **Rheumatoid arthritis.** Rheumatoid involvement of the elbow usually begins with repeated effusions. Control of the effusions may require systemic medications or intraarticular steroid injections. Depending on the severity of disease, there is a gradual loss of motion as the joint surfaces become barren of articular cartilage. The loss of motion becomes more debilitating and self-care more difficult when the adjacent joints become affected. For patients with significant pain and joint destruction, total elbow replacement is often the best option.

G. **Hemophilia.** Recurrent hemarthrosis of the elbow may lead to a gradual loss of elbow function. In the early stages of recurrent hemarthrosis, a mild flexion contracture exists, with little chronic pain. Recurrent bleeds lead to destruction of the articular cartilage and a generalized arthropathy with pain, and fibrosis of the joint ensues.

1. **Medical management.** In the early phases of the bleeds, standard care includes factor VIII or IX infusions with plasma levels monitored. Initially, some restriction of activity is necessary, but when the acute bleed has resolved, motion exercises should be encouraged. Pain control is always difficult.
2. **Surgery.** Synovectomy of the elbow may be indicated for recurrent hemarthrosis unresponsive to medical management. For painful arthropathy, total elbow replacement offers improved function in selected cases.

Bibliography

Hotchkiss RN. Fractures and dislocations of the elbow. In: Rockwood CA, Green DP, Bucholz RW, Heckman JD, eds. *Fractures in adults,* 4th ed. Philadelphia: Lippincott–Raven Publishers, 1996.

Morrey BF. *The elbow and its disorders,* 2nd ed. Philadelphia: WB Saunders, 1993.

17. HAND DISORDERS

Robert L. Merkow and Paul Pellicci

Disorders of the hand are common; the primary physician is frequently called on to evaluate, diagnose, treat, or refer these important problems. The diagnosis of hand disorders can usually be made by appropriate history, physical examination, radiographs, and laboratory data. A knowledge of basic functional anatomy and physiology, together with a systematic approach to examination, will enable the practitioner to arrive at a working diagnosis and plan a rational therapeutic regimen.

I. **Anatomy and function.** Sir Charles Bell, the leading British anatomist, physiologist, and neurologist of the early nineteenth century, was among the first to recognize the unique qualities of the human hand: "It is in the human hand that we perceive the consummation of all; perfection, as an instrument. This superiority consists in its combination of strength, with variety, extent, and rapidity of motion . . . and the sensibility, which adapt it for holding, pulling, spinning, weaving, and constructing; . . . with the hands, the laborer supports a family, the parent loves and cares for a baby, the musician plays a sonata, the blind 'read' and the deaf 'talk.'"[1] The hand is an essential, complex organ comprising many specialized tissues. The hand-wrist unit integrates 27 bones and joints and 36 intrinsic and extrinsic muscles innervated by branches of three major nerves. The hand is supplied by two blood vessels and contains a variety of highly specialized retinacula and cutaneous structures.

A detailed description of hand anatomy and dynamics of function is beyond the scope of this chapter; however, certain generalities deserve emphasis, for they relate directly to the discussion of common hand disorders.

A. The **bones** of the hand are divided into three groups: the carpal bones, metacarpal bones, and phalanges. These are functionally grouped into fixed and mobile units. The hand is not flat but rather is shaped with structurally and functionally important transverse and longitudinal arches.

The fixed unit of the hand is central and consists of the index and long-finger metacarpals and the slightly mobile capitate, trapezium, and trapezoid bones, which form the bony keystone foundation of the hand. The flanking mobile units consist of the strong, mobile thumb on the radial side and the powerful ring and little finger on the ulnar side.

B. The **muscles and tendons** are divided into two groups: the intrinsic muscles (arising from within the hand) and the extrinsic muscles (arising from the forearm and elbow, but inserting into the hand via long tendons). The extrinsic muscles consist of the long flexors and extensors and provide movement and power to the fingers and thumb. The intrinsic muscles are grouped into the thenar and hypothenar muscles, the lumbricals, and the volar and dorsal interosseous muscles. These provide a strong thumb and a fine balance of flexor-extensor mechanisms for the precise and coordinated motions of the fingers.

C. The **three major nerves** supplying the hand are the median, ulnar, and radial nerves. The hand has an enormous share of sensory and motor representation in the brain. It should be appreciated that all purposeful hand function is initiated in the cerebral cortex.

1. The **radial nerve** innervates the extensor muscles in the forearm and provides dorsal sensation to the thumb, first web space, index finger, long finger, and radial half of the ring finger to the level of the proximal interphalangeal (PIP) joint.

[1] Bell, Sir Charles. *The hand, its mechanism and vital endowments, as evincing design.* Philadelphia: Coney, Lea and Blanchard, 1833.

2. The **median nerve** supplies all motor branches in the volar forearm except to the flexor carpi ulnaris (FCU) and the flexor digitorum profundus to the ring and little finger (FDP4+5). The median nerve enters the forearm through the two heads of the pronator teres at the elbow; it courses down the forearm volarly within the deep fascia of the flexor digitorum superficialis (FDS) muscle group. The median nerve enters the hand superficially at the wrist through the carpal canal. It also innervates the thenar muscles, except the adductor (via the recurrent motor branch at the base of the thumb), and supplies the lumbricals to the index and long fingers. The median nerve provides important sensation to the thumb, the index and long fingers, and radial half of the ring finger.
3. The **ulnar nerve** supplies only the FCU and FDP4+5 in the forearm. It runs deep to the FCU, entering the hand via the canal of Guyon between the pisiform and the hook of the hamate bone. In the hand, the ulnar nerve supplies the hypothenar muscles and the remaining intrinsic muscles, and its sensory branches innervate the little finger and the ulnar half of the ring finger.

D. The **blood and lymphatic vessels** supply the hand with two major branches of the brachial artery: the radial and ulnar arteries entering the hand at the wrist. These anastomose in the palm, forming superficial and deep arches that give off arterial branches to the thumb and fingers. The venous and lymphatic networks run from the palmar to the dorsal side of the hand (this, together with the loose dorsal skin, accounts for the prominent dorsal swelling that can occur in the hand and fingers). The dorsal veins coalesce into the cephalic (radial side) and basilic (ulnar side) systems.

II. **History.** Because hand function is integral to all activities of daily living, the patient will usually be able to describe accurately the duration and degree of disability.

A. The **general history** should include the following:
1. The patient's age, occupation, hand dominance, and previous impairment.
2. Activities and hobbies.
3. Medical history, including any underlying systemic disorders, such as diabetes, vascular disease, and endocrine or collagen vascular disorders.
4. The distinction between traumatic and nontraumatic causes is useful; however, disorders may occur concomitantly or be noted after an unrelated injury.

B. The **specific history** regarding dysfunction of the hand should include duration of disability, precipitating causes, and specific loss of function. Cardinal symptoms include pain, swelling, deformity, and alteration in sensation or strength.
1. **Type and severity of pain,** as well as **location and pattern,** are important. What is its onset and progression? Is it constant or intermittent? Does it occur at night? Which specific acts make the pain worse? Is the pain well localized, or does it radiate in a nerve or root distribution? Pain in the neck or other joints may also be helpful in determining a remote or systemic cause. Finally, what treatments or medication have been tried, and what have been the results?
2. **Swelling and deformity** may be subjective. They may be subtle or obvious. Inquiries regarding onset, progression, and response to treatment should be made.
3. **Numbness, weakness, and paresthesia** may indicate neurologic dysfunction. The severity, anatomic distribution, duration, and progression of the symptoms are important. Identifying precipitating activities or positions can be very helpful in localizing neurocompressive problems. A history of neck pain or radiation should also be sought.

III. **Physical examination.** The patient should be sitting, and the entire upper extremity should be exposed and evaluated.

A. **Surrounding joints.** Begin at the neck; check range of motion, and palpate for areas of tenderness.

1. The **shoulder and elbow** should be fully examined because either may be the source of a hand disorder. Assessment of active motion at the shoulder and elbow as well as of forearm pronation and supination is important because motion at these joints is necessary for proper positioning of the hand for function. Note any discrepancy between active and passive motion. Closely examine the shoulder, arm, and forearm for evidence of muscle atrophy.
2. **Wrist.** Evaluate both active and passive range of motion, including supination and pronation. Compare right and left sides. Observe and palpate for localized swelling or tenderness. Note whether areas of swelling appear to arise from the carpal joints *per se,* from the distal radioulnar joint, or from the more superficial dorsal tendons crossing the wrist (in the last case, the swelling may move with digital flexion-extension).

B. Hand. Observe the resting posture of the hand, and record specific areas of muscle atrophy, discoloration, abnormal swelling, or deformity. Comparison with the contralateral hand (if normal) can be helpful. Accurate recording of the findings is important; a simple sketch of the hand with appropriate notations and measurements is often helpful.

1. The **attitude or position** of the hand should be inspected for loss of the normal transverse and longitudinal arches, loss of the flexion cascade of the fingers, abnormal posturing, or deformities of the fingers and thumb.
2. **Circulation** is assessed by observing the color of the skin and fingernails as well as blanching and flush of the nail bed. Patency of the radial and ulnar arteries can be assessed by use of Allen's test. This test can also be applied to the digital vessels.
3. **Skin** is normally thick and moist on the palmar surface and thin and mobile on the dorsal surface. Examine for the presence or absence of swelling, wrinkles, moisture, scars, or cutaneous lesions.
4. **Joints** should be inspected for evidence of effusion, synovitis, osteophytes, or loss of normal alignment and motion.
5. **Motions** of the hand as a unit and individual joints should be checked for stiffness or abnormal mobility. Have the patient make a fist and fully extend the fingers. Evaluate and record action range of motion at the metacarpophalangeal (MCP), PIP, and distal interphalangeal (DIP) joints. Gently check passive flexion and extension of the finger joints and record any fixed contractures.
6. **Flexor tendon function** is evaluated by asking the patient to flex at the DIP joints while holding the MCP and PIP joints in extension. This action evaluates the FDP function. To test the FDS function, hold the other fingers in extension at the MCP, PIP, and DIP joints, and allow free the digit to be tested. Flexion should occur at the PIP joint, and the DIP joint should be flaccid.
7. **Sensation** is best tested for light touch with cotton and for two-point discrimination with the prongs of a paper clip. Measure the distance at which the distinction between one and two points is not accurate, and compare with the other digits and contralateral hand. Normally, a patient can distinguish two points 6 mm apart on the pulp of the fingers.
8. **Grip and pinch** strengths are useful objective measurements and should be recorded and compared with the contralateral side.
9. **Simple functional tasks.** The patient's ability to use the hand for activities of daily living should also be evaluated and recorded.

IV. Diagnostic studies

A. Radiographs should include anteroposterior, lateral, and oblique views of the hand and wrist. Additional cone-down views of an involved digit are often needed to look at specific bones and joints.

B. Nerve conduction and electromyographic studies should be obtained if there is evidence of nerve dysfunction (i.e., significant weakness, atrophy, or sensory abnormality). These studies supplement the clinical history and examination in documenting neurologic dysfunction and evaluating the anatomic location and extent of the process.

C. Joint aspiration should be performed when significant effusion is present (see Chapters 4 and 5). Synovial fluid is examined grossly and sent for cell counts and crystal, biochemical, and microbiologic studies.

V. Inflammatory conditions are common and may be caused by infections, sterile synovitis, tendinitis, or tenosynovitis, sometimes with calcifications. (Specific arthritic conditions are discussed in section **VII.**)

A. Stenosing tenosynovitis is the cause of trigger finger or thumb and de Quervain's disease of the thumb extensors. It is commonly encountered in patients with a history of repetitive manual trauma. The process is caused by tenosynovitis of the tendon, sheath, or synovium with a nodule-like enlargement of the tendons. These may catch on the pulley entrance to cause locking or triggering.

1. In **trigger finger or thumb,** digital motion is restricted when the tendon lesion impinges on the unyielding pulley at the base of the finger. The patient will describe a painful "locking" of the finger in flexion. Extension is often possible only by using the contralateral hand to extend (unlock) the finger forcefully, and this is accompanied by moderate pain. The patient will frequently describe this process as worse in the morning (because of swelling) and "loosening up" as the day progresses.

   a. **Physical examination** demonstrates a tender, palpable nodularity in the palm that moves with the flexor tendon and may catch with passive motion. The best way to demonstrate the locking phenomenon is to have the patient fully flex all fingers actively and then slowly extend; the locking fingers will either remain locked or will "snap" open on extension.

   b. **Treatment**

      (1) **Injection** with 4 mg (1 mL) of aqueous dexamethasone (Decadron) and lidocaine into the inflamed tendon sheath may diminish the inflammatory process and swelling and allow for normal motion in approximately 50% of cases. Unfortunately, in a large proportion of cases, recurrence will be noted after several months.

      (2) **Surgical release** of the tight pulley (and a limited tenosynovectomy, when needed) is indicated for severe cases with painful locking or when conservative treatment fails. This provides safe and effective resolution of symptoms.

2. **De Quervain's stenosing tenosynovitis** is similar in pathogenesis to trigger finger. Pain is the cardinal symptom, and it is located in the area of the anatomic snuffbox at the dorsoradial aspect of the wrist. Inflammation of the tendons and sheaths of the abductor pollicis longus (APL) and extensor pollicis brevis (EPB) may result from repetitive movements of the thumb and wrist. Frequently, pain will radiate up the dorsoradial aspect of the arm along the course of these muscles.

   a. On **examination,** there is swelling and tenderness over the first dorsal extensor compartment along the APL and EPB. Flexion-abduction of the thumb induces the pain, which is aggravated by passive ulnar deviation of the wrist (Finkelstein's test).

   b. **Differential diagnosis** includes arthritic conditions of the wrist or basal joint of the thumb and fracture, instability, or posttraumatic disorders of the carpal navicular bone. Injection of lidocaine into the tendon sheath can help establish the diagnosis.

   c. **Treatment** initially includes immobilization of the thumb and wrist with a splint and antiinflammatory medication [25 mg of indomethacin (Indocin) PO three times daily or 600 mg of ibuprofen (Motrin) PO three times daily] or injection with 4 to 8 mg of dexamethasone and lidocaine into the inflamed tendon sheath. In refractory cases, surgical release of the tight, thickened, inflamed tendon sheath has been uniformly successful.

B. Tendinitis and tenosynovitis with or without calcification. Any of the numerous tendons or sheaths about the hand and wrist may be involved with painful inflammation.

1. **Physical examination.** Localized swelling, tenderness, and crepitus will be present. Tenosynovitis commonly occurs in the extensor digitorum communis (EDC) along the dorsum of the hand or wrist; other extensors occasionally involved include the extensor carpi radialis, extensor pollicis longus, and extensor carpi ulnaris. On the palmar side, the flexor carpi ulnaris or radialis may be involved.
2. **Laboratory studies.** Radiographs may show calcifications along these tendons or in periarticular locations. Aspiration and crystal analysis may in some cases establish a specific diagnosis.
3. **Treatment** should include splinting of the inflamed lesion in a resting position and a course of nonsteroidal antiinflammatory medications such as indomethacin (25 mg PO three times daily). If symptoms are not relieved by these measures, dexamethasone injection and further splinting are indicated. Rarely is surgical treatment needed.

C. **Infections** in the hand are common and can cause significant disability. Most will respond favorably when **general principles of care** are followed. These include rest, elevation, immobilization (with early mobilization), bacterial identification, appropriate antibiotic coverage, and surgical incision, drainage, and debridement when indicated. In cases that do not promptly respond favorably when these principles are followed, specific causes for the increased severity or chronicity should be sought. Predisposing systemic conditions include diabetes, hematologic malignancies, and circulatory disorders such as Raynaud's, Buerger's, or atherosclerotic disease. Predisposing local factors that may be responsible for poorly responding infections include retained foreign body, necrotic or sequestered tissue, or ineffective drainage.

1. **Paronychia,** the most common finger infection, is usually a staphylococcal infection of the soft tissues around the nail. It frequently results from rough manicuring or ill-advised picking of a hangnail.
   a. **Physical examination.** Severe pain, swelling, erythema, and sometimes pus are present, located at the base of and alongside the nail.
   b. **Treatment**
      (1) **Initial treatment** should include warm soaks three times daily, elevation, and oral antibiotics with coverage for *Staphylococcus* [250 to 500 mg of cephradine (Velosef) or dicloxacillin PO q6h].
      (2) If there is no resolution in 24 to 47 hours, or if a visible purulent collection is present, **surgical drainage** is advisable.
2. **Felon** is a painful infection of the distal pulp of the fingertip, with swelling, erythema, tenderness, and deep abscess formation.
   a. **Initial treatment,** including elevation, antibiotics, and protective splinting, may occasionally be successful.
   b. Usually, careful **surgical incision and drainage** of the deep pulp space loculations are needed. Antibiotic coverage and local care with dressing changes are usually followed by rapid healing once effective drainage has been performed.
3. **Cellulitis, lymphangitis, and subcutaneous abscess.** These infectious conditions are frequently seen in a busy emergency department.
   a. They may be caused by a scratch, abrasion, or puncture wound that secondarily becomes infected. Introduction of foreign or contaminated material through intravenous or subcutaneous needles by a drug abuser is another source of these types of infections.
   b. Treatment
      (1) **Initial treatment** should include immobilization with plaster splints, strict elevation, and antibiotics.
      (2) If fever, lymphangitis, and axillary adenopathy are present, **hospital admission** is advisable for intravenous antibiotics and controlled treatment.
      (3) **Surgical incision and drainage** are indicated for well-localized abscess collections after 12 to 36 hours of intravenous antibiotic saturation.

4. **Acute suppurative tenosynovitis** is a relatively rare but dramatic serious infection involving the flexor tendons and sheaths that extend into the palm.
   a. There is usually a **history** of prior puncture. Pain is severe, extending along the palmar aspect of the finger into the palm. Motion of the finger exacerbates the pain.
   b. **Physical examination.** There is marked uniform swelling and erythema of the finger, which is held in partial flexion. Dorsal swelling also occurs because of the venous and lymphatic drainage pattern.
   c. **Kanavel's four cardinal signs**
      (1) Pain with passive extension.
      (2) Flexed position of the finger.
      (3) Uniform swelling into the palm.
      (4) Tenderness along the flexor sheath into the palm.
   d. **Treatment**
      (1) **Initial treatment** should include aspiration of the tendon sheath under sterile conditions. Gram's stain and culture are obtained before intravenous antibiotics are begun. Purulent tenosynovitis is a potentially destructive infection of the tendon sheath that can destroy the flexor tendon and extend into the palm, deep structures of the hand, and other tendons.
      (2) Early surgical decompression, irrigation, and judicious debridement are indicated for this serious infection.
5. **Septic arthritis** is most commonly seen in the MCP joints.
   a. These infections are most often caused by a human or animal bite, tooth abrasion, or clenched "fist in mouth" injury.
   b. The **presentation** is one of severe pain, swelling, and erythema about the wound on the dorsum of the hand. Motion is painful and limited. Seropurulent discharge can frequently be expressed.
   c. **Treatment.** Hospital admission for surgical incision and debridement in addition to immobilization, elevation, and administration of intravenous antibiotics is recommended.

VI. Injuries of the fingers

A. **Subungual hematoma.** This extremely painful condition usually results from trauma to the distal finger (e.g., car door slam, hammer blow).
   1. Immediate elevation and immersion in ice water may reduce the nail pain and bleeding.
   2. Relief of pain is dramatic if the nail bed is carefully punctured over the hematoma area with a paper clip prong that has been inserted in a flame until red hot. Soak the finger in antiseptic solution and then apply a bandage.

B. **Flexor tendon rupture.** Pain in the palmar aspect of the finger can be caused by rupture of the FDP tendon from its insertion into the distal phalanx.
   1. A **history** of sudden pain in the finger while grabbing (e.g., a football jersey, a stumbling child) is classic.
   2. Methodic **testing** of FDP function (see section **III.B.6**) establishes the diagnosis.
   3. **Treatment.** Surgical repair is the treatment of choice.

C. **Mallet finger.** Similar trauma may rupture the terminal extensor tendon to produce a flexed distal phalanx and an inability to extend the DIP joint actively. The pain here is localized over the dorsum of the joint.
   1. **Radiographs** of the affected finger are necessary, as avulsion fractures of the distal phalanx may occur as the tendon ruptures.
   2. **Treatment** consists of application of an aluminum foam splint to the dorsal surface of the finger, immobilizing only the DIP joint in extension (avoid hyperextension). A dorsal splint spares the palmar tactile surface and allows PIP joint motion during the necessary 6 weeks of splinting.

D. **Fractures and dislocations of the hand** are classified by the nature and site of injury and whether the skin surrounding the injury is open or closed.

1. Careful **examination** of the hand for angular or rotational deformities and proper anteroposterior and true lateral **radiographs** are necessary.
2. **Treatment.** Intraarticular, displaced, or potentially unstable fractures usually require reduction and stabilization with Kirschner wires.

VII. Arthritic conditions involving the small joints of the hand and wrist are frequently seen in cases of rheumatoid arthritis (RA), osteoarthritis, or posttraumatic arthritis. Treatment depends on the sites and severity of involvement and is individualized based on the patient's functional disabilities and overall needs. General goals in the care of arthritic hands are to relieve pain, prevent or correct deformity, and maintain or improve function.

A. **Rheumatoid arthritis** is a systemic autoimmune disease that frequently involves the hand and wrist (see Chapter 28).
1. The wrist, MCP, and PIP joints are most frequently involved.
2. Erosive synovitis, pain, stiffness, progressive deformity, and loss of function are the hallmarks of this disease process.
3. **Radiographically,** one sees generalized osteoporosis, joint space narrowing, and periarticular erosions, particularly of the carpal bones and metacarpophalangeal joints.
4. Pain and stiffness are frequently worse in the morning. As the disease progresses, the fingers may become deformed, and the classic ulnar drift may develop. Swan neck and boutonniere deformities are common.
5. Carpal tunnel syndrome, trigger finger or thumb, dorsal wrist synovitis, flexor tenosynovitis, and tendon ruptures are frequently encountered.
6. **Treatment** should be comprehensive. A team approach utilizes the combined expertise of rheumatologists, surgeons, and therapists, as well as psychologists and social workers.
   a. **Initial treatment** should include aspirin or nonsteroidal antiinflammatory medications, occupational therapy for splinting, and judicious functional exercises as indicated. Systemic steroids, intraarticular injections, and surgery are indicated in aggressive or refractory cases.
   b. **Surgery** is primarily indicated for severe pain, chronic aggressive synovitis that is unresponsive to adequate medical treatment, nerve entrapment syndromes, tendon ruptures, and deformities resulting in impaired hand function.

B. **Osteoarthritis** is common in adults (see Chapter 44).
1. It most frequently involves the interphalangeal joints, especially the DIP joints of the fingers and the carpometacarpal (CMC) or basal joint of the thumb.
2. It is caused by repetitive abnormal physical stress with subsequent activation of tissue factors and consequent joint wear, destruction, and juxtaarticular changes.
3. Pain, swelling, stiffness, and joint malalignment are hallmarks of the disease.
4. **Radiographically,** one sees joint space narrowing, marginal osteophytes, sclerosis, and subchondral cysts.
5. **Heberden's nodes** (marginal osteophytes), with or without mucous cysts, occur at the DIP joints. These are often inflamed and painful. Initial treatment with topical steroid cream and protective covering may provide a beneficial response in 1 to 2 months. Surgical excision of cysts and underlying osteophytes arising from the arthritic joint can provide relief of symptoms and cosmetic improvement.
6. **Bouchard's nodes** (marginal osteophytes) at the PIP joints and radial dorsal osteophytes at the thumb basal joint are indicators of degenerative arthritis at these joints. Pain, swelling, tenderness, malalignment, and loss of pinch strength are the characteristic clinical findings.
7. **Treatment**
   a. Antiinflammatory medications, occupational therapy, and a supportive abduction thumb splint can provide significant relief of pain and improve function.

b. Surgical debridement of osteophytes, excision of cysts, arthroplasty, or fusion may be indicated for advanced disease.

VIII. Tumor and swelling

A. Ganglions

1. Ganglions are the most common soft-tissue tumor in the hand. They most frequently present as painless, firm dorsal swellings around the wrist. They may also occur over the volar wrist and in the hand near the MCP flexion crease at the base of the fingers. Although their etiology is unknown, ganglions are cystic swellings containing mucinous material that are closely connected to joints or tendon sheaths. They transilluminate in a darkened room.

2. Ganglions rarely interfere with hand function, but on occasion, particularly after strenuous activity, they may become painful.

3. Radiography may reveal underlying pathology (i.e., dorsal spurs of the carpal bones).

4. Treatment. Ganglions may be aspirated, providing diagnostic confirmation, and injected with a steroid suspension; however, recurrence is common. Aspiration, if attempted, should be performed with an 18-gauge needle, as ganglionic fluid is extremely viscous. Surgery is indicated for painful ganglion, symptomatic recurrence, and cosmetic complaints.

B. Giant cell tumor of the tendon sheath (pigmented villonodular synovitis) is a locally aggressive, benign tumor arising from synovium and periarticular tissues. It is the second most common tumorous growth in the hand. It is usually painless but may cause mild pain or local nerve compression. Joint motion is occasionally impaired when impingement is caused by the size or location of the growth. Generally, these reactive lesions are slow-growing, but they may invade tendon or bone. They are solid tumors and therefore do not transilluminate. Surgical excision is warranted to confirm the diagnosis and to relieve pain and nerve compression and improve cosmesis. Recurrence after excision is common.

C. Synovitis of rheumatoid disease may present as swelling over the PIP, MCP, and wrist joints and over the dorsum of the hand. Swelling over the dorsum of the hand should not be confused with an infectious process. Motion of the fingers and wrist may be limited.

1. Aspiration may be attempted if the diagnosis is doubtful, but care should be taken not to convert a synovial swelling into an iatrogenic infection.

2. Treatment. Immobilization by splinting, together with an appropriate antiinflammatory medication, is indicated for therapy of the acute attack. Tenosynovectomy may be indicated in selected patients with refractory dysfunction.

D. Swelling of disuse. Normally active hand motion is essential to promote venous and lymphatic drainage. Any condition that causes an absence or decline of hand motion will promote the collection of edematous fluid and lead to diffuse hand swelling, stiffness, and ultimately loss of function. Bed rest and inactivity resulting from an unrelated condition (myocardial infarction, skeletal traction, sciatica) may lead to this potentially disabling condition. Physician awareness of the problem and the services of a trained therapist are essential to manage the problem.

E. The **carpometacarpal boss** is a bony prominence involving the CMC joints of the index and long fingers. It may appear in conjunction with a ganglion.

1. Pain and tenderness are caused by underlying arthritis of the CMC joints.

2. Treatment with antiinflammatory medications and a short period of immobilization may provide symptomatic relief. If surgical treatment is indicated (rarely, for refractory pain), the underlying CMC joint arthrosis should also be addressed when the dorsal bony prominence is excised.

IX. Hand deformities may be associated with previous traumatic injuries to joints, tendons, or nerves, with arthritic conditions, or with progressive fascial contracture.

A. **Dupuytren's contracture** is a process of painless thickening and contracture of proliferative longitudinal bands of the palmar aponeurosis, which lies between the skin and flexor tendons. The tendons are not primarily involved. Dupuytren's contracture occurs most commonly in male subjects (90%), is often bilateral, and frequently is associated with diabetes, heavy alcohol consumption, seizure disorders, repetitive trauma, and a family history of the disease.

1. **History.** Patients complain of thickened bands, inability to open their hands fully, and difficulty with handshakes or grasping large objects. The ring and little fingers are most often involved.
2. **Physical examination** reveals the fixed flexed position of the finger, palpable nodules, and thickened longitudinal cords in the palm extending into the fingers.
3. **Treatment.** Surgical excision is recommended if the contracture impairs function or if fixed metaphalangeal and PIP contractures are progressive.

B. **Swan neck.** This abnormality consists of hyperextension of the PIP joint and flexion of the DIP joint. It may occur following trauma or, more commonly, in RA.

1. Anatomically, synovitis causes erosion of the volar stabilizing elements, allowing PIP hyperextension and dorsal displacement of the extensor apparatus. With contracture of the joint and extensor apparatus, PIP flexion is impossible, and deformity can be severe.
2. **Treatment.** In the early posttraumatic condition, splinting may be attempted with the deformity reversed (PIP flexed and DIP extended) for a 6-week period. Surgical correction is necessary if hand function is sufficiently impaired.

C. **Boutonniere.** Disruption of the extensor mechanism over the PIP joint from trauma, laceration, or synovitis will produce flexion of the PIP joint and extension of the DIP joint. The deformity is not as functionally disabling as swan neck deformity because grasp function is still possible. Acute **therapy** consists of splinting the finger with the PIP joint extended and the DIP joint flexed. Surgical reconstruction may be necessary if disability is marked.

D. **Extensor tendon ruptures** without laceration are uncommon except in patients with chronic RA. Rupture probably results from multiple factors, notably compromise of the tendon blood supply as a result of florid tenosynovitis. Rupture of EDC4+5 is common at the site of dorsal dislocation of the distal radioulnar joint from rheumatoid synovitis. The presenting complaint of inability to extend the thumb or finger should alert the examiner.

1. **Examination** of the resting posture of the hand will demonstrate increased flexion of the digit or digits; active extension of the digits will not be possible. These extensor tendon ruptures are usually painless and may go unnoticed by the patient.
2. **Treatment.** Early surgical consultation is advised because single extensor tendon rupture puts more strain on the remaining tendons and often heralds a chain of tendon ruptures across the dorsum of the hand.

E. **Claw hand** is a deformity manifested by flattening of the hand arches, hyperextension of the MCP joints, and flexion of the interphalangeal joints. It may be caused by ulnar or combined nerve paralysis, brachial plexopathies, or central nervous disorders. It results from an imbalance of the intrinsic and extrinsic muscles. In the presence of intrinsic weakness, overpull of the long extensors causes MCP hyperextension and clawing of the fingers as a consequence of powerful interphalangeal flexion from the long flexors.

X. **Abnormalities of sensation**

A. **Carpal tunnel syndrome** is produced by compression of the median nerve at the wrist. As the nerve passes through the unyielding carpal tunnel, it is at risk for compression by the transverse carpal ligament. In most patients, no specific etiology can be determined, but thickening and proliferation of the peritendinous synovium is seen. This condition is very common in RA, in diabetes, during or after pregnancy, and after wrist fracture. It is also seen in postmenopausal women and in patients with the myxedema of thyroid disease.

1. A **history** of wrist pain and paresthesias in the thumb, index finger, and long finger (the median nerve distribution), frequently occurring at night, is fairly typical. The patient may report being awakened by the pain and paresthesias and needing to shake the hand for relief. The lack of muscle activity at night allows fluid accumulation, and wrist flexion during sleep is thought to account for this exacerbation of symptoms. Patients may also report daytime paresthesias, clumsiness or dropping of objects, and weakness of pinch or grasp.
2. **Physical examination** may demonstrate a mild flattening of the thenar eminence. Light touch with a cotton applicator along the radial border of the ring finger and both sides of the index finger and thumb will demonstrate a decrease in sensation. Care must be taken to apply the applicator along the palmar surface of the digit, as the dorsum of the fingers is supplied by the radial and ulnar nerves. A decrease in two-point discrimination occurs late in the neuropathy. Thumb opposition, the ability to draw the thumb away from the palm and oppose the thumb pulp to the pulp of the little finger, may be diminished. Tapping the volar surface of the wrist over the median nerve may produce **Tinel's sign,** which appears as shooting pain in the long or index finger and indicates median nerve compression. **Phalen's sign,** also helpful, is performed by flexing both wrists for 30 to 60 seconds to elicit median nerve numbness in the affected hand.
3. **Electromyography and nerve conduction studies** may confirm a delay in nerve conduction across the carpal canal and denervation of thenar musculature.
4. **Treatment**
   a. **Splints** to hold the wrist in slight extension during sleep.
   b. A 40 mg dose of **methylprednisolone** injected into the area of the carpal canal provides some relief in early cases. Care must be exercised to avoid injuring the median nerve and flexor during injection.
   c. **Surgical release** of the transverse carpal ligament is indicated if the response to local measures is poor or if the neurologic deficit progresses.

B. **Ulnar nerve entrapment** may occur at the wrist as the ulnar nerve passes through the tight canal (of Guyon). It may be seen after wrist trauma, in patients with RA, and in jackhammer workers.

1. **History.** Symptoms include weakness of the intrinsic muscles of the hand and numbness in the ulnar nerve distribution.
2. **Laboratory studies.** Diagnosis is confirmed with nerve conduction studies and electromyography.
3. **Treatment** is usually local injections of methylprednisolone and surgical decompression if symptoms persist or neurologic dysfunction progresses.

Bibliography

Burton RI, Littler JW. Nontraumatic soft tissue afflictions of the hand. *Curr Probl Surg* 1975;July:1.

Burton RI, et al. *The hand, examination and diagnosis,* 2nd ed. American Society for Surgery of the Hand. New York: Churchill Livingstone, 1983.

Kleinart HE. Trauma of the hand. *Curr Probl Surg* 1978;10:1.

Lampe EW, Netter FHL. Surgical anatomy of the hand, with special reference to infections and trauma. *Found Clin Symp* 1969;3.

Lister G. *The hand, diagnosis and indications.* New York: Churchill Livingstone, 1983.

18. LOW BACK PAIN

Daniel J. Clauw and John F. Beary, III

Low back pain is an extremely common condition, affecting 80% of persons at some point in their lifetime, which makes this complaint second only to the common cold as a reason for outpatient physician visits. Most episodes of acute low back pain resolve spontaneously, regardless of the type of therapy chosen. However, a small percentage of these acute cases, 5% to 10% in most series, progress to chronic low back pain. It is this latter group of patients that primarily accounts for the enormous amount of disability caused by low back pain, estimated to cost more than $20 billion annually and completely disable more than 2.5 million persons in the United States alone.

Epidemiologic studies have established demographic characteristics and risk factors for the development of low back pain. First episodes of low back pain typically occur between the ages of 20 and 40, with a relatively equal sex ratio. Well-established risk factors for the development of low back pain include heavy manual work, especially when twisting while lifting is involved; poor job satisfaction; exposure to vibration (especially while driving motor vehicles); and cigarette smoking. A sedentary lifestyle and pregnancy are possible but unproven risk factors. The emphasis in this chapter is to guide the physician into a directed history and physical examination that will allow differentiation of the common causes of low back pain from the more serious, uncommon causes. Once these salient differences in presentations are understood, it becomes clear that the majority of patients who present with low back pain need no diagnostic tests and will respond to conservative management.

I. Etiology. Any of the components of the lumbosacral process may be responsible, alone or in combination, for low back pain, or pain may be referred to this area from a distant site. The history, physical examination, and diagnostic studies will allow the formation of a **differential diagnosis** from the list below.

- **A. Vertebral body** (e.g., metastatic disease, metabolic bone disease, fracture).
- **B. Intervertebral disk** (e.g., infection).
- **C. Joints** (e.g., ankylosing spondylitis, osteoarthritis)
  - **1.** Apophyseal joints.
  - **2.** Sacroiliac joints.
- **D. Ligaments**
  - **1.** Anterior and posterior longitudinal ligaments.
  - **2.** Interspinous and supraspinous ligaments.
  - **3.** Iliolumbar ligaments.
  - **4.** Apophyseal ligaments.
- **E. Nerve roots** (e.g., herniated nucleus pulposus, spinal stenosis).
- **F. Paraspinous musculature** (e.g., fibromyalgia, myofascial pain).
- **G. Pain from adjacent structures or referred pain**
  - **1.** Kidney (e.g., pyelonephritis, perinephric abscess, nephrolithiasis).
  - **2.** Pelvic structures (e.g., pelvic inflammatory disease, ectopic pregnancy, endometriosis, prostatic disease).
  - **3.** Vascular (e.g., aortic aneurysm, mesenteric thrombosis).
  - **4.** Intestinal (e.g., diverticulitis).
- **H. Malignancy** (involving any of the above structures).
- **I.** Miscellaneous conditions (e.g., sickle cell disease).

II. History. The history is of the utmost importance to obtain **associated symptoms** and establish a **pattern** of pain.

- **A. Associated symptoms.** A thorough review of systems is required to establish concomitant symptoms that would suggest a nonmechanical cause of low back pain.
  - **1. Fevers or chills** would raise the possibility of an infectious process.

2. **Weight loss, chronic cough, change in bowel habits, night pain, or other constitutional symptoms** may suggest an **underlying malignancy.**
3. Similar pain or morning stiffness in other areas of the body would increase the suspicion that this represents a more generalized rheumatologic condition (e.g., ankylosing spondylitis, psoriatic arthritis, or endocrine disorder, such as hypothyroidism, hyperthyroidism, or hyperparathyroidism).
4. If **fatigue** or a **sleep disturbance** is present, the diagnosis of fibromyalgia should be considered.
5. **Morning stiffness** or back pain that **improves with exercise** should prompt consideration of a seronegative spondyloarthropathy.

B. **Pain.** The quality of pain, its distribution, and modulating factors are helpful in determining etiology.
1. **Onset of pain**
   a. **Sudden onset,** particularly if associated with trauma, suggests bony or soft-tissue injury.
   b. **Indolent onset** suggests a nonmechanical cause.
   c. **Episodic or colicky pain** suggests an intraabdominal or pelvic etiology.
2. **Localization of pain**
   a. Localized.
   b. Radicular, suggesting nerve root impingement.
3. **Modulating factors**
   a. **Exercise.** Pain that worsens with exercise, especially walking, suggests osteoarthritis or spinal stenosis, whereas morning stiffness and improvement with exercise suggest a seronegative spondyloarthropathy.
   b. **Valsalva maneuvers.** Radicular pain worsened by coughing or sneezing suggests nerve root impingement.

C. **Neurologic symptoms.** The presence of neurologic symptoms should be specifically sought in patients with low back pain. Their presence not only can help delineate the site of the abnormality but also may prompt more rapid intervention.
1. **Weakness, numbness, or paresthesias in a dermatomal distribution** suggest nerve root impingement (Table 18-1).
   a. The most common cause of nerve root impingement in persons between ages 20 and 50 is a **herniated nucleus pulposus;** this condition is rare under age 20 because the disk is well hydrated and resilient.
   b. Radicular symptoms in persons over age 60 are more likely to be secondary to **spinal stenosis** resulting from degenerative arthritis.

Table 18-1. Signs and symptoms of common disk lesions

Site	Pain	Sensory findings	Motor weakness	Reflexes
L3-4	Anterolateral thigh, medial knee	Anterolateral thigh	Knee extensors	Patellar decreased
L4-5	Posterior thigh, lateral calf, dorsum of foot, great toe	Posterolateral calf, dorsum of foot, web of great toe	Ankle dorsiflexors, extensor of great toe	No specific reflex change
L5-S1	Buttock, posterior, thigh, calf, heel, ball of foot, lateral toes	Buttock, posterior thigh, calf, lateral foot or lateral two toes	Normal or weak plantar flexors of ankle	Achilles decreased

L3-4 disk affects the L-4 nerve root.
L4-5 disk affects the L-5 nerve root.
L5-S1 disk affects the S-1 nerve root.

c. Be aware that neoplasm or infection that causes expansion or dislocation of any of the elements of the spinal cord can likewise lead to radiculopathy.

2. **Bowel or bladder dysfunction** suggests the presence of cauda equina syndrome and should prompt emergent investigation.

III. **Physical examination.** In addition to a general examination, patients with low back pain should be examined for specific abnormalities and undergo provocative maneuvers specifically designed to elicit pain in certain syndromes.

A. **Patient standing**

1. Note alignment of the spine, looking for a pelvic tilt that may indicate paravertebral spasm, for loss of normal lumbar lordosis that could indicate either spasm or ankylosis, and for evidence of structural scoliosis.
2. Evaluate gait, station, and posture.
3. Evaluate the patient's ability to flex, hyperextend, rotate, and tilt the spine.

B. **Patient supine**

1. **Straight leg raising (SLR).** Flex each leg at the hip with the knee extended and record the angle at which pain occurs and whether it causes pain to radiate below the knee.
   a. A true **positive SLR test,** defined as **radicular pain radiating below the knee,** is a sensitive indicator of nerve root impingement and should be confirmed by extending the knee while the patient is sitting to eliminate malingering.
   b. A **crossed SLR test** (radicular pain contralateral to the leg being raised) is highly predictive of nerve root compromise.
2. Evaluate hip and knee range of motion to eliminate these areas as a source of pain.
3. Carry out thorough neurologic (see Table 18-1) and vascular examinations.

C. **Patient prone**

1. Look for evidence of sciatic notch tenderness, sometimes seen in sciatica.
2. Results of the femoral stretch test (extending the hip) may be positive in L-4 radiculopathy.
3. Palpate bony structures, especially vertebral bodies, for localized tenderness, and examine for presence of trigger points, not only in the low back but also in other areas of the body.

IV. **Diagnostic studies**

A. **Imaging studies.** These studies are not performed until the patient fails a trial of conservative therapy or unless neurologic or constitutional symptoms are present. Because all of these studies have a high incidence of false-positive results, it is imperative that the history and physical examination correlate with the detected abnormality.

1. **Plain films** should be taken as an **initial study** in the evaluation of low back pain.
   a. Anteroposterior, lateral, and cone-down views of the lower two interspaces are standard; oblique views will identify subtle spondylolysis but are not routinely necessary.
   b. Flexion and extension views may be obtained to document instability.
2. **Bone scintigraphy (bone scan)** is useful as a screening study when malignancy (other than multiple myeloma) or infection is suspected.
3. **Diskography** is performed by injecting dye into the disk space. The incidence of false-positives is high unless symptoms are reproduced during diskogram injection. It is performed primarily when the results of other studies are negative or equivocal.
4. **Computed tomography (CT).** When used without intradural contrast, CT is the study of choice for delineating the bony structures of the spine (e.g., spinal stenosis). With the addition of intrathecal metrizamide, the sensitivity for detecting neural involvement is enhanced. Pitfalls are that CT does not detect intraspinal pathology (e.g., tumors) and that the rate of false-positives is high in certain populations, especially older patients.

5. **Myelography** outlines the dural theca and its contents after injection of a contrast medium into the dural sac. This is a good study to delineate neural compression (it remains the study of choice when metal hardware is present or when arachnoiditis is a consideration) and is still required by many surgeons contemplating intervention. However, myelography is slowly falling from favor because of its side effects and because of improvements in MRI and CT.
6. **Magnetic resonance imaging (MRI)** is the newest diagnostic modality for the spine. The newer scanners have excellent resolution and can visualize both bony and soft-tissue structures well. MRI is now the study of choice for imaging intraspinal pathology (e.g., tumors). The principal problem with MRI is the high rate of false-positive examinations; up to 30% of asymptomatic persons will have significant abnormalities on this study.
7. **Electrodiagnostic testing.** Electromyography and nerve conduction studies are sometimes useful in the evaluation of low back pain. With acute nerve entrapment, results of these studies may be normal, but in chronic cases, they are often abnormal and can be used to corroborate findings from imaging studies and so help to eliminate false-positive results.

B. Radiologic signs

1. **Degenerative disk disease.** Radiographic abnormalities correlate poorly with symptoms.
   - **a. Narrowing** of the intervertebral disk.
   - **b. "Vacuum phenomenon."** Radiolucency in the disk space.
   - **c.** Traction osteophytes.
2. **Osteoarthritis**
   - **a.** Osteophyte formation.
   - **b.** Facet joint destruction.
   - **c.** Spinal stenosis.
   - **d.** Acquired spondylolisthesis (see section **3.b**).
3. **Congenital and developmental defects.** Many are asymptomatic and are incidental findings detected on plain radiographs.
   - **a.** Spondylolysis (defect in pars interarticularis) is located in the "neck of the Scotty dog" on oblique views.
   - **b.** Spondylolisthesis is slippage of one vertebral body on another. It can be a consequence of spondylolysis or acquired conditions.
   - **c.** Transitional vertebrae, with lumbarization of S-1 or sacralization of L-5.
   - **d.** Schmorl's nodes are defects in the vertebral end plates that allow vertical disk herniation.
   - **e.** Scoliosis or kyphosis.
4. **Seronegative spondyloarthropathies** (ankylosing spondylitis, Reiter's syndrome, psoriatic arthritis, inflammatory bowel disease).
   - **a. Erosions or sclerosis of the sacroiliac joints** are best seen in a Ferguson view of the pelvis, a special view that allows better visualization of the entire length of the joint.
   - **b. Syndesmophytes.** Calcification of ligamentous structures leads to bridging of adjacent vertebral bodies.
5. **Neoplasm**
   - **a.** Destruction of vertebral body.
   - **b.** Loss of outline of pedicle on anteroposterior films.
   - **c.** Pathologic fracture.
6. **Infection** should be suspected when destruction of adjacent vertebral end plates is present or bony destruction is accompanied by constitutional symptoms.
7. **Miscellaneous**
   - **a. Osteoporosis.** Loss in mineralization, compression fractures with characteristic anterior wedging, "fish mouth" appearance to intervertebral spaces.
   - **b.** Metabolic bone disease.
   - **c.** Sickle cell disease.

C. Laboratory studies should be performed as indicated by the history and physical examination, age of patient, and chronicity of symptoms.

1. The erythrocyte sedimentation rate and C-reactive protein reflect acute-phase reactants and will usually be elevated in infection, inflammatory joint disease, and metastatic malignancies.
2. Determinations of calcium, phosphorus, and alkaline phosphatase levels screen for metabolic bone diseases.
3. Serum and urine protein immunoelectrophoreses should be performed if multiple myeloma is suspected.

V. Treatment. Because more than 90% of cases of low back pain are self-limited and resolve spontaneously, any treatment algorithm must account for this and avoid laboratory or imaging studies unless constitutional symptoms, weakness, or neurologic dysfunction suggests an urgent problem.

A. Acute treatment

1. **Bed rest.** The exact length of bed rest has yet to be established, but recent studies suggest that 2 to 3 days may be adequate for most patients who have no neurologic deficit, slightly longer if a deficit is present. Bed rest for longer than 1 week should generally be avoided because muscle weakness quickly develops.
2. **Spinal traction.** Although still used frequently, its only therapeutic value is to enforce bed rest, as the amount of traction that must be applied actually to affect pressure within disks is excessive.
3. **Pharmacologic treatment**
   - a. **Pain control.** Antiinflammatory drugs (e.g., 400 to 800 mg of ibuprofen four times daily or 250 to 500 mg of naproxen twice daily) or analgesics (325 to 650 mg of acetominophen q4h) as needed to control pain. Narcotics should be used with caution if at all.
   - b. **Muscle relaxants.** The mechanism of action of these drugs is not entirely clear, but they are helpful in some patients with acute low back pain. Examples include cyclobenzaprine (10 mg q6h), methocarbamol, and chlorzoxazone. Benzodiazepines such as diazepam may also be used for a limited period (long-term use can decrease the pain threshold).
4. **Physical measures**
   - a. Moist heat.
   - b. Massage, ultrasound.
   - c. The use of bracing for any extended period is ill-advised, as it may lead to muscle weakness.

B. Failure of conservative therapy as outlined above, when followed for 4 to 6 weeks, is generally considered an indication to initiate a diagnostic workup and consider surgical intervention. The workup should include plain radiographs of the lumbosacral spine in addition to any other imaging or laboratory studies deemed necessary based on the history and physical examination (see section **IV**).

C. Other treatment modalities

1. **Injection of trigger points** may be useful if the patient exhibits only a few specific "trigger points" and local pressure elicits pain in that area or is referred to another area (myofascial pain). Inject these areas with a corticosteroid and local anesthetic (e.g., 40 mg of methylprednisolone and 1 mL of 1% lidocaine without epinephrine).
2. **Facet block.** The true incidence of pain originating from facet joints is controversial, but injection of these joints in patients demonstrating facet abnormalities on imaging studies should certainly be considered before surgery is contemplated. In some centers, if this initial injection is successful in reducing pain, a more permanent surgical procedure such as rhizotomy may be performed.
3. **Transcutaneous electrical nerve stimulator (TENS) therapy** is helpful in some cases.
4. **Physical therapy.** Physical therapists who specialize in back problems (e.g., those involved in "back-hardening" programs) can make a major contribution to therapeutic success.

D. Invasive intervention should be contemplated when there is a failure of conservative therapy *and* there is a radiographically demonstrable anatomic defect that could explain the pain, or when malignancy or infection cannot be excluded with noninvasive techniques. The timing of surgery is critical; it should rarely be performed before 2 months of conservative therapy (except in circumstances noted above that require urgent intervention, such as persistent or worsening neurologic deficit). However, a delay of more than 6 months can lead to the development of a chronic pain syndrome and decrease the likelihood of a good surgical outcome. Types of surgical intervention include the following:

1. **Laminectomy or hemilaminectomy.** Removal of all or part of the lamina while preserving the apophyseal joints, or in the case of spinal stenosis, trimming the joints to decompress the neural tissues.
2. **Laminotomy or hemilaminotomy.** An opening is created in the lamina without its being totally removed.
3. **Diskectomy.** Removal of the nucleus pulposus from the intervertebral space and from any other ectopic location in the epidural space. This can be accomplished in one of the following ways:
   - **a.** Standard surgical approach.
   - **b.** Fiberoptic scope.
4. **Spinal fusion.** This is performed when instability is present, usually in combination with one of the above operations.

E. Chronic pain arises from a failure of standard therapy, and patients with this problem are a very difficult group to treat. A subset of this group has fibromyalgia, and these patients are identified by poor sleep, fatigue, and widespread pain and tender points. They may respond well to low doses of tricyclic antidepressants at bedtime (e.g., begin 10 mg of amitriptyline nightly, and escalate the dose by 10 mg once weekly to 50 to 70 mg nightly). In general, however, these patients are best managed by a multidisciplinary approach that combines psychosocial evaluation with one or more of the modalities discussed above.

VI. Rehabilitation and exercise. Flexibility and strengthening exercise is frequently recommended for patients with low back pain, although objective data supporting benefits are sparse. Nonetheless, there are some basic principles regarding rehabilitation in these patients that should be followed. Physical therapists are helpful in instructing patients in these programs.

A. Postsurgical patients

1. Ambulation is encouraged early, and prolonged sitting is avoided.
2. Lifting should be avoided.

B. Exercises for low back pain (see Chapter 56) should not be initiated until the acute phase of recovery has been completed and the patient can move freely without pain (approximately 2 weeks). Patients should be instructed to begin with only three to five repetitions of each exercise and proceed slowly.

1. **Pelvic tilt.** Buttocks are tightened, and the lumbar spine is flattened isometrically.
2. **Modified sit-ups.** With the patient supine, knees bent and arms at the side, the head and shoulders are lifted off the ground and held for 5 seconds.
3. **Knee-chest stretch.** Both knees are brought to the chest and held with the arms for 5 seconds; then, one at a time, the knees are extended and the legs are slowly brought to the ground.
4. **Back extension.** While lying prone with the arms at the sides, lift the chin and shoulders upward and hold for 5 seconds. Then, in the same position, lift one leg at a time upward and hold for 5 seconds.

C. Other recommendations

1. **Weight reduction** for obese patients.
2. **Aerobic fitness should be increased,** whenever possible, with walking, swimming, or other low-impact activities. Before one of these activities is performed, the patient should do **stretching** exercises to warm up properly.
3. **Life-style modifications**
   - **a. Proper lifting techniques.** While lifting, the knees should be flexed and the back straight. Twisting while lifting should be avoided.

b. A **firm mattress** should be used.
c. Vocational training may be helpful.

Bibliography

Borenstein DG, Wiesel SW. *Low back pain medical diagnosis and comprehensive management.* Philadelphia: WB Saunders, 1995.
Frymoyer JW. Back pain and sciatica. *N Engl J Med* 1988;318(5):281.
Kelsey JL, Golden AL, Mundt DJ. Low back pain/prolapsed lumbar intervertebral disk. *Rheum Dis Clin North Am* 1990;16(3):699.
Porter RW. Mechanical disorders of the lumbar spine. *Ann Med* 1989;21(5):361.

19. HIP PAIN

Thomas P. Sculco and Paul Lombardi

I. Etiology. The bone and soft-tissue structures around the hip joint, thigh, and low back should be considered in evaluating the patient's symptoms.

A. Hip joint

1. Proximal femur and acetabulum.
2. Articular surfaces.
3. Synovium.

B. Periarticular soft tissues

1. **Bursae.** Greater trochanteric, iliopsoas, ischial.
2. **Tendons.** Hip abductor, adductor, internal-external rotators, extensors, flexors, and hamstrings.
3. **Acetabular labrum.** Soft-tissue rim surrounding the acetabulum.
4. **Herniae.** Inguinal, femoral.

C. Referred pain

1. **Lumbosacral.** L-1 and L-2 dermatomes traverse the proximal thigh.
2. **Visceral.** Ovarian and prostate disorders.
3. **Knee symptoms.** Obturator nerve supplies sensory innervation to the hip and knee. Hip pathology can present as knee pain.

II. History. Patients with hip pain usually complain of limitation of hip motion and a painful limp. Careful history taking may reveal childhood hip disorders such as Legg-Calvé-Perthes disease, slipped capital femoral epiphysis, developmental dysplasia of the hip, and septic arthritis. Concomitant disorders such as osteoarthritis, rheumatoid arthritis (RA), malignancy, or low back pain may provide insight into the etiology of the hip pain. A history of alcohol or steroid use is pertinent in patients suspected of having osteonecrosis. Response to prior therapies, including physical therapy, antiinflammatory medications, modification of activity, or use of assistive devices, helps one to assess the severity of the pain.

A. Duration and location of pain

1. Pain of short duration is usually posttraumatic or inflammatory.
2. Pain that is chronic and progressive may indicate mechanical joint incongruity related to an underlying arthritis. The pain of osteoarthritis is usually alleviated with rest. Constant hip pain is characteristic of an inflammatory or neoplastic process. The presence of morning stiffness and its duration are important aspects of RA.
3. Groin pain with radiation into the buttock indicates hip joint dysfunction. Pure buttock or back pain without a groin component is usually back in origin. When patients say their hip hurts, they mostly point to the buttock. Lateral hip pain with radiation to the lateral thigh may be related to greater trochanteric bursitis or abductor tendinitis. Discomfort over the anterior superior iliac spine extending down the anterior thigh is associated with meralgia paresthetica (inflammation of the lateral femoral cutaneous nerve).
4. Buttock pain may be related to ischial tuberosity bursitis or spinal disorders such as spinal stenosis, ruptured intervertebral disk, and instability.

B. Relation of pain to activity

1. Pain from the hip joint and surrounding soft tissues is usually aggravated by weight bearing and relieved by rest.
2. Patients will usually describe a specific position of the limb that exacerbates or relieves their symptoms.

C. Decreased function. Patients complain of progressive decrease in maximum walking distance and exercise tolerance. Ability to perform activities of daily living is decreased. These decreases can be quantified with functional assessment scores such as WOMAC, the Harris Hip Score, and SF-36.

III. Physical examination

A. Gait. Observe the patient entering the examination room, and note the presence of a limp or expressions of pain.

1. **Abductor lurch (Trendelenberg gait).** The patient shifts the center of gravity over the affected limb during the stance phase of gait to unload weakened abductors and avoid pain production.
2. **Coxalgic gait.** The patient quickly unloads the painful leg while bearing weight. Decreased stance phase of gait and stride length on the affected side will be seen.
3. **Stiff hip gait.** Patient will walk by rotating the pelvis and swinging the legs in a circular fashion.

B. Patient standing

1. Measure unequal leg lengths by balancing the pelvis with calibrated blocks, if necessary. Note a fixed pelvic obliquity if present.
2. Evaluate the spine for scoliosis or kyphosis.
3. Trendelenburg's sign. While bearing weight with one leg on the affected side, the patient will drop the opposite side of the pelvis because the hip abductor, which normally elevates the pelvis, is weakened. This may take 30 to 45 seconds to become apparent.

C. Patient supine

1. Record active and passive range of motion, and compare with values of the opposite side.
   - **a.** Note flexion, extension, abduction, adduction, and internal-external rotation in both flexion and extension. Internal rotation is usually most affected in osteoarthritis.
   - **b.** Snapping hip (coxa sultans) can be elicited with range of motion (see section **V**).
   - **c.** Thomas test for hip flexion contracture. Flex the contralateral knee and hip; extend the affected hip while keeping the lower back flat on the examination table. Note the amount of affected hip flexion present against the horizontal.
   - **d.** Patrick's test for sacroiliac joint symptoms. While the patient is supine, place the affected side in a figure 4 position with knee flexed and ankle on opposite knee. Apply pressure to the knee. Positive result if significant pain is present in the contralateral sacroiliac joint.
   - **e.** Hip apprehension test for acetabular labrum pathology. Flex, adduct, and internally rotate the affected limb while looking for pain.
2. Palpate the anterior hip capsule by applying pressure just inferior to the inguinal ligament over the femoral triangle, and evaluate the degree of tenderness.
3. Palpate the groin in supine and standing positions, searching for femoral or inguinal herniae.
4. Measure thigh circumference bilaterally to assess muscle atrophy.
5. Measure leg lengths with a tape measure, recording from umbilicus to medial malleolus and from anterior superior iliac spine to medial malleolus. Note whether a fixed pelvic obliquity is present.
6. Perform a complete neurovascular examination.
7. Examine the knee and ankle. Patients with RA will often present with polyarticular involvement.

D. Patient lying on unaffected side

1. Palpate the greater trochanteric area for bursal tenderness.
2. Assess abductor muscle power.
3. Ober's test for iliotibial band tightness. With the patient in the lateral position, extend the affected hip and attempt adduction. If you are unable to do this, the test result is positive.

E. Patient lying prone

1. Palpate the lumbosacral area to evaluate the low back as a potential source of pain.
2. Evaluate hip extensor power.

3. Palpate the sciatic notch for tenderness.
4. Ely's test for hamstring tightness. With the patient prone, extend the knees until the buttocks are raised involuntarily. Positive result if this happens.

IV. Laboratory and radiographic studies

A. Radiographs should include an anteroposterior view of the pelvis, and anteroposterior and lateral views of the affected hip. Lumbosacral films should be obtained if spinal pathology is present. Current films should be compared with prior ones, if available, to look for progression of disease. In osteoarthritis, patients' symptoms may often not correlate with the degree of radiographic involvement of the affected hip.

1. Degenerative changes in the hip joint, with osteophytes, subchondral sclerosis, and cyst formation, is consistent with osteoarthritis.
2. Periarticular osteoporosis and global joint space narrowing is seen in RA. Osteophytes are not typically present.
3. In cases of bone involvement by a neoplastic process, tissue erosion of 50% can occur before being detected on radiographs.
4. Computed tomography (CT) may be used to visualize complex acetabular pathology, and to determine the degree of bone involvement in a neoplastic or fracture process.
5. Magnetic resonance imaging (MRI) is the most sensitive tool for diagnosing occult hip fractures and osteonecrosis.

B. Laboratory studies. Directed by physical examination and history.

1. A complete blood cell count with differential, measurements of erythrocyte sedimentation rate or C-reactive protein, and hip aspiration should be performed if infection is suspected.
2. Serum and urine immunoelectrophoreses should be performed to rule out multiple myeloma in patients with bone pain in the setting of anemia and an elevated ESR.

V. Differential diagnosis

A. Hip joint

1. Acetabulum and proximal femur

a. **Fractures** may occur in the femoral neck or intertrochanteric region. Fractures may also occur to the acetabulum after trauma. Stress fractures of the femoral neck or acetabulum, particularly in runners and patients with osteoporosis, may be seen.

b. **Primary or metastatic tumors** may infiltrate the femoral head and acetabulum, and pathologic fractures may occur. The most common tumors to metastasize to bone are breast, lung, prostate, kidney, and thyroid. The most common primary tumor of bone is multiple myeloma.

c. **Osteonecrosis of the femoral head** with or without collapse may produce severe hip pain, especially in alcoholics, patients taking steroid preparations and steroid-treated patients with systemic lupus.

2. Articulating surfaces

a. Osteoarthritis, RA, ankylosing spondylitis, or septic arthritis may cause hyaline cartilage destruction with resultant hip joint incongruity and pain.

b. Incongruity of the femoral head and subsequent arthritis can be seen in osteonecrosis with segmental collapse, or in the adult manifestations of pediatric hip disorders such as Legg-Calvé-Perthes disease, slipped capital femoral epiphysis, and developmental dysplasia of the hip.

3. Synovium

a. **Synovitis of the hip joint** may result from RA, seronegative spondyloarthropathies such as ankylosing spondylitis, viral infections, and hemophilia.

b. **Tuberculosis** may lead to a proliferative synovitis and severe joint destruction. Hip aspiration, acid-fast stain, and histologic assessment culture confirm the diagnosis. **Pigmented villonodular synovitis** may lead to cyst formation in the femoral neck or joint destruction. The radiographic changes seen in these two conditions are present on both sides of the joint.

c. **Synoviochondromatosis** is a benign cartilage tumor of the synovium that usually presents with pain and a decreased range of motion.

d. **Pigmented villonodular synovitis** is a synovial proliferation in the hip joint characterized histologically by hemosiderin-stained synovium and giant cells.

B. Periarticular soft tissues

1. Bursae

a. Greater trochanteric bursitis is common and produces acute pain over the lateral thigh, which usually radiates distally. Swelling and pain with weight bearing are often present, and a limp may result. Pain is present when the patient is lying on the affected side and often awakens the patient from sleep.

b. Iliopsoas bursitis is uncommon. It may communicate with the hip joint in 15% of patients.

2. Tendons and fascia

a. **Hamstring, adductor, abductor, and rotator tendons** may become inflamed at their insertions into bone. Piriformis syndrome is diagnosed by pain in the sciatic notch with palpation and resisted external rotation.

b. The **fascia lata** is quite taut as it passes over the greater trochanter and may produce a snapping sensation and pain, particularly on hip flexion and adduction. Other causes of a "snapping hip" (coxa sultans) include a tight iliopsoas tendon and hypertrophic fovea.

3. Herniae

a. **Inguinal herniae,** if symptomatic, may produce severe groin pain and limitation of hip motion.

b. **Femoral herniae** with prolapse may produce severe groin pain and limping. However, pain is intermittent until incarceration occurs.

4. Referred pain

a. **Lumbosacral.** Osteoarthritis involving the lumbosacral apophyseal joints can produce buttock pain. Radicular pain from nerve root irritation may be manifested in the lateral thigh or groin. Disk herniations involving L1-2 and L2-3 may produce these symptoms. Pott's disease, tuberculous infection of the intervertebral disks and vertebral bodies, may spread to the hip joint via the psoas muscle insertions along the anterior portion of the lumbar spine.

b. **Visceral origin**

(1) Renal colic can radiate to the groin. Ovarian or prostate disorders may mimic hip pathology.

(2) Vascular occlusive disease of the aorta can produce buttock pain; femoral vein phlebitis can present with thigh and groin pain.

VI. Therapy. (For therapy of specific disease entities, see the appropriate chapters.)

A. Rest

1. **Joint rest** may be accomplished by unloading the affected hip with various forms of external support.

a. **Cane.** It should be held in the contralateral hand to assist weakened abductors and to unload the hip. Forearm crutches or axillary crutches can be used in more severe disease or bilateral involvement.

B. Compresses

1. If an acute inflammatory condition involves a tendon or bursa, ice compresses are useful.

2. For chronic pain, moist heat improves local blood supply and relaxes spastic musculature.

C. Medications

1. **Antiinflammatory medications** are useful for arthritic problems involving the hip joint. Nonsteroidal antiinflammatory drugs such as ibuprofen 600 mg to 800 mg three times daily can be helpful. These medications are contraindicated in patients taking anticoagulants or who have peptic ulcer or renal disease. Cox-2 specific antiinflammatory agents may offer relief to patients who are currently unable to take traditional NSAIDs.

2. **Analgesics.** Darvocet-N 100 (100 mg of propoxyphene napsylate and 650 mg of acetaminophen) may be used in conjunction with an antiinflammatory drug. The dosage is one to two tablets q4h as needed.
3. **Soft-tissue injections.** For bursitis or tendinitis, local injection with 40 mg of methylprednisolone acetate (Depo-Medrol) and 3 to 5 mL of 1% lidocaine is effective. If no improvement occurs after one injection, two more weekly injections may be given.

D. Exercises

1. Attempts should be made to maintain passive and active hip motion without aggravating the underlying pain.
2. Gentle isometric exercises for the quadriceps and hamstrings and antigravity exercises as tolerated for hip flexors, extensors, abductors, adductors, and rotators are recommended. See Chapter 56 for specific exercise prescriptions. Weight reduction is an important aspect of the treatment of hip disorders. The prognosis in many hip disorders is guarded if aggravating factors such as obesity are not addressed. Ideal patient weights are listed in Appendix C.

20. KNEE PAIN

Norman A. Johanson and Paul Pellicci

I. Anatomy

A. Joints. There are three articulations in the knee, referred to as compartments. They can be affected separately or together as part of a single process.

1. Patellofemoral compartment.
2. Medial tibiofemoral compartment.
3. Lateral tibiofemoral compartment.

B. Ligaments. The knee ligaments are specially designed to accommodate a wide range of motion and flexibility while providing essential stability for weight bearing.

1. Medial collateral ligament.
2. Lateral collateral ligament.
3. Anterior cruciate ligament.
4. Posterior cruciate ligament.

C. Menisci are crescent-shaped fibrocartilaginous structures that are peripherally situated in the medial and lateral tibiofemoral compartments. They share in weight bearing and augment the stability of the knee.

D. Periarticular structures. Several musculotendinous structures pass across the knee to insert at or near the joint. Injury or inflammation of any of these structures can result in knee pain.

1. Quadriceps mechanism (quadriceps tendon, patellar tendon).
2. Pes anserine tendons (sartorius, gracilis, semitendinosus).
3. Semimembranosus.
4. Biceps femoris.
5. Iliotibial band.
6. Popliteus.
7. Gastrocnemius (medial and lateral heads).

II. Causes of knee pain

A. Traumatic. The mechanism of injury is important in formulating a differential diagnosis; however, components of several mechanisms may be present in a given injury.

1. **Hyperextension** (anterior cruciate tear).
2. **Varus** (lateral collateral ligament tear, anterior cruciate tear).
3. **Valgus** (medial collateral ligament tear, anterior cruciate tear).
4. **Torsion** (meniscal tears).
5. Axial impact on femur and posterior displacement of tibia (dashboard injury), patellar fracture, posterior cruciate ligament tear, femoral shaft fracture, fracture dislocation of hip.

B. Spontaneous

1. **Inflammatory** (synovitis, tendinitis).
2. **Vascular disorder** (osteonecrosis, sickle cell crisis).
3. **Degenerative** (meniscal tear, articular erosion).
4. **Neoplastic** (primary or metastatic bone tumors near the knee; soft-tissue tumors around the knee).
5. **Referred pain** from hip or spine disorder.

III. Common presenting symptoms associated with knee pain

A. Swelling. Enlargement of the knee with loss of normal contour.

B. Locking or severe stiffness (meniscal tear, chondromalacia patellae).

C. Giving way or buckling (anterior cruciate tear or patellofemoral disorder).

D. Clicking or crackling sound in the knee (meniscal tear or chondromalacia patellae).

E. Audible pop at the time of knee injury (cruciate or meniscal tear).

IV. Physical examination

A. Observation

1. **Contour** of the knee.
2. **Alignment** of the knee while patient is standing (varus, valgus, flexed, or hyperextended).
3. **Gait.**

B. Palpation

1. **Effusion.** Fluid in the knee may be demonstrated by sweeping the hand distally to empty the suprapatellar pouch. Medial and lateral bulging of the capsule can be felt and sometimes seen (distinguish from synovial thickening).
2. **Popliteal fullness** is suggestive of Baker's cyst.
3. **Joint line tenderness** exacerbated by tibial rotation (Steinmann test) is suggestive of meniscal tear.
4. **Tenderness on patellofemoral compression** with the knee slightly flexed is suggestive of chondromalacia patellae.

C. Range of motion (active and passive flexion and extension, fixed flexion deformities)

1. Note presence of **patellofemoral crepitus** throughout the range of motion.
2. **McMurray test.** With the knee at first in full flexion, the tibia is rotated internally and externally while the knee is brought slowly into extension. A palpable jumping at the joint line sometimes accompanied by an audible click is suggestive of a meniscal tear.

D. Strength

1. **Thigh circumferences** are measured and compared (10 cm above patella).
2. **Quadriceps** strength. Note whether an apparent weakness is secondary to pain, stiffness, or actual muscle dysfunction. Note the presence of thigh atrophy.
3. **Hamstring** strength.

E. Stability

1. **Varus and valgus** stability is best demonstrated by cradling the knee with one hand and, with the knee in extension, applying a medial or lateral knee stress. Any more than a jog of motion is suggestive of medial or lateral collateral ligament laxity.
2. The **anterior and posterior cruciate ligaments** are tested with the knee in flexion and extension. While sitting on the patient's foot with the knee flexed to 90 degrees, the examiner applies anterior and posterior displacement force on the proximal tibia. A firm end point should be present in each direction (anterior drawer test). With the knee in extension, the tibia is lifted anteriorly on the femur (Lachman test). Minimal excursion and a firm end point should be noted.

V. Diagnostic tests

A. Radiography should be performed while the patient is standing (anteroposterior and lateral views) to demonstrate joint space narrowing. Tangential patellar views (Merchant views) are obtained to assess the patellofemoral compartment. A tunnel view is obtained to assess the contour of the intercondylar notch.

B. Screening blood tests such as complete blood cell count and measurement of differential, erythrocyte sedimentation rate, biochemistry profile, and rheumatoid factor should be performed if systemic disease is suspected.

C. Aspiration of synovial fluid for analysis of cells and crystals is helpful in rheumatoid arthritis, gout, and pseudogout. Culture and sensitivity are definitive in infectious arthritis.

D. Arthrogram is helpful to confirm meniscal and cruciate tears and to demonstrate a popliteal cyst or nodular synovitis. This test has generally been supplanted by the MRI.

E. Bone scan is helpful in demonstrating early osteonecrosis (increased or decreased uptake in subchondral bone) when radiographic findings are still normal or when there is the presence of a stress fracture. It can also define the diffuse increased uptake in RA or medial uptake in OA.

F. **Magnetic resonance imaging (MRI)** has become the imaging procedure of choice for evaluating torn menisci and ligaments.

VI. **Principles of treatment**

A. **Acute phase**

1. **Rest** through decreased activity and weight bearing (crutches, cane if needed).
2. **Antiinflammatory medications.**
3. **Therapeutic aspiration of synovial fluid** (or blood in traumatic effusion) often relieves pain. This can be supplemented by injection of a local anesthetic into the joint.
4. **Injection of a steroid preparation** into the knee is recommended for older patients with arthritic changes on radiography or in patients with inflammatory joint disease in whom infection is not present.

B. **Convalescent phase**

1. **Quadriceps and hamstring exercises** are frequently used for many knee disorders. Straight leg raising without weights is helpful in arthritis patients because it minimizes patellofemoral stress. Exercises with weights are more effective in rehabilitation after athletic injuries.
2. **Progressive activities** (e.g., swimming and bicycle riding) preserve knee motion and strength without excessive impact loading.
3. **Braces** are used according to the condition being treated (usually not effective in arthritis, but beneficial in chondromalacia patellae and mild ligament injuries).

VII. **Common causes of knee pain**

A. **Chondromalacia patellae** is a spectrum of knee disorders resulting from excessive pressure on the patellar cartilage and the subsequent softening and fibrillation of the articular surface. Increased pressure may be caused by an abnormality of patellar tracking during knee motion. Associated conditions include femoral anteversion, external tibial torsion, valgus knee alignment, a hypoplastic high-riding patella, or foot pronation. Excessive malalignment may cause subluxation or dislocation of the patella.

1. **History**
   a. **Anterior knee pain** is felt during climbing or descending stairs, sitting for long periods of time, or squatting.
   b. There may be a history of **direct trauma** to the patella (dashboard injury).
   c. Sports that may cause overloading of the patellofemoral joint (jogging, basketball, gymnastics, dancing) are associated with chondromalacia.
2. **Physical examination**
   a. **Mild peripatellar swelling** may be present, but joint effusion is rare.
   b. **Crepitus of the patellofemoral joint** is usually palpable during range of motion. Full flexion may elicit an increase in pain.
   c. In cases of **patellar malalignment or recurrent subluxation/dislocation,** the patella may exhibit mediolateral hypermobility, and when the patella is displaced laterally, significant apprehension may be elicited.
3. **Radiographic findings**
   a. **Tangential view** of the patella (Merchant view) may demonstrate lateral displacement or tilt of the patella. Narrowing of the joint space is suggestive of patellofemoral arthritis.
   b. **Lateral view** of the knee may demonstrate a high-riding patella (patella alta), which has been associated with patellofemoral pain. Patella alta is defined as a ratio of the length of the patellar tendon to the length of the patella greater than 1.2 : 1.0.
4. **Differential diagnosis.** Chondromalacia patellae must be distinguished from **meniscal tears.** Meniscal tears are more frequently associated with a specific traumatic event and even more likely to result in a knee effusion, locking, and a reduction of range of knee motion. Meniscal tears may be ruled out by an arthrogram, MRI, or arthroscopic evaluation.
5. **Treatment**
   a. Temporarily discontinue or reduce those activities that exacerbate pain.

b. **Quadriceps muscle strengthening** is the most important objective. This is accomplished through quadriceps exercises in the range of 90 to 30 degrees or through straight leg raising.
c. In some cases, **nonsteroidal antiinflammatory medications** are necessary to control acute pain in chondromalacia. Ibuprofen in a dosage of 600 mg four times daily may be effective.

B. **Meniscal tears.** Traumatic tears of the medial and lateral menisci are common causes of knee pain, particularly in athletic persons. The medial meniscus is by far the most frequently affected.

1. **History**
   a. A **twisting injury** is often the cause of a meniscal tear.
   b. **Swelling** of varying severity is often reported.
   c. Knee **stiffness, pain, and limitation of motion** are frequent complaints. A history of locking is less common.
2. **Physical examination**
   a. Swelling and knee effusion are frequently present.
   b. Tenderness is present along the medial or lateral joint line.
   c. Range of motion may be limited in extension and flexion, or the knee may be locked in one position.
   d. Result of the McMurray test or Steinmann test (tibial rotation) is often positive with meniscal tears.
3. **Diagnostic studies**
   a. **Radiographic findings** in the knee are usually normal except for the demonstration of a knee effusion.
   b. **Arthrography or MRI** will demonstrate meniscal tears in most cases.
   c. **Arthroscopy** is an important therapeutic modality for meniscal tears.
4. **Differential diagnosis**
   a. **Medial collateral ligament sprains** may produce medial joint line pain and tenderness with a limp and an effusion. Locking is not present. Arthrography is negative or demonstrates leakage of dye in the area of the ligament injury. MRI is diagnostic.
   b. **Acute chondromalacia patellae** may produce anteromedial pain. An effusion is rarely present, and locking is also very uncommon. Findings on arthrogram or MRI are negative.
   c. **A pes anserine bursitis** presents with pain and tenderness over the proximal medial tibia just below the joint line without effusion, limitation of motion, or locking. Direct tenderness is present over the bursa, and the arthrographic or MRI findings are negative.
   d. **Medial compartment tibiofemoral osteoarthritis** may produce an effusion with medial joint line pain, tenderness, and a limp. Radiography will demonstrate sclerosis and joint space narrowing in the medial aspect of the knee joint.
5. **Treatment.** In patients with a locked knee or recurrent symptoms from a torn medial meniscus, **surgical removal** is the treatment of choice. If the tear is longitudinal, simple excision of the injured segment may be performed. Arthroscopic techniques are the preferred method of treatment.

C. **Tibial tubercle apophysitis (Osgood-Schlatter disease)** occurs primarily in adolescents and presents as pain located at the insertion of the patellar tendon into the tibial tubercle. Some investigators believe the syndrome represents an injury to the apophysis that is similar to mild avulsion.

1. **Physical examination.** There is localized pain on palpation of the tubercle.
2. **Radiography** often shows a displaced ossicle of bone anterior to the tubercle within the tendinous insertion.
3. **Treatment.** The pain usually disappears when the ossicle fuses to the underlying tibia. Until that time, the patient's activity level must be monitored. Depending on the severity of the pain, some or all athletic activity must be discontinued. A cylinder cast for 4 to 6 weeks may be necessary in resistant cases. Ibuprofen 600 mg three times per day or other NSAIDs may be used during the acute phase.

21. ANKLE AND FOOT PAIN

David S. Levine and Gordon A. Brody

I. Anatomy

A. The **joints** of the foot and ankle can be divided into two groups: essential joints, whose motion is required for normal foot function, and nonessential joints, which have little appreciable motion and are largely responsible for providing stability.

1. **Essential joints**
   - **a.** The **tibiotalar (ankle) joint** maintains an axis through the malleoli such that dorsiflexion and external foot rotation are coupled. Similarly, plantar flexion and internal foot rotation are coupled motions. Surrounding ligamentous structures limit inversion or eversion through the ankle joint.
   - **b.** The **talocalcaneal (subtalar) joint** is responsible for hindfoot inversion and eversion. Motion occurs around an axis inclined 15 degrees lateral to the longitudinal axis of the foot. Along with the ankle joint, the subtalar joint forms a "universal" joint enabling the hindfoot to accommodate to uneven ground.
   - **c.** The **talonavicular and calcaneocuboid (transverse tarsal) joints** function to link the mobile hindfoot to the mobile forefoot.
   - **d.** The **metatarsophalangeal (MTP) joints** of the forefoot have significant dorsiflexion and plantar flexion capability, which enables the center of gravity of the body to be propelled forward efficiently in terminal stance phase.
2. Nonessential joints such as the **navicular-cuneiform, intercuneiform,** and **tarsometatarsal** joints have little motion as a consequence of stout ligamentous reinforcement. These joints serve to provide a rigid lever during weight transfer from the hindfoot to the forefoot.

B. Ligaments

1. The **deltoid ligament** is the prime stabilizer of the medial side of the ankle joint. It runs from the medial malleolus to the talus, calcaneus, and navicular. Its deep portion resists lateral translation of the talus within the ankle joint. The superficial portion blends with other capsular and ligamentous structures over the medial hindfoot.
2. The **lateral collateral ligaments** consist of the anterior and posterior talofibular ligaments and the calcaneofibular ligament. As a group, these ligaments are the prime stabilizers of the lateral side of the ankle joint. The anterior talofibular is the most frequently injured ligament, especially during plantar flexion of the foot. With increasing energy or when the foot is in a neutral position or in slight dorsiflexion, the calcaneofibular ligament may also be injured.
3. The **medial talocalcaneonavicular (spring) ligament** has been increasingly noted to be important in supporting the head of the talus and preventing loss of medial longitudinal arch height.
4. The **plantar intertarsal (interosseous) ligaments** stabilize the bones of the midfoot, thereby maintaining their static contribution to the medial longitudinal arch.

C. Muscles. Dorsiflexion of the foot and ankle (tibialis anterior, extensor digitorum longus, extensor hallucis longus, peroneus tertius). Plantar flexion of the foot and ankle (gastrocnemius, soleus). Hindfoot inversion (posterior tibialis, gastrocnemius). Hindfoot eversion (peroneus brevis, peroneus longus). The intrinsic muscles of the foot contribute to the bulk and padding of the sole, help to maintain the architecture of the transverse and longitudinal arches, and influence the alignment of the toes. The toes are flexed and extended by their long flexors and extensors.

D. Fascia. The plantar fascia originates on the posteromedial tubercle of the calcaneus and inserts into the bases of the proximal phalanges via the plantar plate and flexor tendon sheaths. It maintains a static support of the longitudinal arch via a "windlass" mechanism.

E. The **blood supply** of the ankle and foot comes principally from the dorsalis pedis artery (an extension of the anterior tibialis artery), which is palpable between the first and second metatarsal bases on the dorsum of the foot, and the posterior tibialis artery, palpable about one finger's breadth posterior and inferior to the medial malleolus. Communicating branches from the peroneal artery provide an inconsistent anastomosis with the above-named arteries.

F. Innervation of the foot and ankle is from the superficial and deep peroneal nerves, which supply the dorsum of the foot. The medial and lateral plantar nerves provide sensation to the plantar surface of the foot and innervate the intrinsic muscles. The sural nerve provides sensation to the outer border of the heel and the dorsolateral border of the foot. The saphenous nerve, a terminal branch of the femoral nerve, provides sensation to the medial border of the ankle and foot.

II. History

A. Pain

1. Exact localization, radiation.
2. Aggravating, alleviating factors.
3. Associated findings.
4. Acute or insidious onset (traumatic or atraumatic).
5. Intensity.
6. Quality. Radiating pain with an "electric" quality may be consistent with neuroma.

B. Footwear

1. Recent alterations in usual footwear.
2. Attitude toward footwear influences expectations.
3. Barefoot activities associated with increased or decreased symptoms.

C. Past medical history. Numerous conditions, including gout, rheumatoid arthritis (RA), neoplasm, peripheral vascular disease, diabetes mellitus, congenital deformity, and neurologic conditions, can all contribute to foot or ankle dysfunction. Similarly, the altered gait pattern related to foot and ankle dysfunction can contribute to other musculoskeletal complaints, such as low back pain and medial knee pain.

D. Past surgical history. Any prior history of surgical procedures on the foot and ankle should be thoroughly discussed.

III. Physical examination

A. Gait and alignment should be evaluated with the patient in shoes and barefoot.

1. At heel-strike, the hindfoot should assume a valgus attitude, allowing shock absorption through the flexible hindfoot. Weight is transferred forward during foot-flat. At heel-rise, the hindfoot is inverted (by the tibialis posterior muscle). The transverse tarsal joint becomes rigid when the hindfoot is inverted, enabling the body weight to be transferred via the rigid midfoot to the metatarsophalangeal joints preparing for toe-off. The swing phase then completes the gait cycle.
2. An **antalgic gait** involves a shortened stance phase, which signifies a painful limb.
3. A **steppage gait** involves hip and knee flexion to clear the foot during swing phase in the setting of a "drop foot" (e.g., after a peroneal nerve palsy).
4. Observe the **patient from behind.** Physiologic hind foot valgus should be readily apparent. Excessive valgus (as in a flat foot) or hindfoot varus (as in clubfoot sequelae or cavovarus foot) should be noted.
5. Heel-rise should be associated with hindfoot inversion (tibialis posterior).
6. Total limb alignment should be evaluated from the hips to the toes.
7. Rotational deformities such as internal tibial torsion or excessive femoral anteversion are best evaluated with the patient prone.

B. Range of motion should be compared with that of the contralateral extremity. Both active and passive range of motion should be evaluated.

1. **Ankle dorsiflexion** must be examined with the hindfoot in the neutral position. Dorsiflexion with the knee in extension versus flexion should be noted to differentiate tendoachilles from gastrocnemius contracture.
2. The **subtalar joint** is assessed by inverting and everting the heel while stabilizing the tibia.
3. **Forefoot inversion** (supination) and **eversion** (pronation) as well as **abduction** and **adduction** are assessed by holding the heel in the cup of the hand to lock the subtalar joint and grasping the forefoot.
4. **Active and passive motion of the MTP and interphalangeal joints**
   a. **Hammertoes** are lesser toes having a fixed or flexible flexion contracture of the proximal interphalangeal (PIP) joints.
   b. If MTP hyperextension coexists, the term **claw toe** is used.
   c. A **mallet toe** exists with a fixed or flexible flexion contracture of the distal interphalangeal (DIP) joints of the lesser toes.

C. Tenderness. The point of maximal tenderness is of critical importance to establishing a correct diagnosis. Systematically palpate the foot to localize tenderness and evaluate bony and soft-tissue asymmetry.

1. Tenderness over a prominent medial eminence of the hallux MTP joint is commonly seen in hallux valgus.
2. Tenderness over the lateral ankle ligaments is seen commonly after an inversion ankle sprain.
3. Tenderness over the MTP joint of the hallux may be seen in gout and degenerative arthrosis.
4. Metatarsalgia is signified by tenderness along the plantar surfaces of the metatarsal heads.
5. Medial hindfoot or posterolateral hindfoot tenderness is often associated with acute or chronic posterior tibial tendon insufficiency, respectively.

D. Swelling may be nonspecific or the manifestation of a systemic disease (i.e., RA, congestive heart failure or venous obstructive outflow disease).

1. **Dorsal forefoot** swelling together with pain on weight-bearing suggests a metatarsal stress fracture.
2. Swelling anterior to the **distal fibula** indicates an anterior talofibular ligament sprain.
3. Swelling distal to the **medial malleolus** along with inability to invert the heal is consistent with posterior tibial tendon insufficiency.
4. Swelling, especially when associated with pain and **erythema,** is consistent with musculoskeletal infection, or it may be seen in severe flares of inflammatory disease such as RA or gout.

E. Skin

1. **Callosities** (keratoses) are areas of thickened skin that reflect areas of increased weight-bearing. Calluses under the second and third metatarsal heads may represent lesser metatarsal overload secondary to a hypermobile first ray.
2. **Corns.** A hard corn (clavus durum) is frequently seen over the dorsolateral aspect of the PIP joint of the fifth toe where it contacts the shoe upper. A soft corn (clavus mollum), caused by moisture, is most frequently seen in the fourth web space.
3. **Ulceration** may be the consequence of underlying bony prominences, altered protective sensation as in diabetic neuropathy, or systemic vascular insufficiency.

F. Neurologic and vascular examinations, including evaluation of sensation, motor function, reflexes, position sense, skin temperature, pulses, and capillary refill, should be performed carefully.

1. **Charcot's arthropathy** may develop in diabetics with peripheral neuropathy. The resulting destruction of normal foot architecture leads to deformity and ulceration.
2. **Skin breakdown** resulting from vascular disease with arterial insufficiency may be amenable to vascular bypass surgery to improve inflow.

G. **Footwear** should be examined. Insufficient insole support may contribute to posterior tibial tendinitis. The wear pattern of the sole of the shoe may provide insight into the overall alignment of the foot. A constrictive toe box may aggravate a hallux valgus or deformity of the lesser toes. Insole wear patterns can provide insight into points of high pressure during weight-bearing.

IV. **Additional investigations**

A. **Results of blood testing** to evaluate the white cell count, erythrocyte sedimentation rate, and C-reactive protein level may support a diagnosis of infection or RA. Measurements of rheumatoid factor and uric acid levels and human leukocyte antigen (HLA) testing may be helpful in suspected cases of inflammatory arthropathies.

B. **Joint aspiration** in the presence of an effusion with culture, cell counts, and analysis of glucose, protein, and crystals should be performed to rule out a septic joint, RA, or a crystal-induced arthropathy such as gout or pseudogout.

C. **Radiographs** provide a confirmation of the suspected diagnosis after the history and physical examination have been performed. All radiography should be performed during weight-bearing whenever possible.

1. The **ankle series** consists of anteroposterior, mortise (30-degree internal rotation), and lateral views of the ankle. The joint space, alignment, and distal tibia-fibula syndesmosis as well as bony structures themselves should be carefully evaluated. Contralateral radiographs are often useful for evaluating asymmetries.

   a. **Ankle fractures** are usually readily apparent. The presence of a medial malleolar fracture without a concomitant lateral malleolar fracture necessitates a full-length radiograph of the fibula.

   b. **Osteochondral fractures** of the talar dome are often not visible on films of initial injuries. Repeated films obtained when symptoms persist should be carefully scrutinized.

   c. **Chronic lateral ankle instability,** seen after 20% of ankle sprains, may be further assessed with stress radiographs. Talar tilt (mortise) and anterior drawer (lateral) views must be compared with those of the contralateral, uninjured limb.

2. The **foot series** consists of weight-bearing anteroposterior and lateral radiographs. Joint spaces, bone density, alignment, and presence of deformity should be noted.

   a. **Forefoot, midfoot, and hindfoot relationships** cannot be evaluated in the non–weight-bearing condition.

   b. An **oblique radiograph** may provide additional information about the midfoot bony architecture (e.g., Lisfranc's fracture-dislocation) and about a suspected tarsal coalition (calcaneonavicular).

   c. Broden's views (taken with the ankle in 30 degrees of internal rotation and in a neutral position, with varying degrees of tilt to the x-ray beam) provide information about the congruity of the posterior talocalcaneal facet after calcaneus fractures.

   d. Canale's view (taken with the ankle in plantar flexion, the foot internally-rotated 15 degrees, and the x-ray beam tilted 15 degrees cranially) profiles the talar neck after talus fractures.

   e. A sesamoid view of the forefoot demonstrates the sesamoid-first metatarsal articulation for arthrosis, fracture, and subluxation.

D. **Computed tomography (CT)** provides high-resolution anatomic detail of the cortical and cancellous structures of the foot and ankle. Computer-assisted reconstruction can provide images in planes other than that actually imaged. Arthrosis of the tarsal bones, coalitions, and osteochondral lesions are well seen with this modality. In addition, the complex fracture patterns of the talus, calcaneus, and midfoot structures are well delineated on CT, which enables improved preoperative planning and management.

E. **Magnetic resonance imaging (MRI)** provides exquisite anatomic detail of the soft-tissue elements of the foot and ankle, such as the ankle ligaments (after suspected talofibular ligament tear), tendons (e.g., a diseased posterior tibial tendon), skin, and subcutaneous structures. In addition, the condition of the articular chondral surfaces can be well visualized on certain sequences. The extent of soft-tissue involvement of a neoplastic lesion can be more accurately assessed on MRI.

F. Technetium bone scanning provides information about the metabolic activity of the bones of the foot and ankle. Increased activity as seen diffusely in RA and locally in a stress fracture is visualized as a "hot spot." However, low specificity makes the differentiation of the multiple diagnostic possibilities difficult without additional clinical information.

V. Common foot problems

A. Achilles tendinitis is a common condition of the Achilles tendon that presents with pain either at or just proximal to its insertion into the calcaneal tuberosity. It is frequently caused by overuse related to athletic participation. Degenerative changes within the tendon itself may be the cause in older persons. Occasionally, inflammatory disorders such as gout or Reiter's syndrome may precipitate such a condition.

1. **Physical examination.** The tendon itself may be thickened approximately 2 to 3 cm proximal to the insertion. Local tenderness is frequently present. A palpable bony prominence may be noted at the calcaneal insertion. An overlying adventitial bursa may be present as well. Active ankle plantar flexion may reveal subtle weakness in comparison with the contralateral extremity. The Thompson test (squeezing the calf) causes ankle plantar flexion, thereby ruling out a rupture of the tendon.
2. **Radiography** may demonstrate a soft-tissue thickening at the level of the tendinopathy. Alternatively, a degenerative spur may be seen "growing" up into the tendon at its insertion.
3. The **treatment** of an acute tendinitis revolves around reducing the associated inflammation. A brief period of rest in a walking boot or cast may result in significant resolution of symptoms. Antiinflammatory medications, judicious use of cryotherapy, and gentle physiotherapy on the resumption of athletic activity are valuable adjuncts. Steroid injection can lead to tendon rupture. Particular attention should be paid to gastrocnemius equinus contracture, which is frequently present in recalcitrant cases. Chronic tendinitis unresponsive to conservative measures frequently will benefit from surgical debridement of the diseased tendon with excision of a bony spur, if present. Should considerable weakness exist in the degenerative condition or if insufficient tendon remains after debridement, augmentation with the flexor hallucis longus tendon is particularly useful.

B. Plantar heel pain is one of the most common disorders seen by physicians who manage foot and ankle problems. Plantar fasciitis, an irritation of the plantar fascia at its origin on the posteromedial tubercle of the calcaneus, is the most common cause of plantar heel pain. Atrophy of the normal plantar fat pad may result in difficulty walking because of plantar heel pain. Entrapment of branches of the posterior tibial nerve as they cross in close proximity to the heel may also result in plantar heel pain. Inflammatory arthropathies (psoriatic arthritis and Reiter's syndrome $\gg$ RA) frequently present with plantar heel pain, often before the systemic nature of these diseases is appreciated.

1. **Physical examination** may reveal tenderness at the origin of the plantar fascia. Dorsiflexion of the MTP joints may exacerbate the tenderness because this stretches the fascia. "Start-up" pain during the first step in the morning or after prolonged sitting is common. Gastrocnemius equinus contracture (continuous with the plantar fascia) is frequently present.
2. **Radiographic findings** are frequently normal. An incidental traction spur at the origin of the flexor digitorum brevis muscle may be present. This is rarely, however, the source of the discomfort.
3. **Treatment** should be directed at unloading the heel with soft cushioning in the shoe, vigorous stretching of the plantar fascia-gastrocnemius complex, and administering nonsteroidal antiinflammatory medications. Occasional night splinting is helpful in the persistent case. Patients should be counseled

about the often-prolonged nature of the disorder. In more than 95% of cases, symptoms will resolve within 12 months. In the presence of significant tendoachilles or gastrocnemius contracture, tendon release and lengthening are often curative.

C. **Pes planus deformity and posterior tibial tendon insufficiency** have received considerable attention recently. A flat foot, in and of itself, is not pathologic. However, when associated with progressive pain and deformity, it warrants intervention. Static factors contributing to the integrity of the medial longitudinal arch include the plantar fascia, the spring ligament, and the capsular and ligamentous structures associated with the bones of the medial column of the foot. The dynamic factor most commonly associated with the maintenance of the medial arch is the posterior tibial muscle and its tendon. When overloaded (e.g., by a gastrocnemius equinus contracture), the posterior tibial tendon fails. The hindfoot remains in valgus. Eventually, the static supports of the longitudinal arch fail and a sag is noted in the midfoot. The foot assumes a pronated posture and exacerbates the hindfoot valgus, which increases the gastrocnemius contracture. Eventually, degenerative changes occur in the midfoot and hindfoot joints if the problem is left untreated.

1. **Physical examination** demonstrates a complex deformity with varying degrees of hindfoot valgus and midfoot pronation and abduction. Early on in the disorder, tenderness is noted along the posterior tibial tendon below the medial malleolus. However, in the advanced case, pain along the posterolateral hindfoot predominates because of calcaneofibular impingement. The "too many toes" sign may be viewed from behind with excessive hindfoot valgus. The inability to perform a single-limb heel-rise or invert the heel may be noted. Claw toes and a hallux valgus deformity may develop secondarily.
2. **Radiography** should always be performed during weight bearing. The lateral radiograph will often demonstrate a sag in the longitudinal arch of the foot and an increase in the talocalcaneal angle. The anteroposterior radiograph will similarly demonstrate an increase in the talocalcaneal angle as well as loss of coverage of the talar head by the navicular. In long-standing cases, degenerative arthrosis may be noted in the hindfoot, particularly the subtalar joint.
3. **Treatment** depends on the stage of the disease.
   a. **Stage 1** disease, marked by posterior tibial tendinitis (without deformity), is treated by immobilization of the foot to allow the posterior tibial tendinitis to resolve, followed by use of a supportive insole orthosis. Lengthening of a contracted tendoachilles complex, when present, is particularly helpful in arresting progression.
   b. **Stage 2** disease, marked by tendon insufficiency and flexible pes planus deformity, is best treated surgically with tendoachilles lengthening, posterior tibial tendon augmentation, and medial column stabilization via arthrodesis of the nonessential joints of the midfoot.
   c. **Stage 3** disease is characterized by either fixed pes planus deformity or degenerative arthrodesis of one or more of the essential hindfoot joints (i.e., the subtalar joint). However, the significant limitation of normal gait mechanics that results warrants early, aggressive intervention when the deformity is flexible and hindfoot arthrodesis can be avoided.

D. **Metatarsalgia** represents a condition characterized by pain under the weight-bearing surfaces of the metatarsal heads. Its many causes include hypermobility of the first ray with compensatory overload of the lesser metatarsals, claw toes (in which the plantar fat pad is drawn distally to expose the plantar metatarsal heads), and a rigid cavovarus foot and tendoachilles-gastrocnemius equinus contracture. It may be prominent in RA.

1. On palpation of the plantar forefoot, prominence of the metatarsal heads may be noted. The plantar metatarsal fat pad may be displaced distally in the presence of hammer toe or claw toe deformities. A hypermobile first ray with overload of the lesser toes will present with plantar keratoses beneath the second (and third) metatarsal heads. Gastrocnemius equinus contracture and claw toes routinely coexist in this syndrome.

2. **Radiography.** Claw toe deformities may be demonstrated on weight-bearing lateral radiographs. A forefoot cavus posture may be evident as well. The anteroposterior radiograph will demonstrate a long, hypertrophied second metatarsal in the hypermobile first-ray syndrome.
3. **Treatment** is directed at unloading the excessive plantar pressure beneath the metatarsal heads. Various nonoperative measures that are particularly helpful include placing a metatarsal pad just proximal to the metatarsal heads. Accommodative inserts can also provide unloading of the metatarsal heads. Surgical correction of lesser claw toe deformities can replace the plantar fat pad beneath the metatarsal heads. Stabilization of the hypermobile first ray can redistribute plantar weight-bearing forces. Gastrocnemius equinus contracture can be relieved through tendoachilles or gastrocnemius tendon lengthening.

E. **(Morton's) neuroma** is the presence of pain in the web space between the third and fourth toes caused by irritation of the common plantar interdigital nerve at this location. Many etiologies are thought to contribute to this disorder, including constrictive shoes with a narrow toe box, forefoot overload with metatarsalgia, and gastrocnemius equinus contracture. Patients typically complain of a numbness or burning sensation radiating into the toes that is promptly relieved by removing the shoes and rubbing the feet.

1. **Symptoms** may be reproduced during compression of the metatarsal heads by the examiner. A palpable mass may be appreciated in the appropriate web space.
2. **Radiographic findings** are routinely normal. MRI can be helpful when the diagnosis is uncertain.
3. **Treatment** includes wearing appropriate shoes to accommodate the natural width of the forefoot. A metatarsal pad may serve to splay the metatarsal heads and provide symptom relief. In recalcitrant cases, local steroid injection or surgical excision is warranted.

F. **Inversion ankle injuries (sprains)** are among the most common musculoskeletal injuries seen by the physician. Recall that the talus is wider anteriorly than posteriorly, which renders it particularly susceptible to inversion injury in the plantar-flexed position. Approximately 20% of ankle sprains will progress to varying degrees of chronic ankle instability.

1. **Physical examination** shortly following an inversion ankle injury reveals swelling located over the anterolateral aspect of the ankle joint. Ecchymoses may be present. Tenderness over the anterior talofibular ligament will be noted on palpation. Involuntary guarding and apprehension to attempted inversion maneuvers will be evident. Depending on the severity of the injury, weight-bearing may not be possible. Additional findings on the medial portion of the ankle indicate a higher-energy injury. Manual stress testing with anterior drawer and talar tilt maneuvers, if tolerated, may reveal asymmetry in comparison with the uninjured extremity.
2. **Radiographs** should always be obtained to rule out a fracture of the fibula or medial malleolus. Small avulsion fractures of the distal fibula are frequently seen and require no specific treatment. As mentioned previously, anteroposterior and lateral stress radiographs comparing the injured and uninjured extremities may prove helpful in subtle cases.
3. **Treatment** initially is largely supportive. Immobilization, elevation, cryotherapy, and nonsteroidal antiinflammatory medications are instituted until the patient is comfortable. Organized physical therapy to restore normal muscle strength and proprioception is essential for a good outcome. Weight-bearing in a light-weight orthosis that controls inversion and eversion is particularly helpful. Normal activities can gradually be resumed when strength in the injured ankle is equal to that in the uninjured extremity. Chronic ankle instability is most often associated with premature return to athletic activities and early reinjury. Long-term use of a protective orthosis may provide symptomatic relief to those with chronic ankle instability. Surgical repair or reconstruction of elongated lateral ankle ligaments is helpful in those cases in which nonoperative therapy has failed.

G. **Hallux valgus** is a common condition whose cause is likely multifactorial. Tight and constrictive shoes, ligamentous laxity with muscle imbalance, and hereditary predisposition all contribute to a lateral deviation of the hallux on the first metatarsal. Hallux valgus may often be a part of a larger deformity—namely, the planovalgus foot with a pronated midfoot that gradually stretches the medial capsule of the hallux MTP joint into valgus.

1. **Physical examination** reveals a lateral deviation of the hallux phalanges, often with impingement of the lesser toes that causes an overlapping second-toe deformity (claw toes). Prominence of the medial aspect of the hallux metatarsal head may cause local paresthesias or ulceration of the overlying soft tissues. Bursal swelling can occur and can become infected. Gastrocnemius equinus contracture and a hypermobile first ray may often be present.
2. **Radiography** will demonstrate an increased hallux valgus angle and an increased intermetatarsal angle (metatarsus primus varus). Second metatarsal overload may be present. Lateral radiographs may reveal claw toe deformities of the lesser toes. Loss of medial column height (sag) may be noted as well.
3. **Treatment** should be based on the severity of the deformity and degree of functional limitation and should be directed at the cause of the deformity. Nonoperative measures include accommodative shoes with a wide toe box and insole orthoses to support a flexible pes planus deformity associated with hallux valgus. Operative intervention, when nonoperative measures are not successful, should be directed at the restoration of soft-tissue and osseous stability. Operative intervention is largely successful in appropriately selected patients.

H. **Hallux rigidus** is a painful condition characterized by a limitation of hallux dorsiflexion. It often coincides with degenerative arthrosis to varying degrees. Remote injuries to the hallux MTP joint may be recalled. Alternatively, an elevated first ray causes the hallux proximal phalanx to "jam" into the first metatarsal head rather than "glide" over it in a smooth arc.

1. **Physical examination** reveals restricted dorsiflexion at the hallux MTP joint. Prominent osteophytes may be readily palpable, especially over the dorsolateral aspect of the joint.
2. **Radiography** may reveal varying degrees of osteoarthrosis, from osteophyte formation to joint space narrowing. An elevated first ray may be noted on the lateral radiograph.
3. **Treatment** in which a steel rocker bar is used in the sole of a shoe to relieve motion at the MTP joint can be quite effective. Surgical intervention, including cheilectomy, is of limited short-term value. In intractable cases, arthrodesis of the MTP joint can be quite helpful.

22. SPORTS INJURIES

Riley J. Williams and Thomas L. Wickiewicz

During the past decade, the importance of regular exercise in the maintenance of good health has been well established. Consequently, with increasing attention now focused on personal fitness, the incidence of sports-related injuries has increased significantly. Both primary care physicians and specialists can expect to see a variety of athletic injuries. All clinicians should be able to recognize these conditions and administer appropriate care. A thorough history, physical examination, musculoskeletal imaging, and laboratory testing are all important in arriving at the proper diagnosis. A treatment plan is then developed for the injured athlete based on these objective findings.

I. **Cervical spine.** Injuries to the cervical spine range from mild to severe. Certain athletic activities (football, diving, gymnastics) are associated with an increased incidence of cervical spinal injury in comparison with other sports. Prompt recognition and treatment of persons who suffer cervical spinal injuries may prevent the progression or severity of the associated neurologic injury.

A. **Anatomy.** See Chapter 14.

B. **Classification of cervical spinal injuries.** Neck injuries can be classified according to neurologic sequelae or the type of force acting on the cervical spine at the time of injury.

1. **Cervical spinal injury with minimal, transient, or no neurologic symptoms**
   - a. **Muscle strains.** Pain and neck stiffness with no neurologic findings and negative imaging studies. Usually resolve spontaneously.
   - b. **Brachial plexus injuries ("stingers" or "burners").** Transient symptoms. See below.
   - c. **Bony fracture, ligamentous injury, disk injury without neurologic involvement.**
2. **Cervical spinal injuries accompanied by incomplete or complete spinal cord syndromes**

C. **Classification by mechanism of injury and syndrome**

1. **Flexion without axial load or rotation.** These forces usually cause a compression fracture of the cancellous cervical vertebral body without tearing of the stabilizing ligamentous complex of the facet joints. Avulsion fractures of the transverse processes can also occur. These are stable fractures usually not associated with neurologic loss.
2. **Flexion with rotation.** These forces place high loads on the facet joint capsules and the posterior interspinous ligaments. Unevenly applied forces can cause unilateral facet dislocation resulting from facet capsular rupture. Larger loads can lead to bilateral facet dislocations with associated anterior subluxation of the vertebral bodies and fractures of the facets, laminae, or vertebral bodies. Neurologic injury associated with these injuries is quite variable, ranging from no loss to complete spinal cord injury.
3. **Axial compression.** This type of load usually results when the head strikes a hard object, as when a swimmer dives into shallow water. With forward flexion of the head, cervical lordosis is decreased such that the spinal column is essentially straight. The resultant force is transmitted to the cervical spine and can cause vertebral body fracture with retropulsion of bony elements into the spinal canal. Neurologic loss, including quadriplegia or complete motor paralysis secondary to anterior spinal cord syndrome, is commonly associated with this injury pattern.
4. **Extension.** Extension forces that exceed the normal range of motion of the cervical spinal facet joints can lead to fracture of these elements or an avulsion of the superior margin of the vertebral body. Neurologic loss is vari-

able. Occasionally, the spinal cord impingement occurs between the lamina posteriorly and a disk anteriorly. A complete spinal cord injury or central cord syndrome can result.

D. Spinal cord syndromes

1. **Central.** Extension forces. Injury affects upper more than lower extremities. Motor and sensory loss. Fair prognosis. Most common type.
2. **Anterior.** Flexion-compression. Incomplete motor and sensory loss. Poor prognosis.
3. **Brown-Séquard.** Results from penetrating trauma. Ipsilateral loss of motor function; contralateral pain and loss of temperature sensation. Best prognosis of all syndromes.
4. **Complete.** Spinal canal disruption, canal compression. No function below injury. Poor prognosis.
5. **Single root.** Avulsion or compression (disk). Symptoms related to level. Good prognosis.

E. Physical examination. In suspected cervical spinal injuries, a brief screening examination should be administered to assess the magnitude of the injury at the scene.

1. **Observation.** The position of the head and neck at impact should be noted to categorize the mechanism of injury.
2. **History**
   - **a.** In the on-site evaluation after cervical spinal injury, the examiner must first apply the basic ABCs of resuscitation. When unconsciousness follows neck injury, basic life-support measures should be applied.
     Note: Hyperextension of the neck should be avoided during these efforts.
   - **b.** If the patient is awake and alert, a history is taken to establish whether consciousness was lost (amnesia for the event).
   - **c.** The location and quality of any pain (neck, arms, shoulders, hands, back, or legs) is noted.
   - **d.** Numbness patterns must be defined. In the event of complaints of numbness, the clinician must define whether the pattern is global (all extremities) or partial (upper vs. lower extremities) and whether it was transient or is persistent.
3. **Motion.** If the patient is not amnesic for the event, did not lose consciousness, and has no self-reported neurologic loss, the clinician can then encourage the patient to attempt active range of motion of the neck without assistance. If significant pain is encountered, the neck should be immobilized and the patient further evaluated.
4. **Neurologic examination**
   - **a. Sensory examination.** This portion of the examination should include tests of sharp versus dull discrimination, light-touch sense, deep pressure, vibration, and position sense in all extremities.
   - **b. Motor examination.** Muscular strength should be assessed and graded in all limbs. Reflexes should also be graded in all limbs.
   - **c. Rectal examination.** In cases of spinal cord injury, the rectal examination is the most important part of the examination and can help the clinician discriminate between complete and incomplete spinal cord lesions after the resolution of spinal shock.
     Note: This procedure, although important, is not part of the on-site evaluation.

F. Radiographs

1. **Standard cervical spinal radiographs** include anteroposterior, lateral, oblique, and odontoid views. If there is no evidence of fracture or dislocation, a flexion-extension view of the cervical spine is also obtained. Active neck flexion and extension are always performed by the patient alone and should not exceed the patient's reported comfort level. The spinal column is considered unstable when vertebral body subluxation in excess of 3.5 mm or an angular deformity of 11 degrees or more exists.

2. **Supplemental radiographs** consist of pillar views to evaluate the lateral masses. Computed tomography (CT) can be used to detect subtle fractures and evaluate the spine for rotatory subluxation. Magnetic resonance imaging (MRI) is also very useful in the evaluation of soft-tissue abnormalities (ligamentous disruption, disk protrusion).

G. **Treatment.** The most important aspect of the management of cervical spinal injury is **immobilization.** Neck immobilization should be maintained until a definitive diagnosis has been made. For example, football-related cervical spinal injuries are managed by transporting the patient (with helmet in place) on a backboard. The patient is log-rolled onto a backboard with vigilant head stabilization. The face guard is left in place unless respiratory difficulty is encountered, in which cases it is removed. The neck is never moved passively until a fracture or dislocation is ruled out.

Note: In cases of spinal cord injury, the administration of IV **methylprednisolone** should be strongly considered because this agent has been shown to improve neurologic recovery if given **within 8 hours** of injury.

H. **Common cervical spinal problems**

1. **"Burners" or "stingers."** These injuries represent a stretch of the brachial plexus with a transient loss of motor power and transient pain radiating down the arm(s). This phenomenon usually occurs in football players. Most often, the symptoms are temporary and usually resolve within 1 to 2 minutes. The person can generally return to play the day of injury. With more severe brachial plexus injuries (i.e., persistent pain or weakness), nerve damage may result. Consequently, neurologic loss and pain will persist. These athletes cannot return to play and should be carefully examined in a controlled, off-field setting.
2. **Ligamentous sprain.** These injuries occur when a force moves a joint through an abnormal range of motion. This condition presents with localized neck pain and muscle spasm. The neurologic and radiographic examination findings are usually normal. Treatment consists of immobilization (semirigid collar), local heat, muscle relaxants, antiinflammatory medicines, and restriction of activity. Athletes can return to play when the symptoms resolve.
3. **Cervical spinal fractures—stable.** These types of fractures include C-1 burst fractures (Jefferson fracture), most odontoid fractures, traumatic C-2 spondylolisthesis (hangman's fracture), compression fracture of a vertebral body without comminution, and spinous process fracture (clay shoveler's fracture). Most of these fractures are treated with rigid immobilization (halo vest) until healing is complete.
4. **Cervical spinal fractures and subluxation—unstable.** Cervical spinal subluxation/dislocation usually presents with neurologic loss. These injuries require immediate immobilization and should ultimately be reduced. MRI is useful for assessing soft-tissue damage in these cases. Cervical traction or surgical reduction and stabilization are frequently indicated.
5. **Cervical disk herniation.** This phenomenon is uncommon in young athletes but may be seen in axial compression injuries sustained during rugby or football. Again, MRI is the best diagnostic modality for assessing patients for potential disk problems.

II. **Thoracolumbar spine.** Repetitive stresses to the ligamentous and bony supports of the thoracic (dorsal) spine can result in an overuse syndrome with subsequent acute or chronic back pain. **Spondylolysis** is a unilateral or bilateral fracture of the pars interarticularis. This lesion is frequently nontraumatic and may represent a congenital lesion or stress fracture. However, spondylolysis can occur acutely, especially in gymnasts, weight lifters, and football linemen. **Spondylolisthesis** is a fracture of the pars interarticularis, which is associated with translation of one vertebral body over another. It is frequently observed in the lumbar spine, especially at the L5-S1 junction.

A. **History.** Pain is usually localized to the low back and, less commonly, to the buttocks and posterior thighs. Radicular symptoms are uncommon.

B. Physical examination. Hamstring tightness is common. Point tenderness may be noted along the dorsal thorax.

C. Diagnostic studies. Oblique views of the lumbosacral spine usually demonstrate the spondylolytic lesion (lucency at the neck of the "Scotty dog"). A stress fracture of the pars interarticularis that is not obvious on plain radiographs may be demonstrated by means of bone scintigraphy.

D. Treatment consists of local measures, including heat, nonsteroidal anti-inflammatory drugs (NSAIDs), muscle relaxants, and rest during the acute period. Modification of activity or bracing is usually required. Surgical fusion is indicated only in cases of severe spondylolisthesis or unrelenting pain.

III. Shoulder. Sports that require repetitive overhead arm motion (baseball, racquet sports, swimming) place unusual stresses on the supporting structures of the shoulder. Injuries to the shoulder capsule, rotator cuff musculature, biceps tendon, scapular stabilizers, and shoulder musculature are common. Most of these problems are discussed in Chapter 15. Additional shoulder problems, unique to overhead athletes, are discussed in this section.

A. Little Leaguer's shoulder typically affects adolescents and teen-agers and represents a separation of the proximal humeral epiphysis. The observed physeal abnormality is likely caused by repetitive forces associated with the acceleration phase of the pitching cycle (extreme humeral abduction and external rotation to forward flexion and internal rotation).

1. **History.** These typically young patients complain of arm pain during and after throwing.
2. **Radiographs** reveal widening of the proximal humeral growth plate and demineralization and fragmentation adjacent to the epiphyseal plate. Occasionally, loose bodies are noted in the glenohumeral joint.
3. **Treatment** is conservative. Patients are prohibited from throwing until clinical and radiographic healing has occurred.

B. Rotator cuff tendinitis usually occurs as a result of overuse or in cases of subtle glenohumeral subluxation. It responds well to conservative measures (ice, NSAIDs, rest). Rehabilitation is most effective in relieving symptoms.

C. Posterior capsular tears, which occur in throwers, can result in ossification of the posterior capsule near the glenoid labrum. These lesions occur secondary to traction on the capsule during the acceleration and follow-through phases of the pitching cycle. Treatment initially consists of rest, NSAIDs, strengthening exercises, and restriction of pitching.

D. Internal impingement syndrome typically occurs in baseball pitchers. Lesions occur at the posterosuperior margin of the glenoid in the undersurface of the rotator cuff tendons (partial tears). These lesions are attributed to impingement of the rotator cuff on the bony margin of the glenoid during the cocking phase of the pitching motion (abduction, external rotation). Treatment is conservative (activity modification, NSAIDs). Recalcitrant cases may require debridement of the lesion.

E. Instability. Global instability (anterior, posterior, inferior) of the shoulder can occur in overhead athletes because of microtrauma to the shoulder capsule. The shoulder usually does not frankly dislocate but rather feels "loose" to the patient. Many cases can be treated with physical therapy; surgical stabilization may be necessary in severe cases.

IV. Elbow. The diagnosis and treatment of problems of the elbow require an understanding of the anatomy and function of the joint.

A. Anatomy and function. The elbow is a hinge joint. Elbow flexion and extension occur at the articulation of the humerus and ulna. Rotation takes place at the proximal radioulnar and radiocapitellar joints.

B. Joint stability. During valgus stress, primary stability is derived from the bony fit of the ulnohumeral and radiocapitellar joints. Secondary stability is derived from the restraint provided by the medial (ulnar) collateral ligament. The lateral (radial) collateral ligament and the anconeus muscle provide some resistance to varus loads; however, bony constraint is much more important in resisting these forces. Most throwing activities subject the elbow to valgus stress.

C. **Common elbow problems.** Overhead athletes (throwers, tennis players) place tremendous, repetitive valgus forces on the medial side of the elbow. These forces result in the application of compressive forces on the lateral elbow during the acceleration phase of throwing. Forceful extension during follow-through (extension overload) leads to posterior compartment lesions (loose bodies, osteophytes). Medial elbow tension-overload injuries include acute valgus instability and chronic valgus instability, both of which can be complicated by ulnar neuropathy.

1. **Acute valgus instability**
   a. **Flexor mass tears.** These lesions occur at the elbow in association with sudden forced wrist flexion and pronation. Tenderness and pain at the point of the tear are noted with resisted wrist or finger flexion. Partial tears are initially treated with rest, ice, and NSAIDs. This is followed by resistive exercises at the wrist. Complete tears present with a palpable soft-tissue defect distal to the flexor muscle origin and may require surgical reattachment.
   b. **Medial (ulnar) collateral ligament tears (acute).** These lesions present with pain and tenderness during valgus stress of the elbow. Laxity with valgus testing at 30 degrees of flexion confirms the diagnosis. MRI is useful in distinguishing between complete and partial medial collateral ligament injuries. Partial tears are treated with ice, rest, early motion, and a gradual return to full activity. Complete tears require surgical repair/reconstruction in high-level athletes who wish to continue throwing.
   c. **Little Leaguer's elbow.** Repetitive valgus stresses in children can cause epiphyseal avulsion of the medial epicondyle rather than ligamentous rupture. Treatment is usually conservative (ice, rest, early motion).
   d. **Athletes at risk** are pitchers, catchers, and javelin throwers.
2. **Chronic valgus instability** is common in athletes involved in throwing sports. Medial collateral ligament laxity develops slowly over time and occurs secondary to the microtrauma associated with repetitive throwing. Traction spurs at the distal insertion of the medial collateral ligament and calcification within the ligament can occur. Chronic ligamentous laxity may require surgical excision of calcified deposits and spurs, debridement, and reefing of the medial collateral ligament or reconstruction with use of the palmaris longus tendon. Loose bodies can also form within the elbow joint as a result of this condition, so that elbow arthroscopy is generally performed on patients undergoing reconstruction of the medial collateral ligament.
3. **Ulnar neuropathy** can develop secondary to ulnar nerve compression at or near the elbow (cubital tunnel). Affected patients present with pain along the ulnar groove, with radiation of pain and paresthesias into the fourth and fifth fingers. In most patients, Tinel's sign is positive at the elbow. Electromyographic and nerve conduction studies may be required to confirm the diagnosis. Studies have demonstrated that this condition often accompanies chronic laxity of the medial collateral ligament of the elbow. Initial treatment consists of rest and NSAIDs. Decompression of the cubital tunnel and nerve transposition may be required.
4. **Lateral compartment injuries**
   a. **Osteochondritis dissecans.** Valgus forces at the elbow result in compressive loading of the lateral side. Osteochondritis dissecans of the humeral capitellum frequently occurs in male adolescents 12 to 14 years of age.
      (1) **History.** The thrower presents with pain, motion loss, and catching or locking symptoms.
      (2) **Radiographs** usually reveal flattening of the capitellum (most common site) or fracture.

(3) **Differential diagnosis** includes Panner's disease, which has a similar radiographic appearance but is found in younger patients (6 to 9 years) and is not related to trauma.

(4) **Treatment** of osteochondritis dissecans depends on the size of the lesion. Small osteochondral lesions are managed by activity modification and antiinflammatory medications. Large lesions or loose bodies may require surgical debridement (elbow arthroscopy).

b. **Lateral epicondylitis (tennis elbow)** causes pain at the lateral humeral epicondyle. Although commonly found in participants in racquet sports, this malady also occurs in persons who do not play tennis.

(1) **Pathogenesis.** The site of pathology is generally found at the origin of the extensor muscle (extensor carpi radialis brevis) at the lateral epicondyle. The period of peak incidence is the fourth decade of life. This finding suggests a degenerative process in the tendon aggravated by repetitive stress, which leads to macroscopic and microscopic tears of the extensor origin. Approximately 40% of these patients will have other sites of soft-tissue degenerative problems (shoulder bursitis, rotator cuff tendinitis).

(2) **History.** Patients typically present with lateral elbow pain that is exacerbated by wrist extension. They commonly complain of pain while they are using a screwdriver, shaking hands, making a fist, or lifting a weight. The pain radiates from the dorsum of the forearm to the fingers. Tennis players often complain of accentuated pain during backhand strokes. Numbness or paresthesias may occur. Such complaints should alert the physician to consider other causes of elbow pain (i.e., cervical radiculopathy). A history of fluoroquinolone antibiotic (i.e., ciprofloxacin) use may also be reported.

(3) **Physical examination.** Point tenderness at the lateral epicondyle is typical. Tenderness may also be present distally along the extensor muscle sheaths. Resisted wrist extension with the elbow straight and the hand and forearm pronated should reproduce symptoms.

(4) **Radiographs.** Calcification may be seen in the region of the lateral epicondyle, but the elbow joint itself is normal.

(5) **Differential diagnosis**

(a) **Medial epicondylitis (golfer's elbow)** is an inflammatory condition that leads to pathology within the origin of the flexor pronator muscle group and pain at the medial epicondyle.

(b) **Intraarticular pathology.** A patient with elbow pathology (loose bodies, RA, osteoarthritis) may present with lateral elbow pain. Limitation of elbow motion and radiographic changes can clarify the diagnosis.

(c) **Gout.** Differentiation is not difficult because the acute, inflammatory signs of gout (erythema, swelling) are not usually present in tennis elbow. Crystals found on joint aspiration will confirm the diagnosis of gout.

(d) **Cervical spinal disease** may cause referred pain to the elbow. MRI of the cervical spine can be useful.

(e) **Posterior interosseous nerve (branch of radial nerve) entrapment** may mimic lateral epicondylitis. Tenderness is more volar over the entrance of the nerve into the supinator muscle.

(6) **Treatment** is initially conservative. Activities that accentuate the pain are avoided for 8 to 12 weeks. Oral NSAIDs should be given acutely for pain relief. Should symptoms persist, injection of 40 mg of methylprednisolone acetate (Depo-Medrol) with 1 mL of 1% lidocaine into the point of maximum tenderness usually provides some relief. When the acute pain has subsided, exercises directed at strengthening the extensor muscles are started. A flexibility program is also started, and ice is used judiciously. A forearm band

may reduce tension on the extensor muscle origin and provide relief in some patients. A volar wrist splint may also be helpful. Surgical excision of the degenerative tissue at the origin of the extensor carpi radialis brevis may be necessary in patients who fail conservative treatment.

(7) Prevention

(a) Awareness. Warm-up, stretching, exercise, and weight-lifting programs serve as prophylactic measures and should be encouraged.

(b) Warm-up. Abrupt physical stresses may predispose certain muscle groups to injury. Appropriate warm-up activity should precede vigorous racquet sports. For example, the first 15 to 20 minutes of tennis should consist of low-intensity volleying. Speed and duration should be gradually increased. Stretching and ice application for 15 minutes should follow all activities.

(c) Technique. Poor technique is one of the main causes of tennis elbow. Patients with lateral epicondylitis should pay specific attention to grip and the technique of backhand strokes. Lighter racquets, large grip size, and less taut stringing (52 pounds) have all been reported to be helpful. Clay is a better surface, and opponents should be selected who hit at lower speeds.

V. Hand. The hand is exposed to many forces that may result in significant injury in the course of athletic activity.

A. Bennett's fracture is a fracture of the base of the first metacarpal.

1. **History.** The mechanism of injury is a direct blow against a partially-flexed metacarpal or a fall on an outstretched hand while a ski pole is clutched.
2. **Physical examination.** Swelling and tenderness are present at the carpometacarpal joint, and deformity of the thumb is present, particularly if the joint is dislocated.
3. **Radiographs.** The fracture line characteristically separates the major part of the metacarpal from a small volar lip fragment, disrupting the carpometacarpal joint.
4. **Treatment.** Closed or open reduction with pinning is required to reestablish articular congruity.

B. Ulnar collateral ligament insufficiency (gamekeeper's thumb). Rupture of the ulnar collateral ligament of the metacarpophalangeal (MCP) joint of the thumb can be acute or chronic.

1. **History.** A sudden valgus (abduction) stress applied to the MCP joint of the thumb results in partial or complete disruption of the ulnar collateral ligament. Falling with a ski pole in one's hand predisposes a skier to this injury.
2. **Physical examination.** The patient presents with a painful, swollen MCP joint of the thumb. An abduction stress (45 degrees of flexion) should reveal laxity in comparison with the normal side. The stress test may also be performed under local anesthesia in more severe cases.
3. **Imaging.** An avulsion fracture from the base of the proximal phalanx may be associated with the injury. A stress test with radiographs confirms the diagnosis. MRI can also aid in the diagnosis and confirm the presence of a Stener's lesion (interposition of the adductor aponeurosis) between the free ends of the torn ulnar collateral ligament.
4. **Treatment.** Partial tears are treated nonoperatively with a molded thumb spica cast/splint. Complete tears are surgically repaired.

VI. Knee (ligamentous injuries)

A. Anatomy. Stability of the knee occurs in several planes: anteroposterior, medial, lateral, and rotational. Medial and lateral stability is imparted by the medial collateral ligament, lateral collateral ligament, and anterior cruciate ligament. Anteroposterior stability is imparted by the anterior cruciate and posterior cruciate ligaments. Other structures that contribute to knee stability include the knee joint capsule, menisci, and surrounding muscles.

1. The **medial collateral ligament** prevents medial opening of the knee with valgus stress. The anterior cruciate ligament and posterior capsule are secondary stabilizers against medial opening with valgus stress.
2. The **lateral collateral ligament** prevents lateral opening with varus stress. Secondary stabilizers against varus stress are the anterior cruciate ligament, posterior cruciate ligament, and popliteus muscle.
3. The **anterior cruciate ligament** prevents anterior displacement of the tibia relative to the femur. Secondary stabilizers are the medial meniscus and medial collateral ligament.
4. The **posterior cruciate ligament** prevents posterior displacement of the tibia relative to the femur. Secondary restraint to posterior displacement is imparted by the medial collateral ligament.

B. Classification of ligamentous injuries of the knee

1. **Grade 1 (first-degree/mild) sprain.** Characterized by local pain and swelling, without instability. Joint opening of 0 to 5 mm is found on examination. This injury is represented microscopically by a mild tear in the collagen fibers of the ligament; however, full continuity of the ligament is maintained.
2. **Grade 2 (second-degree/moderate) sprain.** Characterized by pain, swelling, and minimal to moderate instability. Joint opening of 6 to 10 mm is found on examination. A more substantial tear of collagen fibers is found, with some loss of continuity in the ligament.
3. **Grade 3 (third-degree/severe) sprain.** Characterized by swelling and marked instability. Joint opening of more than 10 mm is noted at examination. There is complete disruption of ligament continuity.

C. History

1. **History of prior injury.** An apparent acute tear of a ligament may actually represent the last of many recurrent episodes, each of which has damaged the involved ligament.
2. **Mechanism of injury.** Determine the nature of the knee injury. Valgus versus varus stress? Hyperflexion versus hyperextension injury? If a ski injury, ask the patient in which direction the ski pointed at the time of injury. If a football injury, determine how the foot was planted at the time of impact and the site and direction of the injury force.
3. **Pain.** Collateral ligament injuries are most painful at the site of damage. Cruciate ligament injury usually results in capsular distension (hemarthrosis) and vague knee pain.
4. **Ability to continue sports.** An athlete who, at the time of injury, could not resume activity as a result of pain or instability usually has more severe pathology than one who was able to continue.
5. A **"pop" or "snap"** immediately followed by swelling is characteristic of anterior cruciate ligament injuries.
6. **Swelling** that occurs immediately following injury usually indicates acute hemorrhage into the joint (hemarthrosis) and should raise suspicion of intraarticular fracture or cruciate ligament damage. Swelling that appears during the first 24 hours is more common in grade 1 or 2 collateral ligament injuries. Often, less joint swelling will occur in a grade 3 collateral ligament injury because the complete disruption allows joint fluid to escape into the periarticular soft tissues.
7. **"Giving way"** is typical in patients with clinically significant knee instability (i.e., anterior knee instability secondary to anterior cruciate ligament insufficiency). "Locking" or "catching" is more representative of meniscal pathology.

D. Physical examination

1. **Inspection**
   a. **Gait.** Patients with an acute ligamentous injury often walk with a limp, a flexed knee, or both.
   b. **Swelling/effusion.** Is there suprapatellar fullness in the standing or prone position? Is the joint taut with fluid?

c. **Ecchymosis.** Collateral ligament injuries often show external signs of hemorrhage into soft tissue, which can present along the calf or ankle secondary to gravitational flow along muscle sheaths.

2. **Range of motion** is frequently limited secondary to pain. Lack of extension secondary to effusion should not be confused with the locked knee of meniscal etiology. Palpate for intraarticular effusion by compressing the suprapatellar pouch and ballottement of the patella.
3. **Neurovascular status.** A knee evaluation must include an assessment of popliteal and distal pulses as well as a thorough neurologic examination. The peroneal nerve is particularly susceptible to damage, especially in varus stress injuries that stretch the lateral structures of the knee.
4. **Ligament stress testing.** The patient should be supine and must be relaxed, as spasm and apprehension can obscure the diagnosis. The collateral ligaments should be tested with the knee in 0 and 30 degrees of flexion. At 30 degrees, the test is more specific for the collateral ligaments. During full extension, secondary stabilizers tighten to stabilize the joint; if the knee should "open" in extension, the injury is severe. Occasionally, 1% lidocaine injected into the site of pain or even general anesthesia may be needed to evaluate the knee properly.
   a. The **medial collateral ligament** stabilizes the joint against medial opening and thus protects against a valgus stress. To test this ligament, the limb is grasped with one hand while the femur is stabilized with the other, and a valgus stress is applied. Instability, if present, is more often sensed than seen. If the ligament has torn completely, the usual firm, abrupt end point will be absent. If the ligament is injured but not completely torn (grade 2), the end point from the remaining intact fibers is present; however, excursion may be increased.
   b. The **lateral collateral ligament** should be tested with a varus stress in the same manner. Additionally, the lateral collateral ligament can be palpated easily with the leg crossed in a figure 4 position.
   c. The **anterior cruciate ligament** is tested by translating the tibia anteriorly versus the femur.
      (1) The **Lachman test** is easily performed with the knee at approximately 30 degrees of flexion by stabilizing the femur and distal thigh with one hand while an anterior force is applied to the back of the tibia. The examiner notes both the amount of excursion and the sense of end point. The absence of a normal crisp end point, even in the face of only minimal excursion, is usually indicative of an anterior cruciate ligament tear.
      (2) The **anterior drawer test** is performed with the hip flexed 45 degrees and the knee flexed 90 degrees with the patient's foot flat on the table. The examiner sits on the foot and places the hands around the proximal tibia and, ensuring hamstring relaxation, applies an anterior force to the tibia, noting both the amount of excursion and quality of end point. This test is difficult to perform in the acute setting with associated knee swelling and is less accurate than the Lachman test.
      (3) The **pivot shift test** notes anterior and rotational translation of the lateral tibial plateau with respect to the lateral femoral condyle. It is performed by having the patient relax fully and applying a valgus force to the knee with varying degrees of internal and external rotation of the tibia with respect to the femur. As the knee is brought from an extended to a flexed position, a sense of movement or jump takes places that in a chronic setting will reproduce the patient's sense of instability. Grading of the pivot shift is as follows: absent, 1+ (slide); 2+ (jump); 3+ (lock). It is very difficult to perform a pivot shift maneuver in an acute setting without sufficient anesthesia. Similarly, if a patient is apprehensive, it is a difficult maneuver to reproduce even in chronic settings.

d. The **posterior cruciate ligament** is the primary restraint to posterior translation of the tibia with respect to the femur. The posterior drawer test is performed with the patient's hip flexed at 45 degrees and the knee flexed at 90 degrees. First visual inspection from the side may note less prominence of the tibia tubercle on the affected side with more prominence of the distal femoral condyles. On a posteriorly applied force to the tibia, the examiner will sense increased translation and absence of an end point. This is interpreted as a positive posterior drawer test.

Note: When examiners perform a Lachman maneuver with the knee at 30 degrees of flexion and sense a large increase in amount of translation but a normal end point associated with a normal anterior cruciate ligament, they should suspect that they are really feeling a knee that has suffered a posterior cruciate ligament tear. What the examiner is actually doing is bringing the tibia back to its normal position under the femur.

e. An evaluation of rotational stability includes an assessment of the **popliteal tendon and lateral collateral ligament complex.** These tests are performed at both 30 and 90 degrees of knee flexion. The patient lies prone and the degrees of external rotation of the affected and unaffected sides are compared. Increases in amount of external rotation are noted.

E. Diagnostic studies

1. **Radiographs.** Standard knee radiographic findings are usually negative but are useful to exclude a fracture. Avulsion fractures can sometimes be seen at ligamentous insertions (e.g., the tibial spine for anterior cruciate ligament injuries).
2. **Stress radiographs.** The joint opening is best viewed anteroposteriorly by applying mild stress.
3. **Arthrograms** are most useful for definite meniscal tears but may also demonstrate tears of the cruciate ligaments and more severe tears of the collateral ligaments. Leakage of dye from the joint usually indicates a complete collateral ligament disruption. This test is mostly of historical significance because of the ascendency of the MRI.
4. **Magnetic resonance imaging** has become increasingly accurate in the diagnosis of knee injuries and is easier for the patient to undergo in the acute setting. This is the study of choice for delineating soft-tissue injuries.

F. Differential diagnosis

1. **Meniscus tear.** The history of a twisting injury followed by swelling, locking, medial or lateral pain, and a limp suggests a collateral ligament injury; however, the Lachman or anterior drawer test findings are negative. Tenderness is usually along the joint line; patients are usually unable to perform a deep knee bend. The combination of meniscal damage with collateral or cruciate ligament injuries is common and should always be suspected when an acute knee injury is evaluated.
2. **Patellofemoral subluxation or dislocation** will often present as acute knee pain. Inherent abnormalities of the patellofemoral mechanism usually result in most patellofemoral injuries. These patients will complain of patellar apprehension and usually respond to physical therapy. However, surgical realignment of the extensor mechanism may be necessary in recurrent cases.

G. Treatment

1. **Collateral ligament injuries** without cruciate involvement are treated according to the degree of injury. However, most isolated injuries of the medial collateral ligament are treated in a conservative fashion.
   a. **Grades 1 and 2.** Protected weight-bearing based on the degree of the pain followed by early range of motion and rehabilitation of quadriceps musculature is indicated. Bracing is also used. MRI may be indicated to rule out concomitant meniscal pathology.
   b. **Grade 3.** These injuries seldom occur as an isolated event but still can be treated in a conservative manner. Attention should be directed at

range of motion, as flexion contractures will easily develop in the immediate post-injury period in patients with significant medial collateral ligament pathology. Collateral hinge bracing is indicated. Early range of motion of the knee is instituted. If concomitant cruciate injury dictates surgical repair, surgery should be delayed until range of motion, specifically restoration of full extension, is obtained.

2. **Cruciate ligament injury**
   a. **Injuries to the anterior cruciate ligament,** when complete, usually lead to anterior instability in the knee. Whether patients are affected by that instability is dictated by their activity level and age. For a person whose life-style places high demands on the knee, surgical treatment is indicated. If a patient is willing to avoid activities that involve deceleration and cutting and jumping maneuvers, then anterior cruciate ligament injuries may be treated in a conservative fashion. MRI or arthroscopic investigation should be performed to rule out concomitant meniscal pathology.
   b. **Injuries to the posterior cruciate ligament,** although they leave the knee with a characteristic instability, are often tolerated on a functional basis and are treated in a conservative fashion, with attention directed primarily at restoration of quadriceps muscle power.
   c. Cruciate injuries that have an associated injury to the posterolateral structures of the knee (**popliteus, lateral collateral ligament, joint capsule**) will lead to functional disability even in day-to-day activities in sedentary persons. These injuries are also very difficult to treat when they become chronic. The best results are obtained with early surgical reconstruction of the cruciate ligaments and repair of the posterolateral corner.

H. **Resumption of athletics.** Patient should not be allowed to resume their usual athletic activities until the knee is stable, pain minimal, and the range of motion adequate. They should be able to run in place, hop on the affected leg without difficulty, run figure of 8 patterns in both directions, and start and stop quickly. Muscle strength should be 80% or more of that of the opposite extremity, and muscle atrophy should be less than 1 cm (comparative circumference).

VII. **Running injuries.** Most running injuries to the musculoskeletal system are overuse-type problems that are typically preventable. A proper therapy program for any specific injury should include a conditioning regimen to prevent the recurrence of such injuries.

A. **Etiology of injury**
1. **Biologic fatigue.** Jogging or running requires repetitive motion that exposes the musculoskeletal system to severe stress. Even the most conditioned runner reaches a point of fatigue and biologic failure. Limitations and proper preparation are important in preventing running injuries.
2. **Improper training.** The "once-a-week" runner is the perfect candidate for a running injury. When muscle groups are inadequately conditioned, the repetitive forces associated with running can lead to injury. Excessive mileage, a sudden increase in mileage, and inadequate warm-up can lead to overuse injuries.
3. **Anatomic variability.** Patients with increased ligamentous laxity may be susceptible to sprains while running. The abnormal distribution of stresses on the feet of runners with flat feet or high arches makes them prone to particular problems. The likelihood of patellar problems is increased in a person with congenital abnormalities of the patellofemoral joint. The "Q angle" of the female hip may also predispose women to certain overuse running injuries.

B. **History**
1. **Important questions**
   a. Weekly mileage?
   b. Type of shoe worn—any change in shoe type recently?
   c. Duration, location, and quality of pain?

C. **Physical examination**

1. **Medical examination.** A complete respiratory and cardiovascular examination is mandatory for all patients, particularly those over 40 years of age.
2. **Musculoskeletal examination**
   a. **Observation** for joint swelling, muscular atrophy, ecchymosis.
   b. **Joint alignment**
      (1) In runners, it is important to evaluate the foot and ankle. Flat feet (pes planus) and high-arched feet (pes cavus) will be subjected to different stress patterns that predispose to different injuries. The knee examination should include an assessment of ligamentous stability and patellar tracking.
      (2) Always watch the patient walk or run. Such activity will best demonstrate overall joint alignment in a functional, weight-bearing position.
   c. **Palpation.** Areas of maximum tenderness should be noted.
   d. **Range of motion** (active and passive) of the involved joint should be compared with that of the contralateral limb.
   e. **Neurovascular status.**
3. **Type of shoe.** If available, the runner's shoe should be examined.
   a. **Fit.** The shoe should be both wide and long enough to allow space for the toes. This reduces blistering and the formation of subungual hematomas. The tongue should be well-padded to prevent extensor tendinitis and irritation of the dorsum of the foot.
   b. **Cushioning** should be thick enough to reduce impact stresses.
   c. The **heel** should be wide, thick, and soft. Many runners use a "heel-toe" type of gait. Impact concentrates on the heel. Increasing the width of the heel increases the contact area and decreases the transmitted stresses.
   d. **Rigidity** is needed for support and flexibility for foot motion. The shoe should be flexible at the metatarsophalangeal region, where "push-off" occurs, but rigid at the arch (midfoot).
   e. The **counter** must be high enough to avoid injury to the Achilles tendon and long enough medially to prevent hindfoot valgus and counteract forefoot pronation.

D. **Imaging studies**

1. **Radiographs.** Many running injuries involve the soft tissues. However, stress and avulsion fractures, which occur quite frequently in runners, may be visualized on routine films. Joint alignment is best visualized with weight-bearing films.
2. **Bone scans** may afford the earliest diagnosis of a stress fracture, which may not be apparent on routine films for several weeks.
3. **Magnetic resonance imaging and ultrasound** can aid the clinician in chronic cases of refractory Achilles tendinitis (tendinosis).

E. **Specific injuries**

1. **Foot and ankle problems**
   a. **Corns, calluses, and blisters.** Painful, hypertrophic skin changes are caused by abnormal pressures and stresses. Pain is usually centered on the plantar surface of the metatarsal heads or the dorsum of the interphalangeal joints of toes. There are usually underlying structural foot deformities, including pes planus (flat foot) or pes cavus (high arch).
      (1) **Treatment** is directed toward obtaining proper footwear, including padding to reduce stress on the area.
      (2) **Prevention.** A gradual increase in running distance is recommended.
   b. **Subungual hematoma** is a traumatic hemorrhage under the nail bed with associated severe pain. Clotted blood under the nail causes it to lift off. Subungual hematoma is caused by poorly fitting footwear with a tight toe box. It is often noted in long-distance runners (marathon).
      (1) **Treatment.** Therapy ranges from observation to decompression (placement of a hot wire through the nail to evacuate the hematoma). Removal of the nail may be needed secondarily.

(2) **Prevention.** Well-fitting footwear with sturdy, high, wide toe boxes will prevent the injury.

c. **Metatarsalgia** is a syndrome of pain under the metatarsal heads, with the first to third most commonly involved. Pain usually follows an episode of prolonged running. Tenderness is noted directly under the involved metatarsal head, and an underlying structural deformity (pes cavus, hammertoes) may be present.

(1) **Radiographs** may reveal the underlying foot deformity.

(2) **Treatment** consists of a modification of footwear to include adequate cushioning and insertion of orthotics to redistribute weight from the metatarsal heads (metatarsal pad/bar).

(3) **Prevention.** The running gait should be changed to a heel-toe pattern.

d. **Stress fractures,** which are fatigue fractures of bones secondary to repetitive stresses, are common in runners. There is a sudden or gradual onset of pain with swelling and tenderness at the site. The condition is often confused with "shin splint." The tibial shaft and the first to third metatarsals are most commonly involved. A recent change in distance or running terrain is commonly reported.

(1) **Radiographs** may demonstrate periosteal callus 7 to 14 days after the appearance of symptoms, and the bone scan will demonstrate increased uptake within 3 to 5 days.

(2) **Treatment** consists of abstaining from running until symptoms cease. This is followed by a gradual increase in mileage. Stress fractures of the tarsal navicular and the base of the fifth metatarsal present unique problems and often require more aggressive forms of treatment.

(3) **Prevention** includes an adequate stretching program, avoidance of hard surfaces, no abrupt changes in running technique, and adequate footwear.

e. **Plantar fasciitis** is inflammation of the plantar fascia, usually at its medial calcaneal origin. It is the most common cause of heel pain in runners. The patient usually experiences pain with the first few steps taken in the morning. There is usually tenderness at the anteromedial calcaneal margin, and tightness of the Achilles tendon may be present.

(1) **Radiographs** may reveal a calcaneal spur, but this is not diagnostic.

(2) **Treatment**

(a) Achilles tendon stretch program.

(b) Heel pads and/or heel cups.

(c) NSAIDs.

(d) Application of ice after running.

(e) Adhesive strapping.

(f) Injection of 20 to 40 mg of methylprednisolone acetate at the site of maximum tenderness.

(g) In rare cases, surgical release of the plantar fascia at the heel with removal of the spur may be needed.

(3) **Prevention** includes an adequate stretching program, avoidance of hard surfaces, no abrupt changes in running technique, and adequate footwear.

f. **Achilles tendinitis** is a painful inflammation of the Achilles tendon resulting from repetitive stresses. Pain is present near the insertion of the Achilles tendon. Tenderness may be noted along the length of the tendon. Increased warmth and swelling are often present, and in severe cases, crepitus and a tendon nodule may develop.

(1) **Predisposing factors** include tightness of the Achilles tendon, cavus foot, functional talipes equinus, or a pronated foot secondary to forefoot or hindfoot varus or tibia vara. Running on hills and uneven terrain inflicts small cumulative tears in the tendon that produce the inflammatory response seen clinically.

(2) **Treatment.** Acute symptoms are treated by limitation of running, ice, and NSAIDs. A gradual return to running with a vigorous stretching program before and after running is essential. Local steroid injection may lead to tendon rupture. Rarely, surgical tenolysis or excision of a tender nodule is indicated.

(3) **Prevention**

(a) The runner should avoid hills and banked roads.

(b) The running shoe must have a flexible sole, a well-molded Achilles pad, a heel wedge at least 15 mm high, and a rigid heel counter.

(c) An aggressive Achilles tendon stretching program should be undertaken.

2. Leg problems

a. Shin splint, characterized by pain along the inner distal two-thirds of the tibial shaft, is an overuse syndrome of either the posterior or anterior tibial muscle-tendon units.

(1) **History.** The patient experiences aching pain after running, usually in the posteromedial aspect of the leg; pain may be severe enough to prevent running.

(2) **Physical examination.** Tenderness is present along the involved muscle unit, and no neurovascular deficits are found on examination.

(3) **Predisposing factors** include poor conditioning, running on hard surfaces, and abnormal foot alignment, including hyperpronation.

(4) **Treatment.** Ice and rest are the initial measures. Alternating hot and cold soaks are helpful.

(5) **Prevention** includes avoidance of hard surfaces, a warm-up and stretching program, and, if needed, orthotic devices to prevent hyperpronation.

b. Stress fracture. Tibia and fibula stress fractures present as sudden or gradual onset of pain in the leg. These fractures usually are a result of excessive training. Other etiologic factors include running too far and too fast, often with improper shoes on hard surfaces. A history of a recent increase in mileage is common. Point tenderness is noted at the site of fracture. The proximal posteromedial tibia and the distal fibula are two common sites.

(1) **Radiographs.** A stress fracture may not appear on a radiograph for 3 to 4 weeks after the onset of symptoms. Results of a bone scan will be positive within 3 to 5 days.

(2) The **treatment** of all stress fractures is the avoidance of running. Running is resumed gradually after the patient has been asymptomatic for at least 6 weeks and radiographic healing has occurred.

(3) **Prevention** includes gradual changes in running regimens, a vigorous stretching program, and orthotics for underlying structural foot problems.

c. Exertional (chronic) compartment syndrome. This malady represents a common cause of leg pain in young persons. It is caused by a transient increase in muscular compartment pressure in response to exercise. The anterior and lateral compartments of the leg are most commonly involved.

(1) **History.** Increasing and progressive pain in the anterior or lateral aspect of the leg is reported with varying levels of exercise. Rest relieves symptoms. Numbness and paresthesias in the foot are common.

(2) **Physical examination.** Before exercise, findings are normal. Exercise causes the onset of symptoms. Occasionally, neurologic symptoms and signs become evident during the examination.

(3) **Compartmental pressure measurement** represents the mode by which a definitive diagnosis is made. An absolute value above 30 mm Hg or a relative increase in pressure of at least 20 mm Hg, after exercise, is usually diagnostic.

(4) **Treatment.** Conservative measure are always indicated initially (activity modification, orthotics, stretching). Surgical decompression (fasciotomy) of the compartment may be needed in refractory cases.

3. Thigh and hip problems

a. Hamstring strain (pull) represents an injury to the musculotendinous unit. Symptoms may occur suddenly or develop slowly and are usually caused by inadequate stretching of these muscles before running activities. Patients with tight hamstrings are at an increased risk. Tenderness is present in the region of the hamstring in the back of the thigh or at the hamstring origin from the pelvis. Ecchymosis may be noted in more severe injuries.

(1) **Radiographic findings** are usually negative but may show an avulsion fracture or periosteal reaction at the origin of the hamstring.

(2) **Treatment**

(a) **Acute.** Ice, rest, and modification of activity.

(b) **Chronic.** Stretching program, heat therapy, and ultrasound.

(3) **Prevention** includes a warm-up and stretching program.

b. Stress fracture of the femoral neck presents as acute or insidious onset of pain in the hip or pelvis. Running accentuates the pain. Tenderness is usually present over the pubis or ischium in patients with pelvic stress fractures. Pain on hip motion (particularly internal rotation) may indicate a stress fracture of the femoral neck. The fracture occurs in novice runners or in runners whose training regimen is changed abruptly.

(1) **Radiographs.** A stress fracture may not appear on radiographs for 3 to 4 weeks after the onset of symptoms. Results of a bone scan will be positive within 3 to 5 days.

(2) **Treatment** consists of a reduction in activity and no weight bearing for a hip stress fracture, with a gradual return to normal activity after 6 to 8 weeks. In refractory cases, surgical fixation may be required to protect the femoral neck (pinning).

(3) **Prevention** includes proper training, a stretching program, avoidance of abrupt changes in training habits and assessment of bone density, if indicated.

c. Iliotibial band friction syndrome is an overuse injury involving the iliotibial band and lateral femoral condyle. Pain is noted during knee flexion over the lateral condyle, where the friction occurs. Excessive iliotibial band tightness is prevalent in these patients; excessive foot pronation, genu varum, and tibial torsion may also be found. Climbing stairs and running (especially downhill) cause symptoms.

(1) **Physical examination.** Point tenderness is noted over the lateral condyle and sometimes the greater trochanter. Ober's test should be performed to assess iliotibial band tightness. Patients lie on their side with the unaffected limb flexed at the hip and down on the table, and the involved knee is flexed to 90 degrees and the hip extended. An excessively tight iliotibial band will prevent the affected limb/knee from dropping below the horizontal plane between the two limbs.

(2) **Radiographs.** There are no significant findings.

(3) **Treatment** consists of rest, ice, NSAIDs, and stretching of the iliotibial band. Equipment change (i.e., shoes, bicycle seat) or foot orthotics may be helpful. More resistant cases may require ultrasound treatment or steroid injection. Surgical excision is performed only in the rarest of circumstances.

(4) **Prevention** consists of thorough iliotibial band stretching before activities.

23. BURSITIS AND TENDINITIS

Paul Pellicci and Richard R. McCormack

Bursitis

I. **Anatomic considerations.** A bursa is a closed sac containing a small amount of synovial fluid and lined with a cellular membrane similar to synovium. Bursae are present in areas where tendons and muscles move over bony prominences; they facilitate such motion. Approximately 160 formed bursae are present in the body, and others may form in response to irritative stimuli. Descriptions of the clinically important bursae follow.

   A. **Shoulder**
      1. The **subacromial** bursa lies between the acromion and the rotator cuff.
      2. The **subdeltoid** bursa lies between the deltoid muscle and the rotator cuff.
      3. The **subcoracoid** bursa lies at the attachment of the biceps, coracobrachialis, and pectoralis minor tendons to the coracoid process.

   B. **Elbow**
      1. The **olecranon** bursa lies over the olecranon process.
      2. The **radiohumeral** bursa lies between the common wrist extensor tendon and the lateral epicondyle.

   C. **Hip**
      1. The **iliopsoas** bursa may communicate with the hip joint and lies between the hip capsule and the psoas musculotendinous unit.
      2. The **trochanteric** bursa surrounds the gluteal insertions into the greater trochanter.
      3. The **ischiogluteal** bursa separates the gluteus maximus from the ischial tuberosity.

   D. **Knee**
      1. The **prepatellar** bursa lies between the skin and the patellar tendon.
      2. The **infrapatellar** bursa lies deep to the insertion of the patellar ligament.
      3. The **popliteal** bursae are numerous. The largest lies between the semimembranous muscle and the medial head of the gastrocnemius muscle.

   E. **Foot**
      1. The **Achilles** bursa separates the Achilles tendon insertion from the posterior aspect of the calcaneus.
      2. The **subcalcaneal** bursa is located at the insertion of the plantar fascia into the medial tuberosity of the calcaneus.

II. **Etiology**

   A. **Direct trauma** to a bursal area may lead to an inflammatory response in the bursa of hyperemia and the exudation of fluid and leukocytes into the bursal sac. Bursal fluid can be clear, hemorrhagic, or xanthochromic.

   B. **Chronic overuse or irritation** of a bursal area.

   C. A **systemic disorder,** such as rheumatoid arthritis or gout.

   D. Septic bursitis may occur secondary to **puncture wounds** from trauma or an overlying rash such as psoriasis, a surrounding cellulitis, or after a **local therapeutic injection.** The organisms most frequently responsible are staphylococci (*S. aureus, S. epidermidis*) and streptococci.

III. **Diagnosis**

   A. **Localized pain** is the presenting complaint, with radiation into the involved limb as an occasional feature.

   B. **Swelling** is common in olecranon bursitis but is usually not seen in subdeltoid bursitis.

   C. **Erythema** may be present and does not necessarily indicate sepsis.

   D. **Tenderness** is always present.

   E. Pain is usually elicited when the patient is asked to execute a maneuver that stresses the involved motor unit; for example, abduction of the hip against gravity will cause pain in trochanteric bursitis.

IV. Radiographs may, on occasion, demonstrate deposits of calcium in the region of the bursae. Calcific bursitis and calcific tendinitis may be indistinguishable, both clinically and radiographically.

V. Treatment

A. Rest

1. The region should be immobilized for 7 to 10 days.
2. The patient should be told to discontinue activities that aggravate the symptoms for 1 to 2 weeks.

B. Ice compresses to the acutely inflamed area reduce swelling and provide relief from pain.

C. Antiinflammatory medications

1. For **mild** symptoms, 650 mg of aspirin PO four times daily, either buffered or with food or other NSAIDs.
2. For **moderate** symptoms, 600 mg of ibuprofen PO three times daily with food.
3. For **severe** symptoms, 25 mg of indomethacin PO four times daily with food. This treatment should not be continued for more than 5 to 7 days.

D. Swollen subcutaneous bursae, such as the olecranon bursa, should be **aspirated.** Reaccumulation is common, and it is not unusual for two or three aspirations to be required to resolve the problem. The fluid should be cultured and a crystalline evaluation performed. Incision of the bursa may lead to prolonged drainage or infection and is rarely indicated.

E. Injection of the offending bursa with 3 mL of 1% lidocaine mixed with 40 mg of methylprednisolone acetate (Depo-Medrol) is usually successful in relieving symptoms.

F. Surgery to excise a bursa is rarely necessary. However, if the procedures outlined in **A** through **E** have been repeatedly unsuccessful and the disability is significant, surgery may provide relief.

G. If **infection** is suspected (i.e., red, warm bursa yielding cloudy or purulent fluid associated with a cellulitis and/or fever) the bursa must be aspirated and the fluid smeared for direct Gram's stain and sent for microbiologic culture. Pending results, patients with mild symptoms may be treated as outpatients with 500 mg of dicloxacillin or cefalexin PO four times daily. Patients who demonstrate no improvement or worsening on oral antibiotics with bursal aspirations, have more severe infections or who are markedly symptomatic should be hospitalized and treated with nafcillan or cefalexin IV. In chronic cases refractory to antibiotics, bursectomy may be indicated.

Tendinitis

Tendinitis is a general term used to describe any inflammation associated with a tendon. The inflammation may occur within a substance of the tendon (intratendinous lesion) or be associated with the tenosynovial sheath (tenosynovitis). Because bursae are often located near tendons, the terms tendinitis and bursitis are often used interchangeably to represent the same affliction (see preceding discussion of bursitis). Together, these entities are the most common causes of soft-tissue pain.

I. Pathogenesis

A. Intratendinous lesions occur primarily later in life as the vascularity of the tendon diminishes. They are usually associated with repetitive motion and are felt to represent microtrauma or limited macrotrauma short of rupture within the substance of the tendon. Local signs and symptoms of inflammation are caused by the reparative process of vascular infiltration with acute and chronic cellular responses. During the reparative process, calcium salts, which are visible on radiographs, may be deposited in degenerated portions of the tendon—hence the term calcific tendinitis. Tennis elbow, calcific tendinitis in the supraspinatus, and trochanteric tendinitis are examples of intratendinous lesions.

B. Acute or chronic paratendinous inflammation or tenosynovitis may have several etiologies.

1. **Repetitive motion with injury** is by far the most common etiology. Synovial tendon sheaths are located in areas where tendons pass over bony surfaces and where large tendon excursions are found, most commonly above the wrist and ankle. Repetitive motion causes inflammation with edema and a decrease in the fine tolerances already present in these gliding areas. The result is decreased excursion and painful motion of the affected tendon, often with signs of mechanical blocking, such as may be seen with de Quervain's disease and trigger finger.
2. These paratendinous inflammations may also be triggered by **direct or microtraumatic intratendinous injuries** and result from the reparative process initiated in the tenosynovium.
3. Systemic inflammation disorders such as RA may be associated with prominent tenosynovitis of the hands and feet.
4. Acute tenosynovitis may also be of **septic origin.** Most commonly, this disorder involves a direct wound contaminating the sheath. Alternatively, it may result from a generalized sepsis, especially in a compromised host, and may be multifocal. Neisserial organisms such as gonorrhea typically can cause this type of inflammation. Because vascular supply is poor, infection due to nongonococcal organisms is not well controlled with antibiotics alone, and surgical drainage is usually necessary.

II. Physical examination

A. The classic sign of inflammation within the tendon or tendon sheath is **pain on motion,** especially with passive stretch or contraction of the affected motor tendon unit against resistance.

B. Local **swelling, warmth, and tenderness** are usually present. Tenderness may be palpated along the course of the tendon. On deep structures, such as the supraspinatus or gluteus medius tendons, deep-point tenderness in a specific and reproducible location may be elicited.

C. **Erythema** may or may not be present, depending on the depth of the structure and the acuteness of the process. Because most tendons cross joints, tendinitis must be distinguished from acute **inflammatory or septic arthritis.** In the latter case, range of motion will be more severely restricted. Systemic signs may be present, and capsular tenderness should be distinguished from tenderness directly over the tendon. In doubtful cases, diagnostic arthrocentesis will resolve the matter.

III. Treatment. The treatment of tendinitis is similar to that of bursitis.

A. **Immobilization** is the most important therapy. Methods are as follows:

1. A **splint** or cast for the affected region in the distal upper and lower extremities.
2. A **sling** for lesions of the proximal upper extremity.
3. **Crutches** for lesions of the proximal lower extremity.

B. **Gentle physical therapy** within the limits of pain should be started as the inflammation resolves to avoid permanent stiffness.

C. **Local heat** is helpful in relieving symptoms and in alleviating painful muscle spasm associated with tendinitis. Hot packs, warm soaks, skin counterirritants (e.g., balms, ultrasound), or hot wax treatments are equally effective and should be utilized.

D. **Antiinflammatory medications**

1. **Ibuprofen** may be given in dosages of up to 600 to 800 mg three times per day as needed.
2. **Nonsteroidal antiinflammatory medications** in appropriate doses are used for acute inflammation.
3. **Corticosteroids,** given systemically or locally as injections with a local anesthetic, can also be beneficial in certain cases. The injected area should be cooled with ice for 24 hours after injection, and adequate analgesics should be prescribed to counteract the pain experienced when the local anesthetic wears off. The use of a long-acting local anesthetic such as **bupivacaine** can minimize the pain associated with corticosteroid injection. A suspension of

20 to 40 mg of methylprednisolone acetate is the most frequently used preparation. No more than three weekly injections should be administered. Steroid preparations are contraindicated in the presence of infection.

E. Surgery is the treatment of choice when nonoperative therapy has failed. It involves repair of a degenerative tendon, as in tennis elbow; release of fibroosseous tunnels, as in de Quervain's disease; and tenosynovectomy for chronic wrist tenosynovitis, a common manifestation of rheumatoid arthritis.

III. DIAGNOSIS AND THERAPY

24. ANTIPHOSPHOLIPID ANTIBODY SYNDROME AND LUPUS PREGNANCY

Lisa R. Sammaritano

Antiphospholipid Syndrome

Antiphospholipid antibodies (aPL) are antibodies directed at phospholipids. The aPL family includes anti-cardiolipin antibodies (aCL), lupus anticoagulant (LAC) antibodies, and antibodies causing both true-and false-positive tests for syphilis. Autoimmune aPL are associated with arterial and venous thrombosis, midpregnancy fetal loss, thrombocytopenia, stroke, cardiac valvular disease, and other, less common complications. The aPL syndrome may be seen in patients with systemic lupus erythematosus (SLE) or in otherwise healthy persons (as primary antiphospholipid syndrome, or PAPS). The presence of aPL is necessary but not sufficient for the diagnosis of the aPL syndrome (APS); the syndrome requires the presence of aPL in the setting of typical complications (precise definitions vary).

Wasserman first described a type of aPL in 1906, the "reagin" associated with syphilis. It later became clear that there were biologic false-positive serologic tests for syphilis (BFP-STS) of two types: acute, usually associated with viral or other infections (e.g., tuberculosis, leprosy, endocarditis, malaria), and chronic, often associated with the presence of collagen vascular disease.

The LAC was described by Conley and Hartman in two patients with hemorrhagic complications; later work showed a paradoxical association with thrombosis. The LAC prolongs phospholipid-dependent coagulation steps *in vitro* by competing with coagulation factors for binding to phospholipid. Because of the numerous assays used for diagnosis with varying sensitivities, difficulty with definition of the LAC arose. This lack of standardization, and increasing interest in aPL and the clinical associations, prompted Harris and colleagues in 1983 to develop a solid-phase radioimmunoassay using cardiolipin (CL) as antigen.

I. Immunology

A. **Concordance/discordance of lupus anticoagulant and anti-cardiolipin antibody.** Autoimmune aPL represent a spectrum of autoantibodies including BFP-STS, LAC, and aCL. Although LAC and aCL are often present in the same patients, concordance is only about 80%. This depends partly on the assay used for LAC, which varies widely. The most sensitive assays seem to be the kaolin clotting time (KCT) and the dilute Russell viper venom time (dRVVT). Controversy exists as to which test, LAC or aCL, provides greater predictive value for thrombosis. The presence of both does not seem to confer a greater risk. Antibodies that test positively in both aCL enzyme-linked immunosorbent assay (ELISA) and LAC assay have been purified from patient plasma, but at least two groups have separated such plasma chromatographically into fractions with specific reactivity in one or the other assay. The newly recognized anti-β_2-glycoprotein I (anti–β_2-GPI) antibodies, found in some but not all patients with traditional aPL, may be the most specific marker in predicting risk for complications. BFP-STS alone does not have significant predictive value in non-SLE patients.

B. **Characteristics of antiphospholipid antibodies.** aPL of the immunoglobulin M (IgM), IgG, and IgA isotypes are detected in autoimmune, infectious, and drug-induced conditions; however, only the autoimmune aPL appear to be closely associated with clinical complications. Infection- and drug-induced aPL differ from autoimmune aPL in important antibody characteristics: autoimmune aPL are generally IgG2 subclass and lambda light chain-predominant, have high avidity, and require the presence of a phospholipid-binding protein such as β_2-GPI for binding in routine ELISA. Common infections that may induce aPL include syphilis and a number of transient and chronic viral infections, including those caused by adenovirus, human immunodeficiency virus (HIV), and hepatitis C virus. These infection-induced antibodies show IgG1 and IgG3 subclass and kappa light chain predominance, low avidity, and lack of requirement for a phospholipid-binding protein cofactor. All aPL appear to bind (directly or indirectly) to anionic (negatively charged) phospholipids. β_2-GPI is a requirement for binding of autoimmune but not infection-induced aCL to CL in ELISA. Although the precise function of this protein is not clear, β_2-GPI may function as a natural anticoagulant. The presence of anti–β_2-GPI antibodies has been demonstrated in sera that possess aCL activity, and these antibodies may bind to a cryptic epitope exposed when the protein is bound to negatively charged surfaces. Anti–β_2-GPI antibodies have been suggested to be more specific than aCL in predicting thrombosis. The presence of the IgG2 subclass of both autoimmune aCL and anti–β_2-GPI antibodies has been associated with an increased risk for clinical complications. Infection- and drug-induced aPL, usually not pathogenic, is likely to bind directly to anionic phospholipid without requirement for a serum cofactor.

Animal models of aPL do exist. In MRL/lpr mice (one of several autoimmune strains), high levels of aPL are seen. Other murine models of APS may be induced through passive immunization with purified human aPL IgG, or through active immunization with a monoclonal human aCL; the latter is presumably an anti-idiotype response.

C. Mechanisms of pathogenicity. Any or all of the major components of the clotting system may be involved in aPL pathogenesis, and it is likely that more than one mechanism may be at work, even within the same individual. These components include the coagulation cascade, which contains many phospholipid-dependent steps, and activation of the endothelial cell or platelet. It is clear that β_2-GPI is not the only phospholipid-binding protein involved in aPL binding because convincing evidence exists for prothrombin as a cofactor in some sera with LAC activity. Other potential phospholipid-binding cofactor proteins include thrombomodulin, antithrombin III, protein C, protein S, or other natural anticoagulant proteins, including annexin V. The presence of multiple mechanisms may explain the relative heterogeneity of APS presentations, including the variable involvement of the vascular bed (venous vs. arterial) and the location and timing of thrombosis.

II. Clinical aspects (Table 24-1)

A. Epidemiology of anti-phospholipid antibodies

1. **Prevalence.** aPL are present in 25% to 54% of SLE patients. In the general population, the accepted range is 2% to 4%. Infections such as syphilis, HIV, Lyme disease, and common viral infections may cause transient aPL that are not associated with thrombosis. Drug-induced aPL are not usually associated with complications, although thrombosis has been rarely reported. Common drugs associated with aPL induction include chlorpromazine, procainamide, quinidine, and phenytoin. aPL present in other rheumatic diseases are generally infrequent, of low titer, and not clinically significant.

   Familial occurrence of aPL has been reported. Suggested associations include HLA-DR7 and C4 null allele; however, none of these data are as yet compelling for a strong genetic predisposition. Genetic backgrounds of patients with primary versus secondary (i.e., secondary to SLE) APS may fall into different patterns.

2. **Primary anti-phospholipid antibody syndrome.** As suggested above, not all patients with aPL and associated complications have SLE. PAPS patients may have high-titer aPL with complications similar to those seen with SLE-associated (secondary) aPL. Antinuclear antibody (ANA) is usually negative or low positive (11% to 47%) in PAPS patients, without other serologic abnormalities. The male-to-female ratio in these patients, unlike that in SLE, is close to 1 : 1.

B. Clinical complications

1. **Recurrent thrombotic events** include arterial thrombosis, as in cerebrovascular disease (stroke and transient ischemic attack), peripheral arte-

Table 24-1. Clinical manifestations of antiphospholipid antibody syndrome

1. Arterial occlusion:
   - extremity gangrene
   - stroke
   - myocardial infarction
   - aortic occlusion
   - other visceral infarct
2. Venous occlusion:
   - peripheral venous and pulmonary emboli
   - visceral venous occlusion (e.g., Budd-Chiari syndrome, portal vein)
3. Recurrent fetal loss: recurrent unexplained first trimester or single unexplained second or third trimester fetal loss
4. Hematologic:
   - thrombocytopenia
   - Coombs'-positive hemolytic anemia
   - thrombotic microangiopathic hemolytic anemia
5. Cutaneous:
   - livedo reticularis
   - pyoderma-like leg ulcerations
   - distal digital cyanosis
   - distal gangrene
6. Nonstroke neurologic abnormalities:
   - chorea
   - multiple sclerosis-like syndrome
   - transverse myelitis
   - seizure
   - migraine
7. Renal insufficiency:
   - arterial or venous occlusion
   - microangiopathic glomerular disease
8. Cardiac disease:
   - valvular abnormalities
   - early myocardial infarction
9. Catastrophic APS: sudden multisystem arterial occlusion

APS, antiphospholipid antibody syndrome.

rial disease, and ocular occlusive disease. Venous thrombosis, often recurrent, is frequently accompanied by pulmonary embolism. Pulmonary hypertension has been associated with aPL; this may represent either recurrent pulmonary embolism or small-vessel thrombosis.

Cerebrovascular accident and transient ischemic attack may be recurrent, and may lead to multi-infarct dementia in relatively young patients. The wide spectrum of thrombosis in APS may result in unusual presentations, including gangrene, mesenteric ischemia, adrenal insufficiency, Budd-Chiari syndrome, and occlusive ocular vascular disease. Thrombosis may be acute in onset, affect multiple systems, and be fatal. A marked decrease in aPL titer has been reported in several known aPL-positive patients during fulminant occlusive episodes.

2. **Cutaneous manifestations.** Most common is livedo reticularis, a lattice-like pattern of superficial veins that is strongly associated with aPL in SLE. Other cutaneous manifestations include pyoderma-like leg ulcers, distal digital cyanosis, widespread cutaneous necrosis, and Degos' disease.
3. **Fetal loss** in women with aPL is common; the rate of pregnancy loss in patients with high-titer antibody and a history of prior fetal loss may approach 80% (untreated). Two factors, high-titer IgG aPL and previous fetal loss, are the most sensitive predictors of fetal distress or death. Women with

habitual abortion should be screened for aPL even in the absence of other symptoms or serologies; cross-sectional studies suggest that 13% to 42% will be aPL-positive. Although aPL-related fetal loss is a more significant etiology in the middle and late trimesters, as many as 51% of aPL-associated losses may occur in the first trimester. Placental microthrombosis is the presumed etiology.

Screening for aPL in asymptomatic pregnant women is not indicated. aPL has been suggested as an etiology for a small proportion of infertility cases; recent data from a murine aPL model suggest normal fertilization but impaired implantation and blastocyst development.

4. **Hematologic manifestations** are generally thrombocytopenia and hemolytic anemia which is Coombs'-positive ("Evans' syndrome" when these occur together). IgG aPL has been detected in up to 72% of SLE patients with thrombocytopenia and in 30% of patients with primary autoimmune thrombocytopenia. An association of aPL with microangiopathy has been reported in a number of settings, from severe preeclampsia associated with HELLP syndrome (**h**emolysis, **e**levated **l**iver enzymes, and **l**ow **p**latelets) to a thrombotic microangiopathic hemolytic anemia.
5. **Cardiac disease** is well recognized in APS. An association with valvular heart disease (aortic and mitral insufficiency) is well established and may be severe enough to require valve replacement. Libman-Sacks endocarditis is commonly seen in both aPL-positive SLE and PAPS patients. Coronary artery thrombosis may also represent a significant complication: 21% of young survivors of myocardial infarction have been reported to be aPL-positive.
6. **Neurologic manifestations other than stroke.** Although less common than stroke, transient ischemic attack, multi-infarct dementia, and other neurologic complications may be significant. These include chorea, transverse myelitis, multiple sclerosis-like syndrome, epilepsy, and migraine.
7. **Renal insufficiency** caused by aPL (and not the glomerulonephritis of SLE) has been increasingly recognized. Thrombosis may develop at any location within the renal vasculature, including the renal artery, intrarenal arteries or arterioles, glomerular capillaries, and renal veins. The aPL-associated glomerular disease is strikingly similar in pathologic features to the thrombotic microangiopathy seen in thrombotic thrombocytopenic purpura and usually presents with a decrease in creatinine clearance, proteinuria, and hypertension.
8. **Catastrophic antiphospholipid antibody syndrome** is characterized by multisystem vascular occlusion and often manifested by renal dysfunction with hypertension, central nervous system involvement, respiratory insufficiency with possible adult respiratory distress syndrome (ARDS), and ischemic cutaneous lesions with gangrene.

C. **Treatment options.** aCL, LAC, and BFP-STS are not identical. If the clinical history is supportive of an APS (whether or not the ANA test result is positive), tests for all three should be performed.

1. **Thrombotic events.** Treatment of aPL-associated complications has not been well defined in clinical prospective studies. Retrospective studies suggest that lifelong anticoagulation with warfarin at an international normalized ratio (INR) of 3.0 or greater after a clearly documented thrombotic complication is most likely to prevent recurrent thromboembolic events. Reports suggest an especially high risk for recurrent thrombosis in the 6 months following discontinuation of warfarin. Fulminant multisystem thrombotic episodes have been treated with prednisone, cytotoxic therapy, intravenous immunoglobulin, and plasmapheresis, in addition to anticoagulation, in an effort to suppress or remove antibody. No clear evidence exists as yet to support these therapies.
2. **Recurrent fetal loss.** Treatments for recurrent fetal loss have included prednisone, low-dose (81 mg) aspirin, and heparin, alone or in combination. Although success has been reported with each of these therapies, it is now clear that high-dose prednisone alone worsens fetal outcome and, even in a

more efficacious combination with low-dose aspirin, increases maternal morbidity. The currently recommended treatment for aPL-positive women who have a history of prior fetal loss is 5,000 units of unfractionated heparin administered subcutaneously twice daily with daily low-dose aspirin. This regimen is as effective as low-dose aspirin with higher doses of heparin and more effective than low-dose aspirin alone. If patients fail this regimen, a common next step is the addition of intravenous immunoglobulin, shown to be efficacious with combination therapy in case reports.

3. **Prophylactic treatment.** There is no clear evidence to support the prophylactic treatment of asymptomatic patients with known aPL, although some of these patients, especially those with high titers, will be treated empirically with low-dose aspirin. A change in aPL titer has not been clearly shown to predict a clinical event or remission.

Lupus Pregnancy

SLE is most often diagnosed in women in their childbearing years. Fertility is generally unimpaired unless the patient has been treated with cyclophosphamide or chlorambucil. SLE patients have a high risk for miscarriage or fetal loss, largely because of the presence of aPL. If disease is quiescent for at least 6 months before conception, pregnancy outcome is improved.

I. **Risk for lupus flare.** Early (uncontrolled) studies suggested an increased risk for disease flare during pregnancy and the immediate postpartum period. Recent case-control studies, however, support little or no increased risk for flare during these periods. The definition of lupus flare at any time is not uniform; however, this issue is more complicated in pregnancy because physiologic changes in normal or complicated pregnancy can mimic symptoms of SLE flare. Some standard measures of lupus activity are invalid in the pregnant patient.

Normal pregnancy may be associated with palmar and facial erythema, chloasma gravidarum, anemia, mild thrombocytopenia, edema, and an increased erythrocyte sedimentation rate. Pregnancy-induced toxemia may present with hypertension, renal insufficiency, proteinuria, generalized edema, marked thrombocytopenia, disseminated intravascular coagulation, and seizures. Eclampsia may also be associated with decreased complement levels. Changes felt to represent SLE activity and not pregnancy include an increase in anti–double-stranded DNA antibody level, lymphadenopathy, true lupus rash, inflammatory arthritis, fever, and renal sediment abnormalities of microscopic hematuria with erythrocyte casts.

II. **Antiphospholipid antibody** (Table 24-2). As described in detail in the first section of this chapter, "Antiphospholipid Syndrome," high-titer IgG aPL and history of pregnancy loss are strong predictors of fetal distress or loss in a current pregnancy. Complications of aPL occur independently of clinical SLE activity and do not generally respond to high-dose corticosteroid therapy. Although aCL and LAC antibodies are strongly associated with fetal loss, women with an isolated BFP-STS in the absence of aCL, LAC, or a diagnosis of SLE are not at increased risk for fetal death.

III. **Neonatal outcome** depends on several factors: presence of aPL, presence of anti-Ro/SS-A and anti-La/SS-B auto-antibodies, and current maternal medications. The risk for development of SLE in a child of an SLE mother is small; the risk for positive auto-antibodies in the child is about 10%, and the risk for development of clinical SLE is about 1%.

A. **Antiphospholipid antibodies.** The primary complication of aPL is fetal loss or premature delivery with fetal distress. aPL appear to act on the placenta rather than on the fetus itself, although antibody does cross the placental barrier and several case reports describe thrombotic complications in newborns of aPL-positive mothers. The major risks to the newborn are those of prematurity, which entails pulmonary insufficiency and neurodevelopmental delay. Thrombocytopenia, whether associated with aPL or another etiology, may be found in the fetus if present in the mother. If sampling of fetal scalp blood indicates that the fetus has a low platelet count, delivery is by cesarean section.

Table 24-2. Estimated prevalence of aPL and LAC in various patient populations

	aPL (% positive)	LAC (% positive)
Normal	<2	<1
Normal pregnancy	<2	<2
SLE	30–40	10–20
SLE with livedo	80	n.d.
Non-SLE recurrent fetal death	10–20	10–20
RA	10[a]	<5
HIV	60–90[a]	20–40
Stroke, myocardial infarction <40 years old	10–20	n.d.

SLE, systemic lupus erythematosus; n.d., not done; RA, rheumatoid arthritis; aPL, antiphospholipid antibody; LAC, lupus anticoagulant.
[a] Low titer.
From Sammaritano et al. Antiphospholipid antibody syndrome: immunologic and clinical aspects. *Semin Arthritis Rheum* 1990; 20:81.

B. Anti-Ro/SS-A and anti-La/SS-B antibodies. Offspring of mothers positive for anti-Ro/SS-A and anti-La/SS-B (and very rarely anti-U1RNP) are at risk for **neonatal lupus erythematosus syndrome,** consisting of rash, thrombocytopenia, abnormal results on liver function tests, and congenital heart block. The risk for any manifestation of neonatal lupus erythematosus syndrome in the offspring of a mother positive for anti-Ro/SS-A is about 25%; however, the risk for cardiac involvement with irreversible congenital heart block and myocarditis is significantly smaller, estimated at less than 3%. A specific pattern of reactivity on Western blot may be associated with an increased risk for congenital heart block. Because of the low overall risk for congenital heart block in the offspring of mothers positive for anti-Ro/SS-A, however, prophylactic treatment is not generally indicated. Careful monitoring for fetal bradycardia and echocardiographic abnormalities, especially in the critical gestational period between 20 and 24 weeks, is routine. Treatment of an abnormality with high-dose dexamethasone (which easily crosses the placenta) or even plasmapheresis has been suggested and may be helpful, although no large experience supports this.

C. Maternal medications. Commonly used medications in SLE include aspirin, prednisone, hydroxychloroquine, and immunosuppressive agents such as azathioprine, cyclophosphamide, methotrexate, and, rarely, chlorambucil.

1. **Aspirin.** Commonly prescribed for APS, aspirin has been reported to have adverse hemostatic effects on mother and fetus, including prolonged bleeding at labor and prolonged duration of labor. Premature closure of the ductus arteriosus in the neonate is a theoretical concern, but this complications has not been reported with the low-dose aspirin used in APS therapy.
2. **Heparin.** Limited almost exclusively to aPL pregnancies or to pregnancies of women with prior thrombosis irrespective of aPL status, heparin is generally used for the full 8 to 9 months of gestation. Maternal complications may include excessive bleeding and risk for osteoporosis, although these seem to be less frequent with the newer, low-molecular-weight heparins. Both fractionated and unfractionated heparins are too large to pass through the placenta and so do not reach the fetal circulation.
3. **Prednisone.** Used for SLE activity (and not for aPL prophylaxis), the major risk to the fetus is adrenal insufficiency at birth. Prednisone and prednisolone, unlike some other corticosteroid preparations, are largely metabolized by the placenta with few, if any, fetal effects.
4. **Antimalarial agents.** Data are incomplete, and many rheumatologists will discontinue these medications during pregnancy because of theoretical risks for ear and eye toxicity. Some small series of lupus patients main-

Table 24-3. Valid and invalid measures of lupus activation in the pregnant patient

Valid measures	Invalid measures
Inflammatory arthritis	Arthralgia, bland joint effusion
True lupus rash	Palmar or facial erythema
High anti–ds-DNA antibody titers	Hypocomplementemia
Microhematuria, RBC casts	Proteinuria
Fever	Elevated ESR
Mucosal ulcers	Thrombocytopenia
Lymphadenopathy	AC, aCL levels

ds-DNA, double-stranded DNA; RBC, red blood cell; ESR, erythrocyte sedimentation rate; LAC, lupus anticoagulant; aCL, anticardiolipin antibody.
From Lockshin MD et al. Pregnancy in systemic lupus erythematosus. *Clin Exp Rheumatol* 1989;S3:S195.

tained on hydroxychloroquine throughout pregnancy have shown no adverse effects. There may be a risk for flare associated with discontinuation before pregnancy.

5. **Cytotoxic agents.** Chlorambucil, cyclophosphamide, and methotrexate are known teratogens; the safety of azathioprine during pregnancy is uncertain, although it is continued in many patients, especially in the renal transplant population, with few reported complications.

IV. **Evaluation and management of the lupus pregnancy** (Table 24-3). Both the rheumatologist and an experienced, high-risk obstetrician should participate in the evaluation and management of these patients.

A. **Initial evaluation.** Assessment of disease activity, review of current medications, and discussion with the patient and her partner of specific risks as outlined above.

B. **Laboratory evaluation.** Complete blood count with platelet count, biochemical profile with blood urea nitrogen and creatinine, urinalysis, 24-hour urine for creatinine clearance and total protein, aPL (including both aCL and LAC assays), and anti-Ro/SS-A and anti-La/SS-B antibodies. Regular (monthly) follow-up of each of these is helpful, with the exception of the aPL and the anti-Ro/SS-A and anti-La/SS-B antibodies. Complement levels are sometimes but not always helpful; erythrocyte sedimentation rate is generally not useful in monitoring disease activity.

C. **Fetal monitoring.** Antepartum testing of the fetal heart rate ("non-stress test") is usually initiated at about 26 weeks because abnormal findings on this test may precede a decrease in fetal movement by several weeks. If fetal distress is noted and the fetus is considered viable, early delivery may prevent fetal death. Doppler studies may be similarly useful. Fetal echocardiography, generally at weeks 20 through 24, should be performed in mothers positive for anti-Ro/SS-A and anti-La/SS-B antibodies.

Bibliography

Asherson RA, et al., eds. *The antiphospholipid syndrome.* Boca Raton, FL: CRC Press, 1996.

Harris EN, et al. Anticardiolipin antibodies: detection by radioimmunoassay and association with thrombosis in systemic lupus erythematosus. *Lancet* 1983;3:1211.

Lockshin MD, et al. Pregnancy in systemic lupus erythematosus. *Clin Exp Rheumatol* 1989;S3:S195.

Lockshin MD, Sammaritano LR, Schwartzman S. Pregnancy and SLE. In: Lahita R, ed. *Systemic lupus erythematosus,* 3rd ed. Briarcliff Manor, NY: Hermitage Publishing, 1998.

Sammaritano LR, et al. Antiphospholipid antibody syndrome: immunologic and clinical aspects. *Semin Arthritis Rheum* 1990;20:81.

Sammaritano LR. Update: antiphospholipid antibodies. *JCR J Clin Rheumatol* 1997; 3:270.

25. CHILDHOOD RHEUMATIC DISEASES

Thomas J. A. Lehman

I. Etiology and pathogenesis. The rheumatic diseases of childhood represent a diverse group. Their etiologies are varied and their pathogenesis unclear. Lyme disease and acute rheumatic fever result from exposure to known infectious agents, but the majority of childhood rheumatic diseases result from the combination of genetic predisposition, "autoimmunity," and unknown environmental factors.

II. Prevalence. Reactive arthritis (acute episodes of arthritis and arthralgia following an infectious illness) is common in childhood, but chronic rheumatic disease is infrequent. Nonetheless, there are more than 250,000 children with arthritis in the United States. [Prevalence estimates are confused between the number of children with juvenile rheumatoid arthritis (100,000) and the number of children with any form of arthritis (250,000).] This dichotomy is responsible for an ongoing process of redefinition. The term juvenile rheumatiod arthritis (JRA) is being discarded. It is to be replaced by idiopathic childhood arthritis (ICA). At present, eight distinct subtypes of ICA have been described, and it is expected that more subtypes will be delineated before the full redefinition is completed. With this new definition, the spondyloarthropathies and many other subtypes that currently fall outside the spectrum of JRA will be included in ICA. Spondyloarthropathies, for example, will be termed enthesitis-associated arthritis, which will be a subtype of ICA.

ICA (including what was previously termed JRA and spondyloarthropathies), Henoch-Schönlein purpura, Kawasaki disease, systemic lupus erythematosus (SLE), dermatomyositis, and scleroderma are the most common forms of chronic arthritis in childhood.

III. Differential diagnosis. A careful history and physical examination are key to the proper diagnosis of childhood arthritis. The examining physician must have a clear knowledge of the differential diagnosis because children are often poor historians. A useful algorithm is illustrated in Table 25-1. The examining physician must determine whether inflammation is present (objective pain, swelling, warmth, or limitation of motion), whether the inflammation is articular or periarticular, and whether the inflammation is acute or chronic.

A. No inflammation present

1. **Growing pains.** This is the most common and most misused diagnosis for musculoskeletal pain in childhood. The true syndrome of "growing pains" occurs in young children, peaking at 4 to 5 years of age. The pain classically occurs in the popliteal fossa. It is relieved by gentle massage or reassurance and occurs *only* at night. Pain during the day does not represent growing pains. Growing pains are benign and self-limited. Often, there is a family history of similar complaints, which may aid in the diagnosis. Growing pains are typically relieved by acetaminophen and do not require specific therapy.
2. **Psychogenic rheumatism.** Joint pains and fatigue occur frequently as "somatization" disorders. The child who is unable to attend school or participate in normal activities despite an unremarkable physical and laboratory evaluation is worrisome. Some will respond to gentle reassurance, but for others, the complaints mask a significant psychological disorder. Children with persistent complaints despite normal findings should be evaluated carefully by an experienced pediatric rheumatologist to exclude undiagnosed illness. However, once this has been completed, the physician should be aware that the complaints may stem from problems within the family. These families are "troubled" but usually reject an immediate recommendation of psychological counseling. However, physicians who

Table 25-1. Common forms of chronic synovitis in childhood

I. **Idiopathic childhood arthritis-ICA** (previously Juvenile Rheumatoid Arthritis, JRA)
   - A. **Oligoarticular-onset ICA** (typically 2- to 5-year-old girls with fewer than four joints involved *at onset.* Note: Children with a family history of psoriasis, a positive RF, or enthesitis are automatically excluded from this category.
      1. ANA-positive with high risk for iridocyclitis
      2. ANA-negative
      3. Extended oligoarticular-onset-fewer than four joints at onset with progression later
   - B. **Polyarticular-onset ICA**
      1. RF-negative with at least five joints involved during the first 6 months
      2. RF-positive on at least two occasions 3 months apart. Adolescent girls with typical adult-type RA
   - C. **Systemic-onset ICA**
      1. Definite-quotidian fever for at least 2 weeks, evanescent rash and arthritis
      2. Probable-quotidian fever for at least 2 weeks, evanescent rash and any two of generalized lymphadenopathy, hepatomegaly or splenomegaly, or serositis

II. **Spondyloarthropathies-enthesitis-associated arthritis.** Arthritis and enthesitis or arthritis plus two of the following: SI joint tenderness; HLA-B27; uveitis; inflammatory spinal pain; family history of either uveitis; spondyloarthropathy, or inflammatory bowel disease.
   - A. Ankylosing spondylitis (AS).
   - B. Juvenile Spondyloarthropathy
   - C. Reiter's syndrome/Reactive Arthritis—full combination of arthritis, urethritis and conjunctivitis occurs infrequently in childhood
   - D. Psoriatic arthritis-subset with psoriasis-associated ICA-dactylitis, asymmetric joint inflammation and typical skin lesions or a family history of psoriasis (first or second degree relative)
   - E. Inflammatory bowel disease

III. **Arthritis associated with primarily vasculitic conditions**
   - A. Systemic Lupus Erythematosus
   - B. Dermatomyositis
   - C. Kawasaki disease involving small joints
   - D. Sarcoidosis
   - E. Henoch-Schönlein Purpura

IV. **Miscellaneous**
   - A. Plant thorn synovitis (typically 1 to 5 years old)
   - B. Benign hypermobile joint syndrome
   - C. Immunization-associated arthritis
   - D. Arthritis associated with immunoglobulin deficiency
   - E. Linear Scleroderma

V. **Arthritis associated with metabolic and inherited conditions in childhood**
   - A. Marfan syndrome
   - B. Ehlers-Danlos syndrome
   - C. Cystic Fibrosis

establish a trusting relationship with the family may be able to bring about gradual resolution or an acceptance of the need for psychological intervention.

3. **Reflex neurovascular dystrophy** represents an extension of psychogenic rheumatism in which the somatization has progressed to include hyperesthesias, often with mottled skin coloring and vascular instability. The condition often begins with a well-documented injury that fails to improve. The syndrome typically occurs in "perfect" children under excessive parental pressure. Any psychological stress may initiate this syndrome. Excessive pressure to perform and sexual abuse are well-recognized causes. Although the specific complaints may be resolved with intensive physical and occupational therapy, failure to resolve the underlying psychological issues often results in recurrence of similar problems within a short time period.

B. **Periarticular inflammation.** Children with periarticular (i.e., soft tissue, tendon, ligamentous bursal) inflammation must be carefully evaluated for osseous disorders.

1. **Orthopedic disorders.** Acute periarticular pain may result from a stress fracture or osteomyelitis. Small children with fractures may not report trauma. Battering must be considered when a child presents with unsuspected fractures. Bone scan may be helpful in the evaluation of these entities.
2. **Neoplastic disorders** associated with infiltration of the bone marrow include leukemia, lymphoma, and neuroblastoma. All may present with difficulty walking or "joint pains." Disproportionate anemia, thrombocytopenia, hyperuricemia, lymphadenopathy, or hepatosplenomegaly should prompt further investigation and bone marrow aspiration.
3. **Rheumatic disorders.** The juvenile spondyloarthropathies often present with both periarticular and articular inflammation. The periarticular manifestations may predominate, but articular inflammation is usually present. Lumbar stiffness, enthesitis, and heel pain should be specifically sought. Often, these children are thought to have recurrent sprains or strains. The possibility of arthritis is often incorrectly dismissed by inexperienced physicians because the erythrocyte sedimentation rate (ESR) is normal.

C. **Articular inflammation.** Children with true articular inflammation must be subdivided according to whether they have inflammation that is acute or chronic (of more than 3 months' duration).

1. **Acute articular inflammation**

a. **Infection.** An acutely inflamed joint must be considered septic until proved otherwise. Staphylococci, streptococci, and *Haemophilus influenzae* are frequent causes of septic arthritis in childhood. Lyme disease is a frequent infectious arthritis in areas where *Ixodes* ticks are endemic.

Septic arthritis typically presents with a single inflamed joint accompanied by fever and an elevated ESR. It is less common but not impossible for other infectious agents to involve multiple joints. Not infrequently, Lyme disease may involve several joints simultaneously.

b. **Reactive arthritis** may accompany or follow bacterial, viral, or fungal infection. Toxic synovitis is the most common reactive arthritis in childhood. The typical child with toxic synovitis is 3 to 5 years of age. Classically, they have been well except, perhaps, for symptoms of an upper respiratory infection the prior evening. The following morning, the child awakens unable to walk, with a decreased range of motion in one hip. There is only low-grade or no fever, without significant elevation of the white blood cell count or ESR. Unless an experienced physician is comfortable with the clinical picture, the joint must be aspirated to rule out bacterial infection. The joint symptoms of a child with toxic synovitis typically begin to improve within a few hours; in contrast, those of a child with a truly septic hip often rapidly worsen.

c. **Post-streptococcal reactive arthritis** deserves special consideration. This disorder is not classified as acute rheumatic fever because it does not fulfill two of Jones' major criteria. Nonetheless, children with arthritis and elevated ESRs following a documented streptococcal infection should receive rheumatic fever prophylaxis. Cardiac damage has been recorded with subsequent streptococcal infections in some children who did not receive such long-term prophylaxis.

d. **Acute expression of a collagen vascular disease.** Serum sickness, acute rheumatic fever, Henoch-Schönlein purpura, and the "chronic" collagen vascular diseases (e.g., SLE) may present with acute arthritis. Most are discussed elsewhere in this manual; only those that are unique to childhood or that have unique manifestations in children are discussed in this chapter.

2. **Chronic articular inflammation**

a. **Infection.** Chronicity does not exclude infection. Tuberculosis is a frequent cause of smoldering septic arthritis, but other bacterial infections, including staphylococcal arthritis, may present with such a clinical picture. Additionally, physicians must remain aware that in children with known collagen vascular disease, especially those on immunosuppressive drugs, complicating septic arthritis or osteomyelitis may develop.

b. **Collagen vascular diseases.** All the chronic collagen vascular diseases may occur in children. Most are discussed elsewhere.

IV. **Diseases with unique manifestations in childhood**

A. **Idiopathic childhood arthritis (previously called juvenile rheumatoid arthritis).** As noted above, ICA is replacing the term JRA. Although many will be confused by this new term, it should be appreciated that its use has arisen because of the many children with arthritis who do not fulfill the classic criteria for JRA. ICA is used to describe any noninfectious or traumatic arthritis in childhood. There are currently eight recognized subtypes, and it is expected that there will be more. It should be appreciated that ICA is an umbrella term and does not refer to a "specific" disease. Each subtype of ICA is distinct, most likely with a distinct etiology, pathogenesis, prognosis, and optimal therapy. Because the subtypes represent different diseases, it is very important that the subtypes be properly differentiated from one another. Oligoarticular onset (four or fewer joints involved) and polyarticular onset are defined on the basis of the number of joints involved *during the first 6 months after disease onset—not the number of joints involved at the time the child is first seen by the physician.*

1. **Oligoarticular-onset ICA** involves four or fewer joints. It most commonly occurs in young girls but may affect persons of either sex. This group is divided between the subset that is antinuclear antibody (ANA)-positive and at greater risk for complicating eye disease (iridocyclitis) and the subset that is ANA-negative. Young girls with early involvement of small joints (i.e., finger and toe joints) are at high risk for progression to polyarticular involvement and have a poor prognosis. The condition of a child who has fewer than four joints involved during the first 6 months of disease, but who progresses to have more than four involved joints later, is termed extended oligoarticular disease in the new nomenclature.

Some children have "sausage digits" and probably "psoriasis-associated arthritis" (psoriatic arthritis *sine* psoriasis). Children with a close family history of psoriasis or "nail pitting" may be differentiated as having psoriasis-associated arthritis. However, other children, who have neither a family history of psoriasis nor nail lesions, have arthritis with an identical appearance.

Adolescents with involvement of four or fewer large joints are more likely to have a spondyloarthropathy (now called enthesitis-associated arthritis) (see section **IV.B**).

2. **Polyarticular-onset idiopathic childhood arthritis** has at least two distinct subtypes. Rheumatoid factor (RF)-positive adolescent girls have typical adult-type RA. Young children with polyarticular ICA are typically RF-negative. Both of these entities carry a guarded prognosis. Some chil-

dren previously labeled as having polyarticular ICA may in fact have the psoriasis-associated subtype of ICA.

3. **Systemic-onset idiopathic childhood arthritis** presents with high spiking fever, rash, and variable joint involvement. It occurs with a more equal sex ratio than the other forms of ICA, which have a female predominance. Children with systemic-onset ICA are striking for their ill appearance during episodes of fever, with a relatively benign appearance between episodes. The fleeting salmon pink rash and a temperature that falls to normal or below at least once each day are characteristic. Although many children with systemic-onset ICA do well, significant internal organ involvement develops in others, or they progress to chronic destructive arthritis.

B. **Spondyloarthropathies.** The spondyloarthropathies, occurring in both male and female patients, are now defined as enthesitis-associated arthritis. Their hallmark is asymmetric large-joint arthritis associated with limited lumbar flexion and tenosynovitis. These children are ANA-and RF-negative. They are at risk for acute, painful iritis but in general not chronic iridocyclitis. HLA-B27 is present in about half of these children.

1. **Ankylosing spondylitis (AS)** is the "classic" spondyloarthropathy. It occurs predominantly in male patients positive for HLA-B27 who have limited lumbar flexion. Because definite AS cannot be diagnosed in the absence of radiographic sacroiliitis, many children who are "suspect" fail to fulfill the diagnostic criteria. These children should be given a diagnosis of juvenile spondyloarthropathy.
2. **Juvenile spondyloarthropathy (seronegative enthesopathy/arthropathy syndrome).** These are children with asymmetric large-joint arthritis and enthesopathic findings who do not meet the criteria for AS. They are easily differentiated from patients with other forms of ICA by their later age at onset (usually age 10 or older), the early presence of back or hip involvement, and the frequent occurrence of asymmetric metatarsal joint pain or Achilles tendinitis. Although many of these patients are boys positive for HLA-B27, girls and HLA-B27–negative persons of either sex may also be affected. It was initially thought that classic AS would develop in most of the boys when they reached adulthood. It is presently thought that significant disease will develop in many of the HLA-B27–positive boys, but in only a small percentage of the others.
3. **Reiter's syndrome.** The full combination of arthritis, urethritis, and conjunctivitis occurs infrequently in childhood. When it does, its manifestations are the same as in adults. It is not important to differentiate children with "incomplete" Reiter's syndrome from others with juvenile spondyloarthropathy because the therapy and prognosis are similar.
4. **Psoriatic arthritis/"psoriasiform" arthritis, subset with psoriasis-associated idiopathic childhood arthritis.** True psoriatic arthritis with typical skin lesions and bony changes is infrequent in childhood. However, a subgroup of children without psoriatic skin changes present with asymmetric dactylitis (sausage digits), a family history of psoriasis in a first-or second-degree relative, and variable degrees of asymmetric joint inflammation. In contrast to the other spondyloarthropathies, this constellation of findings affects not only adolescents but also young girls who would otherwise be labeled as having oligoarticular ICA. The proper nomenclature for this group is currently psoriasis-associated ICA.
5. **Inflammatory bowel disease.** The arthritis accompanying inflammatory bowel disease is expressed as a typical spondyloarthropathy. Because arthritis may be the initial manifestation of inflammatory bowel disease, any child with a spondyloarthropathy in whom chronic or recurrent abdominal pain or persistent unexplained anemia develops should be carefully evaluated for the presence of Crohn's disease or ulcerative colitis.

V. **Miscellaneous conditions.** Several forms of arthritis that occur predominantly in children are not easily characterized. Recognition of these conditions is important to prevent their being confused with more serious entities and ensure proper therapy and counseling.

A. **Plant thorn synovitis** results from retention of a fragment of plant material within the joint following a puncture injury. When the injury is recalled and the condition suspected, it is easily diagnosed. Confusion arises when a small child falls and the parents are unaware that foreign matter may have entered the joint. The onset of joint swelling and limitation is usually delayed by 4 to 6 weeks. The arthritis is often quite painful and unresponsive to normal measures. The proper diagnosis is often made following surgical biopsy of patients with intractable synovitis. The pathologic specimen reveals plant fibers under polarized light microscopy. Synovectomy is the treatment of choice.

B. **Benign hypermobile joint syndrome** typically occurs in girls during or just before early adolescence. They are most often gymnasts who practice extensively and have great flexibility that can be attributed to marked ligamentous laxity. As a result of their athletic activities and ligamentous laxity, their joints are subjected to repeated episodes of "microtrauma." Acute episodes may be treated with nonsteroidal antiinflammatory drugs (NSAIDs), but more prolonged difficulty should prompt review of the athletic program. Osteochondritis dissecans (particularly of the knee) may present in this group of patients. In rare cases, children who have continued their activities despite chronic pain have suffered permanent disability.

C. **Immunization-associated arthritis.** The development of a benign polyarthritis affecting primarily the small joints of the hands 10 to 14 days following rubella immunization is well documented. The arthritis is typically mild and resolves during 7 to 10 days with only symptomatic therapy. Similar episodes have been reported less frequently with other viral immunizations.

D. **Arthritis associated with immunoglobulin deficiency.** Children with IgA deficiency are most often asymptomatic, but this immunodeficiency occurs with a greater than expected frequency in populations of children with arthritis. The arthritis commonly consists of benign recurrent joint effusions; however, some children present with typical erosive ICA. A benign arthritis may also occur in children with mild transient hypogammaglobulinemia. This arthritis may recur with viral infections, but ultimately it resolves as the child's immune system matures and the immunoglobulin levels normalize. IgA deficiency will be detected only if quantitative immunoglobulins are routinely measured. Pan-hypogammaglobulinemia may be suspected if the total protein is decreased with a normal serum albumin.

E. **Linear scleroderma** occurring in childhood is a gradually progressive, bandlike tightening of the skin that may occur over the face, trunk, or an extremity. It typically does not cross the midline. There may be progressive loss of underlying muscle and bony tissue with markedly disturbed growth when a limb is involved in a young child. Findings on laboratory evaluation are usually entirely normal. Physical therapy may be beneficial, but surgical intervention is required in extreme cases. Medical therapy with low-dose methotrexate has been beneficial for more severe cases in which the skin involvement crosses a joint line, but its efficacy remains anecdotal.

F. **Linear scleroderma *en coup de sabre*.** This entity is a variant of linear scleroderma characterized by primary involvement of one side of the scalp. It is incompletely differentiated from the Parry-Romberg syndrome of progressive facial hemiatrophy. Recognition of Parry-Romberg syndrome is important because affected children may be afflicted with neurologic disorders, including learning disability and seizures—findings that are not normally associated with linear scleroderma.

VI. **Arthritis associated with primarily vasculitic conditions.** Arthritis is a well-recognized complication of many forms of vasculitis that occur in childhood, including SLE, Wegener's granulomatosis, Takayasu's arteritis, and Henoch-Schönlein purpura. These diseases are not unique to childhood and are discussed elsewhere.

Kawasaki disease and juvenile-onset dermatomyositis are vasculitic diseases with unique manifestations in childhood.

A. **Kawasaki disease** typically affects children in the first 5 years of life. It presents with fever accompanied by a pleiomorphic rash, conjunctivitis, and cervical adenopathy. As the disease progresses, changes in the oral mucosa become evident, with dryness and cracking of the lips. Indurative edema of the hands and feet followed by peeling of the skin from the tips of the fingers or toes (but sometimes beginning in the perineal region) is characteristic. An acute arthritis may accompany the disease, but most often there is diffuse swelling of the hands or feet. Marked elevations of the ESR, white blood cell count, and platelet count evolve during the first 10 days of illness. Prompt recognition and echocardiographic evaluation are desirable. Untreated Kawasaki disease is associated with a 1% to 3% mortality rate caused by aneurysmal dilatation of the coronary arteries with subsequent thrombosis and myocardial infarction. The illness should be suspected whenever the characteristic findings are present. Early intervention with large doses of intravenous gamma globulin has been shown to decrease the frequency of aneurysms and improve outcome. For children who fail to respond after two courses of intravenous gamma globulin, the diagnosis should be reevaluated and consideration given to corticosteroid therapy.

B. **Childhood-onset dermatomyositis** most often presents with the gradual onset of weakness and fatigue but may have an explosive onset with fever, weakness, and vascular collapse. A heliotropic rash, although not always present, is characteristic of the disease. Childhood-onset dermatomyositis is divided into three subtypes.

1. **Unicyclic disease** usually presents with the gradual onset of proximal muscle weakness, responds well to prednisone, and disappears completely within 1 year.
2. **Polycyclic disease** is similar to unicyclic disease but recurs whenever the corticosteroids are tapered. It may be associated with a poor prognosis secondary to chronic skin manifestations, subcutaneous calcification, or vasculitic involvement of internal organs.
3. A third form of childhood dermatomyositis consists of prominent skin manifestations and muscle enzyme elevation in children who are not strikingly weak. These children often have persistent vasculitis. Children with any evidence of dysphonia or cough when eating are at high risk for aspiration.

VII. **Arthritis associated with metabolic and inherited conditions in childhood.** Many inherited disorders, such as hemophilia, sickle cell disease, mucopolysaccharidoses, sphinoglipidoses, and epiphyseal dysplasias, may present with arthritis or periarticular pain in childhood. Characteristic nonarticular manifestations usually predominate.

A. **Marfan syndrome.** Children with Marfan syndrome characteristically are tall with arachnodactyly. They typically exhibit ligamentous laxity and present with complaints similar to those of the hypermobile joint syndrome. Characteristic findings are an arm span greater than the height and a leg length greater than trunk length. Recognition is important because these children are vulnerable to dissecting aortic aneurysms. Aortic root dilatation may be evaluated by routine echocardiography.

B. **Ehlers-Danlos syndrome.** Children with Ehlers-Danlos syndrome suffer from an extreme form of joint hypermobility associated with abnormal connective tissue. Recurrent joint injury secondary to chronic subluxation is common. In typical cases, marked cutaneous laxity is present with characteristic "cigarette paper" scarring. However, milder cases that lack the cutaneous manifestations occur.

C. **Cystic fibrosis** in childhood will be recognized by the pulmonary and gastrointestinal manifestations. Occasionally, however, benign effusions of the large joints or immune complex-related synovitis develops in these patients, which will prompt rheumatologic referral. Hypertrophic osteoarthropathy may also occur in children with cystic fibrosis.

VIII. **Treatment**

A. **Nonsteroidal antiinflammatory drugs** are the first-line agents of choice for children with chronic synovitis. Although these drugs are often criticized because they are not "disease-modifying agents," this criticism is unjustified. NSAIDs directly modify disease outcome by reducing pain and inflammation. As a result of decreased pain and inflammation, the patient is better able to preserve strength, range of motion, and endurance, which in turn preserve function. Preservation of function has a definite positive impact on outcome. Thus, NSAIDs definitely are disease-modifying agents, but they are not remission-inducing agents.

1. **Aspirin** remains the nominal drug of first choice because of its cost advantages, but it has been supplanted by naproxen and tolmetin in many centers because of less frequent dosing and reduced risk for both hepatotoxicity and Reye's syndrome. The dosage schedules and pharmacologic characteristics of the NSAIDs are discussed in Appendix E.
2. **Indomethacin** deserves special mention in childhood because it was regarded as unsafe for children under 12 years of age for many years. This restriction has been removed from recent issues of the Physicians' Desk Reference. Indomethacin is a potent NSAID that is very effective for childhood rheumatic diseases. It is frequently effective in children with severe, systemic-onset ICA or spondyloarthropathies that have not responded to other NSAIDs. Care must be taken in its use because of potential hepatotoxicity and gastric irritation. Headaches are a frequent side effect during the initial stages of therapy but usually respond to symptomatic therapy. The accepted dosage in childhood is 1 to 3 mg/kg daily.

B. **Slow-acting antirheumatic drugs (SAARDs)** provide useful adjunctive therapy in children with chronic rheumatic disease.

1. **Gold salts.** There is an extensive literature regarding the long- and short-term efficacy of gold salts. Although the patient must be monitored carefully for evidence of toxicity, injectable gold salts (aurothioglucose and gold sodium thiomalate) are highly effective for children with specific subtypes of ICA. The accepted dosage of injectable gold salts in childhood is 1 mg/kg weekly after initial evaluation of the response to a series of gradually increasing "test doses."
2. **Auranofin** has been demonstrated to be effective in JRA but is less effective than injectable gold salts, which are preferred.
3. **Methotrexate** is frequently used in the therapy of childhood rheumatic disease. The short-term effectiveness of methotrexate is quite good, but it is difficult to wean patients from this agent. Long-term studies of efficacy and toxicity in childhood have not been completed. The accepted dosage regimen for methotrexate in childhood is 10 mg/M^2 per week up to a maximum of 20 mg/M^2 per week. Hematologic toxicity and hepatic toxicity require close monitoring. The long-term risks for hepatic cirrhosis or pulmonary fibrosis in childhood appear low. The major concern with methotrexate therapy is that in up to 50% of children, the disease flares when the methotrexate is withdrawn. Furthermore, a significant subset of these children does not improve when the methotrexate is reinstituted.
4. **Hydroxychloroquine (Plaquenil)** has been used with success in children with chronic arthritis. However, the onset of efficacy is extremely slow. The accepted dosage regimen is 7 mg/kg daily up to 200 mg/day. Children receiving Plaquenil require ophthalmologic examinations every 6 months to monitor for evidence of retinal toxicity.
5. **Enternacept (Enbrel),** a recombinant tumor necrosis factor-alpha blocker, has recently become available for use in children with severe arthritis. Early results have been extremely promising in children with systemic-onset disease. Administered at a dose of 0.4 mg/kg as a subcutaneous injection twice weekly, Enbrel has not been associated with significant toxicity. At present, long-term efficacy and toxicity are unknown, and the drug is being used primarily in those who have not responded adequately to methotrexate. The full potential and proper utilization of Enbrel in childhood should become apparent within the next few years.

C. Surgery. Replacement of severely damaged and painful hip, knee, and elbow joints is now routinely performed in adolescents at larger orthopedic centers. For younger and smaller patients, the procedures require a center with extensive surgical expertise, the ability to manufacture custom prostheses, and extensive rehabilitation facilities. Although there is a risk that further replacements may be required in the future, the physical and psychological benefits of maintaining independent function throughout adolescence far outweigh the risks associated with the potential need for subsequent surgery. Soft-tissue releases and synovectomies have been performed on many children with ICA. The loss of function associated with postoperative pain and loss of strength that accompanies these procedures generally outweigh the transient gains in alignment and range of motion. However, the ability to perform arthroscopic synovectomy has led to renewed interest in this technique.

D. Physical and occupational therapy are vital components of the care of children with rheumatic disease. Appropriate exercises to maintain strength and range of motion coupled with splinting to maintain proper alignment are important to the ultimate outcome.

E. Family support remains a major component of the overall program of care for children with chronic disease. The primary burden of family support may be carried by social workers, nurse clinicians, or psychologists in different institutions. Each group has different strengths to bring to these families, and optimally all will be available for the families. The presence of a child with chronic disease in the family creates profound stress in even the "best-adjusted" families. A program of care that does not provide for the emotional needs of the affected child's parents and siblings may result in profound psychological scarring.

F. Ophthalmologic evaluation. The ophthalmologist is a major participant in the care of children with rheumatic disease. All children with JRA are at risk for the development of iridocyclitis. Those with ANA-positive pauciarticular onset require slit-lamp evaluation every 4 months, and those who are ANA-negative should be checked every 6 months.

Bibliography

Cassidy JT, Petty RE. *Textbook of pediatric rheumatology,* 3rd ed. New York: Churchill Livingstone, 1994.

Hicks RV. *Vasculopathies of childhood.* Littleton, MA: PSG, 1988.

Southwood TR. Classifying childhood arthritis. *Ann Rheum Dis* 1997;56:79.

26. POLYMYALGIA RHEUMATICA AND TEMPORAL ARTERITIS

Richard Stern

Polymyalgia Rheumatica

Polymyalgia rheumatica (PMR) is a descriptive term that was first suggested by Barber in 1957 to denote a syndrome of aching, usually in elderly patients with an elevated erythrocyte sedimentation rate (ESR), that could not be attributed to more defined rheumatic, infectious, or neoplastic disorders.

PMR is estimated to affect approximately 1 in 1,000 persons in the U.S. population over 50 years of age. Sixty percent of the patients are female. Most patients present after their fiftieth year, and the peak incidence is between ages 60 and 80. However, there are well-documented reports of PMR (usually in association with temporal arteritis) in patients in their forties. Rarely, cases have been observed in younger patients.

I. Clinical presentation

A. Proximal myalgias. PMR is characterized by chronic, symmetric aching and stiffness of the proximal muscles. These symptoms are most prominent in the shoulder and pelvic girdles and neck, but distal muscle groups may also be involved. Aching and stiffness are worse in the morning and on exertion and may be severe and incapacitating. Muscles may be tender; disuse may lead to atrophy, and contractures occasionally may develop. Muscle strength is often difficult to evaluate because pain is present; however, it should be normal.

B. Constitutional symptoms. Patients with PMR frequently complain of malaise and fatigue. Fever is usually low-grade, but temperature may occasionally reach 102°F. Night sweats may occur. PMR may rarely present as a fever of unknown origin. Anorexia and weight loss may be prominent features and suggest malignancy; however, no direct association of PMR with neoplastic disease has been proven.

C. Neuropsychiatric manifestations, such as depression, dementia, acute disorientation, and amnesia (without focal neurologic disease), may be seen and occasionally are the presenting manifestations of PMR.

D. Joints. The majority of patients have poorly localized tenderness over their joints, especially prominent over the shoulders and hips. The original description of the syndrome excluded synovitis as a feature, but moderate bland effusions can be seen in the knees and occasionally other joints, such as the wrists. Carpal tunnel syndrome has also been noted. The presence of synovitis may make differentiation from rheumatoid arthritis difficult. Interpretation of radionuclide scans has suggested the presence of synovitis in proximal joints.

E. Temporal (cranial) arteritis (TA). A detailed discussion of this syndrome and its relationship to PMR can be found in the second section of this chapter.

The incidence of association of the two syndromes is a subject of controversy; however, in some series, 30% to 50% of patients with PMR have had TA, and 60% to 70% of patients with TA have had PMR.

II. Laboratory studies

A. Blood studies

1. An elevated **Westergren sedimentation rate** is the laboratory hallmark of PMR; it is usually in excess of 50 mm/h and may exceed 100 mm/h.
2. **Normocytic normochromic anemia** is seen in approximately 50% of patients.
3. **Immunologic studies.** The frequency of rheumatoid factors, antinuclear antibodies, and other autoreactive antibodies is not higher than that of age-matched controls.
4. **Muscle enzyme levels** (creatine kinase, serum glutamic-oxaloacetic transaminase, lactic dehydrogenase, aldolase) are normal.

B. Radiographic findings are nonspecific, although erosive lesions in the symphysis pubis and the acromioclavicular and sacroiliac joints have been observed.

C. **Electromyographic findings** are within normal limits.
D. **Muscle biopsy histology** is nondiagnostic; type 2 muscle fiber atrophy probably represents disuse.
E. **Synovial fluid and tissue studies**
   1. **Leukocyte counts** in joint fluid range between 1,000 and 8,000, with a preponderance of lymphocytes.
   2. **Synovial biopsy specimens,** when available, reveal mild synovial proliferation with slight lymphocyte infiltration.

III. **Differential diagnosis.** PMR should be considered in patients over 50 who complain of proximal arthralgia and myalgia. The Westergren ESR is usually elevated above 50 mm/h. Central to the diagnosis of PMR is a rapid dramatic response to low-dose corticosteroid therapy (see section **IV.A**). The diagnosis requires exclusion of other syndromes associated with aching, ESR elevation, or both, such as the following:
A. **Neoplasia.**
B. **Infectious syndromes.**
C. **Other rheumatic conditions,** such as rheumatoid arthritis and systemic lupus erythematosus.
D. **Muscle disease,** such as polymyositis or thyroid myopathy.
E. **Plasma cell dyscrasias.**
F. **Fibromyalgia** (an ill-defined syndrome of aching *not associated* with an elevated ESR; see Chapter 49).

IV. **Treatment**
A. **Prednisone.** Initial therapy for PMR is usually 10 to 15 mg of prednisone daily. A prompt and dramatic clinical response is considered by some to be an absolute criterion for the diagnosis. Most symptoms resolve in 48 to 72 hours, and the ESR should normalize after 7 to 10 days. Unusually, a patient who fails to respond to prednisone may respond to another corticosteroid, such as methylprednisolone or dexamethasone. If a dramatic response does not occur after several days, steroids should be discontinued. Following control of symptoms, the dose of corticosteroids should be reduced to the lowest level required to suppress symptoms, as the morbidity associated with therapy often exceeds that of the underlying disease. The dose of prednisone should be increased only for a recurrence of symptoms, not for an elevation of the ESR alone. Consideration should be given to ensure an adequate calcium intake in these elderly patients on corticosteroids who are at risk for corticosteroid induced osteoporosis (see Chapter 46).

   Low-dose corticosteroid therapy for PMR is not appropriate for patients with features suggestive of TA (see second section of chapter).
B. **Nonsteroidal antiinflammatory agents** may suppress rheumatic symptoms, but they do not reduce the risk for blindness if TA is present.

Temporal Arteritis

Also known as giant cell or cranial arteritis, TA is a vascular syndrome that affects predominantly cranial arteries. In the late nineteenth century, Jonathan Hutchinson reported the first case, of a man who had difficulty wearing a hat because his temporal arteries were tender. Since that time, the clinical spectrum of TA has broadened (see section **I**). Its incidence is unknown but is probably about half that of PMR. TA occurs about equally in men and women. The age distribution of TA is similar to that of PMR, with a peak incidence from 60 to 80 years of age, and it rarely occurs in patients less than 50 years old.

I. **Clinical presentation.** TA is a strikingly heterogeneous syndrome. All the features of PMR (myalgia, arthralgia, fatigue, malaise, fever, weight loss, and depression) are common. Whether PMR and TA represent different parts of a single disorder is a subject of continuing debate (see section **I.D**).

   Earlier descriptions of TA emphasize manifestations attributable to involvement of the ophthalmic artery and branches of the external carotid system, but it is now recognized that arterial lesions may be widespread. The varied expressions of the syndrome can be analyzed according to the anatomic patterns of affected arteries.

A. **Symptoms related to involvement of branches of the external carotid artery**

1. **Headache** is probably the most frequent symptom of TA, occurring in 50% to 75% of patients; it is often the first manifestation of disease. It is described as extracranial, dull, boring, and burning. Classically, patients complain of temporal headaches, and the temporal arteries on physical examination may be prominent, beaded, tender, and pulseless. Patients with occipital artery involvement may have difficulty combing their hair or experience discomfort from the pressure of a pillow on their head.
2. **Jaw claudication** occurs infrequently in TA, but its presence is highly suggestive of the syndrome. Patients with involvement of the maxillary or lingual arteries may have jaw or tongue pain on chewing or talking. There are rare case reports of tongue gangrene.
3. **Pain in the ear canal, pinna, or parotid gland** may be secondary to involvement of the posterior auricular artery.
4. **Temporomandibular joint pain** may be secondary to temporal artery involvement.

B. **Symptoms related to involvement of the internal carotid artery**

1. **Ocular damage** secondary to arteritis is the most common serious consequence of TA. Although it occurs in 20% to 50% of patients and is the presenting symptom *at diagnosis* in 60% of patients with TA in whom visual loss develops, ocular damage is rarely the earliest symptom. In most patients with visual loss, a careful history will reveal that headache, usually specific enough to suggest the diagnosis, preceded blindness in about 40% of cases. Symptoms characteristic of PMR are early manifestations in about 30% of patients.

   Because loss of vision in TA is often irreversible unless treatment is initiated within several hours following the onset of ocular symptoms, special attention must be directed toward early recognition of the syndrome. Ocular manifestations vary according to the pattern of arterial branch involvement. The retina is supplied by the central retinal artery, which is the terminal branch of the ophthalmic artery. Also derived from the ophthalmic artery are the posterior ciliary arteries, which supply the optic nerve, and the muscular branches, which supply the extraocular muscles. Because the posterior ciliary arteries are the most frequently involved arteries in TA, ischemic optic neuritis is by far the most common lesion. Occlusion of the central retinal artery or its branches occurs in fewer than 10% of patients with eye involvement. Therefore, retinal changes such as exudates, hemorrhages, or vasculitis are infrequent. Results of the funduscopic evaluation will often be normal, or the examination will show only mild edema of the nerve head several days after the onset of symptoms. Optic atrophy is a late finding.

   a. **Amaurosis fugax** occurs in about 10% of patients with TA, and permanent visual loss will develop in 80% of these if they are not treated.
   b. **Unilateral or incomplete blindness** occurs in about 30% to 40% of patients and, if untreated, may progress to complete blindness over a period of several days.
   c. **Bilateral blindness** occurs in 25% of patients with TA and, as noted in **a** and **b,** is often preceded by amaurosis fugax or partial blindness.
   d. **Diplopia secondary to ischemic paresis** of the extraocular muscles occurs in about 5% of patients with TA.
2. **Central nervous system disease** can occur in TA secondary to involvement of any of the intracerebral arteries and produce seizures, cerebral vascular accidents, or abnormal mental status. Peripheral nerve involvement is rare. As a result of the relative inaccessibility of intracranial vessels and the high prevalence of arteriosclerotic vascular disease in older patients, the frequency with which TA leads to significant ischemic central nervous system disease is not known.

C. **Symptoms related to involvement of large arteries**

1. **Aortic arch and thoracic aorta.** Careful physical examination in patients

with TA often reveals bruits over the carotid, axillary, or brachial arteries. Limited pathologic studies have shown giant cell arteritis in such vessels; however, because bruits secondary to arteriosclerotic vascular disease are common in elderly subjects, the frequency of aortic and aortic root involvement in TA is not known. Nevertheless, giant cell arteritis has been documented as a basis for aneurysms, dissections, and stenotic lesions of the aorta and its major branches. In isolated cases, coronary artery disease and a variety of aortic arch syndromes secondary to giant cell arteritis have been demonstrated.

2. **Abdominal aorta.** Involvement of the abdominal aorta, like that of the thoracic aorta, can produce symptoms secondary to aortic aneurysms and intestinal infarction. For unknown reasons, renal involvement is rare. There are some definite examples of leg claudication secondary to giant cell arteritis, but the relevance of this finding is not clear. There is no indication to use steroids to treat peripheral vascular disease in the usual elderly patient with leg claudication who may, for some other reason, have an elevated ESR. As will be discussed later, even in the patient with known TA, steroids should not be used to treat large-vessel disease without evidence that vasculitis, rather than atheromatous disease, is the cause of symptoms.

D. **Symptoms related to polymyalgia rheumatica.** The clinical picture of PMR has already been described in detail (see first section of chapter). Patients with TA, with or without PMR, may have similar systemic complaints, such as fatigue, malaise, fever, weight loss, depression, and arthralgias or transient arthritis. Still at issue is how to predict which patient with PMR has TA. Some physicians advocate treating all patients with PMR as if they had TA. However, this approach involves unnecessary treatment of a large group of patients with high-dose steroids. Because a temporal artery biopsy is a relatively benign procedure, having all patients with suspected PMR undergo a biopsy, rather than treating them all as if they had TA, would clearly be preferable. If a patient with polymyalgia has the classic signs or symptoms of TA, a biopsy should be performed. A temporal artery biopsy can be accomplished on an ambulatory basis and, if the results are positive, can dramatically diminish the number of diagnostic studies that are otherwise needed to evaluate systemically ill patients with an elevated ESR. Several clinical studies have demonstrated that the chance of a positive result in a temporal artery biopsy in PMR patients is greatly enhanced if temporal artery pulses are absent or diminished, even without other localizing signs. Even the presence of a nonspecific headache may increase the yield. No differences have been demonstrated among PMR patients with and without TA in regard to degree of ESR elevation, presence of minor visual symptoms, sex, age, and duration of symptoms. Furthermore, about 10% of patients with PMR and localized temporal artery signs have negative biopsy results (see section **IV.A.**). In conclusion, PMR patients without signs or symptoms of TA or histologically demonstrated arteritis should not be empirically treated with steroid regimens that are appropriate for TA.

II. **Laboratory studies**

A. **Erythrocyte sedimentation rate.** As in PMR, the laboratory hallmark of TA is the elevated ESR. The ESR (Westergren) is usually between 50 and 100 mm/h, rarely below 40 mm/h, and commonly above 100 mm/h. A normal ESR does not exclude TA. A mild normocytic, normochromic anemia may be present. As in PMR, muscle enzyme levels are normal. Rheumatoid factor, antinuclear antibodies, and anti-DNA antibodies are negative. Complement levels are normal, and cryoglobulins and monoclonal immunoglobulins are absent.

B. **Radiographs.** Temporal artery arteriography has no value. However, arteriography of the aorta may be useful in differentiating giant cell arteritis from arteriosclerotic vascular disease. In the former, the vessels often show slowly tapering stenotic lesions, in contrast to the "cobblestone" pattern of arteriosclerotic disease. Unfortunately, most TA patients are elderly persons who also have arteriosclerotic disease, which makes this differentiation difficult.

III. **Pathologic findings.** The biopsy specimen should always be taken from the temporal artery on the symptomatic side of the head. If a specific part of the artery is tender, beaded, or inflamed, the biopsy specimen should include that area. There is no information as to whether the artery trunk or a distal branch specimen is best. At least 1 cm of the artery should be taken. Because the process may be segmental, multiple sections should be taken. Histologically, the following are seen:

A. **An inflammatory infiltrate,** predominantly of mononuclear cells, usually involving the entire vessel wall. Fibrinoid necrosis is not a feature of the lesion.

B. **Fragmentation** of the internal elastic lamina.

C. **Giant cells** are almost always present and often seem to engulf parts of the internal elastic lamina. They are difficult to find in some cases, and their absence does not rule out the diagnosis.

D. **Intimal proliferation** is often marked, is a nonspecific feature in this age group, and cannot, if found alone, be considered evidence of past or present arteritis. These findings are in contrast to those of the lesions of polyarteritis nodosa, which are characterized by fibrinoid necrosis of the vessel and neutrophil infiltration. When TA involves larger vessels, the lesions are indistinguishable from those seen in Takayasu's arteritis (see section **IV.B**).

IV. **Differential diagnosis.** The diagnosis of TA is made in a patient with a compatible history and physical findings (see sections **I** through **III**). Polymyalgia need not be present, but the ESR should be above 50 mm/h. A definite diagnosis requires a biopsy specimen showing the histologic changes described in section **III.** Finally, all symptoms should dramatically improve on steroids; the exception is loss of vision, which is usually irreversible.

A. **Arteriosclerotic vascular disease** may be responsible for some clinical signs of TA, including a decrease in the temporal artery pulse, temporal artery thickening, and acute visual loss. Patients have been described with loss of vision, elevated ESR, and absent temporal pulses who had only arteriosclerotic changes on temporal artery biopsy and did not respond to steroid therapy. Similarly, in patients with previously documented and treated TA, symptoms may develop suggesting relapse that are actually secondary to arteriosclerotic vascular disease (see section **VI.E**).

B. **Takayasu's arteritis** is a large-vessel disease and does not directly involve the temporal artery or other arteries of medium and small size. Although Takayasu's arteritis is pathologically indistinguishable from TA involving large vessels, its clinical picture is different. Female patients predominate, and patients are usually 20 to 50 years old. Although symptoms of arteritis may be preceded by a "pre-pulseless" stage (arthralgias and fatigue), the characteristic PMR symptoms are not common. Finally, the ESR has no consistent pattern, and the response to steroids is unpredictable.

C. **Systemic necrotizing vasculitis.** The temporal arteries may occasionally be histologically involved in patients with polyarteritis (see Chapter 32); however, these arteries are rarely abnormal on physical examination, and clinical signs of TA are rarely seen, even in patients with involvement of the temporal arteries. Finally, kidney and peripheral nervous system involvement is rare in TA, even when large vessels are involved.

V. **Treatment.** The management of uncomplicated TA is 40 mg of prednisone PO daily in divided doses. However, when acute visual changes thought to be secondary to TA are present, patients should be started on 80 to 100 mg of methylprednisolone IV daily and then tapered to the conventional 40-mg oral dose of prednisone after 7 to 10 days. Alternate-day therapy is not effective in preventing visual loss. Symptoms (e.g., PMR, headache, and lethargy) should disappear in 36 to 72 hours. Elevated ESR and ischemic manifestations, such as temporal headache, jaw claudication, and localized temporal artery inflammation, should diminish in several days. The temporal artery pulse may not return, and visual loss may be permanent. High-dose steroids should be maintained only as long as necessary for symptoms to resolve and then should be tapered during several weeks to a maintenance dose of 5 to 10 mg of prednisone daily. Both clinical signs and ESR may be used to follow the response. In patients with visual involvement, tapering should be slower. The average patient will require continued maintenance therapy with 5 to 10 mg of prednisone daily for 2 years, but some patients may need treatment for as long as 5 years. Because the incidence of new visual damage appears to decrease with duration of disease, patients who relapse after 18 to 24 months should probably undergo a repeated temporal artery biopsy before being restarted on high-dose corticosteroids.

VI. Summary of diagnostic and therapeutic approach to temporal arteritis

A. Temporal arteritis suspected in a patient with no evidence of ocular involvement. Obtain a biopsy specimen from the symptomatic artery, and if findings are positive, treat with high-dose steroids. If the findings are negative, do not treat with steroids unless clinical suspicion is very strong; in that case, obtain a specimen from the contralateral artery. If the result is still negative but clinical suspicion remains very strong, a short clinical trial of oral prednisone may be warranted. If clinical and laboratory parameters improve, continue therapy (see section **V**). If they do not improve dramatically, discontinue the treatment.

B. Temporal arteritis suspected in a patient with acute visual loss. Immediately institute treatment with IV high-dose steroids (80 to 100 mg of methylprednisolone or equivalent). If subsequent biopsy findings are positive, continue therapy as outlined in section **V.** If the biopsy result is negative and the picture is strongly suggestive of TA, obtain a specimen from the contralateral artery and proceed as described in **A.**

C. Polymyalgia rheumatica

1. **Temporal arteritis not suspected.** Do not perform a biopsy. Treat with low-dose steroids (10 to 15 mg of prednisone daily).
2. **Temporal arteritis suspected.** Follow the procedure described in **A;** however, if the biopsy result is negative, low-dose steroids (10 to 15 mg of prednisone daily) should be instituted.

D. Large-vessel involvement suspected

1. **Patient with previously proven temporal arteritis**
   - **a.** If involvement is clinically insignificant (bruits or diminished pulses), no therapy is indicated.
   - **b.** If involvement is clinically significant (claudication, coronary artery disease, or other occlusive arterial disease) and if there is other evidence of active TA, treat as described in section **V.** Arteriography of the involved artery may be helpful; if it suggests that the vascular symptoms are secondary to arteritis, treat as described in section **V.**
2. **Patient with suspected temporal arteritis.** Obtain biopsy specimens from temporal arteries as described in **A.** If findings are negative, do not institute therapy. If positive, treat as outlined in section **V.**

E. Suspected relapse of temporal arteritis

1. If the presentation is similar to that of the original episode, re-treat as outlined in section **V** with 40 mg of prednisone daily.
2. If the presentation is not similar, perform another biopsy and proceed as described in section **A.**

Bibliography

Fauchald P, Rygvold O, Oystese, B. Temporal arteritis and polymyalgia rheumatica: clinical and biopsy findings. *Ann Intern Med* 1977;77:845.

Hamilton CR, Shelley WM, Tumulty PA. Giant cell arteritis and polymyalgia rheumatica. *Medicine* 1971;50:1.

Hollenhorst RW, et al. Neurological aspects of temporal arteritis. *Neurology* 1960; 10:490.

Klein RG, et al. Large artery involvement in giant cell (temporal) arteritis. *Ann Intern Med* 1975;83:806.

Klein RG, et al. Skip lesions in temporal arteritis. *Mayo Clin Proc* 1976;51:504.

27. POLYMYOSITIS AND DERMATOMYOSITIS

J. Robert Polk and Lawrence J. Kagen

Polymyositis (PM) is an inflammatory disease of striated skeletal muscle. In some patients, a characteristic skin rash is present, thus the term dermatomyositis. Dermatomyositis (DM) was described by Unverricht in 1887. PM occurs at any age, but most cases occur between the fourth and sixth decades of life, with a mild female preponderance. A childhood form of DM has been recognized. Estimates of the prevalence of PM range from 0.2 to 0.6 cases per 100,000 population. DM may be associated with malignancy.

I. Disease classification. Various classification systems have been proposed. It should be remembered that not all patients who are weak have PM. The following is a useful classification system:

- **A.** Dermatomyositis
  - **1.** Childhood.
  - **2.** Adulthood.
- **B.** Polymyositis.
- **C.** Myositis associated with other connective tissue and inflammatory disorders (e.g., systemic lupus erythematosus, rheumatoid arthritis, scleroderma, sarcoidosis).
- **D.** Myositis associated with malignancy.
- **E.** Inclusion body myositis.
- **F.** Myositis secondary to infectious agents.
- **G.** Drug- and toxin-induced myositis.

II. Pathogenesis

A. The **etiology** of PM is unknown. Current thoughts relate to possible aberrations in the immune system that give rise to an increased susceptibility to infectious agents, and to modifications of cellular immunity that lead to the development of mononuclear cells capable of injuring muscle. Complement may play a role in tissue injury in DM. Evidence of infection has been sought. At present, the best candidates are viruses and *Toxoplasma gondii.*

Certain viruses, such as those of the influenza virus and coxsackievirus groups, may produce myopathy, and serologic evidence of recent viral infection has been found in some patients. Serologic evidence of recent *Toxoplasma* infection has also been demonstrated in some groups of patients with PM. This organism can produce myopathy in humans and experimental animals.

B. The **histologic appearance of muscle** among these seven groups by ordinary light microscopy is quite similar. The principal feature is an inflammatory cellular infiltrate in muscle, with an associated degeneration and necrosis of muscle fibers. Regeneration of fibers and a perivascular inflammatory infiltrate may be seen. A later finding is interstitial fibrosis. Calcinosis may be seen, especially in the childhood form. Not all the changes of degeneration, inflammatory infiltrate, regeneration, necrosis, and fiber size variation need be present. In 10% to 20% of muscle biopsies, the findings may be normal. The vasculopathy of childhood myositis may be seen in small arteries of muscle, skin, and the gastrointestinal tract. Inclusion body myositis is characterized by the presence of eosinophilic inclusions in the sarcoplasm, nucleus, or both. Rimmed vacuoles filled with basophilic granules are seen on frozen sections. The inclusions appear as masses of filamentous material by electron microscopy.

The infiltrates in PM and inclusion body myositis contain mainly CD8+ T lymphocytes and macrophages. B cells are more common in biopsy specimens of muscle tissue in DM.

C. The **skin findings** are marked by an infiltrate of CD4+ T lymphocytes.

III. Clinical presentation

A. General diagnostic considerations. Pearson has defined several criteria for classifying patients with PM. The diagnosis of PM is definite when four criteria are present, probable with three, and possible with two. DM must include the characteristic rash, and the diagnosis is definite with three or four criteria present, probable with two, and possible with one. The criteria are as follows:

1. **Symmetric proximal muscle weakness** with or without dysphagia or respiratory muscle involvement.
2. **Elevation of serum enzymes:** creatine kinase (CK), aldolase, lactic dehydrogenase, and serum aspartate aminotransferase.
3. **Typical electromyographic triad**
   - **a.** Small-amplitude, polyphasic motor unit potentials.
   - **b.** Pseudomyotonic high-frequency pattern.
   - **c.** Spontaneous fibrillation and positive sharp waves (sawtooth pattern) in resting muscle.
4. **Typical histology in muscle specimens,** as described in section **II.B.**
5. **Characteristic skin rash of dermatomyositis,** consisting of a lilac discoloration of the upper eyelids with periorbital edema (heliotrope rash) and an erythematous or atrophic scaling, patchy, or linear rash involving the extensor surfaces of the joints, face, neck, back, and chest in a V-shaped pattern.

   Erythematous scaling (Gottron's) papules occur over the metacarpophalangeal and proximal interphalangeal joints.

B. Diagnostic characteristics of polymyositis types

1. **Childhood myositis**
   - **a.** Childhood DM-PM appears most commonly between ages 7 and 10 years. It occurs slightly more often in girls than in boys. Most patients have the characteristic rash of DM at presentation. About 90% present with proximal muscle weakness. Raynaud's phenomenon is said to be less common in childhood DM-PM, but up to 18% of patients may have it.
   - **b.** Distinctive features of the myopathy are atrophy, contractures, and tissue calcifications. Calcifications usually appear after the disease has been present for a year or more.
   - **c.** Visceral involvement is probably more frequent in the childhood than in the adult form. Abnormal pulmonary function, esophageal motility, and gastrointestinal absorption have been reported. Some patients may present with an acute myositis with accompanying fever, malaise, and abdominal pain. Gastrointestinal ulcerations caused by a diffuse necrotizing arteritis (which may also be seen in skin and muscle) may occur and lead to hemorrhage.
2. **Dermatomyositis in adults.** Rash is the primary presenting feature of DM and is present initially in about 95% of patients. Only 50% to 60% of patients have proximal muscle weakness at presentation. Follow-up of patients with a rash is therefore essential, as it is a rare patient who will not eventually manifest proximal weakness. Arthralgia, Raynaud's phenomenon, and dysphagia are seen in 10% to 25% of DM patients. As in PM, interstitial pneumonitis, cardiomyopathy, and heart block have been reported but are rare manifestations.
3. **Polymyositis in adults.** Proximal muscle weakness is the presenting feature in 90% to 95% of patients with PM. Myalgia is common. Arthralgia, Raynaud's phenomenon, and dysphagia are seen in 10% to 15%. Patients usually have an insidious onset of proximal weakness and their condition may remain undiagnosed for several months because their complaints are vague. They may note gradually increasing difficulty in climbing steps or getting out of a chair. They may complain of not being able to comb their hair or reach above their heads. Eventually, patients may become bedridden and be unable to raise their head from a pillow.
4. **Myositis associated with other connective tissue diseases.** Overlap syndromes as defined here consist of PM or DM that fulfills the previously mentioned criteria and another connective tissue disease that fulfills a sep-

arate set of diagnostic criteria. These patients present more commonly than other PM patients with Raynaud's phenomenon, sclerodactyly, arthralgia, and myalgia (about 50%). Proximal muscle weakness is seen in 40% at presentation, and the characteristic rash of DM in 20%. The presenting features reflect the underlying connective tissue disease; systemic sclerosis, systemic lupus erythematosus, and rheumatoid arthritis are the diseases most commonly associated with PM features. Sicca syndrome and necrotizing vasculitis are also associated with PM-DM.

5. **Inflammatory myositis associated with malignancy.** Controversy exists concerning the true association of PM and DM with malignancy. Most reports indicate that DM has a higher association with malignancy than does PM. Between 10% and 20% of patients with PM-DM may have an underlying malignancy. It is said that the possibility of malignancy in an elderly patient with PM-DM is four times greater than in an age-matched control. Dysphagia occurs in 15% of patients. In PM-DM of malignancy, myositis precedes malignancy by an average of 1 to 2 years in 70% of patients and follows it in 30%. In some of the patients, neuropathy may also be associated.
6. **Inclusion body myositis** is typically a disorder of older men. Progress of disease is often insidious, with only borderline elevation of enzymes. Neuropathic features may be noted, and response to therapy is poor.
7. **Infectious agents.** History and serologic findings often provide clues to the diagnosis. The following categories should be considered:
   a. Viral infection (e.g., influenza virus, coxsackievirus, human immunodeficiency virus).
   b. Toxoplasmosis.
   c. Bacterial pyomyositis.
   d. Lyme myositis.
8. **Drug- and toxin-induced myositis.** Penicillamine employed to treat rheumatoid arthritis may be the cause of a syndrome indistinguishable from naturally occurring PM. In addition, myositis-like states have been noted in patients treated with propylthiouracil and azathioprine. Other agents (e.g., lovastatin and other statins, gemfibrozil) may rarely cause painful myopathy and rhabdomyolysis. Zidovudine [formerly called azidothymidine (AZT)] also has produced myopathy and myositis.

   Certain toxins (i.e., alcohol, cocaine) may also produce severe acute or chronic myopathy.

IV. Laboratory studies

A. White blood cell count and **hemoglobin level** are generally normal.

B. Erythrocyte sedimentation rate may be elevated or normal.

C. Creatine kinase, aldolase, serum aspartate aminotransferase, and lactic dehydrogenase are elevated, with decreasing sensitivity as listed.

D. Serum myoglobin is elevated.

E. Urine may contain myoglobin but is otherwise usually normal.

F. Antinuclear antibodies may be present.

G. Total hemolytic complement is normal, except in childhood DM, where it may be low.

H. Anti-tRNA synthetase may be present, especially in association with pulmonary disease.

I. Electromyographic triad

1. Short-duration, small-amplitude, and polyphasic potentials appear on voluntary contraction.
2. Spontaneous high-frequency potentials (pseudomyotonic discharges) can be triggered by movement of the electrode.
3. Spontaneous fibrillation and positive sharp waves (sawtooth pattern) are identical to the denervation pattern.

J. Muscle biopsy reveals inflammatory cellular infiltration of muscle with degeneration, necrosis, and regeneration of muscle fibers.

K. An age-appropriate evaluation for malignancy is appropriate in PM and DM patients over the age of 50.

V. Differential diagnosis

A. Hypothyroid myopathy. Features such as weight gain, constipation, hoarseness, anemia, and a slow relaxation of deep tendon reflexes suggest this disorder. Serum CK and cholesterol may be elevated.

B. Myasthenia gravis. Ocular symptoms and swallowing difficulties are prominent. Patients complain of increasing weakness with use of muscles and restoration of strength after rest. Muscle enzymes are normal, the result of the edrophonium test is positive, and the electromyogram has a characteristic pattern (see Chapter 10).

C. Muscular dystrophies. A positive family history gives a clue to these disorders, and the average age at onset is younger than in PM. Electromyographic findings and muscle enzyme levels may be similar to those of PM; however, muscle biopsy usually serves to make the distinction, especially in children (see Chapter 10).

D. Polymyalgia rheumatica. Levels of serum muscle enzymes are normal, the erythrocyte sedimentation rate is elevated, and malaise and proximal myalgia are prominent complaints (see Chapter 26).

E. Fibromyalgia. Pain in muscles is a prominent complaint and multiple tender points are present, but weakness cannot be demonstrated clinically and muscle enzyme levels are normal (see Chapter 49).

F. Alcohol abuse may be associated with acute rhabdomyolysis or chronic wasting myopathy.

G. Trichinosis. The periorbital swelling and erythema may mimic those of DM. Distinguishing features include a history of ingesting undercooked pork, nausea, vomiting, abdominal pain, and eosinophilia.

H. Electrolyte disturbances (especially of calcium, magnesium, phosphorus, and potassium) may be associated with myopathic symptoms and should be looked for, especially in patients on parenteral fluid replacement therapy.

I. Metabolic disorders of carbohydrate and lipid metabolism (e.g., McArdle disease, carnitine palmityltransferase deficiency) may be associated with exertional myalgia and myoglobinuria.

VI. Treatment

A. Supportive therapy. Patients may be hospitalized for diagnostic tests and initiation of rehabilitation. Range of motion and passive exercises should be performed to prevent contractures, especially in childhood myositis. However, active exercises are not tolerated well early in the course of severe disease.

B. Corticosteroids. Once a firm diagnosis has been established, prednisone in a dosage of approximately 40 to 60 mg daily is begun. Clinical experience suggests that alternate-day steroid therapy is not as effective as initial therapy but may be used as the dosage is tapered. IV bolus steroids may also be used.

Controversy exists concerning the best indicators of clinical response. Some experts believe that improvement in serum enzymes is the best indicator of response. The CK level will usually decrease to half its original value by 1 month but may not normalize for an average of 3 months. Because muscle strength often improves as CK levels return to normal, steroids may be tapered in small decrements with both muscle strength and serum enzyme levels used as guides. If relapse occurs, then a 60- to 80-mg daily dose of prednisone should be resumed immediately and tapering deferred until serum enzyme values approach normal. The goal is a daily dose of 5 to 15 mg of prednisone. This low dose of corticosteroid should be continued for 6 to 12 months to allow an adequate period of observation while some antiinflammatory effect is maintained. Discontinuation of steroids should then be attempted by slowly decreasing the dosage. A few patients may never be able to discontinue steroids because disease activity remains constant. If no clinical improvement occurs after 3 months of daily high doses of prednisone, cytotoxic drugs may be used.

C. Cytotoxic drugs. See Appendix E for detailed drug information, including toxicity. The two most frequently used are methotrexate and azathioprine.

1. **Methotrexate** is given PO at weekly intervals in doses from 7.5 to 30.0 mg. IV methotrexate in similar schedules has also been employed. Prednisone is also continued. As strength improves, prednisone may be slowly tapered and methotrexate continued. A response to methotrexate should be seen in about 12 weeks. Methotrexate may be tapered when clinical and laboratory parameters have improved. Hepatic fibrosis may develop with daily methotrexate therapy but is very rare in patients receiving the drug on a weekly schedule.
2. **Azathioprine** (150 mg PO daily) may be used along with prednisone. Response may be noted after 1 to 3 months. Care should be taken to monitor frequently for side effects and to check blood counts regularly.

D. Other therapies. A number of other agents have been used for patients who have not done well on the regimens described above. Among these agents have been cyclosporine and cyclophosphamide. Excellent results have recently been noted in certain patients given IV gamma globulin. Gamma globulin may be used early in therapy for selected patients.

VII. Prognosis. About 75% of patients respond to steroid therapy with improved muscle strength. About 90% of patients survive for long periods. The worst prognostic indicator is the presence of malignancy. Patients with myositis and malignancy have a poor 10-year survival. These data were collected retrospectively; some neoplasms may have been missed in this series because autopsies were not performed in all deceased patients. Patients with myositis of malignancy do not respond to steroid therapy as well as do other patients with PM. The leading cause of death, excluding malignancy, is sepsis. Patients treated early in the course of myositis seem to respond better than do those treated late in their illness. Myositis may occasionally improve during treatment of the underlying malignancy.

Bibliography

Kagen LJ. Management. In: Klippel JH, Dieppe PA, eds. *Inflammatory muscle disease in rheumatology.* London: Mosby, 1994:14.1.

Medsger TA, Oddis CV. Clinical features. In: Klippel JH, Dieppe PA, eds. *Inflammatory muscle disease in rheumatology.* London: Mosby, 1994:12.1.

Miller FW. Inflammatory myopathies: polymyositis, dermatomyositis, and related conditions. In: Koopman WJ, ed. *Arthritis and allied conditions.* Baltimore: Williams & Wilkins, 1997:1407.

Plotz PH, Miller FW. Etiology and pathogenesis. In: Klippel JH, Dieppe PA, eds. *Inflammatory muscle disease in rheumatology.* London: Mosby, 1994:13.1.

Spiera RF, Kagen L. Collagen vascular disease: polymyositis, dermatomyositis and inclusion body myositis. In: van de Putte DE, et al., eds. *Therapy of systemic rheumatic disorders.* New York: Marcel Dekker, 1998:547.

Wortman RL. Inflammatory disease of muscle and other myopathies. In: Kelley W, et al., eds. *Textbook of rheumatology.* Philadelphia: WB Saunders, 1997:1177.

28. RHEUMATOID ARTHRITIS

Dror Mevorach and Stephen A. Paget

Rheumatoid arthritis (RA) is a chronic, systemic, autoimmune, inflammatory disorder in which an erosive, symmetric joint disorder maintains the center stage accompanied by a variable, but at times prominent, degree of extraarticular involvement. The term was introduced by Garrod in 1859 and relates today to a disorder occurring in about 1% of the world's population, with a twofold to threefold female predominance before 60 years of age and greater equity between the sexes thereafter. Rheumatoid factor (RF), an immunoglobulin M (IgM) auto-antibody against the Fc portion of an IgG molecule first described by Waaler in 1940, is the main serologic marker, found in 75% to 80% of patients.

During the past 10 years, epidemiologic studies have unearthed disturbing information about the true potential of this disease, which now guides our modern therapeutic approach; RA is a chronic disease that leads to joint damage within the first 2 years, causes marked functional limitation and a 30% loss of work within the first 5 years, and shortens life by 5 to 7 years. This aggressive disorder demands the early institution of an equally aggressive therapeutic approach. A treatment plan should be individually crafted that is based on patient-specific clinical and functional parameters and employs a wide range of effective medications and physical therapeutic modalities aimed at altering the disease course and maintaining function.

As our concepts about the pathogenesis and clinical realities of RA have crystallized and been coupled with refined methods derived from biotechnology, promising biologics have been developed. Monoclonal antibodies, recombinant cytokines, cytokine receptor fusion proteins, and other biologics have moved from the status of novel reagents studied in phase I trials to validated therapeutic tools in widespread use. With the development of these extraordinary agents, a new era in the focused treatment of RA has begun.

I. Epidemiology. Whereas the worldwide prevalence rate of RA is about 1%, higher rates are found in certain groups, such as 5.3% in certain Native-American tribes. RA is two to three times more common in women than in men, but in persons over 50 years of age, the disease frequency becomes more equal. Although the onset of disease is most common between the ages of 40 and 60, in one-third of patients, RA develops after the age of 60.

II. Genetic factors in RA are important in defining disease susceptibility and severity.

- **A. Family studies** have demonstrated an increased risk for disease in siblings of persons affected with RA. Concordance has been found to be 12% to 15% in monozygotic and 4% in dizygotic twins, strong evidence for a major influence of genetic factors in disease causation.
- **B.** The **major histocompatibility complex (MHC)** is a region of genes whose MHC I and II products provide a system for displaying antigenic peptides to T cells. RA was shown to be associated with the HLA-DR4 and -DR1 haplotypes; on further molecular characterization, the association was confined to a short sequence in the HLA-DRB1 gene that codes for the RA epitope in amino acid positions 67 through 74. Some of the HLA-DRB1 alleles (HLA-DRB1*0401, *0404, and *0408 in general populations and some others in specific ethnic populations) are RA-associated alleles. These MHC genes are related not only to the initiation of the disease but also to its course and severity. For instance, patients with non-DR4 disease-associated genes have milder, seronegative disease, and patients with two (homozygous) DRB1*04 alleles have more severe and extraarticular disease.
- **C. Other genetic factors** are not as well defined, but because the HLA association represents less than 30% of the genetic risk, several candidate genes coding for cytokines, chemokines, and signal transduction factors may influence disease initiation, severity, and progression.

III. Pathogenesis

A. No clear **etiology** has been defined. Although there are no convincing studies demonstrating a specific infectious etiology in RA, some studies support the possibility that an infectious agent may be responsible for the disease in a genetically predisposed host. Immune responses initially generated against such immunogens would be sustained by cross-reactivity to host antigens within the synovial joints, leading to a breakdown of normal immunologic tolerance and a chronic destructive autoimmunity. Candidate infectious agents include viruses (e.g., parvovirus B19, Epstein-Barr virus), *Mycoplasma,* and other bacteria (e.g., streptococci). Possible auto-antigens include type 2 collagen, proteoglycan, chondrocyte antigens, heat shock proteins, and immunoglobulins.

B. **Histopathology.** In the early months of RA, edema, angiogenesis, hyperplasia of synovial lining, and inflammatory infiltrate are already present. Once the disease enters a more chronic phase, massive hyperplasia, mainly of type A synovial cells, and subintimal mononuclear cell infiltration are prominent. The synovium of RA assumes the appearance of a reactive lymph node because of the extensive infiltration by plasma cells, macrophages, and lymphocytes in the form of large lymphoid follicles. The histologic appearance of the synovium in RA, however, is not specific, as a similar picture is seen in other inflammatory arthritides, such as psoriatic arthritis and Reiter's syndrome. One characteristic feature of RA is the invasion of and damage to cartilage, bone, and tendons by an infiltrating inflammatory synovial tissue mass called the pannus.

C. **Cellular immunity.** CD4+ T lymphocytes in the form of aggregates or diffuse infiltrates are found in the subintimal area. B cells, although in low numbers, evolve into plasma cells and produce RF. Activated macrophages and dendritic cells are intermixed with other immunoreactive cells and are thought to be important in antigen presentation. Neutrophils, mainly localized to the synovial fluid and not the synovial membrane, are prominent effectors of inflammation, and cartilage is damaged by the various enzymes they release.

D. **Cytokines, chemokines, growth factors, enzymes, and other soluble mediators.** Cytokines and growth factors bind to cell surface receptors and transmit a signal to the cell, with a resultant shift in activation. In this way, they play an integral role in the initiation and perpetuation of synovitis. Interleukin-1 (IL-1), IL-6, tumor necrosis factor-alpha (TNF-α), and colony stimulating factor-1 (CSF-1) are produced by macrophages and fibroblasts; they have broad effects on many cells that lead to cell proliferation, increased release of prostaglandins and matrix-degrading proteases, fever, and bone resorption. IL-2, IL-3, IL-4, IL-6, and interferons are produced in T cells and lead to activation and amplification of cellular and humoral immune responses. Enzymes such as metalloproteinases (collagenase, stromelysin), which degrade matrix proteins, and complement proteins, which participate in acute inflammation, are effector molecules and as such have the ability to alter the environment directly. The relative contribution of each arm probably depends on the degree of chronicity, extent of therapeutic interventions, and other poorly defined factors. Because of the highly complex interrelationships between these cells, it is unlikely that therapies aimed at only one aspect of the axis will succeed in all patients.

E. **Auto-antibodies.** RFs are anti-globulin antibodies that bind to the Fc portions of IgG. The mechanisms initiating RF secretion and its exact role in disease pathogenesis have not been established. RF is found in the serum of 75% to 80% of RA patients, is locally produced in rheumatoid synovial tissue, and may be present in the serum of patients with other disease characterized by B-cell or immune hyperreactivity, such as systemic lupus erythematosus (SLE) and bacterial endocarditis. The presence of high RF titers is associated with severe, erosive disease, a worse functional outcome, rheumatoid nodules, other extraarticular disease manifestations, and HLA-DR4 positivity.

IV. Clinical presentation

A. Disease criteria. The 1987 revised American Rheumatology Association criteria for the classification of RA were developed for epidemiologic purposes. However, because of the high sensitivity and specificity of these criteria in the classification of RA, they are useful to consider at the time of diagnosis. Of the seven criteria, the presence of four is sufficient for classifying a patient as having RA. The first four criteria must be present for at least *6 weeks.* They include the following:

1. Morning stiffness or stiffness after rest lasting longer than 1 hour.
2. Polyarthritis of at least three joints in 14 areas, including right and left proximal interphalangeal (PIP) joints, metacarpophalangeal (MCP) joints, wrists, elbows, knees, ankles, and metatarsophalangeal (MTP) joints.
3. Arthritis of hands, wrists, MCP joints, or PIP joints; symmetric arthritis.
4. Simultaneous arthritis in both sides of the body.
5. Subcutaneous rheumatoid nodules.
6. Serum RF.
7. Hand radiographic changes typical of RA, including erosions or periarticular osteoporosis.

B. Joint, tendon, and bursal involvement. *Symmetric* polyarthritis with variable degrees of damage and inflammation of the hands and feet, mainly the wrists, MCP joints, PIP joints, MTP joints, elbows, knees, ankles, and shoulders is characteristic of RA. Early changes include ulnar styloid prominence, and later deformities resulting from combinations of joint and tendon damage may evolve, including ulnar deviation, boutonniere and swan neck deformities. Flexor tenosynovitis can lead to triggering of the fingers and may eventuate in rupture of tendons. Extensor tenosynovitis is seen as swelling over the dorsum of the wrist, and flexor tenosynovitis can lead to carpal tunnel syndrome from median nerve entrapment. Olecranon bursitis often presents as swelling at the tip of the elbow; synovial extensions, known as Baker's cysts, appearing from the knee to the medial calf region may mimic phlebitis. Spinal disease is limited to the cervical region and, in patients with severe disease, may lead to atlanto-axial subluxation and even cord compromise.

C. Disease presentation and course. The gradual onset of symmetric polyarthritis is most common, occurring in at least 50% of patients; a sudden onset is seen in 10% to 25% of patients. Other patterns of presentation include monarticular disease; palindromic (short-lived and episodic) disease; extraarticular features, such as nodules; and a proximal type resembling polymyalgia rheumatica. Whatever the onset is, the subsequent course may be brief or episodic, prolonged and progressive, or something intermediate. A monocyclic course is a single cycle with remission for at least 1 year, seen in 10% of patients. A polycyclic course is seen in 70% of patients, with either intermittent or continuing subtypes. The latter group shows smoldering activity with incomplete remission or progression. A progressive pattern with increasing joint damage and extraarticular manifestations is seen in about 10% of patients. Included in this group are patients with malignant RA, a polyarteritis nodosa-like disorder.

D. Extraarticular presentation. Although the joint disease dominates the clinical picture, constitutional symptoms such as fatigue and extraarticular features such as serositis, sclerosis, subcutaneous nodules, and rheumatoid vasculitis may be prominent, dominant, or life-threatening. Subcutaneous nodules appear in 20% to 30% of seropositive patients. Nodules develop mostly in pressure areas such as the elbows, finger joints, Achilles tendon, and occipital scalp and are associated with active and more severe disease. Interestingly, methotrexate treatment may cause an increase in nodulosis, especially in the fingers. Nailfold infarcts may be seen when rheumatoid vasculitis develops. Pulmonary involvement is common, with pleurisy, pleural effusion, parenchymal nodules, interstitial alveolitis, fibrosis, and bronchiolitis obliterans organizing pneumonia. Cardiac manifestations include pericarditis, myocarditis, valvulitis, nodule formation with arrhythmia, amyloidosis, and vasculitis. Ocular keratoconjunctivitis sicca is the most common eye abnormality, but sclerosis and scleromalacia may be associated with extensive disease activity. The median, ulnar, and posterior tibial nerves may become entrapped by neighboring sites of joint inflammation or damage. Peripheral neuropathies and central nervous system disease can be manifestations of rheumatoid vasculitis. Felty's syndrome (granulocytopenia, splenomegaly, recurrent infection) and Sjögren's syndrome may coexist with RA and often occur in patients with active, systemic disease.

V. Laboratory studies and imaging

A. Laboratory studies. IgM RF is detected in the serum of about 75% to 80% of RA patients. High titers are associated with more severe and extraarticular disease. The fact that 20% of RA patients are seronegative highlights the fact that the diagnosis of RA is based on clinical, not laboratory, data. An elevated erythrocyte sedimentation rate (ESR) and levels of C-reactive protein are commonly found in RA and correlate well with disease activity in most patients. Normochromic normocytic anemia of chronic disease is frequently seen in active RA; it may be complicated, however, by other conditions, such as drug-induced suppression of bone marrow and blood loss. Thrombocytosis is a frequent correlate of active RA; thrombocytopenia and leukopenia may be seen in drug-induced bone marrow suppression or in Felty's syndrome. Elevated alkaline phosphatase is common in severe disease, but elevation of other liver enzymes more likely is related to treatment with nonsteroidal antiinflammatory drugs (NSAIDs), steroids, or methotrexate.

B. Imaging techniques are employed in defining the diagnosis, severity, progression, extent of disease, response to therapy, and presurgical state of RA patients. The most common plain radiographic findings are soft-tissue swelling, periarticular osteoporosis, marginal erosions, joint space narrowing, and joint deformities.

VI. Diagnosis. A careful clinical examination (history plus physical examination) is a powerful diagnostic tool; it should focus on the pattern and severity of joint inflammation and damage, the presence and extent of constitutional and extra-articular manifestations, modifying medical and psychosocial factors, coexistent medical illnesses, and family history.

A. Differential diagnosis

1. **Systemic lupus erythematosus and other connective tissue disorders.** The symmetric joint inflammation of RA and SLE may be indistinguishable. However, in SLE, erosions do not develop, and the joint disease is commonly accompanied by such manifestations of SLE as fever, serositis, nephritis, dermatitis, cytopenias, and antinuclear antibody (ANA) and anti-DNA seropositivity. Other connective tissue disorders, such as scleroderma and the vasculitides, may present with an RA-like polyarthritis, or this may develop later.
2. **Polymyalgia rheumatica.** Especially in the elderly, it is at times very difficult to differentiate between late-onset (>60 years) RA that is seronegative and polymyalgia rheumatica. At times, RA may present with prominent soreness and stiffness in the shoulder and pelvic girdles. The presence of temporal arteritis symptoms or signs supports the diagnosis of polymyalgia rheumatica.
3. **Seronegative spondyloarthropathies** characteristically present with asymmetric inflammatory disease of the large joints of the lower extremities, often with low-back disease and telltale manifestations such as psoriasis, urethritis, uveitis, or inflammatory bowel disease.
4. **Crystal deposition arthritis.** Both gout and pseudogout may present in a polyarticular, RA-like fashion. Careful history, radiographs, and joint fluid analysis are helpful in defining these diagnoses.
5. **Osteoarthritis.** In the setting of severe, RA-related joint damage, secondary osteoarthritis may develop and be a contributing factor to joint dysfunction and the need for hip or knee replacement. Osteoarthritis itself can easily be differentiated from RA by a late age of onset, localization in

the distal and proximal interphalangeal joints, monarticular involvement of a single hip or knee, the propensity to involve the neck and low back, and the absence of joint inflammation and constitutional features.

6. Infectious arthritis

a. Viral arthritides may present as a self-limited, RA-like disorder. This is particularly true in the setting of rubella infection or immunization and parvovirus B19 infection. Associated symptoms and signs, serologies, and course establish the diagnosis. Hepatitis C-associated RA-like disease is another consideration. The finding of RF in hepatitis C-associated cryoglobulinemia makes it distinguishable only on documentation of hepatitis C infection. Early hepatitis B may present as a self-limited RA-like disease in the pre-icteric phase.

b. Spirochetal arthritis. Lyme disease rarely presents in an RA-like fashion. Early Lyme disease may present with arthralgias and myalgias in the setting of the erythema chronicum migrans rash and history of tick bite. Late (tertiary) Lyme presents with a waxing and waning monarticular synovitis or oligoarthritis (four or fewer joints) that often involves the knees.

c. Bacterial arthritides. Whipple's disease may present as a peripheral, symmetric, migratory, non-deforming seronegative polyarthritis, simultaneously with or long before gastrointestinal manifestations and lymphadenopathy.

d. Reactive arthritis associated with group A β-hemolytic streptococcal infection. Rheumatic fever must be considered in children and adults of all socioeconomic strata. The telltale clinical presentation is a *migratory* polyarthritis, particularly in the setting of a recent sore throat. Almost invariably, the patient will have an elevated anti-streptolysin O titer and sedimentation rate.

VII. Global assessment of functional status and disease. To craft an optimal therapeutic plan and establish baseline data for later comparison, the initial collection of pertinent clinical, laboratory, and functional information is mandatory. Apart from the traditional detailed history and clinical evaluation, a number of self-report questionnaires [Health Assessment Questionnaire (HAQ), Arthritis Impact Measurement Scale (AIMS)], as well as physician joint count and radiographic scores, have been developed to assess functional capacity, performance of daily activities, disease severity and progression, and response to therapy. Clinical evaluation of the amount of joint damage is based on range of motion, instability, mal-alignment, subluxation, crepitus, and radiographic changes. Negative prognostic markers (e.g., high RF titers; development of erosions, particularly early in the disease course; early or severe functional limitation; family history of severe RA; development of extraarticular disease) should be entered into the clinical and therapeutic equations.

VIII. Treatment

A. Treatment goals in rheumatoid arthritis

1. Control of the immunologic and inflammatory disease process.

2. Prevention of joint damage and normalization of function and life span.

3. Complete relief of symptoms and return to normal performance of activities of daily living.

4. Avoidance of complications of the disease and its treatment.

5. Education, counseling, and physical and occupational therapy.

B. General approach to the patient with rheumatoid arthritis

1. Patient and family education is important in the management of rheumatoid disease. Strong emphasis must be placed on the crucial role played by the patient in minimizing disability. Both the patient and the family must be taught what RA is and how it differs from other forms of arthritis. The patient should be told that RA can be a chronic, lifelong disease but that a variety of measures can lead to disease control. Such emotional support may help the patient to maintain employment or an optimal activity schedule. In addition to familiarizing patients with the concepts of chronic disease and its management, specific points must be stressed regarding individual drug and physical medicine therapies used, nutritional information, quackery, and the social services available to the patient with arthritis. Such an education program can take the form of frank discussions between the physician and the patient and family, supplemented by literature dispensed by the doctor. An optimal setting is an established patient education program that employs lecture and audiovisual material. Sex and vocational counseling should be part of the comprehensive approach to the RA patient.

2. **Exercise and rest.** It is important for the RA patient to maintain a balance between resting and exercising joints that falls short of causing significant pain or fatigue. Systemic and articular rest are both important. Although the classic recommendations for short rest periods during the day (1 hour of bed rest at mid-morning and mid-afternoon) remain, they are incompatible with the work requirements of most people. At times, hospitalization may become necessary to impose a strict balance of rest and activity that cannot be followed by the patient at home. Articular inflammation may be decreased by adequate rest of the affected joints with either bed rest or splints. The purpose of splints is to provide rest for inflamed joints, relieve spasm, and prevent deformities or reduce deformities already present. Wrist splints are particularly useful during bouts of acute wrist synovitis and for the management of carpal tunnel syndrome.
3. **Regular active exercise** with instructions by the physician or physical therapist is important. Exercise is most successful after heat application. A 15-minute early-morning shower or a bath at 98° to 100° will help decrease morning stiffness. Unless advanced deformity, significant joint pain, or muscle wasting is present, slow and deliberate active or active-resistive exercises should be performed twice daily for approximately 15 minutes. These exercises should involve the fingers, wrists, shoulders, and knees, which are the areas most vulnerable to deformity and functional disability (see Chapters 56 and 57). As tolerance for exercise increases and the activity of the disease decreases, progressive resistive exercises are indicated for the improvement of muscular function. Static quadriceps exercises should be performed to strengthen the muscular, ligamentous, and tendinous support of the knees. Initial therapy is 10 to 20 exercise sets in each thigh twice daily.
4. **Principles of joint protection** include maintenance of muscle strength and range of motion, avoidance of positions of deformity, use of the strongest joints possible for a given task, utilization of joints in the most stable anatomic planes, avoidance of continuous use of muscles and joints in a fixed position, and avoidance of activities beyond the patient's muscular capacity. Active exercises in the form of activities that interest the patient should be provided (e.g., sculpting, clay modeling, weaving).
5. **Activities of daily living.** Instruction by the occupational therapist should include self-help devices, resting and functional splints, and the demonstration of alternate methods for task performance aimed at avoiding positions that cause joint deformity. This often includes the use of simulated kitchens, bathrooms, and workplace environments that allow for improvement in functional capacity in sites germane to the patient's life-style.

C. Medication and therapy with biologics: general information

1. Rationale for the modern therapeutic approach

- **a.** RA is an aggressive disorder that demands equally aggressive and early treatment.
- **b.** A lack of evident joint inflammation (e.g., no evidence of disease) is highly correlated with an absence of joint damage.
- **c.** Disease- and damage-modifying medications with acceptable safety profiles are available.
- **d.** Early treatment can prevent joint damage, maintain function, prolong life, and alter the natural history of RA.

e. Combination therapy is usually both effective and safe and is focused on multiple pathogenetic sites.
f. Careful clinical profiling can effectively guide therapy.
g. Careful choice of medications and monitoring for side effects improves outcome.

2. **General therapeutic concepts**
a. A well-crafted treatment regimen should begin soon after the diagnosis and be guided by the patient profile.
b. The regimen, its rationale, potential side effects, and monitoring must be discussed with the patient.
c. The aggressiveness of the regimen should match that of the disease.
d. Patient comorbidities should be factored into the choice of medications.
e. Disease activity and severity and the patient's functional status should be measured at baseline and at regular intervals.
f. Lack of reasonable disease control demands a change in the treatment regimen.
g. Multidrug regimens are state-of-the-art and include the following:
(1) A nonsteroidal antiinflammatory drug (NSAID).
(2) One or more disease-modifying antirheumatic drugs (DMARDs) or biologic agents.
(3) Short courses of an oral or intraarticular steroid, as needed to reset the level of inflammation, improve function, and act as a bridge for other treatments. Regular monitoring is mandatory for each medication and drug combination. Side effects or drug intolerance demands a change in the treatment approach. Collaboration with other professionals should be sought as needed to improve the outcome.

3. **Definition of the patient profile.** This should be established at baseline and at regular intervals. Initial and future therapeutic decisions should be based on the following data:
a. **Quantification of the level of inflammation**
(1) Intensity and extent of joint inflammation (i.e., number and intensity of red, warm, tender, swollen joints).
(2) Duration of morning stiffness, in minutes or hours.
(3) Severity of constitutional symptoms (fatigue and weight loss can be quantified).
(4) Determination of ESR, levels of C-reactive protein and hemoglobin, platelet count.
(5) Presence or development of manifestations of extraarticular disease.
b. **Measurement of functional limitation.** Use of functional instruments, including the HAQ and the AIMS2, can accurately measure function (see Chapter 7), as can use of a simple visual analog scale in which 0 represents full function and 10 the worst possible functional limitation.
c. **Measurement of joint damage.** New erosions or joint deformity, as defined by physical examination and plain radiography.

4. **Treatment regimens.** All regimens should include physical therapy, an educational program, optimal drug-specific monitoring, and prevention of side effects (protective medication for the stomach for patients on NSAIDs, if indicated by past medical history).

5. **Patient profile for mild disease.** Mild joint inflammation (5 to 10 joints mildly swollen and tender), 20 minutes of morning stiffness, minimal functional limitation or still working full-time, no manifestations of extraarticular disease, mild elevation of ESR to 20 to 30 mm/h without anemia or thrombocytosis, no erosions or joint deformities.
a. **Recommended treatment regimen**
(1) NSAID.
(2) DMARD: antimalarial drug (Plaquenil), sulfasalazine (Azulfidine), or IM gold. Some rheumatologists might add minocycline in early disease.

b. Follow-up

(1) Assessment of disease activity and response to treatment regimen every 1 to 2 months.

(2) Lack of a 75% or better improvement or clear worsening of disease parameters within 3 months demands a reassessment of the treatment approach and possible movement to the regimen for moderate disease.

6. Patient profile for moderate disease. Moderate joint inflammation and some limitation in range of motion (20 to 30 joints with moderately severe swelling, tenderness with some erythema), 1 hour or more of morning stiffness, moderate functional limitation with threatened loss of work, moderate fatigue that limits function, rheumatoid nodules, ESR over 50 mm/h with anemia and thrombocytosis, high RF titers, marginal erosions in hands and feet.

a. Recommended treatment regimen

(1) NSAID.

(2) Combination DMARD: methotrexate (MTX) plus hydroxychloroquine, or IM gold plus hydroxychloroquine. Short courses of low-dose prednisone to reset the level of inflammation (e.g., 10 to 20 mg of prednisone daily in divided doses, tapered to zero over 3 to 5 days). If the patient fails to show a 75% or better improvement in response to a combination of hydroxychloroquine plus full-dose MTX (i.e., 20 to 25 mg/wk) or a 3-month course of parenteral gold, consider the following therapeutic alternatives, as guided by prior drug usge, comorbidities, and patient choice.

(3) At times, a change from oral to SC, IM, or IV routes of administration of MTX can improve the clinical response.

(4) Addition of sulfasalazine (SSZ) to MTX plus hydroxychloroquine.

(5) Addition of low-dose cyclosporine (CyA) (1 to 2.5 mg/kg daily) to 15 mg of MTX per week. Hydroxychloroquine can be continued or stopped.

(6) Addition of parenteral anti-TNF therapy to 15 mg of MTX per week, or discontinuation of MTX and use of anti-TNF therapy alone.

(7) Discontinuation of MTX and institution of 2 mg of azathioprine (AZA) per kilogram daily.

(8) Discontinuation of MTX and institution of 100 mg of leflunomide daily for 3 days, then 20 mg PO daily or combination therapy with both.

b. Follow-up. Assessment of disease activity and response to treatment regimen every month, with changes in therapy as noted above.

7. Patient profile for severe disease. Severe joint inflammation and deformities (20 to 30 or more red, warm, swollen, tender joints with ulnar deviation, swan neck deformities, and moderate to severe limitation in range of motion), morning stiffness lasting most of the day, loss of work, severe fatigue with weight loss, rheumatoid nodules, and possibly other extra-articular manifestations, such as sclerosis, serositis, ESR between 50 and 100 mm/h with significant anemia (hemoglobin, 9.5 g%) and thrombocytosis (platelet count, 500,000 to 600, 000/mm^3 or higher), many erosions, joint space narrowing, and joint deformities noted on plain radiography.

a. Recommended treatment regimen

(1) NSAID.

(2) DMARD combination

(a) MTX plus hydroxychloroquine plus SSZ.

(b) MTX plus CyA.

(c) MTX plus anti-TNF agent.

(3) Short courses of prednisone (as above) *or* daily low-dose prednisone (5 mg/d), *or* intermittent minipulses of IV Solu-Medrol (250 mg/d for 1 to 2 days).

(4) If improvement is no better than 50% to 75% or if disease worsens despite the above regimens, consider the following:
   (a) AZA (2 mg/kg daily) in combination with hydroxychloroquine or an anti-TNF agent.
   (b) Leflunomide (100 mg daily for 3 days), then 20 mg PO daily in combination with hydroxychloroquine or MTX.

(5) In the *setting of severe, refractory disease* unresponsive to the above regimens, or of systemic, necrotizing vasculitis, consider the following:
   (a) Cyclophosphamide (CTX) (2 mg/kg PO daily), with steroids or
   (b) CTX (monthly IV dose of 0.5 g/m^2).
   (c) Until disease control is attained, (a) or (b) can be given for 3 to 4 months, then one can switch to 20 to 25 mg of MTX per week or to alternative immunosuppressive agents such as AZA, CyA, or leflunomide.

b. Follow-up
(1) Close follow-up monthly or more often.
(2) Vigorous program of physical therapy, emotional and vocational support.
(3) Hospitalization may be needed to balance activity and therapy optimally, institute new medications, and consider parenteral steroid treatments.

D. Medications and biologic agents

1. Nonsteroidal antiinflammatory drugs. NSAIDs do not appear to alter the natural history of RA, but they can contribute to control of a component of the inflammatory process. NSAIDs are appropriately used early in the course of the disease to relieve pain and decrease the amount of inflammation while the diagnosis is established. Later in the course of the disease, NSAIDs are used in combination with DMARDs. The choice of NSAIDs is quite individual, and most rheumatologists employ traditional nonacetylated salicylates and nonsalicylate NSAIDs or COX-2-specific NSAIDs rather than aspirin. This system has evolved because of the ease of dosing and despite the higher costs of non-aspirin NSAIDs. The side effect profile of some of the NSAIDs has been shown to be higher than that of some of the DMARDs. This is particularly true in the elderly. All NSAIDs can lead to gastrointestinal ulceration and renal injury, but in general, COX-2-specific NSAIDs appear to cause significantly fewer gastrointestinal problems.

a. Indications. Although these drugs do *not* appear to have the capacity to induce a disease remission or prevent the formation of joint erosions, they can decrease pain and inflammation, so that the patient is better able to preserve function and range of motion.

b. Mechanism of action. Although their dominant action relates to the ability to inhibit the cyclooxygenase enzyme and thus pro-inflammatory prostaglandins, NSAIDs also inhibit lipoxygenase and lysosomal enzyme release, antagonize kinins, and induce apoptosis. Cyclooxygenase-1 (COX-1) is present in many tissues and is responsible for the production of prostaglandins in the gastric mucosa, endothelium, platelets, and kidneys. COX-1 inhibition by NSAIDs is linked to known adverse effects, such as gastric ulceration and renal toxicity. Cyclooxygenase-2 (COX-2) is an inducible, pro-inflammatory enzyme. Although different NSAIDs vary in the degree to which they inhibit both enzymes, in many cases, both COX-1 and COX-2 are inhibited at the high doses used for clinical purposes. Two new COX-2-specific inhibitors are now in widespread use (Celebrex and Vioxx); although similar in effectiveness to other NSAIDs, they appear to cause significantly less gastrointestinal toxicity.

c. Therapeutic approach. NSAIDs are often used in combination with one or more of the DMARDs, and at times with DMARDs and steroids. All salicylate and nonsalicylate NSAIDs share a similar toxicity profile.

The elderly, however, are more vulnerable to all types of side effects in view of age-related alterations in metabolism and excretion. The presence of preexisting gastric, hepatic, or renal disease in any patient is particularly important and may predispose to increased tissue injury. Thus, if NSAIDs are needed in this group of patients, they should be used with great caution, in the lowest dose possible, and with close monitoring for adverse drug effects. Note that elderly women on NSAIDs have the highest likelihood of developing potentially life-threatening gastric ulcer disease with bleeding. Gastric protection is not indicated in every patient; however, it should be considered in high-risk patients. The use of COX-2-specific NSAIDs will protect all patients.

d. Cost. All the non-aspirin NSAIDs are very expensive, at times costing more than $1.00 a day. This needs to be factored into the therapeutic equation when the physician is deciding on which NSAID to choose. This is particularly true in patients on a fixed budget who are taking multiple medications. However, although plain aspirin is much cheaper, the cumbersome regimen of 12 to 16 tablets per day taken in four doses must be appreciated.

e. Routine use and dosage regimen. The choice of NSAID is quite individual, varies greatly from physician to physician, and often depends on the presence of preexisting medical problems. The general approach is to choose an NSAID and treat for 3 to 4 weeks, the usual time period needed to define the efficacy and side effect profile of a drug. If there is no clinical response, or if the patient cannot tolerate the drug, an alternative NSAID is started. Often, four to five such cycles are carried out, and then the patient is placed on the most effective of the drugs tried. Patients vary greatly with regard to their propensity to improve clinically or suffer side effects. The physician's choice should be guided by an appreciation of the patient's age and medical history. Patient compliance is highest with once-daily dosing or a twice-daily regimen.

f. Specific agents. Carboxylic acids, enolic acids, and non-acidic compounds are the three chemical classes of NSAIDs. Carboxylic acids comprise the largest family, and salicylates (aspirin), acetic acid (diclofenac, indomethacin), proprionic acids (ibuprofen, naproxen), enolic acids (piroxicam), and substituted pyrozoles (celecoxib, rofecoxib) are commonly used.

(1) Salicylates were, historically, the initial treatment of choice for RA. Aspirin (acetylsalicylic acid) is antiinflammatory in therapeutic dosages of 3.6 to 6.0 g/d (12 to 16 300-mg tablets per day; serum salicylate levels of 15 to 25 mg/dL) and analgesic at lower dosages (fewer than eight 300-mg tablets per day). Salicylates are administered at dosages of 600 to 1,200 mg every 4 to 6 hours, usually with meals or with antacid to minimize gastric irritation. Constant serum drug levels can be achieved in most patients with this dosage interval. The dosages needed to achieve therapeutic concentrations vary widely, especially in the elderly. Salicylate levels can be used to monitor compliance. Hepatic metabolic pathways may become saturated at higher levels. Therefore, a small dosage increase can result in a very large elevation of the serum salicylate level and salicylism. Similarly, when the dose is decreased, small decreases may bring about rapid decreases in the salicylate level. The maximum tolerated dosage should be approached slowly because it may take as long as a week after each dosage change to achieve a new, steady level. Rectal suppositories are available; however, rectal absorption is incomplete.

(2) Other nonsteroidal antiinflammatory drugs. These agents are equipotent to aspirin and are thought to exert their antiinflammatory action by modifying prostaglandin metabolism. Most rheumatologists use nonsalicylate NSAIDs rather than plain aspirin. Major attributes of this class of drugs include ease of administration (especially in the once- or twice-daily regimens), the potential for improved compliance, and COX-2 specificity. This has to be balanced against their high cost relative to aspirin. More than a dozen NSAIDs are available. The complete list is found in Appendix E. The agents listed below have been successfully used at our institution.

(a) **Celecoxib.** The first of the class of COX-2-specific inhibitors, it is well tolerated and indicated for treatment of RA in a dosage of 200 to 400 μg/d (tablet sizes of 100 μg and 200 mL). As discussed below, the COX-2-specific inhibitors offer analgesic and antiinflammatory efficacy comparable to that of the older NSAIDs but are significantly safer with regard to the GI tract.

(b) **Naproxen.** Well tolerated; twice-daily regimen or slow-release tablets for once-a-day use encourage compliance; tablet sizes are 250 mg, 375 mg, and 500 mg; the dosage schedule is defined by the severity of joint disease.

(c) **Piroxicam.** Generally well tolerated; once-daily dosage schedule encourages compliance; capsule sizes are 10 mg and 20 mg; usual dosage is 20 mg/d PO (sometimes taken as an evening dose for patients with severe morning stiffness or 10 mg PO twice daily); doses larger than 20 mg/d are probably associated with increased gastrointestinal toxicity. NSAIDs with a long half-life, such as piroxicam (Feldene), should be used with greater caution in elderly patients because of the increased propensity for side effects.

(d) **Sulindac.** Generally well tolerated; twice-daily regimen encourages compliance; tablet sizes are 150 mg and 200 mg; usual dosage is 150 to 200 mg PO twice daily.

(e) **Indomethacin** is effective in the control of acute flares of RA. Capsule sizes are 25 mg and 50 mg; the usual dosage regimen is 25 mg three to four times daily. A slow-release preparation is available; the 75-mg dose is equivalent to 25 mg three times daily; two 75-mg doses are equivalent to 50 mg three times daily.

(f) **Ibuprofen.** 200 to 800 mg. The therapeutic dosage is usually 300 to 800 mg three to four times daily. Shorter-acting NSAIDs may be safer in the elderly. A 200-mg tablet is available over the counter.

(g) **Diclofenac** is available as 25- to 75-mg tablets, as 100-mg extended-release tablets, and in combination with misoprostol (arthrotec). The usual effective dosage is 50 to 100 mg twice daily.

g. Common side effects

(1) **Gastrointestinal effects.** The most common side effects of NSAIDs include dyspepsia, peptic ulceration (gastric more often than duodenal), hemorrhage, and perforation. Protective techniques include the following:

(a) **Avoidance of nonsteroidal antiinflammatory drugs and treatment with alternative modalities** (i.e., oral or intraarticular steroids, pain medications, physical therapy, DMARDs). This is particularly true in high-risk patients, including the elderly, those with a past history of peptic ulcer disease or significant NSAID-related dyspepsia, patients on steroids, and those with comorbidities such as cardiac disease.

(b) **Taking nonsteroidal inflammatory drugs with meals** will reduce the incidence and severity of dyspepsia but does not reduce occult bleeding (2 to 10 mL/d in 70% of patients taking usual aspirin doses). Guaiac-positive stools (trace to 1+) are common during aspirin therapy. A gastrointestinal evaluation is performed when clinically indicated by persistent gastrointestinal reflux, abdominal discomfort, significant decrease in hemoglobin levels, syncope, or melena.

(c) **Use of medications to protect the stomach.** Misoprostol, a synthetic prostaglandin E_1 analog, acid pump inhibitors, and histamine$_2$ inhibitors have all been shown to protect the gastric mucosa from the irritative effects of NSAIDs. The first two medications are probably the most effective. The main side effects of misoprostol include the potential to cause abortion, teratogenicity (congenital facialis), and diarrhea and bloating soon after institution. These agents should be employed only in those high-risk patients noted above.

(d) **Use of cyclooxygenase-2-specific inhibitors.** These drugs may be employed first, especially in higher-risk patients. It must be noted that although they are safer, these drugs do not appear to be more effective than other NSAIDs.

(2) **Tinnitus or deafness** is usually the earliest indication of salicylate toxicity in adults and is reversible with a small (one or two tablets) decrease in daily dosage. There is an inverse relationship between plasma salicylate levels at which auditory symptoms appear and the age of the patient. Other NSAIDs can also cause tinnitus.

(3) **Central nervous system symptoms** such as headache, vertigo, nausea, vomiting, irritability, and even psychosis can occur, especially in the elderly. These symptoms can be quite severe with indomethacin treatment. NSAID-induced aseptic meningitis has been reported.

(4) **Hepatic abnormalities.** Transient and asymptomatic transaminase elevations are commonly seen in patients on NSAIDs and often resolve with or without drug discontinuation. The drug should be stopped if the serum level is more than three times the upper limits of normal. Significant hepatitis may also occur, especially in patients with juvenile RA and active SLE. Acute hepatic cellular injury can occur, particularly when aspirin is taken in the setting of a viral illness (Reye's syndrome).

(5) **Platelet and hematologic abnormalities.** Platelet adenosine diphosphate release, adhesiveness, and aggregation are inhibited for as long as 72 hours after a single 300-mg dose of aspirin, probably as a result of irreversible acetylation of platelet membrane proteins. COX-1 is also found on platelets, and inhibition of COX-1 by the nonspecific NSAIDs will inhibit platelet aggregation. This side effect should be taken into consideration before and after surgery and in the final weeks of pregnancy. This effect does not occur with salsalate and is reversible with other traditional NSAIDs. NSAIDs should be stopped at least 3 to 5 days before surgical procedures. COX-2-specific NSAIDs do not cause these platelet effects but can increase the prothrombin time (international normalized ratio) via protein binding effects. Other, less common adverse hematologic effects include aplastic anemia and neutropenia. The presence of unexplained anemia should stimulate an assessment for blood loss.

(6) **Acute bronchospasm** can be induced by aspirin and other NSAIDs in asthmatic patients and patients with nasal polyposis. Patients in whom this problem develops with one NSAID should avoid others.

(7) **Dermatologic abnormalities.** A wide spectrum of skin lesions can be caused by the broad array of NSAIDs, including exfoliative dermatitis.

(8) **Drug interactions.** These occur either through competition for albumin binding or overlapping drug effects. With oral anticoagulants, the effect of warfarin (Coumadin) can be increased, and an NSAID-induced platelet defect can further increase the risk for bleeding. Gastrointestinal bleeding can occur in the setting of

NSAID-related gastric mucosal defects. Decreased renal clearance resulting from NSAIDs and albumin-binding competition can lead to increased levels of lithium and an increased risk for hypoglycemia in patients taking oral hypoglycemic drugs.

2. **Corticosteroids.** Although these drugs are highly potent antiinflammatory agents, they are associated with a high incidence of cumulative toxicity when administered on a long-term basis. It is for this reason that the physician and patient must be aware that optimal therapy in RA involves the lowest dose for the shortest period of time. Steroids can be used in short courses systemically or intraarticularly to control acute disease flares, as bridge therapy until DMARDs begin to act, or on a long-term basis.
   a. **Indications.** The indications for corticosteroids in RA include the following:
      (1) **Active synovitis** in a single joint out of proportion to all others: intraarticular steroids are quite effective in this setting. The dose of Depo-Medrol (40 mg/cc) is proportional to the size of the joint. The full 40 mg is injected into knee joints in the same syringe with 1 cc of 1% xylocaine without epinephrine. Note: Steroids should *not* be injected if there is a possibility of joint infection.
      (2) **Multiple joints are inflamed and markedly limited in function despite the active use of nonsteroidal antiinflammatory drugs and disease-modifying antirheumatic drugs.** In this setting, a short course of oral prednisone (a 4-day course beginning with 20 mg and tapered by 5 mg/d to zero over 4 days) may be very helpful in rapidly resetting the level of inflammation and improving function. At times, minipulses of IV Solu-Medrol (250 mg/d for 1 to 3 days) are needed to bring severe disease under control rapidly.
      (3) **Bridge therapy** is needed to control disease until a recently started DMARD begins to work. This can be in the form of short (2 to 4 days) courses of prednisone or a daily, low-dose (5 mg/d) regimen. The physician should attempt to taper the steroids once the DMARD begins to control the disease.
      (4) **Severe flares of polyarthritis with any attempt to taper steroids** may occur while a patient appears to be doing well on a combination drug regimen of NSAIDs and DMARDs. At times, these patients will be relegated to long-term steroid therapy. If that is the case, the safest dose is 5 mg or less daily. This possible scenario must be appreciated when steroids are started. Long-term steroid use requires increased monitoring for and prophylaxis against side effects such as osteoporosis.
      (5) **Prominent constitutional or extraarticular manifestations.** At times, manifestations such as fatigue, weight loss, serositis (pleurisy or pericarditis), or a polyarteritis nodosa-like vasculitis dominate the clinical picture. Although DMARDs will be employed to control these problems in the long run, steroids are often needed acutely to regain disease control and function.
      (6) **Fatigue, weight loss, fever.** (Note: Fever is *not* a common manifestation of active RA.) Low doses of prednisone (10 to 20 mg initially, then 5 mg/d) are often sufficient to control these problems that have not been suppressed by NSAIDs. DMARDs are also aimed at such problems but take longer to act.
      (7) **Rheumatoid vasculitis (malignant rheumatoid arthritis).** Fortunately rare, rheumatoid vasculitis is a polyarteritis nodosa-like disorder that occurs in patients who have had chronic, severe, deforming, seropositive, nodular RA. Presentations might include fever, neuropathy, leg ulcers, and ischemic disease of the intestines, heart, and nerves. This is often an organ- or life-threatening disorder and thus demands aggressive treatment. Steroid dosage varies and is guided by the severity of the disorder. Prednisone (40 to 60 mg/d in divided doses; 20 mg three times daily with meals) or

pulses of Solu-Medrol (250 to 1, 000 mg/d for 1 to 3 days) followed by prednisone are employed and titrated in proportion to disease control. Steroids are commonly employed along with immunosuppresive agents such as cyclophosphamide in the setting of active, systemic vasculitis.

b. **Mechanism of action.** Corticosteroids attach to cell membrane receptors and trigger an increased synthesis of lipocortin. This substance inhibits the release of phospholipase A_2 and therefore the production of pro-inflammatory prostaglandins, leukotrienes, and oxygen radicals. Corticosteroids inhibit cytokines such as IL-I, IL-2, TNF, and α-interferon as well as some pro-inflammatory enzymes such as elastase and plasminogen activator. Corticosteroids induce apoptosis of lymphocytes *in vitro* and *in vivo* and inhibit lymphocyte proliferation and delayed-type hypersensitivity *in vitro.* Inhibition of antigen presentation and reduced expression of Fc receptors may represent additional mechanisms of action.

c. **Therapeutic approach.** Steroids continue to be the most powerful antiinflammatory agents available today. However, because of their well-defined side effects, one should always try to taper steroids as much as possible and use alternative disease-controlling, steroid-sparing agents (i.e., NSAIDs, DMARDs, physical and occupational therapy, and intraarticular steroids). Remember that starting a patient on steroids does not commit the physician to continuing it forever. And, with an understanding of other medications in the RA armamentarium, the physician can prescribe steroids in an enlightened manner and prevent their long-term side effects.

d. **Steroid preparations and administration**

(1) **Prednisone** is the preferred oral agent because its cost and mineralocorticoid activity are low. Scored tablets come in many sizes, so that the patient can mix and match them as disease control is attempted and the dose is tapered. Tablet sizes include 1 mg, 2.5 mg, 5 mg, 10 mg, and 20 mg. For suppression of disease manifestations, the optimal and safest maintenance regimen is no more than 5.0 to 7.5 mg of prednisone, preferably in a single morning dose. In patients with severe disease and incapacitating morning symptoms, the dose can be taken with dinner, or a split schedule with dosing at breakfast and dinner may be best. The total dose should be the smallest possible needed to relieve symptoms. At times, a severe and incapacitating acute flare of RA may require ambulatory or in-hospital management with the institution of 20 mg of prednisone per day for 3 to 5 days and tapering thereafter. Rheumatoid vasculitis, if manifested by mesenteric and other internal organ ischemia, is an indication for 40 to 60 mg of prednisone per day because of its malignant, life-threatening nature.

(2) **Prednisolone and methylprednisolone** are alternative types of steroids. Some physicians favor these because of the fact that prednisone is metabolized in the liver to prednisolone, the active steroid agent. These drugs are a bit more expensive than prednisone but have less mineralocorticoid effect (i.e., less fluid and salt retention), and they may be absorbed better and work effectively in some patients. Four milligrams of these agents equals 5 mg of prednisone. "Pulse," high-dose Solu-Medrol (250 to 1,000 mg/d for 1 to 3 days IV) is sometimes administered to patients with severe, active disease unresponsive to other treatment modalities, or patients with rheumatoid vasculitis. At times, this therapy can bring about disease control, which can then be maintained with low-dose oral steroids, DMARDs, and NSAIDs. Particular surveillance for hypertension, arrhythmia, hyperkalemia, serum glucose elevation, and infection is indicated in patients receiving this form of treatment. This should not be considered part of the routine management of RA patients.

(3) Administration of **intraarticular corticosteroids** is a highly effective way of controlling a disease flare concentrated in a single joint and avoids the need for systemic oral steroids. A single joint flare, out of proportion to all others, is common in RA. However, the physician must consider and rule out the possibility of infection in that single joint before injecting steroids, especially in patients who have fever or prior infections. The risk for introducing infection, although slight, is always present; thus, careful aseptic technique is required. (For technique, dosage, and preparations, see Chapter 20.) An evanescent flare in a joint after injection may occur because of inflammation induced by leukocyte ingestion of corticosteroid ester microcrystals. This possibility should be brought to the patient's attention, and the patient should be told to treat this with a pain medication and an ice pack. Within 12 to 24 hours, the injection-induced joint pain should improve, and relief may persist anywhere from a month to forever. If the initial joint pain was primarily mechanical in origin (i.e., resulting from joint damage), the improvement may be very short-lived. Frequent intraarticular corticosteroid injections (more than once in a 2- to 3-month period or more than three times a year) are not advised because there is evidence that they may lead to accelerated cartilage damage.

e. Common adverse effects. Fifty years ago, steroids were first used for the treatment of RA. Since that time, steroids have been the model of a "double-edged sword," one edge representing the most powerful anti-inflammatory agent and the other a wide array of dose-related side effects. A recent study evaluated RA patients who were treated with oral steroids for more than 1 year and compared them with patients who had never received them. An average of 5 mg or less of prednisone was not associated with a higher risk for peptic ulcer, infection, or osteoporosis. However, the incidence of these side effects increased significantly as the mean steroid dosage increased, with the highest likelihood at dosages above 15 to 20 mg/d. The problem of using steroids in a chronic disorder such as RA is that the dose often has to be increased as the disease progresses. A more complete list can be found in Appendix E.

(1) **Osteoporosis.** In patients with RA, the combined effects of cytokine-induced bone resorption, long-term steroid therapy, the postmenopausal state, and decreased mobility can lead to severe osteoporosis. Thus, for any RA patient who is placed on steroids for more than 1 month and in whom long-term treatment is anticipated, a bone protection monitoring and treatment program should be instituted. This includes an initial bone density test (dual-energy x-ray absorptiometry), calcium and vitamin D_3 supplements, and antiresorptive medications (e.g., estrogens, bisphosphonates) if osteopenia or osteoporosis is defined by density testing. This protocol should be followed for both women and men, the latter assessed for androgen deficiency in the face of low bone density or fragility fractures. Optimal RA control is mandatory because it improves mobility, decreases levels of bone-depleting, disease-related cytokines, and allows doses of steroids to be decreased.

(2) **Risk for infection.** The use of steroids clearly increases the risk for all types of infection, most prominently in those patients treated with mean doses above 10 mg PO daily. RA patients are particularly prone to *Staphylococcus aureus* infections. Influenza and pneumococcal immunization are strongly recommended, and the presence of fever in an RA patient should always stimulate the search for an infection. Bacterial infections are particularly problematic in patients with joint replacements because of the possibility of seeding of the artificial joint.

(3) **Miscellaneous.** The following selected steroid-related adverse effects can further exacerbate functional limitation or shorten life:
(a) Diabetes mellitus.
(b) Hypertension.
(c) Premature atherosclerosis.
(d) Cataracts.
(e) Steroid myopathy.

3. **Disease-modifying antirheumatic drugs.** Drugs in this class differ from NSAIDs and steroids in that they **act slowly,** during a period of 1 to 3 months. This trait has led to use of the term slow-acting antirheumatic drugs. In addition, they appear to **alter the natural history** of RA by causing erosions to heal and preventing new ones from developing, controlling the inflammatory state, and improving function. Many of the so-called DMARDs fall short of fulfilling this difficult-to-achieve definition, especially the ability to control the development of erosions. This general class of drugs includes gold (oral and IM), hydroxychloroquine, sulfasalazine (SSZ), D-penicillamine, immunosuppressive agents [methotrexate (MTX), azathioprine (AZA), leflunomide (LEF), cyclosporine (CyA), and cyclophosphamide (CTX)], and biologic agents. These drugs differ greatly in chemical structures and pharmacokinetics, presumed modes of action, clinical indications, positions in the treatment algorithm, and toxicity profiles. MTX, as a single agent or in combination with other DMARDs, has had a profound effect on our ability to control this aggressive disease. Its effectiveness and safety have established its central position in treatment plans, particularly in patients with moderate to severe disease. The fact that 60% of RA patients are still on MTX after a 5-year period, as opposed to only 20% on other DMARDs, attests to the excellent track record of MTX in regard to effectiveness and patient tolerance.

a. **Gold salts.** Injectable (IM) gold is a slow-acting DMARD that can prevent disease progression and, in a small percentage of patients, lead to an impressive, albeit short-lived, degree of disease control. However, gold as a single drug has fallen out of favor because of the effectiveness, safety profile, and ease of administration of MTX. Because of a high rate of toxicity (minor and reversible in most patients), the need for repeated visits to the physician's office for IM injections, and a variable clinical response, most patients discontinue gold within 1 to 2 years after initiation of treatment. However, some may greatly benefit for many years from the safe weekly and eventually monthly treatment. Oral gold, although associated with fewer side effects than IM gold, is less effective, especially in patients with severe disease and functional limitation.

(1) **Indications.** Despite the fact that IM gold has been relegated to a secondary role in the treatment of RA, it is a useful option, and along with NSAIDs and antimalarial drugs could be an early choice in established RA. It is contraindicated in patients with a history of previous severe skin, bone marrow, or renal reactions to gold. Significant functional impairment of the kidneys or liver is a relative contraindication to gold therapy, but toxicity to these organs is rare, and with careful clinical and laboratory monitoring, serious problems can be avoided. Leukopenia was previously considered a relative contraindication, but gold-induced improvement of leukopenia has been demonstrated in patients with Felty's syndrome (RA, granulocytopenia, and splenomegaly).

(2) The **mechanism of action** of gold is not completely understood. At physiologic concentrations, aurothiomalate inhibits the binding of transcription factors such as AP-1, which is a dimer of jun and fos. The possible consequence is a reduction of expression of cytokines, metalloproteinases, and adhesion molecules. Another cellular action of injectable gold may be related to the formation of monomeric aurocyanide during phagocytosis.

(3) **Therapeutic approach.** Clinical response occurs after a cumulative dose of 400 to 600 mg and often plateaus after 800 to 1,000 mg. If toxicity occurs, it usually appears after 300 to 700 mg of gold has been administered; however, undesirable reactions may occur at any time during the course of therapy. Although the incidence of adverse reactions varies, some toxicity develops in 30% to 40% of patients receiving gold salts.

(a) **Parenteral gold.** Aurothioglucose (Solganal, our recommended IM gold preparation) and gold thiomalate (Myochrysine) are given by deep IM injection. The initial dose should be small (10 mg) to test for drug idiosyncrasy (e.g., rash, thrombocytopenia). If this dose is tolerated, 25 mg should be given 1 week later, and then 50 mg weekly if tolerated. Improvement is gradual and continues over a period of several weeks to months. When improvement levels off, usually at doses ranging from 800 to 1,000 mg, the frequency of administration can be decreased to 50 mg once every 2 weeks for 1 to 2 months, then gradually to 50 mg once a month. If gold is discontinued, the condition flares in some patients within several months. Therefore, if gold is tolerated, the patient is advised to continue gold injections indefinitely (some physicians reassess gold therapy at the 5-year level). The degree of improvement is proportional to the duration of treatment. However, if improvement does not occur after a total dose of 1,000 mg, the drug should be discontinued. Future courses of gold salts in such patients are unlikely to be effective. Close monitoring of the urinalysis and complete blood counts with platelet and differential evaluation is mandatory.

(b) **Oral gold (auranofin).** Although parenteral gold therapy has played an important role in the treatment of RA, alternative, less toxic gold preparations have been sought. Auranofin, a unique, synthetic oral gold compound, has been used in the treatment of mild RA. Although the overall toxicity of oral gold is lower, the effectiveness of parenteral gold is significantly higher. Auranofin can produce all the same toxicities as parenteral gold (skin rash, stomatitis, proteinuria, thrombocytopenia); diarrhea develops in 40% of patients, and 6% of patients discontinue the drug because of this toxicity. Auranofin comes in 3-mg capsules, and the dosage is one capsule twice a day. Toxicities other than diarrhea should be addressed by immediate drug discontinuation, just as with parenteral gold. If diarrhea is mild, a decrease in dosage to 3 mg/d may relieve the gastrointestinal complaint; if severe, discontinuation is indicated. Although the drug manufacturer recommends only monthly complete blood cell counts, platelet counts, differential counts, and urinalysis, we recommend studies at least every 2 weeks for the first 3 to 4 months of therapy with close observation for cytopenias, proteinuria, and hematuria.

(4) Common **side effects** include the following:

(a) **Skin and mucous membrane reactions.** The most common gold toxicity is dermatitis, which is invariably associated with pruritus and at times with eosinophilia. It is almost always reversible on drug discontinuation. Stomatitis, another mucocutaneous side effect, is frequently painless. The development of these side effects is an indication to withhold gold until the lesions clear. Except in the instance of a severe reaction or exfoliative dermatitis, an uncommon but serious problem, treatment may be reinstituted at a low dose such as 5 mg, with eventual slow escalation of dose. Eosinophilia without rash should alert the physician to watch more carefully for side effects.

(b) **Renal effects.** Because proteinuria is detectable in at least 10% of patients receiving gold therapy, a urinalysis should be performed before each gold injection. Nephritis and the nephrotic syndrome are uncommon. The most common histologic lesion is a membranous glomerulonephritis. Renal failure is rare. If minor urinary abnormalities occur (proteinuria <500 mg/d), therapy should be interrupted until the urine is normal, then reinstituted at low doses. If the abnormalities recur, gold must be stopped. Most skin and kidney reactions, particularly dermatitis and proteinuria, will clear only after discontinuation of the drug. Antihistamines (25 mg of hydroxyzine three times daily) may be useful for pruritus. Corticosteroids (40 to 60 mg of prednisone daily) are beneficial in some instances of severe rash or exfoliative dermatitis or nephritis. Treatment with heavy-metal chelators (dimercaprol or penicillamine) is usually unnecessary.

(c) **Hematologic effects.** The most serious side effects of gold therapy are hematologic and include thrombocytopenia, agranulocytosis, and aplastic anemia. These complications are rare. Granulocytopenia may be noted incidentally on routine blood tests or may present with fever and pharyngitis. Thrombocytopenia is not dose-related and may occur after very low cumulative doses of gold. Aplastic anemia is a rare complication and has been reported even long after the cessation of gold therapy. For the first few months of therapy, complete blood cell and platelet counts should be performed *before* each gold injection is given. If no changes have occurred after 3 to 4 months, the tests can be performed at 2-week intervals and, ultimately, at monthly intervals. A trend toward progressive cytopenias may be observed by making a flow sheet of the patient's laboratory data, including white blood cell count, hemoglobin level, platelet count, polymorphonuclear percentage, and absolute neutrophil count. Management of severe hematologic gold toxicity, such as thrombocytopenia, includes the administration of 60 mg of prednisone daily in three divided doses; 200 mg of anabolic steroids such as testosterone propionate IM three times weekly; and chelating agents such as dimercaprol, penicillamine, and ethylenediamine-tetraacetic acid (EDTA). *N*-acetylcysteine may be employed for the treatment of leukopenia and thrombocytopenia. However, it has not been proven that any of these therapies influence outcome. Granulocyte colony-stimulating factor (G-CSF) has been effective in the setting of gold-induced leukopenia.

(d) A **nitritoid reaction** consisting of hypotension, flushing of the face and neck, shortness of breath, tongue swelling, nausea, and vertigo can sometimes occur after administration of gold compounds, especially gold thiomalate. Management includes switching to another gold compound or decreasing the dosage and administration with the patient supine.

(e) **Miscellaneous.** A number of unusual adverse reactions have been ascribed to gold, including enterocolitis, intrahepatic cholestasis, skin hyperpigmentation, peripheral neuropathy, deposits of gold in the cornea (chrysiasis), and pulmonary infiltrates.

(5) **Repeated treatment.** Patients with severe toxicity, such as thrombocytopenia, aplastic anemia, exfoliative dermatitis, or nephropathy, should not be re-treated with gold. With milder side effects, especially mucocutaneous reactions, it may be possible to reinstitute gold beginning with low doses (e.g., 5 mg) 4 weeks after resolution of the skin reaction.

b. Antimalarial drugs. Hydroxychloroquine (Plaquenil) is an effective, slow-acting, antimalarial DMARD with an optimal balance between positive and negative clinical effects.

(1) Indications. Hydroxychloroquine is commonly employed as a single agent in the setting of mild disease or in combination with other DMARDs in the treatment or more severe or refractory disease.

(2) The **mechanism of action** is probably related to accumulation of the drug in the acid vesicular lysosomal system of mononuclear cells, granulocytes, and fibroblasts. In macrophages, antimalarials may inhibit antigen presentation and IL-1 release.

(3) Therapeutic approach. Studies have demonstrated the effectiveness of hydroxychloroquine in RA following 4 to 6 months of treatment. It is considered a somewhat weaker agent than MTX or gold. However, because of its relatively low toxicity, it is often used in patients with milder courses of RA or in combination regimens. Tablet size is 200 mg. Six weeks to 6 months of therapy may be required before a therapeutic effect is evident. If objective improvement does not occur within 3 to 6 months, the drug should be discontinued or another DMARD should be added.

(4) Dosage and administration. The initial dosage (5 to 6 mg/kg daily) is given with food to decrease gastric intolerance. When a good response is obtained (4 to 12 weeks), maintenance of effect is usually satisfactory at the next lower whole-tablet dosage level. The dose can be adjusted by cutting the tablet in half (the taste can be bitter) or by taking a whole tablet on an every-other-day basis (e.g., 200 mg one day and 400 mg the next gives a mean dose of 300 mg).

(5) Side effects

(a) Eye toxicity. Antimalarial drugs, particularly chloroquine, which is a cousin of hydroxychloroquine, have a history of causing retinal toxicity. The **premaculopathy** phase of retinal toxicity is an "early-warning period" and is completely reversible. The **maculopathy phase** is not reversible. Such retinal changes can occur *after* chloroquine is stopped; this is not true of hydroxychloroquine. Because of this potentially serious retinal side effect, the patient must be seen by an ophthalmologist experienced in the use and surveillance of antimalarial drugs at least every 6 months. At the first sign of visual impairment (especially reduced sensitivity to red light), the drug should be stopped. With such close and conservative ophthalmologic follow-up and appropriate dosing, permanent retinal changes should be either nonexistent or very rare. Adherence to the following rules ensures safety:

(b) Calculation of dosage is needed. The recommended dosage for hydroxychloroquine is 5 to 6 mg/kg daily.

(c) Ophthalmologic evaluation, before initiation of treatment and every 6 months thereafter, helps to prevent visual loss by detecting early disease in a reversible stage. The daily use of a red filter allows for an early warning sign of toxicity.

(d) Normal renal and hepatic function is necessary for safe use. Fixed dosages given regardless of a patient's renal and hepatic function, size, and age are not reasonable and lead to an increased risk for side effects.

(e) Other considerations. This drug is contraindicated in patients with significant visual, hepatic, or renal impairment, or porphyria. In pregnant women, it is traditionally contraindicated; however, the safety of the drug during pregnancy has been defined via experience with patients having SLE. The most common undesirable side effects are allergic skin eruptions and gastrointestinal disturbances, including nausea, diarrhea, and unexplained weight loss.

c. **Sulfasalazine (SSZ),** a compound synthesized through the linkage of 5-aminosalicylic acid (5-ASA) and sulfapyridine, was initially developed in the 1930s for the treatment of RA. Randomized controlled trials have demonstrated significant beneficial effects of this drug in RA. Although the exact mechanism of action in RA is unknown, there is evidence for antiinflammatory and immunomodulatory actions.

(1) **Indications.** Because of its convenient oral dosing, safety profile, and fairly rapid onset of action, SSZ may be an appropriate choice for early and mild cases of RA. It is often used before MTX and with similar clinical indications to those of antimalarial drugs. It is at times employed in combination drug regimens, such as SSZ plus hydroxychloroquine plus MTX.

(2) The **mechanism of action** is unknown, but possibilities include inhibition of prostaglandins, ability to modify pro-inflammatory reactive oxygen species released from activated macrophages, reduction of activated circulatory lymphocytes, and effects on the metabolism of folic acid and adenosine.

(3) **Therapeutic approach.** As a single agent, SSZ is somewhat interchangeable with hydroxychloroquine, primarily in the setting of mild RA. It works rapidly, with clinical benefits becoming apparent at 4 weeks. In studies in which SSZ was used in combination with gold or MTX, effectiveness was increased, but so was discontinuation because of toxicity.

(4) **Dosage.** Begin with a 500-mg enteric-coated tablet with breakfast for 1 week. Then, if laboratory test results are stable on a weekly basis, the dose is increased by 500 mg/wk during 4 weeks to an eventual dose of 1,000 mg with breakfast and dinner. The optimal dose range is between 2 and 3 g/d.

(5) **Common side effects.** SSZ ranks with antimalarial drugs and auranofin as the best tolerated of the DMARDs. Adverse effects primarily occur in the first 2 to 3 months of therapy. The most common side effects are gastrointestinal, mainly nausea and vomiting. This problem is often avoided with the use of enteric-coated tablets and administration with meals. Leukopenia has occurred in 1% to 3% of patients, and agranulocytosis, although rare, may occur early in the course of SSZ treatment. Thus, monitoring should include weekly complete blood counts and differential counts for the first month, then every 2 to 4 weeks for 3 months, and eventually every 6 to 8 weeks. Make sure that your patient is aware of the warning signs of leukopenia, such as fever and sore throat. Note: In RA patients negative for RF and positive for ANA in whom SLE is a possibility, SSZ should be avoided because sulfa drugs may lead to a flare of SLE.

d. **D-Penicillamine** has been shown in controlled studies to be effective in reducing inflammatory synovitis in approximately 50% of patients with RA, a response rate similar to that of gold. Toxic side effects are common (60% of patients) and may be severe, and there is a long time period between drug institution and clinical response. For these reasons and because of the availability of other effective and well-tolerated DMARDs, D-penicillamine is no longer a first- or second-line agent for RA. D-Penicillamine may be of value when extraarticular manifestations of RA dominate the clinical picture.

(1) **Indications.** In the 1980s, D-penicillamine was commonly used to treat moderate to severe RA. Now, it is employed as a third-line agent for patients who have been unresponsive to other DMARDs or in whom extraarticular manifestations are prominent. Close monitoring and an appreciation of the side effect profile of this drug are mandatory.

(2) The **mechanism of action** is not well understood but is believed to be related to immunomodulation via an effect on sulfhydryl reactions in mononuclear cells.

(3) **Therapeutic approach.** A history of allergy to penicillin is not a contraindication to the use of D-penicillamine, but institution of therapy in such patients should initially be carried out under close observation and with low doses, such as 125 mg. Contraindications include pregnancy and renal failure. This drug should not be prescribed for patients who are unreliable, do not have access to a telephone, or who would have difficulty in reporting potential side effects.

(4) **Administration.** D-Penicillamine is available as 125-mg and 250-mg tablets. Up to 12 weeks may elapse between the initiation of D-penicillamine therapy and signs of improvement. Thus, increments in dosage should be made at 12-week intervals. The initial regimen is a single daily dose of 250 mg, which is maintained for 3 months. If no clinical evidence of response is noted, the dose is doubled to 500 mg. Three-monthly increases to 750 mg and then the final dose of 1,000 mg may eventually be needed, with the understanding that higher doses are associated with an increased frequency of side effects. Rarely do patients respond to doses of less than 250 mg, and evidence of improvement usually is seen after the first 3 to 6 months of therapy. One should attempt to reduce the daily dose in decrements of 125 mg at 3-monthly intervals to determine the least amount of drug required to sustain clinical improvement.

(5) **Common adverse effects** include the following:

(a) **Skin and mucous membranes.** Pruritus and skin rash represent the most common side effects, and dermatitis may occur at any time during the course of therapy. These may be controlled by administration of an antihistamine and a moderate reduction in dosage. If rash persists despite these measures, the drug should be stopped for at least 3 months. Repeated administration of low doses (125 mg) may be possible after this. A sudden febrile response, often associated with a generalized rash, may occur within the first 3 weeks of therapy; defervescence occurs when the drug is stopped. However, in this situation, rechallenge is not recommended. Stomatitis has been observed and often clears with decreased dosage. If oral ulcers persist, the drug should be stopped permanently. Blunting or alteration in taste perception (dysgeusia) may occur during the first 6 weeks of therapy. It may gradually disappear despite continuation of therapy or may persist even after therapy is stopped.

(b) **Hematologic toxicity** is potentially dangerous and dictates the need for close follow-up. Mandatory testing includes complete blood cell counts, including platelet count, differential counts, and definition of the absolute neutrophil count, at 2-weekly intervals for the first 6 months of therapy and at least monthly thereafter. Recording laboratory data on flow sheets will permit early detection of downward trends in white blood cell or platelet counts. Hematologic toxicity may be sudden in onset and may occur in the interval between scheduled laboratory studies. Thus, patients must be aware that they need to report the development of sore throat, skin or mucous membrane bleeding, infection, or fever. Downward trends of white blood cell and platelet counts (specifically a white cell count $\leq 3{,}000/mm^3$ or a platelet count $<100{,}000/mm^3$) require immediate and permanent discontinuation of D-penicillamine therapy. Leukopenia associated with thrombocytopenia or thrombocytopenia alone may indicate impending aplastic anemia.

(c) **Renal toxicity.** Proteinuria is encountered in up to 20% of patients on long-term therapy. If proteinuria of 2+ or more has persisted for 30 days and other causes of renal disease have been excluded, a 24-hour urine protein determination should be performed and repeated at monthly intervals. As long as the protein excretion does not exceed 1 g/d and creatinine clearance is stable, the drug may be continued. Proteinuria may clear completely with only a 125-mg reduction in the daily dose. Development of hypoalbuminemia, nephrotic syndrome, or significant hematuria requires discontinuation of the drug. Nephrosis is reversible, but urinary abnormalities may persist up to 1 year. Rechallenge will usually lead to recurrence of proteinuria.

(d) **Miscellaneous.** Uncommon but severe side effects include autoimmune syndromes such as drug-induced lupus, Goodpasture's syndrome, and polymyositis. They require drug discontinuation and at times disease-specific treatment, and they usually resolve after the drug is stopped.

e. **Immunosuppressive and immunomodulatory drugs.** Five classes of immunosuppressive drugs are now being employed in the treatment of RA: the antimetabolite/antiinflammatory drug methotrexate (MTX), the purine analog azathioprine (AZA), the cyclic polypeptide cyclosporine (CyA), the pyrimidine inhibitor leflunomide, and the alkylating agent cyclophosphamide (CTX). Of all the DMARDs and immunosuppressive agents, MTX is now considered the central DMARD in single or multiple drug regimens.

(1) **Methotrexate.** Given its safety profile and tolerance by patients, relatively rapid onset of action in 4 to 6 weeks, effectiveness, and the availability of various routes of administration (PO, IM, IV, or SC), MTX has dominated the therapeutic armamentarium as a first-or second-choice disease-modifying medication in the treatment of RA. Studies have demonstrated that RA patients remain on MTX longer than on other DMARDs (45% to 62% on MTX for 3 years vs. 18% to 32% on IM gold, 35% on hydroxychloroquine, 11% to 39% on SSZ) because of a combination of effectiveness and safety. Evidence that MTX retards bony damage is provided by many of the available studies.

(a) **Indications.** Although MTX does not induce a complete remission, it is a highly effective drug in controlling the inflammatory process and markedly improving function in a majority of RA patients. Its position in the RA armamentarium is either as a first-line agent, started soon after the diagnosis is made, or as a powerful second-line drug added to or used in place of ineffective courses of antimalarial drugs or SSZ.

(b) **Mechanism of action.** MTX inhibits dihydrofolate reductase, thus interrupting purine biosynthesis and synthesis of thymidilic and inosinic acids. However, MTX is metabolized intracellularly to MTX polyglutamates, and these long-lived metabolites inhibit dihydrofolate reductase plus other folate-dependent enzymes. Other antiinflammatory effects include reduced polymorphonuclear chemotaxis and decreased production of IL-1 and IL-2 production. *In vivo* and *in vitro* studies have demonstrated inhibition of intracellular activity of 5-aminoimidazole-4-carboxamidoribonucleotide transformylase. This inhibition is associated with increased release of adenosine into the extracellular milieu. Antiinflammatory properties of adenosine are mediated by specific receptors on the surface of cells. In inflammatory arthritis, the A_3 receptor occupancy inhibits cytokine release. This mechanism may be related to some adverse effects of MTX, such as nodulosis.

(c) **Therapeutic approach.** The antiinflammatory effect of MTX has been repeatedly demonstrated, and one study has shown that the effect is dose-related. Although the initial dose of MTX continues to be 7.5 mg/wk, the dose at which most patients demonstrate a well-defined clinical improvement now ranges between 15 and 25 mg/wk. Most patients will profit from the addition of 1 mg of folic acid daily without any reduction in drug efficacy. The drug appears to have a steroid-like clinical effect with relatively rapid onset (4 to 6 weeks) and offset of action. The latter point must be appreciated because severe disease flares commonly occur when the drug is stopped, and at times it is difficult to regain disease control. If MTX is stopped for only 2 to 3 weeks (e.g., in the perioperative period or because of minor side effects), disease control can be maintained simply with the repeated administration of MTX. However, if MTX must be stopped permanently, an alternative DMARD, such as SSZ, hydroxychloroquine, AZA, or an anti-TNF biologic should be started to avoid disease exacerbation. Other issues that must be appreciated before MTX is started are the following:

(i) **Cost and route of administration.** The cost of the oral medication is high, especially when the expense of monitoring is added. The cost of parenteral MTX is much lower, and many patients are switched from the oral to the SC, IM, or IV route because of lack of response or intolerance to the oral medication. Some physicians give the less expensive parenteral solution orally in orange juice. Bioavailability studies have demonstrated that approximately 80% of the drug is absorbed via the oral route, and more than 90% by other routes. Patient acceptance of the SC route is high, and the ability to inject it themselves at home avoids an office visit.

(ii) **Nodulosis.** In patients both with and without a history of nodular disease, MTX can lead to the development of painful new nodules. This is particularly prominent on the fingers and can further limit function. The fact that a medication that is so effective in controlling the inflammation of RA can stimulate the formation of a characteristic inflammatory symbol of the disease underscores the incompleteness of our understanding of this disease and the actions of MTX.

(iii) **Liver toxicity** in the form of fibrosis or cirrhosis was an early concern and evolved from prior clinical experience with a *daily* regimen of MTX in patients with psoriasis and psoriatic arthritis. However, with the use of *weekly* MTX dosing, the avoidance of MTX in high-risk patients, and an optimal monitoring approach, such liver problems are uncommon in RA patients treated with long-term MTX. Studies of MTX treatment in RA patients quantifying the risk for fibrosis/cirrhosis have shown that this problem occurs in only 1 in 1,000 patients.

(iv) **Oncogenicity.** One of the reasons why MTX has supplanted AZA in the treatment of RA has been its lack of oncogenicity. However, MTX treatment has rarely been associated with the development of non-Hodgkin's B-cell lymphomas.

(d) Common adverse effects

(i) **Gastrointestinal intolerance.** Nausea and vomiting occur in nearly 20% of patients, usually those on oral MTX. This can be avoided in most cases by switching to SC, IM, or IV administration. Diarrhea occurs in 10% of patients and may be avoided by altering the route of administration.

(ii) **Stomatitis** occurs in 6% to 10% of patients and may be avoided with the use of between 1 and 5 mg of oral folic acid daily.

(iii) **Hypersensitivity pneumonitis.** This acute pulmonary disorder, manifested by cough, dyspnea, eosinophilia, and diffuse pulmonary infiltrates, can occur in as many as 5% of MTX-treated patients. It can be quite severe, always requires the discontinuation of MTX, and may necessitate a course of high doses of steroids. Rechallenge is not recommended. This problem may be more common in patients who smoke or have had interstitial lung disease associated with RA.

(iv) **Teratogenicity and induction of abortion.** MTX must be discontinued 3 *months* before any male or female patient attempts to have a child. MTX is an abortifacient, and women taking it should be made aware of this fact and counseled regarding the need to use appropriate birth control techniques while taking this medication.

(v) **Oncogenicity.** Based on longitudinal data from large studies of patients treated with MTX for psoriasis and choriocarcinoma, MTX was not thought to be oncogenic. However, more than 50 cases of non-Hodgkin's B-cell lymphomas have been reported worldwide in patients taking MTX. In eight of these patients, discontinuation of MTX led to spontaneous disappearance of the lymphoma, without a need for chemotherapy. Although the exact incidence of this association is unknown, it is probably low but should be discussed with patients. It must be appreciated that RA patients already have an inherent increased risk for the development of lymphoproliferative disorders. MTX may be a cofactor, along with Epstein-Barr virus, in altering immunosurveillance capability and triggering lymphomas in some RA patients.

(vi) **Bone marrow toxicity.** This can occur on low-dose, weekly MTX but is uncommon. The synergistic toxic effects on bone marrow of taking antibiotics that contain sulfa along with MTX should be appreciated.

(vii) **Hepatic toxicity.** The following information is important in guiding hepatic surveillance in RA patients treated with methotrexate:

Methotrexate is relatively safe for the liver, and SGOT levels correlate with liver biopsy grade. Despite prior concepts regarding the *inability* of liver function test abnormalities to predict MTX-induced liver disease, recent studies in RA patients support the fact that serial elevations of aminotransferases [AST (SGOT) and ALT (SGPT)] and decreases in albumin have been found to correlate with the progression of histologic abnormalities defined by serial liver biopsies. In such liver biopsy studies, Kremer found that the overall hepatic histologic grade does increase with time. In the patients reported, *minimal* fibrosis was developing; however, almost half the patients had fibrosis that was not present at baseline. Among 13 patients with RA treated with MTX in whom Kremer identified fibrosis, some lost fibrosis on follow-up, seven showed fluctuation in grading, and none showed progression of fibrosis. Hence, fibrosis appeared to be an inconsistent and inconsequential feature. There were statistically significant correlations between liver function test abnormalities and liver biopsy grade after approximately 8 years of MTX. It is important to note that the extent of fibrosis correlates poorly with the extent of hepatic dysfunction.

Note: Alcohol should be completely avoided in patients treated with MTX. The use of alcohol adds an unacceptable risk for the development of liver inflammation and damage.

MTX-induced cirrhosis and liver failure are uncommon in RA patients. In a survey of more than 2,200 members of the American College of Rheumatology (ACR) who had treated 16,600 patients with MTX, Walker et al. found 24 cases of cirrhosis and liver failure, giving a 5-year cumulative incidence of approximately 1 in 1,000 treated patients. Late age at first use of MTX and duration of therapy with MTX were independent predictors of serious liver disease.

Given the above data and the risks and cost of liver biopsy, the following **indications for liver biopsy** have been formulated:

The ACR has published a position paper regarding liver biopsy in MTX-treated RA patients. With their interpretation of the above data, they do *not* recommend baseline or follow-up biopsies unless the patient, in every 6-weekly liver function test, demonstrates persistent or recurrent elevations (even minor) of transaminases or decreases in albumin. This is a clear shift in position from prior (not from the ACR) recommendations for a biopsy between a cumulative dose of 1.5 to 5.0 g or after 3 to 5 years of treatment. The physician should be aware that this stance differs greatly from that taken by dermatologists in their treatment of psoriasis with MTX, and also does *not* address similar questions regarding the use of MTX for psoriatic arthritis.

If a patient is an alcoholic or has known alcoholic liver disease and every other drug has failed to control the disease, a biopsy should be performed before initiation of MTX treatment to guide therapeutic decisions.

For patients with baseline abnormal liver function test results of unknown cause, a biopsy would be performed to define the following disorders: hepatotoxin-induced liver disease, liver damage from prior or ongoing viral infections, and "occult" alcoholic liver disease.

(viii) Opportunistic infections have been reported in some RA patients treated with weekly, low-dose MTX. The combined immunosuppression of corticosteroids and MTX may contribute to the risk for such infection. Appropriate immunizations should be offered to RA patients taking MTX.

(ix) Nodulosis. The development of multiple, new, small, painful nodules on the hands and elsewhere can be quite uncomfortable and functionally limiting. These often occur despite excellent disease control elsewhere. The addition of hydroxychloroquine or colchicine has, in rare patients, led to some control of the development of nodules.

(2) Azathioprine. This purine analog has had an excellent track record in terms of both effectiveness and safety in patients with RA. Through the years, it has been used as a second- or third-line drug for the treatment of moderate to severe RA. Presently, it is considered for patients who have failed other DMARDs, such as MTX, and may be used in combination with other medications, such as hydroxychloroquine.

(a) **Indications.** For established RA after failure of several DMARDs, or as a steroid-sparing and disease-controlling agent in rheumatoid vasculitis.

(b) **Mechanism of action.** Reduction in circulating lymphocytes, mixed lymphocyte reactivity, and immunoglobulin synthesis have been demonstrated. These are probably caused by suppression of inosinic acid synthesis and inhibition of IL-2 secretion.

(c) **Therapeutic approach.** AZA is an effective drug in the treatment of RA, with many studies demonstrating its similarity in efficacy to IM gold, D-penicillamine, MTX, and other DMARDs. Its use is somewhat limited by its potential oncogenicity. The long-term experience with AZA in patients with RA has proved that this drug in this population has an acceptable profile of toxicity. However, the overall oncogenic potential of this drug must be considered before it is prescribed to treat a nonmalignant disorder.

(d) **Administration.** AZA is available in 50-mg tablets. Therapy is begun with 50 mg/d, and the dosage is increased by weekly 50-mg increments until a maintenance dose of 2 to 3 mg/kg is reached. The usual daily dose is 100 mg. Close monitoring is indicated and includes complete blood cell counts with platelet and differential counts weekly for 1 to 2 months, then every 2 weeks for 1 to 2 months, and eventually monthly. Liver function tests should be carried out every 1 to 2 months if the patient has excessive nausea or vomiting or if a fever develops. If gastrointestinal symptoms occur following administration of the drug, it may be given in a single daily dose before bedtime to minimize this effect. If a hypersensitivity reaction develops manifested by fever, hypotension, and liver function test abnormalities, the drug should be stopped immediately and never started again. Reinstitution of AZA in this situation can be fatal.

Caution: Allopurinol inhibits the metabolic breakdown of AZA, and if the drugs are used concomitantly, potentially toxic levels of AZA and its metabolites may accumulate. Thus, this drug combination should be avoided because of the potential for severe bone marrow suppression. If it is essential that the drugs be used together, the dose of AZA should be decreased to one-third of the usual dose. Even then, close hematologic monitoring should be carried out.

(e) **Common adverse effects** include the following:

(i) **Dose-related bone marrow suppression** with leukopenia and thrombocytopenia.

(ii) **Increased susceptibility to infection,** primarily viral, such as herpes zoster, but also bacterial, and **gastrointestinal intolerance,** such as nausea and vomiting. AZA can lead to liver enzyme abnormalities and even clinically significant hepatitis. At times, hepatitis may be part of a hypersensitivity reaction with associated fever and hypotension. If this occurs, AZA should be stopped permanently. Pancreatitis may occur and clears when the drug is stopped.

(iii) **Oncogenicity.** A 50-fold increase in relative risk for malignant disease, primarily non-Hodgkin's lymphoma, has been demonstrated in renal transplant patients treated with AZA. In RA, however, the related risk for lymphoma is confounded by an increased relative risk secondary to RA *per se* or the coexistence of Sjögren's syndrome. Overall, there appears to be a small added risk (relative risk, 1.3) for malignancy when AZA is used in patients with RA.

(iv) Teratogenicity. Although there is mounting evidence demonstrating the safe use of AZA during pregnancy in patients with active SLE, the recommendation is that AZA not be used during pregnancy.

(3) Cyclophosphamide. CTX is an extraordinarily effective disease-modifying agent for the treatment of RA. However, because of its significant potential toxicities, its role is now limited to use in the most severe, refractory cases of RA or in those associated with life- and organ-threatening RA vasculitis. Only physicians experienced in the indications for and monitoring of CTX should administer this drug.

(a) Indications. Treatment with CTX should be limited to those clinical situations in which RA continues to be active and destructive despite the use of many DMARDs, including MTX, CyA, AZA, and anti-TNF biologics. It is also an effective disease-modifying agent in patients with active rheumatoid vasculitis. The physician can use CTX initially, for 3 to 6 months, to gain control of the disease, and then switch back to another medication, such as 15 to 20 mg of MTX per week, to maintain disease suppression. In this way, one employs the best possible medication initially, then changes to a safer therapeutic choice. Daily oral CTX may be more effective than monthly IV CTX, but the choice is often dictated by practical clinical considerations and patient comorbidities.

(b) Mechanism of action. The active metabolites of CTX, principally phosphoramide mustard, cross-link DNA so that it cannot replicate. CTX is cytotoxic to dividing and resting lymphocytes. It induces lymphocytopenia, with B cells more affected than T cells. It readily suppresses primary cellular and humoral immune responses. It suppresses many cell-mediated responses and also has antiinflammatory properties.

(c) Therapeutic approach. When CTX is compared with other DMARDs, its clinical effectiveness is equal to that of AZA and IM gold. In two studies, it has been shown to retard bone destruction. Although no placebo-controlled studies have been performed, daily oral CTX is thought to be the drug of choice for the treatment of necrotizing vasculitis associated with RA, so-called "malignant" RA. Intermittent IV CTX is also being used, but this route of administration may not be as effective as daily oral treatment.

(d) Administration. CTX (Cytoxan) tablets are 50 mg in size. The usual oral dose begins with 50 mg/d for 1 week, and then the dose is increased by 50 mg if the complete blood count is stable. The usual oral therapeutic dose is 2 mg/kg daily, or 75 to 125 mg/d. Higher doses may be needed in severe cases. Complete blood count, differential and platelet count, and urinalysis are assessed every 7 to 14 days initially, then every 2 to 4 weeks after 2 to 3 months of stable dosage. The IV regimen is 0.5 to 0.75 g/m^2 monthly. Once the patient has responded to oral and IV CTX, a switch to a less toxic DMARD, such as MTX, is appropriate to decrease the potential for oncogenicity, sterility, and other side effects. Given the renal excretion of CTX metabolites, dose adjustments and careful hematologic monitoring are needed in patients with renal insufficiency.

(e) **Common adverse effects**

(i) **Oncogenicity.** Alkylating agents in general are associated with the highest risk for tumor formation. Kinlen's experience with 643 RA patients suggests a relative risk of 12.8 for all cancers combined, a risk of 10.9 for non-Hodgkin's lymphoma, and a 10-fold increased risk for bladder cancer. There also appears to be an increased risk for acute leukemia. A major deterrent to the use of CTX in RA is the risk for cancer in treating a disease that is nonmalignant. Patients with a history of cancer should avoid CTX.

(ii) **Bone marrow toxicity.** Dose-related marrow suppression is 6% to 32% for leukopenia and 4% for thrombocytopenia. These abnormalities tend to respond quickly to discontinuation or a decrease in dosage of CTX.

(iii) **Risk for infection.** The overall risk is high (22%), and herpes zoster may occur in 30% of treated RA patients.

(iv) **Infertility, azoospermia, and amenorrhea.** The risk for all of these increases with increasing duration of therapy, cumulative doses, and age in women. Once they have appeared, they are usually permanent.

(v) **Bladder disorders.** Hemorrhagic cystitis has been reported in one-third of patients receiving daily oral CTX, and there is a significant but lower incidence of bladder fibrosis and carcinoma. These abnormalities are caused by the CTX urinary metabolite acrolein. IV CTX is associated with a significantly lower incidence of bladder problems. Appropriate hydration, nighttime voiding, and the use of 2-mercaptoethane sulfonate can help to decrease bladder toxicity. In patients on long-term CTX, either oral or IV, monthly urinalysis is needed to monitor for hematuria. The finding of hematuria should be followed by cystoscopy. **Note:** the development of bladder cancer can occur many years after the institution of CTX. Thus, long-term surveillance is needed.

(4) **Cyclosporine (Sandimmune, Neoral).** CyA, an immunomodulating drug previously effective in preventing transplant rejection, has been found to be an effective and safe DMARD when employed in low doses and in a combination chemotherapeutic regimen with MTX. Initial concerns of renal dysfunction can be minimized by close monitoring.

(a) **Indications.** Short-term studies have shown the efficacy of CyA against both placebo and drugs such as AZA, hydroxychloroquine, and D-penicillamine. However, CyA is probably most effective and safest when low doses are added to MTX in treating RA patients with a suboptimal response to MTX alone. Close renal monitoring is necessary at any dose of CyA.

(b) **Mechanism of action.** CyA is a lipophilic cyclic polypeptide isolated from fungi. It has impressive immunosuppressive activity without causing bone marrow toxicity. CyA inhibits the transcription of DNA and thus prevents accumulation of mRNA for several cytokines. It also inhibits T-cell interaction with macrophages, leading to a decreased synthesis of IL-2, and suppresses the synthesis and release of IL-2 by helper T cells, rendering T cells unresponsive to IL-2. CyA blocks the amplification of cellular immune responses in the generation of T-cell effectors and other functions dependent on IL-2. CyA also inhibits the expression of the CD40 ligand, leading to decreased proliferation of B lymphocytes. Myeloid and erythroid lines, however, are not inhibited.

(c) Therapeutic approach

(i) Clinical use. Studies of low (2.5 mg/kg) and moderate doses of CyA have shown the drug to be effective in controlling inflammation, improving function, and retarding radiologic progression in RA. Nephrotoxicity has been the major limiting factor preventing the use of higher doses. Therefore, patients should be treated with doses no higher than 2.5 to 3.0 mg/kg daily. CyA appears to be less effective as a single agent, and when used in this way, it often is instituted as a third-line DMARD. Combination therapy with MTX and CyA is thought to be logical because of the complementary biologic and immunologic effects of the two agents. CyA was shown to be effective when added to the regimen of patients who had shown a suboptimal response to MTX alone. The combination of CyA at a mean dose of 2.97 mg/kg daily plus 15 mg of MTX weekly demonstrated no significant increase in toxicity over that seen with MTX alone.

(ii) Dose initiation and increase. A dosage schedule that can optimize the careful balance between the efficacy and safety of CyA has been sought. The initial dose should be 2.5 mg/kg daily in two divided doses every 12 hours, and dose increases must follow the principle of "go slow, go low." If there is no clinical response after 4 to 8 weeks, the CyA dose should be increased by 0.5 to 1.0 mg/kg at l- to 2-month intervals to a maximum dose of 5 mg/kg daily (unless this is prevented by a rise in serum creatinine ≥30% to 50%). Caution should be exercised with doses above 4 mg/kg daily, and the safest final recommended dose range is 2 to 3 mg/kg daily. Once the largest required dosage has been reached and no further response is expected after a patient has been stable for 3 months, then the dosage can be decreased by 0.5 mg/kg to the lowest effective dose. Lack of response after 3 to 6 months should lead to a reassessment of the drug regimen or drug discontinuation.

(iii) Renal function: dose reduction and monitoring. Blood pressure should be monitored every 2 weeks for the initial 3 months and then monthly if stable. More frequent monitoring will be required if the dosage is increased. If the serum creatinine level increases to 30% above the baseline on two occasions, then the daily dose should be decreased by 0.5 to 1 mg/kg. If after the dosage is lowered the creatinine level remains more than 30% above the baseline, CyA should be stopped and then resumed after 1 month only if the creatinine level returns to less than 15% above the baseline. Treatment for 6 months or 1 year seems safe under strict monitoring; after a longer administration, nephrotoxicity may not be reversible. CyA should be avoided in patients with preexisting renal disease (i.e., creatinine clearance <80 cc/min).

(iv) Blood pressure. If hypertension develops (diastolic >95 mm Hg), the response should be to lower the dose of CyA or use antihypertensive agents that do not interfere with CyA metabolism.

(v) Serum cyclosporine levels. Determination is not required but may be useful to detect noncompliance or drug interactions. Indications for reducing the dose should include a decrease in renal function or an increase in blood pressure, not CyA levels. If serum creatinine increases to more than 30% above baseline, the dose should be reduced by 25% to 50%. Blood pressure and serum creatinine monitoring are indicated throughout the treatment period, with appropriate adjustment of dosage of CsA. When the dose is stable, creatinine levels should be measured every 2 to 4 weeks.

(vi) **Other screening tests.** Liver function tests, complete blood counts, and urinalyses should be performed along with determination of serum creatinine levels.

(vii) **Drug interactions.** CyA serum levels can be increased by drugs that decrease P-450 metabolism, including calcium antagonists, erythromycin, ketoconazole, and histamine$_2$ blockers. Thus, with these medications, the CyA dosage should be adjusted downward. Alternatively, anticonvulsants such as dilantin and rifampicin increase the metabolism of CyA and thus reduce the concentration.

(d) **Contraindications** include current or past malignancy, uncontrolled hypertension, renal dysfunction, and abnormal liver function test results with enzymes at twice baseline value. Caution should be exercised in patients who are over 65 years of age, taking NSAIDs, or lactating, and in those with controlled hypertension. CyA should be avoided during pregnancy.

(e) **Drug preparations.** Two different preparations are available, the initial oil and alcohol-based solutions and the newer microemulsion-based formulation Neoral, recently developed to increase the bioavailability of CyA. Neoral has more predictable absorption. Selection of the appropriate dosage of the microemulsion should take into account the enhanced bioavailability, especially with respect to the possible renal effects. When changing patients to Neoral from alternative preparations, a 1:1 dose-conversion strategy is employed. However, close creatinine and blood pressure monitoring is mandatory before and after this transition.

(f) **Common side effects**

(i) **Renal toxicity.** The renal effects of CyA are thought to be caused by the following mechanisms: vasoconstriction leading to ischemia, disruption of the mitochondrial membranes, increased procollagen synthesis, and possible coagulopathy. CyA toxicity is characterized by interstitial fibrosis, tubular atrophy, and renal arteriopathy. Dose-related decreases in glomerular filtration rate with corresponding increases in serum creatinine are common during CyA immunosuppression. This risk is increased with dosages greater than 5 mg/kg daily or with persistence of serum creatinine levels more than 30% over the baseline values. CyA doses of 10 mg/kg daily for even 2 months may lead to an irreversible loss of more than 10% of renal function in RA patients. In a study by Tugwell, serum creatinine levels failed to return to baseline during the 6-month follow-up period in only 2 of 72 patients treated with CyA at an average of 3.8 mg/kg daily for 6 months. Serum creatinine rose and creatinine clearance decreased during the period of CyA administration; however, this effect stabilized after month 4, with no further changes thereafter. After discontinuation of CyA, serum creatinine fell to within 15% of baseline in all except two patients. The safest CyA regimen consists of administration of low doses for no longer than 1 year and avoidance of the concomitant use of nephrotoxins such as NSAIDs and aminoglycosides.

(ii) **Elevated blood pressure** occurs in one-third of RA or psoriatic arthritis patients treated with CyA. Antihypertensive agents may be needed, but potassium-sparing drugs should be avoided because CyA may increase serum potassium. Calcium channel blockers may increase CyA levels by decreasing its metabolism, and changes in CyA dosage may be needed. This effect can also be employed in an attempt to decrease the CyA dose and its attendant side effects.

(iii) **Oncogenicity.** CyA can potentially increase the relative risk for malignancy via its immunomodulatory effects. This is particularly important when combination drug regimens are employed, such as the use of MTX along with CyA.

(iv) **Other side effects** include hepatotoxicity with higher doses of CyA; nausea or vomiting; and neurologic symptoms such as tremor, paresthesias, and gum hyperplasia. CyA is teratogenic and should be avoided during pregnancy.

(5) **Leflunomide.** This oral immunosuppressive agent demonstrated a combination of effectiveness and safety in uncontrolled and placebo-controlled European studies. On this basis, it has recently been cleared for use in the United States by the Food and Drug Administration and is widely prescribed in the treatment of refractory RA. This drug does not have the track record of MTX, CyA, and AZA, but it will probably attain a similar importance in the RA armamentarium.

(a) **Indications.** Leflunomide will probably be employed as a second-line DMARD, after MTX alone or MTX combinations fail to control the inflammatory process.

(b) **Mechanism of action.** Immunosuppressant effects of leflunomide may be related to blockade of the proliferation of immune cells via inhibition of pyrimidine nucleotide synthesis in T cells. It is a pro-drug and, as such, most of its clinical immunomodulatory activity appears related to an active metabolite. It is chemically unrelated to other immunosuppressants, such as CyA, MTX, and AZA. Leflunomide functions well as an immunosuppressive and antiinflammatory medication. Its ability to decrease the development of joint erosions is at least as good as that of MTX.

(c) **Therapeutic use.** Oral leflunomide is effective for treating patients with RA when given daily or weekly. However, compliance with the weekly regimen is poor, and adverse effects are more frequent than with daily dosing. Once-daily oral dosing of 20 mg has been associated with significant clinical improvement. Initial therapy involves a 100-mg dose daily for 3 days, followed by 20 mg PO daily.

(d) **Common side effects.** Monitoring for side effects includes serial complete blood counts, liver function tests, and observation for weight loss and gastrointestinal complaints. The long half-life of leflunomide may necessitate the use of cholestyramine in patients who have severe side effects or wish to become pregnant.

(i) **Gastrointestinal effects.** Nausea and vomiting may occur in 15% of RA patients and do not appear to be dose-related. Weight loss may be related to these gastrointestinal symptoms. Severe diarrhea can occur.

(ii) **Hepatotoxicity.** Elevations of serum aminotransferases are dose-related and occur in 6% of patients receiving a 25-mg dose. Severe, symptomatic liver toxicity has not been reported. Leflunomide is metabolized in the liver, and so a history of liver disease should be factored into the decision to use it. Renal impairment does not appear to influence the pharmacokinetics of the primary metabolite of leflunomide. The combined use with MTX may lead to an increased incidence of abnormalities.

(iii) **Alopecia.** Reversible alopecia is seen occasionally and is dose-related.

(iv) **Skin rash.** This dose-related side effect can occur in up to 8% of patients treated with the 25-mg dose. Rare anaphylactic reactions have occurred.

(v) **Hematologic effects** have been seen in RA patients treated with the 25-mg dose of leflunomide but are uncommon.

f. **Novel biologic agents and immunotherapy in rheumatoid arthritis.** Impressive research focused on the pathogenesis of RA has discovered many new mechanisms that illustrate the complex and multicellular nature of the disease. Potential sites for therapeutic intervention include cells such as T and B lymphocytes, macrophages, fibroblasts, endothelial cells, and dendritic cells, and their many products such as cytokines and adhesion molecules. The development of these agents have already revolutionized the treatment possibilities for patients with RA. How such agents will be merged with presently accepted and effective DMARDs such as MTX will be defined by their effectiveness as disease-controlling and disease-modifying agents, their side effect profile, and their cost.

g. **Minocycline.** Tetracycline derivatives have many actions that could contribute to their effectiveness in RA, including their antibiotic activity, immunomodulatory effects, and antiinflammatory and metalloproteinase inhibitory capacity. Many well-designed trials have demonstrated a significant clinical improvement in early RA patients treated with minocycline in comparison with placebo, but not with other DMARDs. Side effects include dizziness, skin rashes, gastrointestinal symptoms, and headaches. Of note is the development of SLE-like manifestations in adolescents and young adults receiving minocycline for acne. *Place of minocycline in the RA armamentarium:* Minocycline should not be considered a first- or second-line DMARD to be used alone in the treatment of early RA. Pending the results of ongoing trials and studies comparing minocycline with other DMARDs, some rheumatologists are using minocycline at a dosage of 100 mg twice daily for patients with early, mild disease who refuse DMARDs such as hydroxychloroquine or as part of a combination regimen in patients with severe, refractory disease.

h. **Combination disease-modifying antirheumatic drug regimens.** Combinations of DMARDs are now used by most rheumatologists in the United States to treat an estimated 24% of all RA patients. This trend is increasing because (a) the effectiveness of a single DMARD often wanes with time, (b) minor clinical improvements with single DMARD regimens are unacceptable, and (c) some combinations can be given safely with greater effectiveness than monotherapy. Combination regimens have evolved in parallel with our appreciation of the aggressive nature of RA and the need to intervene quickly and effectively to prevent joint damage, normalize function, and prolong life. This approach is similar to that employed by oncologists in their “war on cancer.” The groupings of medications that are now used by rheumatologists have been crafted either via a knowledge of their synergistic biologic effects (e.g., MTX plus CyA) or by admixing multiple safe and effective DMARDs with the eventual aim of finding a regimen that is more effective, but not more toxic, than each individual agent. However, certain basic beliefs have guided the most commonly used regimens; MTX is considered the best single DMARD and should be a component of any multiple drug regimen, and multiple DMARD regimens should be started after the RA patient has failed to respond to a single DMARD regimen. The cost of multiple drugs and their monitoring has to be factored into these therapeutic decisions. The clinical decision to employ combinations rather than the individual drugs within them should be based on the physician's clinical experience, the patient's prior response to medications, disease severity, and the presence of comorbidities. Some rheumatologists begin these combinations at a single point; most add drugs one by one as defined by the clinical response to the prior regimen. Almost all possible combinations of DMARDs have been employed, but the regimens most commonly used include the following:

(1) **Methotrexate-hydroxychloroquine.** This safe regimen combining two well-known and well-tolerated medications may lead to a moderate improvement over that noted when they are given singly. The dosages are similar to those for each drug alone: an initial dose of MTX of 7.5 mg/wk, increased to 15 to 20 mg/wk, plus 200 mg of hydroxychloroquine twice daily.

(2) **Methotrexate-sulfasalazine.** Initial concerns about possible synergistic toxicity with these two agents have not been supported by clinical studies. Because both are folic acid inhibitors, folic acid supplementation is needed in addition to monitoring for possible bone marrow depression. Dosages are similar to those used in monotherapy.

(3) **Sulfasalazine-hydroxychloroquine.** This is a safe regimen with minimal additive toxicity and moderate effectiveness. Dosages are similar to those used with monotherapy. Trials have demonstrated that this combination appears to be equal in effectiveness to MTX alone.

(4) **Methotrexate-sulfasalazine-hydroxychloroquine.** In a study that followed 60 patients for 3.3 years, therapy with all three active drugs provided substantially greater benefit than did therapy with MTX alone. Of these patients, 73% maintained a 50% improvement, 17% failed to maintain improvement, and 10% had side effects that led to withdrawal. Although 13% of the patients fulfilled criteria for remission, in most cases no drug in their three-DMARD was tapered and withdrawn. The MTX median dosage in the study was 17.5 mg/wk; for SSZ it was 1 to 2 g/d, and for hydroxychloroquine it was 400 mg/d.

(5) **Methotrexate-cyclosporin A.** The evidence from combination trials suggests that CyA can be considered in patients who have exhibited a suboptimal clinical response to MTX alone. The MTX dose at which CyA was added was 15 mg/wk; the CyA dosage should start at 2.5 mg/kg daily and increase to a maximum of 3.5 mg/kg daily, as noted above. Close monitoring is mandatory.

(6) **Role of biologic agents in combination DMARD regimens.** Biologic agents, described below, have been released and are widely used for the treatment of RA. The ultimate place of these agents in the armamentarium remains to be elucidated. Cost and convenience will be major considerations; however, their eventual disease-modifying potential and side effect profile will define their place in the treatment protocol. Initially, they will probably be employed in RA patients unresponsive to full-dose MTX or in DMARD combination failures. They may eventually play a key role in the induction of disease control and then be balanced with less expensive and more convenient DMARDs. The most promising biologic agents now involve cytokine-based therapies and are discussed above.

(a) Elimination of lymphocytes and subsets of T cells and inhibition of cellular function. Antibodies targeted at lymphocytes (CDw52) were associated with some clinical improvement but also serious side effects resulting from cytokine release and prolonged lymphopenia. Monoclonal antibodies aimed primarily at CD4+ T cells had variable results, but the degree of clinical improvement was disappointing and the profound lymphopenia needed for minimal improvement did not justify the treatment. Future therapies targeted at the "arthritogenic" clones or co-stimulatory molecules may modulate T lymphocytes and be more specific and less toxic. Therapies directed toward molecules involved in the trimolecular complex (MHC plus T-cell receptor plus processed peptide antigen) will probably become increasingly important.

(b) Blocking adhesion molecules. Blocking leukocyte migration may be an important intervention at the effector phase. Initial trials with anti-ICAM-1 monoclonal antibody were reported to be encouraging.

(c) Blocking cytokine and receptor function. Blockade of cytokines or their receptors with anti-TNF-α, soluble TNF-α receptors, and anti-IL-1, or immune deviation with IL-10 and IL-4, are examples of current research directions. TNF-α inhibitors: TNF-α is a critical initiating and perpetuating pro-inflammatory molecule in rheumatoid synovitis. Two different approaches have been taken to inhibit the action of this molecule:

Soluble tumor necrosis factor receptor fusion protein (enbrei, etanercept). Soluble TNF receptors are the shed extracellular portion of the membrane-bound molecule. Such shed receptors work as antiinflammatory molecules because they bind with and competitively inhibit the binding of the pivotal pro-inflammatory cytokine TNF-α to the cell surface TNF receptor. Two human soluble TNF receptors were linked to the Fc portion of an IgG molecule, resulting in an immunoglobulin-like molecule. This molecule had not only a high affinity for TNF-α but also a half-life that made it an ideal therapeutic agent. This agent acts as both a cytokine "carrier" or decoy and a TNF antagonist, rendering TNF biologically unavailable. Phase III placebo-controlled studies have demonstrated a rapid (steroid-like), significant, and prolonged clinical improvement with a significant decrease in erosion development in RA patients with active disease refractory to MTX. Seventy-one percent of patients had a 20% improvement, 39% a 50%, and 15% a 70% improvement. This was particularly impressive given the severity of the patients studied. Side effects have included development of local erythema at the site of the twice-weekly SC injection in 20% of patients, mild upper respiratory tract symptoms, and some more severe systemic infections. Six episodes of fatal sepsis occurred in the 25,000 patients treated, a number not thought to be above that expected. However, since these six patients had active infections and skin ulcers, at times in the setting of diabetes, the use of this drug in high risk patients with active infection is not recommended.This treatment has been evaluated in combination with MTX in refractory RA patients and is presently being compared with MTX in early RA. The results of these trials, long-term data regarding side effects, and the apparent capacity of this therapy to reduce or eliminate the development of joint erosions has already defined its importatnt role in the treatment if RA.

Anti-TNF-α monoclonal antibody therapy. This is a chimeric monoclonal antibody that consists of the variable regions of a murine anti-TNF-α monoclonal antibody engrafted onto a human IgG1 kappa molecule (Remidade, infliximab). The resulting construct is two-thirds human and has a high affinity for TNF-α. Although the clinical effectiveness of this chimeric molecule administered as a monthly IV infusion has been well defined in placebo-controlled trials, clinical benefit was transient when it was used as monotherapy. When added to 7.5 mg of MTX per week, the clinical response was sustained and the immunogenicity of the chimera was decreased. During infusion of this monoclonal antibody, minor side effects developed in some patients, including headache, fever, nausea, vasovagal reactions, and urticaria. Minor infections such as bronchitis have also occurred, but no substantial increase in infection risk has been demonstrated. Antibodies to DNA developed in nearly 10% of patients, but clinically evident SLE occurred in only one patient. Although a few cases of hematologic malignancy have occurred after treatment, the relationship of the malignancy to the monoclonal antibody has not been defined. The Food and Drug Administration has approved this new therapy for the treatment of Crohn's disease of the rectum, but, as of the time of this printing, not RA. How this drug will be employed in the treatment of RA depends on the results of further assessment and its long-term safety profile and cost. As with Enbrel, disease-modification has been demonstrated and clinical improvement impressive.

(d) **Induction of oral tolerance.** Type 2 collagen is one of many candidate auto-antigens that might stimulate T lymphocytes and lead to the self-perpetuating inflammatory disorder known as RA. The oral administration of type 2 collagen to animals with experimentally induced arthritis leads to suppression of the disease. One mechanism thought to be involved in this suppression of inflammation is collagen type 2-induced dormancy of T cells. The results of studies in which various doses of oral type 2 collagen were given to RA patients and compared with placebo indicated an excellent safety profile but only modest clinical improvement. *Place of chicken collagen in the RA armamentarium:* The theoretical aspects are interesting, but such therapy should not be considered a disease-modifying modality in RA patients, either as a single treatment or in combination with other DMARDs.

(e) **Effector function blockade.** Metalloproteinase inhibitors and blockade of metalloproteinase production.

(f) **Modulation of growth control, apoptosis, and angiogenesis.** This includes induction of apoptosis genes and gene products and inhibition of growth factors or receptors promoting angiogenesis and cellular proliferation.

E. Surgical treatment. Orthopedic surgeons play a major role in the management of RA patients, particularly those in whom joint damage has developed. Although traditional techniques of joint fusion and synovectomy remain in the orthopedist's armamentarium, total joint arthroplasty has achieved a high level of acceptance. Surgical reconstruction in RA patients must be regarded as part of a comprehensive care plan and judiciously balanced with medical management. The pattern of joint involvement and eventual functional goals of the patient must be considered.

1. **Criteria for surgery.** Many factors enter into the choice and timing of an operation. More than 40 years ago, Dr. Philip Wilson, Sr. of the Hos-

pital for Special Surgery listed these questions to assist in forming a surgical plan:

a. Is the arthritis still active?
b. Is the patient in adequate physical condition to permit extensive surgical procedures?
c. Considering the age and physical state of the patient, and the number of operations required, is the expected gain in function from the operation worth the effort and risk?
d. Should the operation be delayed so that other therapy may be instituted?
e. Will the patient cooperate with the proper postoperative care on leaving the hospital?
f. Are the comprehensive facilities necessary for successful treatment available in the hospital?
g. Will the patient be able to receive proper postoperative care on leaving the hospital?
h. Will the patient's financial status permit independent undertaking of the entire treatment, or have community resources been mobilized to care for such treatment?
i. In the final analysis, either intractable pain or disability requires the patient to request the operation.

2. **Surgical procedures**

a. **Cervical spine.** Cervical spinal instability should be considered in all patients with neck pain, occipital or lower cervical radiculopathy, patient-reported neck crepitation, instability on active motion, or signs of cervical myelopathy. Radiographic signs of cervical spinal instability may be seen in 40% of RA patients, but neurologic symptoms develop in only 10% of these.

Important lesions include atlanto-axial subluxation, superior migration of dens, and subaxial subluxation. Subluxation of lower cervical vertebrae is most common at the C3–4 level. These lesions can be expected to progress in 30% of patients. Lateral cervical spinal films in extension and flexion are mandatory for evaluation of instability, and magnetic resonance imaging (MRI) can best define the anatomic abnormalities. Cervical orthotics can serve as temporary stabilizing devices, but little evidence exists to suggest that they enhance autofusion. Surgical intervention is reserved for those with incapacitating pain related to spinal instability or neurologic signs of cord or root entrapment. All levels of instability should be included in a posterior cervical fusion procedure. Along with traditional wiring and autogenous bone grafting techniques, methylmethacrylate cement has proved of great value in achieving stabilization of osteoporotic bone, especially when long fusions are needed for multiple levels of instability. Postoperative care should include a rigid orthotic device until bony consolidation appears on radiography.

b. **Shoulder.** Evaluation of shoulder pain in RA requires differentiating soft-tissue pain from that of articular origin. Bursitis, bicipital tendinitis, and rotator cuff tears can be discerned with a careful history, examination, diagnostic xylocaine injections, and MRI when indicated (see Chapter 13). Rotator cuff tears are difficult to repair in this group because of degenerated tissue. The presence of severe articular destruction and refractory pain and disability is an indication for total joint replacement. Shoulder prostheses are in a state of evolution, as problems of restoring rotator cuff power in the face of degenerated tissue and loosening of the glenoid component have required design adjustment.

c. **Elbow.** Elbow synovectomy and radial head excision can be expected to provide good pain relief in those with persistent elbow synovitis and minimal bone loss. Total elbow replacement is reserved for patients with severe articular destruction and moderate activity expectations. It should be kept in mind that complication rates and loosening rates are relatively high in total elbow arthroplasty.

d. Wrist and hand. Severe wrist synovitis and bony destruction are amenable to surgical therapy; the degree of involvement dictates the choice of a synovectomy and ulnar head resection (dorsal stabilization procedure), a total wrist arthroplasty, or wrist fusion. Total wrist arthroplasty retains wrist motion while providing pain relief. Wrist synovitis can attenuate and rupture extensor tendons. Wrist synovectomy is indicated in the presence of persistent boggy, dorsal swelling to prevent rupture of extensor tendons. Implants continue to play an important role in the management of thumb and MCP joint disease. Critical to success are soft-tissue balancing and prolonged dynamic postoperative splinting to prevent recurrence of ulnar drift. This procedure results in pain relief with only a slight decrease in grip strength. Although fusions are not indicated for finger MCP joints, they are often useful in advanced proximal PIP joint disease to reestablish a functional hand. Cemented PIP joint arthroplasty may prove useful in augmenting finger function. Thumb reconstruction requires careful consideration of tendon imbalance and articular destruction. A combination of tendon repositioning and joint fusion is often needed.

e. Hip. Total hip replacement has provided consistent success in treating end-stage RA hip disease. Early problems with materials and designs, infections, and pulmonary emboli have diminished, and clinical results are excellent. The osteoporosis often found in RA patients makes the challenge of long-lasting implant fixation a formidable one.

f. Knee

(1) Arthroscopic knee synovectomy can be expected to provide pain relief in those with persistent boggy synovitis, recurrent large painful effusions unresponsive to medical therapy, and minimal articular destruction. Long-term studies have shown that although pain relief is good, synovectomy does not prevent progression of cartilage loss. Regrowth of the synovial membrane often occurs within 3 to 5 years. Synovectomy with use of radioisotopes has been studied as a potential replacement for surgical methods.

(2) Total knee replacement can give results as good as those in total hip replacement if patients are properly selected. A variety of nonarticulated condylar prostheses are available and allow for resurfacing of the femoral, tibial, and patellar surfaces. Preexisting alignment deformities (varus-valgus) or flexion contractures require experienced surgical attention for soft-tissue balancing, proper bony cuts, and component choice.

g. Ankle and foot. Ankle pain may be caused by talotibial or subtalar disease. This differentiation is important in selecting the proper surgical procedure.

(1) Talotibial pain that is intractable is treated by ankle fusion. Rates of latent loosening in total ankle replacements have been too high to gain general acceptance.

(2) Subtalar pain, elicited by hindfoot inversion or eversion, is a result of destructive changes in the talocalcaneal, talonavicular, and calcaneocuboid joints. Triple arthrodesis, which fuses three joints, is a highly successful procedure.

(3) Forefoot pain in RA is the result of synovitis, capsular destruction, and joint subluxation giving rise to hallux valgus (bunion) or metatarsalgia. Carefully placed shoe inserts can redistribute weight and provide pain relief (see Chapter 20) Surgery is reserved for those who fail conservative treatment. Excision of the first metatarsal exostosis and the proximal half of the proximal great toe phalanx (Keller procedure) is a time-honored procedure for correction of hallux valgus in RA. Excision of the metatarsal heads (Hoffman procedure) is successful in relieving plantar metatarsal pain.

Bibliography

Day RO. SAARDs. In Klippel JH, Dieppe PA, eds. *Textbook of rheumatology,* 2nd ed. Philadelphia: Mosby, 1998:8.1.

Goronzy JJ, Weyand CM. Rheumatoid arthritis: epidemiology, pathology, and pathogenesis. In: Klippel JH, ed. *Primer on the rheumatic diseases,* 11th ed. GA: Arthritis Foundation, 1997:155.

Kelley WN, et al., eds. Rheumatoid arthritis. In: *Textbook of rheumatology,* 5th ed. Philadelphia: WB Saunders, 1997:851.

Klippel JH, Dieppe PA, eds. Rheumatoid arthritis. In: *Textbook of rheumatology,* 2nd ed. Philadelphia: Mosby, 1998.

Koopman WJ, ed. *Arthritis and allied conditions,* 13th ed. Baltimore: Williams & Wilkins, 1996:979.

Paget SA. Rheumatoid arthritis: treatment. In: Klippel JH, ed. *Primer on the rheumatic diseases,* 11th ed. GA: Arthritis Foundation, 1997:168.

29. SJÖGREN'S SYNDROME

Stuart S. Kassan

Sjögren's syndrome (SS) is a chronic inflammatory disease associated with lymphocytic infiltration of exocrine glands. Certain clinical, serologic, and genetic differences are found among patients with SS alone, also called primary SS (patients with keratoconjunctivitis and xerostomia in the absence of any other definable connective tissue disease). These differences suggest varying etiologies for similar clinical manifestations of disease. The most commonly accepted definition of SS has been the presence of two of the following findings: (a) keratoconjunctivitis sicca (dry eyes), (b) xerostomia (dry mouth), and (c) one of the connective tissue disease syndromes. Secondary SS is defined as keratoconjunctivitis and xerostomia as features of a connective tissue disease. Rheumatoid arthritis (RA) is the most common connective tissue disease seen in association with secondary SS, but others have been well-documented and include systemic lupus erythematosus (SLE), scleroderma, polymyositis, mixed connective tissue disease, and juvenile rheumatoid arthritis. As a result of the obvious shortcomings of the above, purely clinical definition, most recent investigators have included pathologic criteria (see section **III**) as supporting evidence of the presence of primary or secondary SS.

The clinical manifestations of the disease were first described in 1888. In 1933, Henrik Sjögren published a monograph describing in great detail the histologic and clinical components of this syndrome, which has often been referred to as Sjögren's syndrome. Confusion later arose between SS and the disease previously reported by Mikulicz in the late 1800s. In 1927, Schaffer and Jacobsen defined two main categories: (a) Mikulicz's disease proper, of unknown etiology and following a benign course, and (b) Mikulicz's syndrome, caused by a variety of disorders such as leukemia, lymphosarcoma, tuberculosis, sarcoidosis, and iodide poisoning. Later, Morgan and Castleman concluded, on the basis of pathologic descriptions, that Mikulicz's disease and SS were identical. Much of the interest in SS during the past decade has focused on the opportunity to study the interrelationships among the autoimmune disorders, lymphoproliferative malignancies, and dysproteinemias, all of which may be features of the syndrome.

I. Prevalence

- **A. Sex.** At least 90% of the patients with SS (primary or secondary) in most studies are women.
- **B. Age.** Most patients with the disease are over 40 years of age, but the disease may be encountered in persons in the second and third decades of life.
- **C. Other connective tissue diseases in patients with Sjögren's syndrome**
  - **1.** When various populations of patients with SS have been evaluated for the presence of other connective tissue diseases, the results have been as follows:
    - **a.** RA, 30% to 55%.
    - **b.** Scleroderma, 5% to 8%.
    - **c.** SLE, 5% to 10%
    - **d.** Polymyositis, 2% to 4%.
    - **e.** Hashimoto's thyroiditis, mixed connective tissue disease, chronic active hepatitis, Raynaud's disease, all with an unknown incidence of SS.
  - **2.** Alternatively, when evidence of SS is specifically sought in patients with other connective tissue diseases, the results are quite different:
    - **a.** SLE, more than 50%.
    - **b.** RA, 20% to more than 50%.
    - **c.** Scleroderma, 40% to 50%.
- **D. Glandular involvement in Sjögren's syndrome**. Eighty percent of SS patients have major salivary gland enlargement. Focal lymphocytic infiltration with linear destruction may be seen in minor salivary glands in labial, nasal, and hard palate mucosa. Involvement of the exocrine glands of the

upper and lower respiratory tracts, gastrointestinal tract, vagina, pancreas, and skin has been found in SS.

E. Extraglandular involvement

1. **Gastrointestinal** disorders in SS have included the following:
   - **a.** Esophageal stenosis.
   - **b.** Atrophic gastritis.
   - **c.** Pancreatitis.
2. **Hepatic** disorders in patients with SS have included the following:
   - **a.** Abnormal liver function tests (especially elevated alkaline phosphatase and γ glutamyl transpeptdase) in 45%.
   - **b.** Primary biliary cirrhosis.
   - **c.** Chronic active hepatitis.
   - **d.** Cryptogenic cirrhosis (15% of SS patients in one study).
3. **Renal** disorders have been found in as many as one-third of SS patients and include the following:
   - **a.** Renal tubular acidosis type 1.
   - **b.** Nephrogenic diabetes insipidus.
   - **c.** Chronic interstitial nephritis.
   - **d.** Immune complex glomerulonephritis.
4. **Pulmonary** disorders may be found in 4% to 15% of SS patients and include the following:
   - **a.** Chronic obstructive pulmonary disease.
   - **b.** Pulmonary infiltrates (e.g., pseudolymphoma).
   - **c.** Fibrosing alveolitis.
5. **Myositis,** often of an indolent nature, may be encountered in SS. Up to 50% of patients have been found to exhibit, on random muscle biopsy specimens, abnormalities consisting of interstitial and perivascular fibrosis, inflammatory infiltrates, or both.
6. **Vasculitis** is present in fewer than 10% of SS patients. It may be seen in association with the following:
   - **a.** Myositis.
   - **b.** Mononeuritis multiplex.
   - **c.** Axonal neuropathy.
   - **d.** Central nervous system involvement (in which immune vasculopathy and anti-SS antibodies may play a pathogenetic role).
   - **e.** Immune complex glomerulonephritis.
   - **f.** Purpura.

F. Malignancy in Sjögren's syndrome

1. **Non-Hodgkin's lymphoma** has been found to occur more often in patients with SS (primary or secondary); the relative risk is 44 times the expected incidence. Patients with a history of parotid enlargement, splenomegaly, and lymphadenopathy are at greatest risk for development of lymphoma.
2. **Waldenström's macroglobulinemia** appears to be more frequent in SS, but the risk is unknown.
3. **Pseudolymphoma** in SS is characterized by extraglandular extension of lymphoproliferation that is clinically and histologically benign. The incidence is not known.
4. **Other malignancies** reported to coexist with SS include Kaposi's sarcoma, immunoblastic lymphadenopathy, and immunoblastic sarcoma.

II. Genetics. Histocompatibility testing of patients with SS has demonstrated a genetic dichotomy between patients with primary SS (SS alone) and those with secondary SS (SS associated with another connective tissue disease, generally RA).

A. Primary sicca syndrome has a significantly increased association with HLA-B8, HLA-DR3, and certain B-lymphocyte allo-antigens.

B. The above HLA associations are usually not found in patients with **secondary sicca syndrome.** In the case of patients with SS and RA, there is an increased incidence of the HLA-DR4 antigen (that antigen found most often in seropositive RA alone).

C. **Family studies** show that relatives of SS patients may have an increased incidence of serum auto-antibodies, positive results on Schirmer's test, elevated gamma globulin levels, and RA. The studies of HLA antigens in primary SS from different ethnic groups show different associations: HLA-DR5 is found in Greeks, HLA-DR11 in Israelis, and HLA-DRw3 in Japanese patients.

III. **Pathogenesis.** Findings in SS pertaining to pathogenesis may be classified as follows:

A. **Abnormalities of humoral immunity**

1. **Anti-salivary duct antibody** is present more frequently in secondary SS (70% positive) than in primary SS (10% positive). No differences in other organ-specific antibodies (e.g., anti-thyroid and anti-gastric parietal cell antibodies) have been found between primary and secondary SS.
2. **Non–organ-specific auto-antibodies**
   a. **Immunoglobulin M (IgM) rheumatoid factor (RF)** is the most common type of RF in all cases of SS.
   b. **Immunoglobulin G and immunoglobulin A rheumatoid factors** seem to be elevated in primary SS more often than in secondary SS.
   c. **Antinuclear antibody (ANA)** positivity was found in 64% to 68% of all SS cases, in which the frequencies of positivity vary between primary and secondary SS. ANA patterns tend to be speckled because of the anti-SS-B antibodies found in SS.
3. **Antibodies to soluble acidic nuclear antigens** extracted from lymphoid cell lines.
   a. **SS-A** (or Ro) antibodies are present in the following percentages:
      (1) Primary SS, 70%.
      (2) SS with RA, 1%.
      (3) SS with SLE, 33%.
   b. **SS-B** (or Ha, La) antibodies are present in the following percentages:
      (1) Primary SS, 50% to 70%.
      (2) SS with RA, 3% to 5%.
      (3) SS with SLE, 73%.

B. **Abnormalities of cellular immunity and immune regulation in Sjögren's syndrome.** There seem to be normal absolute numbers and proportions of peripheral B and T cells. No increase of circulating B cells has been found despite a higher incidence of auto-antibodies, hypergammaglobulinemia, and circulating immune complexes. Evidence suggests the presence of a serum blocking factor that may decrease the percentage of T cells. Natural cell-mediated cytotoxicity is depressed in both primary and secondary SS. The autologous mixed lymphocyte reaction is more depressed in secondary than in primary SS. Studies of T-lymphocyte subsets in SS have yielded conflicting results. A decreased number of helper T cells (CD4+) and suppressor T cells (CD8+) have been reported. Overall, it seems that B-cell activation is the most consistent immunoregulatory aberration in SS patients. It may begin as a polyclonal activation evolving to oligoclonal and monoclonal activation and may end in a transformation to a malignant monoclonal proliferation.

C. **Viral studies.** Tubuloreticular structures have been identified in labial salivary gland tissue and renal endothelium from SS patients. No successful viral isolation from salivary gland tissues has been accomplished. In one study, elevated titers of antibody to cytomegalovirus were found in SS.

D. **Immune complexes.** Elevated levels of immune complexes and abnormal clearance of these complexes by the reticuloendothelial system have been demonstrated in active SS. Their role in the pathogenesis of disease is unclear, but they may be important in vasculitic states and glomerulonephritis.

E. **Graft-versus-host disease.** GVH-initiated SS resembling spontaneous SS suggests a possible pathophysiologic mechanism for the development of SS and other connective tissue diseases in humans and extends previous observations limited to animal models.

F. **Human immunodeficiency virus (HIV) infection.** Patients with HIV infection may manifest a clinical picture indistinguishable from that of SS. These patients usually do not demonstrate antibodies to Ro (SS-A) or La (SS-B) cellular antigens and the intralesional T cells are CD8(+), as opposed to CD4(+) in autoimmune SS.

IV. Clinical features

A. Ocular symptoms may not be present in one-third to one-half of patients at any one time during the course of their disease despite definite pathologic changes. However, approximately 95% of SS patients will have ocular symptoms at some time.

B. Xerostomia is an infrequent presenting sign of SS, but about 90% of patients will have sialographic abnormalities of the parotids. Salivary gland enlargement, primarily of the parotid gland, is present in one-third of SS patients and is usually bilateral. Lacrimal gland enlargement is unusual (4%).

V. Laboratory studies

A. Specific tests

1. Tests of functional abnormalities

a. Schirmer's test. Five millimeters of unstimulated wetting of filter paper in 5 minutes (17% false-positive and 15% false-negative results).

b. Parotoid salivary flow rate.

c. Results of **radionuclide scan** of the parotid glands (pertechnetate Tc 99m) may be falsely abnormal as a result of other abnormalities of the parotid gland (see section **VI**).

d. Parotid gland sialography is performed by introducing radiopaque dye into the parotid duct system. The abnormalities seen in SS include acinar and duct atrophy with puddling of dye, main duct enlargement, and retention of contrast material. All the above may be seen in chronic parotitis with causes other than SS.

2. Tests of anatomic abnormalities

a. Rose bengal staining of the cornea may be helpful in confirming the diagnosis but is not specific (4% false-positive and 5% false-negative results).

b. Parotid gland sialography (see section **V.A.1.d**).

3. Biopsy

a. Minor salivary glands. Abnormalities are nicely demonstrated by lip biopsy.

b. Lacrimal glands and parotid glands. Abnormalities are similar to those found in the minor salivary glands of the lip. Because of the relative lack of morbidity associated with lip biopsies, this procedure is preferred over lacrimal or parotid gland biopsies as a diagnostic tool.

B. Nonspecific laboratory abnormalities. These changes are also often seen in other states of inflammation and in many autoimmune diseases.

1. Elevated erythrocyte sedimentation rate, 80%.
2. Anemia, 40%.
3. Leukopenia, fewer than 30%.
4. Hypergammaglobulinemia, 80%.
5. Positive RF, >90%.
6. Positive ANA, 70%.
7. Circulating cryoglobulins may be 30%.

VI. Differential diagnosis. The salivary gland involvement in SS may be confused with numerous other conditions.

A. Infection of salivary glands

1. **Viral.** Coxsackievirus infection, mumps, cytomegalic inclusion disease, HIV infection.
2. **Bacterial.** Acute sialoadenitis is often seen in dehydrated, debilitated patients. Chronic bacterial sialoadenitis is frequently associated with obstruction of the salivary ducts by inspissated saliva.
3. **Fungal.** Actinomycosis or histoplasmosis.
4. **Tuberculosis.** Rare.

B. Granulomatous disease. Sarcoidosis.

C. Other infiltrative disorders

1. Primary neoplasms of the parotid gland.
2. Leukemia.
3. Amyloidosis.
4. Lymphoma of intraparotid lymph nodes.
5. Burkitt's lymphoma.
6. Pseudolymphoma.

D. Systemic diseases

1. Cirrhosis.
2. Diabetes mellitus.
3. Hyperlipoproteinemias (types 3, 4, 5).
4. Obesity.
5. Pregnancy and lactation.
6. HIV disease.
7. Gouty parotitis (rare).
8. Cushing's disease.
9. Cystic fibrosis.

E. Nutritional deficiency

1. Starvation.
2. Vitamin B_6 deficiency.
3. Vitamin C deficiency.
4. Vitamin A deficiency.

F. Drugs associated with the development of dry mouth

1. Sedatives.
2. Hypnotics.
3. Narcotics.
4. Phenothiazines.
5. Atropine.
6. Propantheline.
7. Antiparkinsonian drugs.
8. Antihistamines.
9. Ephedrine.
10. Epinephrine.
11. Amphetamines.

VII. Treatment. No controlled trials have been undertaken in the therapy of the systemic manifestations of SS. In general, the approach to treatment has been empiric. Vasculitis, renal disease (immune complex-mediated or otherwise), myositis, alveolitis, cryoglobulinemia, and other manifestations have mostly been treated in the past with corticosteroids, immunosuppressive agents, or both, depending on the severity of disease. Because the cytotoxic drugs are immunosuppressive and renal transplant patients and others treated with the agents have an increased incidence of lymphoma (as do untreated SS patients), it is advisable to avoid their use in SS.

A. Ocular abnormalities. Artificial tears are the mainstay of treatment. Solutions consisting of methylcellulose and polyvinyl alcohol are useful. The dosage varies from two drops four times daily to every 15 minutes depending on the clinical state. Inserts placed into the conjunctival sac that release small amounts of methylcellulose during many hours are presently available and may be beneficial in some patients. Lacrimal duct occlusion, temporary or permanent, may enhance local moisture. Bromhexine, a secretagog, is presently being studied in clinical trials for use in the United States.

B. Xerostomia. Salagen (pilocarpine hydrochloride) tablets are indicated for the treatment of symptoms of xerostomia from salivary gland hypofunction. As a cholinergic parasympathetic agent, pilocarpine can increase secretion of the salivary glands. The usual initial dose is 5 mg tid. It is contraindicated in patients with asthma, iritis, and narrow angle glaucoma. Side effects include abdominal cramps and sweating. Lubrication of the mouth and mild secretagogs, such as lemon-flavored juice or lubricating agents proper (water, methylcellulose), are useful. More potent secretagogs may exacerbate the signs and symptoms of parotitis. Prevention of states of dehydration in SS is very important, as dehydration may enhance the formation of parotid ductal calculi. Avoidance of drugs that may aggravate oral dryness (e.g., narcotics, antihistamines, anticholinergics) is also important.

C. **Parotid enlargement.** In the past, numerous modes of therapy have been employed to treat parotid enlargement.

1. **Parotid irradiation** has been associated with an increased incidence of lymphoma in SS patients. Because of its oncogenic potential, this form of therapy should not be used in SS.
2. **Surgical removal** is often technically difficult, and resultant nonhealing fistulae and facial nerve damage preclude this mode of therapy.
3. **Drug therapy** for symptomatic inflammatory parotid enlargement
   a. **Nonsteroidal antiinflammatory drugs.** Useful regimens include 25 to 50 mg of indomethacin four times daily or 400 mg of ibuprofen four times daily.
   b. **Corticosteroid therapy** should be limited to those with severe, recalcitrant disease because of the risk for corticosteroid toxicity. The regimen is 20 to 40 mg/d with dosage tapering as soon as a clinical response is obtained.
   c. **Oral pilocarpine therapy** has been recently approved by the Food and Drug Administration for use in SS. It may be helpful in patients with sicca symptomatology in dosages of 5 mg three or four times daily (see section **VII.B.** above).
   d. **Hydroxychloroquine** has also been studied in SS, and its effects have been very modest in treating sicca symptoms or fatigue symptoms.
4. **Cytotoxic therapy** (specifically azathioprine, cyclophosphamide, chlorambucil, methotrexate) does not seem to offer any significant benefit unless one is treating a true malignancy (lymphoma) or an invasive form of pseudolymphoma in SS.

30. SYSTEMIC LUPUS ERYTHEMATOSUS

Jane E. Salmon and Robert P. Kimberly

Systemic lupus erythematosus (SLE) is a multisystem disease with a spectrum of clinical manifestations and a variable course characterized by exacerbations and remissions. Lupus is marked by both humoral and cellular immunologic abnormalities, including multiple auto-antibodies that may participate in tissue injury. Antinuclear antibodies (ANAs), especially those to native DNA, are common immunologic abnormalities found in the disease. During the nineteenth century, lupus was considered to be a skin disease. By some accounts, the erosive nature of some of the skin lesions seemed to resemble the damage inflicted by the bite of a wolf, which may have led to the name lupus. In 1872, Moriz Kaposi described systemic symptoms in association with cutaneous disease. At the turn of the century, Sir William Osler described arthritis and visceral manifestations in conjunction with polymorphic skin lesions. The presence of circulating immunologic factors became apparent about 50 years later with the discovery of the LE cell phenomenon by Hargraves in 1948, the recognition of the LE factor as an ANA in 1953, and the identification of antibodies to native DNA in 1956. Identification and characterization of abnormal auto-antibodies continue to be major areas of clinical and immunochemical interest. The development of sensitive laboratory tests for auto-antibodies has enabled the recognition of milder forms of SLE, with a consequent change in both reported prevalence and prognosis. The broad clinical spectrum of SLE challenges the diagnostic and therapeutic acumen of the physician.

I. Epidemiology

- **A. Sex.** A female-to-male ratio of 9:1 is seen in most series of adult patients. The female predominance is less striking in childhood SLE (disease onset preceding puberty) and in elderly SLE patients.
- **B. Age.** First symptoms usually occur between the second and fourth decades of life but may be seen in any age group. The presentation of SLE in the elderly (as much as 10% of the total lupus population in some series) may differ from that in younger patients.
- **C. Ethnic distribution.** Although lupus occurs in all races, its prevalence is not equally distributed among all groups. SLE occurs more commonly in the United States than in England and more often in blacks than in whites. Hispanic and black patients have been noted to have more severe disease. The average annual incidence in the United States is approximately 27.5 per million population for female whites and 75.4 per million for female blacks. The reported prevalence figures for women vary widely from 1 in 1,000 to 1 in 10,000.

II. Genetics. The presence of a genetic component in SLE is supported by family studies.

- **A. Clinical disease.** Family members of SLE patients are more likely to have lupus or another connective tissue disease. The risk for development of SLE in a sibling of persons affected by SLE is approximately 20 times that in the general population. Concordance of disease among monozygotic twin pairs may be as high as 50% but is not complete. Fraternal twins, with a concordance rate of 2% to 5%, do not have a higher frequency of SLE than other first-degree relatives do. Asymptomatic (or healthy) family members are more likely to have a false-positive test result for syphilis, ANAs, anti-lymphocyte antibodies, and hypergammaglobulinemia.
- **B. Histocompatibility studies.** Lupus and lupuslike syndromes are associated with inherited abnormalities of the major histocompatibility complex (MHC) class III genes for complement components (most commonly the C4 null allele, but also deficiencies of C2; deficiencies of other complement com-

ponents are rare). Although the strength of the association varies by ethnicity, SLE is associated with the serologically determined MHC class II allo-antigens HLA-DR2 and HLA-DR3. The association with HLA-DR2 reflects the DR2 allele DRB1*1501 in white and Asian populations and the unique DRB1*1503 allele in African Americans. HLA-DR3 is primarily associated with lupus patients of European ancestry.

C. **Non-major histocompatibility complex genes.** Genetic variants of opsonins (mannose binding protein, C-reactive protein, complement components), opsonin receptors (complement receptors, immunoglobulin receptors), lymphocyte cell surface molecules, and cytokine genes (tumor necrosis factor-alpha, interleukin-1, interleukin-10) have been associated with SLE. FcγR are important in immune complex clearance. Allelic variants of FcγR, which differ in their capacities to bind immunoglobulin G (IgG), alter the function of mononuclear phagocytes and thereby provide a mechanism of inherited differences in immune complex handling. The low IgG binding alleles of FcγR have been associated with increased risk for lupus nephritis.

III. Pathogenesis

A. **Pathology.** Although no histologic feature is pathognomonic for SLE, several features are very suggestive: (a) fibrinoid necrosis and degeneration of blood vessels and connective tissue; (b) the hematoxylin body (the *in vivo* LE cell phenomenon); (c) "onion skin" thickening of the arterioles of the spleen; and (d) Libman-Sacks verrucous endocarditis.

1. **Histopathology.** Routine histologic examination of tissue specimens reveals a broad range of findings.
   a. **Skin biopsy** may demonstrate a leukocytoclastic angiitis, especially in palpable purpuric lesions. The typical lupus rash usually shows epidermal thinning, liquefactive degeneration of the basal layer with dermal-epidermal junction disruption, and lymphocytic infiltration of the dermis. Rheumatoid-like nodules with palisading giant cells are uncommon, and panniculitis is rare.
   b. **Synovium.** Synovial biopsies may show fibrinous villous synovitis. The presence of pannus formation or bone and cartilage erosions is rare.
   c. **Muscle biopsies** usually show a nonspecific perivascular mononuclear infiltrate, but true muscle necrosis, as seen in polymyositis, can occur. Muscle biopsy may be helpful in evaluating the possibility of steroid-induced myopathy or chloroquine-induced myopathy, a rare entity in patients taking antimalarial agents.
   d. **Kidney.** The kidney has been the most intensively studied organ in SLE. The entire range of glomerulonephritis (membranous, mesangial, proliferative, and membranoproliferative) is seen (Table 30-1). Crescentic and necrotizing vasculitic lesions may be found. Interstitial abnormalities are often present. No single renal lesion is diagnostic of SLE. Tubuloreticular structures are not restricted to SLE. In general, renal biopsy provides one indicator of prognosis, characterizing patients with diffuse membranoproliferative lesions as having the poorest 5-year survival (40% to 85% depending on the series). Marked chronic changes (glomerular sclerosis, fibrous crescents, interstitial

Table 30-1. World Health Organization classification of lupus nephritis

Class I	Normal or minimal disease
Class II	Mesangial
Class III	Focal proliferative glomerulonephritis
Class IV	Diffuse proliferative glomerulonephritis
Class V	Membranous nephropathy

From Balow JE, Austin HA. Renal disease in systemic lupus erythematosus. *Rheum Dis Clin North Am.* 1988;14(1):117.

fibrosis, tubular atrophy) indicate a poor prognosis. Recognition that the histologic class of the biopsy specimen may not be static and may either deteriorate or improve has emphasized the need for defining renal disease activity sequentially.

e. **Central nervous system.** Multifocal cerebral cortical microinfarcts associated with microvascular injury are the most common abnormalities associated with neuropsychiatic SLE. Central nervous system lesions usually reflect vascular occlusion as a consequence of noninflammatory vasculopathy, leukoagglutination, thrombosis, vasculitis (rarely), and antibody-mediated neuronal injury. Normal brain tissue is often present despite clinical abnormalities. Cytoid bodies, seen as white fluffy exudates on funduscopic examination, represent superficial retinal ischemia.

f. **Other viscera.** Other visceral pathologic findings include Libman-Sacks verrucous endocarditis with redundant mitral valvular leaflets and lengthened chordae tendineae, pulmonary fibrosis, and nonspecific pleural thickening. Necrotizing vasculitis may be present in the viscera and lead to secondary events, including bowel infarction, myocardial infarction, pancreatitis, and accelerated atherosclerosis. In the spleen, the concentric periarterial fibrosis of small arteries (onion skin lesions) may be an end-stage consequence of earlier vasculitis.

2. **Immunopathology**

a. **Skin.** Immunofluorescence shows deposits of immunoglobulins and complement at the dermal-epidermal junction (lupus band test) in 80% to 100% of lesional and 36% to 100% of nonlesional skin specimens. Attempts to correlate a positive lupus band test result with active SLE or the presence of lupus nephritis have given inconsistent results. Positive lupus band test results are not specific for lupus; they are commonly associated with bullous pemphigoid and dermatitis herpetiformis (IgA). Dermal-epidermal immunofluorescence may also be seen in rheumatoid arthritis, scleroderma, dermatomyositis, lepromatous leprosy, multiple sclerosis, cystic fibrosis, chronic active hepatitis, primary biliary cirrhosis, amyloidosis, and, according to some reports, normal subjects.

b. **Kidney.** Glomerular immunofluorescence to determine the distribution, pattern, and density of immunoglobulin, immunoglobulin class, and complement components does not appear to have prognostic or therapeutic significance. The presence of immunofluorescence for immunoglobulin or complement is not restricted to SLE; it is, however, compatible with immune complex-mediated disease.

B. Immunology

1. **Humoral immunity.** Hyperactivity of the humoral component of immunologic responsiveness is manifested by hypergammaglobulinemia, auto-antibodies, and circulating immune complexes.

a. **Various auto-antibodies** may contribute to tissue injury. Attempts to correlate specific clinical patterns of disease with specific types of auto-antibodies have been partially successful. For example, anti-DNA antibodies have been found in renal glomerular lesions. Sicca syndrome with SLE has been associated with La (SS-B) antibodies. Ro (SS-A) antibodies have been associated with neonatal lupus, congenital complete heart block, and subacute cutaneous lupus. The lupus anticoagulant and anti-cardiolipin antibodies are associated with thrombosis, thrombocytopenia, and increased fetal wastage. Although the titer of ANAs does not necessarily correlate with disease activity, the levels of anti-DNA antibodies may vary with clinical disease. Because results vary, this test cannot be used as the sole guide to therapy.

b. **Circulating immune complexes** are commonly found in active SLE and are often associated with **hypocomplementemia.** Immune complex deposits are found in many tissues. Isolated determinations of circulating complexes do not consistently correlate with disease activity. Sequential patterns of change may be of value in individual patients.

2. **Cellular immunity.** SLE is characterized by lymphopenia and often by monocytosis. The normal complex immunoregulatory balance among cells is lost. Anergy, evidenced by diminished delayed hypersensitivity skin testing reactions, is common. Immunoglobulin-producing B cells are hyperactive. T-cell subsets are altered, and mononuclear phagocytes elaborate increased amounts of various cytokines. The primary defect has not been identified.

C. **Provocative agents.** Although the etiologic agent(s) in SLE have not been identified, several factors that may exacerbate the disease are known.

1. **Ultraviolet light.** Sun exposure may precipitate either the onset or a flare of clinical disease, causing both dermatologic and systemic manifestations in about one-third of patients. Because complete avoidance of the sun is impractical, patients should wear long-sleeved shirts, trousers rather than shorts, and wide-brimmed hats and should use sunscreens. Many effective sunscreens are available commercially; however, none can completely obviate the potential for significant sun exposure to exacerbate SLE (see Appendix E).

2. **Situational stresses.** Some patients may experience increased disease activity during periods of fatigue or emotional stress (e.g., when encountering school examinations or interpersonal conflict). The significance of such factors should not be overlooked, and such stress should be reduced as much as possible.

3. **Infection.** Viral infection has been suggested as an etiologic event in SLE. Although unproven as such, viral infection may provoke a flare of disease by an unknown mechanism, perhaps involving superantigens. Concern that exposure to foreign antigen might be harmful has led to some reluctance to immunize patients with SLE. However, current studies with influenza and pneumococcal vaccines suggest that such vaccination provides protection without causing increased SLE disease activity. Specific antibody responses may be lower than those in normal subjects, especially in patients on immunosuppressive agents.

4. **Drugs.** Many drugs have been associated with the development of ANAs and, in some cases, a clinical lupuslike syndrome (Table 30-2); procainamide and hydralazine are the most commonly implicated. However, the potential to induce such serologic changes in non-SLE patients does not preclude the use of these drugs in SLE patients. Although most physicians prefer to avoid them if an alternative drug is available, the use of these drugs in SLE has not been associated with documented exacerbation of disease activity.

IV. **Clinical presentation.** SLE is a multisystem disease in which the diagnosis rests on the recognition of a constellation of clinical and laboratory findings. No single finding makes the diagnosis, although some findings, such as antibodies to double-stranded DNA or a characteristic malar rash, are more suggestive than others. As a result of the wide spectrum of manifestations and severity of disease, criteria for diagnosis have been devised to ensure at least minimum uniformity for disease classification in clinical studies (Table 30-3). The presence of four criteria (not necessarily occurring simultaneously) is required to classify a patient as presenting with SLE.

A. **Fever** is a common manifestation of active SLE. Although often above 103°F at times, sustained fever of such magnitude is not common and should stimulate a search for infection. Acute severe disease ("lupus crisis") may be accompanied by fever up to 106°F.

B. **Skin.** Facial erythema is more common than the classic "butterfly" eruption as an acute cutaneous manifestation; photosensitivity dermatitis and bullous lesions may also occur. Subacute cutaneous LE includes both annular and papulosquamous lesions. Chronic discoid lesions with central atrophy, depigmentation, and scarring or nonscarring alopecia are common occur-

Table 30-2. Drugs implicated in drug-induced lupuslike syndrome

Anticonvulsants
Carbamazepine[a]
Diphenytoin[a]
Ethosuximide[a]
Mephenytoin
Primidone
Trimethadione
Antihypertensives
Hydralazine[a]
Methyldopa[a]
Captopril
Antibiotics
Isoniazid[a]
Sulfasalazine[a]
Penicillin
Tetracycline
Streptomycin
Sulfonamides
Griseofulvin
Nitrofurantoin
Antiarrhythmics
Procainamide[a]
Quinidine[a]
β-Adrenergic blockers
Atenolol
Acebutolol
Practolol
Antithyroidals
Propylthiouracil
Methylthiouracil
Other drugs
Penicillamine[a]
Chlorpromazine[a]
Phenylbutazone
Thiazides
Oral contraceptive pills
Levodopa
Lithium carbonate

[a]Association is well established.

rences in 20% to 30% of patients. Mucous membrane lesions with ulcers of the hard palate and nasal septal perforations may be present. Raynaud's phenomenon may be associated with acrosclerosis and, uncommonly, digital ulceration. Purpura and ecchymosis may occur as a result of either disease (e.g., thrombocytopenia) or corticosteroid treatment.

C. Musculoskeletal system

1. **Arthritis** is common and affects both small and large joints in a symmetric pattern. The axial spine is not involved. Even in the face of long-standing arthritis, bony erosions are uncommon. Reducible joint deformity is caused by capsular laxity and both tendinous and ligamentous involvement, which lead to partial subluxation. Tendon ruptures may occur. Monarticular or asymmetric joint symptoms may also derive from osteonecrosis, most often in large, weight-bearing joints, or joint infection.
2. **Inflammatory myositis** may occur in 5% to 10% of patients. Muscle weakness may also reflect corticosteroid-induced myopathy, rarely chloroquine-

Table 30-3. Revised American College of Rheumatology criteria for classification of systemic lupus erythematosus

Manifestations	Frequency (%)
Facial erythema (butterfly rash)	40–64
Discoid lupus	17–31
Photosensitivity	17–41
Oral or nasopharyngeal ulcerations	15–36
Nonerosive arthritis	86–100
Renal disease	
Proteinuria >0.5 g/24h	>25
Urinary casts (cellular or granular)	17–48
Pleuritis or pericarditis	30–60
Pericarditis alone	17–23
Psychosis, convulsions	16–20
Hematologic abnormality	
Hemolytic anemia	14–54
Leukopenia <4,000/mL	40–47
Lymphopenia <1,500/mL	>40
Thrombocytopenia <100,000/mL	11–14
Immunologic disorder	
Antinuclear antibody	100
LE cells	49–92
Anti-DNA antibody	90–100
Anti-Sm antibody	30–40
Chronic false-positive serologic test for syphilis	8–20

LE, lupus erythematosus; Sm, Smith antigen.
From Tan EM, Cohen AS, Fries JF, et al. The 1982 revised criteria for the classification of systemic lupus erythematosus. *Arthritis Rheum* 1982;25:1771.

induced myopathy, or a myasthenia gravis-like syndrome associated with SLE.

D. Cardiovascular system. The major cardiovascular morbidity associated with SLE appears to be accelerated coronary artherosclerosis and ischemic coronary disease.

1. **Pericarditis** is the most common cardiovascular manifestation. Pericardial effusions demonstrable by echocardiogram may be present in up to 60% of patients. Symptomatic pericarditis occurs in about 25% of patients. Tamponade is rare.
2. **Myocardial disease,** evidenced by signs ranging from persistent tachycardia to frank myocardial infarction, may also occur. The basis is often unknown but may include primary muscle involvement. Atherosclerosis is the most common cause of coronary artery disease in SLE, but coronary vasculitis may occur. Determination of anti-cardiolipin antibodies may be useful in lupus patients with myocardial infarction.
3. **Verrucous endocarditis** (Libman-Sacks endocarditis) is a pathologic diagnosis, as it rarely causes clinically significant valvular lesions or embolic complications. It most commonly affects the posterior leaflet of the mitral valve and may predispose the patient to bacterial endocarditis.
4. **Peripheral vascular manifestations** include vasculitis that usually affects small arteries, arterioles, and capillaries, especially those of the skin. Phlebothrombosis and thrombophlebitis may occur and recur in some patients as a sign of disease activity and in relation to anti-cardiolipin antibodies. Gangrene is rare. Raynaud's phenomenon may be a feature in up to 25% of patients.

5. **Pulmonary hypertension** may occur without relationship to overall disease activity. The clinical presentation is similar to that of idiopathic pulmonary hypertension, although with a higher incidence of Raynaud's phenomenon.

E. **Pulmonary system**

1. **Pleuritis** is the most common pulmonary symptom. Pleural effusions may occur in up to 50% of patients and pleuritic pain in 60% to 70% of patients. Although it is impractical to analyze the pleural fluid of each patient during each occurrence, effusions may be secondary to processes other than active SLE or infection, and pulmonary emboli should always be considered in the differential diagnosis.
2. **Pneumonitis** as evidenced by rales on physical examination and patchy infiltrates or platelike atelectasis on chest radiography is a diagnostic problem. Because SLE patients are often compromised hosts, infection by either common or uncommon agents must be considered. "Lupus pneumonitis" does occur, but this diagnosis requires exclusion of other processes. Progressive lupus pneumonitis ending in acute pulmonary insufficiency is uncommon. Lung biopsy may be required to establish a diagnosis, especially in the setting of persistent or progressive findings despite therapy. Abnormal findings on pulmonary function tests such as moderate restrictive and obstructive deficits are common, but patients usually have mild or no associated symptoms.

F. **Gastrointestinal systems.** Abdominal pain is a common complaint and may reflect gastrointestinal disorders associated with medications or intrinsic SLE-related pathology. Sterile peritonitis (serositis) and mesenteric vasculitis may be difficult to document. Intestinal perforation, especially in patients on corticosteroids that can mask symptoms, must be considered in addition to spontaneous bacterial peritonitis. Pancreatitis may also occur. Hepatomegaly may occur in one-fourth of patients, but abnormal liver function test findings are often drug-related rather than indicative of intrinsic lupus-associated liver damage. Chronic active hepatitis with positive tests for LE cells or ANAs (lupoid hepatitis) is not part of the spectrum of SLE. Splenomegaly may be found in the setting of active disease and splenic infarcts can occur.

G. **Other systems.** Lymphadenopathy is common but obviously not specific. Conjunctivitis, keratoconjunctivitis sicca, episcleritis, and retinal exudates (cytoid bodies) may be present. Parotid enlargement with or without a dry mouth (xerostomia) is reported in up to 8% of patients.

V. **Laboratory abnormalities**

A. **Auto-antibodies** to nuclear and cytoplasmic antigens occur in SLE. Their detection is diagnostically significant, although the sensitivity and specificity for SLE vary with each specific auto-antibody (Table 30-4). Because these auto-antibodies participate in immunologically mediated tissue damage, correlation between disease activity and antibody titer has been sought with the hope that antibody level (especially anti-DNA antibody level) might provide an index of disease activity and a guide to therapeutics. The utility of this approach, however, is problematic, as severe disease does not develop despite conservative treatment in some patients with persistently abnormal values. Indeed, there are some patients who have had only laboratory abnormalities with no symptoms for many years. The different technologies available for measuring any given auto-antibody do not necessarily provide comparable results. Although both IgM and IgG rheumatoid factors may occur in up to one-third of patients, their presence does not correlate with the presence of articular disease.

B. **Serum complement** is often abnormally low in conjunction with elevated auto-antibody titers. Hypocomplementemia *per se* is not specific for SLE and may reflect any immunologically mediated disease accompanied by complement consumption, a hereditary complement component deficiency, impaired synthesis, or an improperly handled serum sample. In the context of SLE,

Table 30-4. Auto-antibodies in systemic lupus erythematosus

Antigen source	Antibody nomenclature	Incidence in SLE (%)	Specificity for SLE
Nuclear			
All determinants	ANA	100	—
ds-DNA	Anti-DNA (double-stranded or native)	80–90	High
ss-DNA	Anti-DNA (single-stranded)	80–90	—
Acidic nucleoproteins	Sm	30	High
	RNP	30–40	—
	Ro (SS-A)	25	—
	La (SS-B)	15–20	—
Cytoplasmic ribonucleoproteins	rRNA, rRNP, Ro, La, P	Uncertain	—
Cell surface determinants			
RBC	Direct Coombs'	30	—
WBC	Antilymphocyte antibodies	Common	—
	Antineutrophil antibodies	Uncommon	—
Platelets		Common	—
Others			
Clotting factor phospholipids	Lupus anticoagulant	10	—
Cardiolipin	Anti-cardiolipin antibody	10–25	—

ANA, antinuclear antibody; ds-DNA, double-stranded DNA; ss-DNA, single-stranded DNA; RBC, red blood cell; WBC, white blood cell.

hypocomplementemia is often, but not invariably, associated with nephritis. Like anti-DNA antibody levels, complement titers are valuable as a therapeutic guide in some but not all patients.

C. **Routine laboratory examination** may reveal abnormalities.

1. **Hematology**

a. **Anemia** occurs in more than 50% of patients, especially during active disease. Most anemias in SLE are of the chronic disease type (normochromic, normocytic with low serum iron and total iron binding capacity). Results of the direct Coombs' test may be positive in approximately 25% of patients; true hemolytic anemia occurs in 10% of patients. The Coombs' test result may represent cell surface immunoglobulin (IgG), complement (C3, C4), or both. Anemia from blood loss or microangiopathic hemolytic anemia must always be considered.

b. **Leukopenia.** SLE patients are often leukopenic, especially during periods of disease activity. Lymphopenia caused by anti-lymphocyte antibodies is the most common type, but antibody-mediated neutropenia can occur. Anti-stem cell antibodies are rare.

c. **Thrombocytopenia.** Anti-platelet antibodies have been demonstrated by a direct test similar to Coombs' test.

d. **Prolongation of the partial thromboplastin time.** Antibodies to both individual components of the clotting cascade (VIII, IX, XII) and to the prothrombin-converting complex have been described. The lupus anticoagulant is not corrected by addition of normal plasma to the patient's plasma. In the presence of normal platelets, the lupus anticoagulant does not appear to cause clinically significant bleeding, but it does lead to an increased propensity to venous and arterial thrombosis.

e. **False-positive reaction to serologic test for syphilis.** A small percentage of biologic false-positive reactions show a "positive" fluorescent treponemal antibody, which can be distinguished from a true positive by its beaded appearance. Circulating lupus anticoagulants and anti-cardiolipin antibodies are associated with a false-positive reaction to the serologic test for syphilis.

f. The **erythrocyte sedimentation rate** is frequently elevated but is an inconsistent index of disease activity. It is not useful in differentiating active SLE from an intercurrent process, such as infection.

2. **Biochemistry.** Apart from hypergammaglobulinemia, routine biochemical screening reflects the pattern and degree of organ involvement. Mild hyperkalemia in the absence of renal insufficiency may reflect an SLE-related renal tubular defect.

VI. Differential diagnosis. The diagnostic strategy for SLE involves recognition of a multisystem disease, the presence of certain serologic findings, and the absence of any other recognized disease process to explain the findings. Not all clinical and laboratory findings are of equal specificity; acute pericarditis and psychosis, as well as proteinuria and leukopenia, can have many causes other than SLE. Conversely, a discoid lupus rash and high titers of anti-native DNA antibodies or anti-Smith antigen antibodies strongly support the diagnosis. The art of diagnosis rests in recognizing a constellation of findings and giving each the appropriate clinical weight. Because the presentations of SLE are many and varied, the full differential diagnosis includes most of internal medicine.

A. The **most common presentation** is a young woman with polyarthritis; however, SLE is not the most likely cause of her symptoms. Rheumatoid arthritis or an infectious arthritis, such as gonococcal arthritis, must be considered first, as specific or curative therapy is available. Early in the course of uncomplicated lupus polyarthritis, radiographs of the joints are usually not helpful. The single most useful laboratory test to evaluate the possibility of SLE is the ANA determination. Although not completely specific, it is highly sensitive (Table 30-5). A positive test result is a signal to consider the diagnosis further, and a negative test result in a patient not receiving corticosteroid therapy makes the diagnosis unlikely.

B. **Organ systems that may be affected** by SLE include skin and mucous membranes (rash, ulceration, alopecia), joints (nondeforming, often symmetric polyarthritis and periarthritis), kidneys (glomerulonephritis), serosal membranes (pleuritis, pericarditis, abdominal serositis), blood (hemolytic anemia, leukopenia, thrombocytopenia), lungs (transient infiltrates, rarely progressive hemorrhagic pneumonitis), and nervous system (seizures, strokes, psychosis, peripheral neuropathies).

C. **Other rheumatic diseases.** Patients with multisystem disease and ANAs may have a condition other than SLE. Up to 40% of patients with rheumatoid arthritis may have ANAs. Systemic sclerosis (scleroderma), mixed connective tissue disease, and chronic active hepatitis must also be considered.

D. **Drug-induced systemic lupus erythematosus-like syndrome.** See Tables 30-2 and 30-5.

VII. Treatment. The diagnosis of SLE does not mandate the use of corticosteroids. Treatment must be individualized. The therapeutic strategy must consider both the pattern and the severity of organ system involvement. The poor prognosis reported in earlier series has been altered because of an overall improvement in general medical care, an enlightened and balanced use of medications, and the capability to diagnose milder forms of the disease. General measures include adequate rest and avoidance of stress. Descriptions of specific measures follow.

A. **Fever.** Nonsteroidal antiinflammatory drugs (NSAIDs) (e.g., 600 to 900 mg of aspirin four times daily, 25 to 50 mg of indomethacin three times daily) and acetaminophen are effective antipyretics. Corticosteroids are not indi-

Table 30-5. Differential diagnosis of common serologic tests

	Antinuclear antibodies	Anti-DNA antibodies	Low CH50	Rheumatoid factor
SLE incidence	~ 100%	80%	80%	20–40%
Diseases with high incidence	Discoid lupus Drug-induced LE Sicca syndrome Scleroderma	Discoid lupus Drug-induced LE (single-stranded)	Hereditary complement deficiency Hereditary angioedema Membranoproliferative glomerulonephritis Cryoglobulinemia	Rheumatoid arthritis Sicca syndrome
Diseases with occasional incidence	Rheumatoid arthritis Dermatomyositis Idiopathic pulmonary fibrosis Chronic active hepatitis Aging	Chronic active hepatitis Sicca syndrome Rheumatoid arthritis Scleroderma Dermatomyositis	Rheumatoid arthritis Serum sickness Serious infection: gram-negative sepsis, pneumococcal sepsis	Dermatomyositis Juvenile rheumatoid arthritis Scleroderma Sarcoidosis Subacute bacterial endocarditis Idiopathic pulmonary fibrosis Aging
Diseases with rare incidence	Necrotizing vasculitis	Necrotizing vasculitis	Necrotizing vasculitis	Insulin-dependent diabetes Normal subjects

LE, lupus erythematosus; CH50, hemolytic complement.

cated for fever alone. Persistent or high fevers should always stimulate a search for infection, particularly in patients on steroids or immunosuppressive agents.

B. Skin rash. Avoidance of exposure to ultraviolet light to prevent exacerbation of both cutaneous and systemic disease is paramount. Sunscreens, wide-brimmed hats, long sleeves, and long pants should be used by all patients. Highly protective sunscreens should be applied liberally 1 to 2 hours before exposure and reapplied after any swimming or sweating.

1. **Topical therapy.** Active skin disease should be treated with topical corticosteroid preparations (e.g., hydrocortisone, triamcinolone, or fluocinonide two to three times daily; see Appendix E) rather than with systemic corticosteroids. Occlusive dressings with cellophane wrap may be used at night, particularly on the upper extremities.
2. **Systemic therapy.** The antimalarial hydroxychloroquine (200 mg PO twice daily) is used to supplement topical treatment of extensive lesions. Quinacrine (100 mg daily) is also effective. Regular ophthalmologic examinations at 6-month intervals should include a slit-lamp examination and measures of light and color perception thresholds. The drug should be tapered as soon as disease control permits. Systemic corticosteroids are usually not indicated for skin disease alone.

C. Arthritis

1. **Nonsteroidal antiinflammatory drugs** (see Appendix E). Gastrointestinal intolerance and the presence of renal disease may limit therapy with NSAIDs in some patients. Occasionally, large elevations of liver enzymes may occur and require either reduction or termination of therapy. Transient changes in renal function with any NSAID may occur. The experience with NSAIDs other than aspirin includes several apparently idiosyncratic reactions in SLE patients manifested by fever and aseptic meningitis.
2. **Antimalarial drugs,** including both hydroxychloroquine and quinacrine, may be effective in the treatment of joint pain and inflammation, fatigue, and skin rash. These drugs can also be used as steroid-sparing agents.
3. **Systemic corticosteroid.** Oral prednisone (10 to 20 mg daily) is reserved for patients with accompanying constitutional symptoms unresponsive to NSAIDs.
4. **Methotrexate** is a reasonable alternative to antimalarial agents or low-dose glucocorticoids in patients with persistent arthritis, rash, or serositis. Dose reductions are necessary for patients with renal insufficiency.

D. Serositis can be treated with an NSAID as outlined for arthritis. At times, severe pericarditis may require a short course of steroids. Rarely, a large pericardial effusion necessitates therapy with high-dose prednisone (20 mg three times daily). Adverse effects of long-term high-dose corticosteroid therapy are discussed under renal disease (see section **VII.I.1**).

E. Pneumonitis. Transient pulmonary infiltrates that clear spontaneously without therapy may occur. The major significance of the radiologic findings relates to differential diagnosis rather than therapeutics. Infection with routine or opportunistic pathogens must be considered. Infiltrates secondary to SLE may require therapy, especially if they are associated with other signs of disease activity. Fulminant pneumonitis with hemorrhage, which is rare, requires aggressive therapy with high-dose corticosteroids (20 mg of prednisone three times daily) and often cytotoxic agents (1 to 3 mg of azathioprine per kilogram daily, or 1 to 2 mg of cyclophosphamide per kilogram daily).

F. Hematologic abnormalities

1. **Hemolytic anemia** is uncommon but may be severe and require corticosteroid therapy if symptomatic. Young patients can tolerate hemoglobin levels of 7 to 8 g/dL. When required, 40 to 60 mg of prednisone is given daily in two to three divided doses and tapered as quickly as possible with the hemoglobin and reticulocyte count used as guides. Microangiopathic hemo-

lytic anemia (elevated lactate dehydrogenase, schistocytes) may be associated with SLE vasculitis and is often treated with high-dose steroids.

2. **Immune thrombocytopenia** secondary to SLE usually responds to corticosteroid therapy. Platelet counts of 80,000 to 100,000 are considered adequate. Life-threatening thrombocytopenia unresponsive to several weeks of 60 mg of prednisone daily may improve with gamma globulin therapy (400 mg/kg IV daily for 5 days consecutively), which usually leads to an immediate (2 to 3 days) rise in the platelet count. Danazol, azathioprine, vincristine, vinca alkaloid-loaded platelets, and IV "pulse" cyclophosphamide have been used on occasions for steroid-resistant thrombocytopenia.
3. **Leukopenia** in SLE usually represents lymphopenia rather than neutropenia and is not associated with the serious risk for infection that accompanies the leukopenia of cancer chemotherapy. Leukopenia usually does not warrant specific treatment *per se,* but it does improve when steroids are used to treat other disease manifestations.

G. **Vasculitis.** Small-vessel cutaneous vasculitis, usually found on the digits and palm of the hand, may be managed with low-dose prednisone (20 mg/d). Medium-vessel and large-vessel vasculitis, although uncommon, requires 60 mg/d in divided doses.

H. **Neurologic disease**

1. **Seizures** require the use of anticonvulsant drugs. Initial therapy is 300 to 400 mg of phenytoin daily, with monitoring of serum drug levels. If needed to achieve seizure control, 20 to 60 mg of phenobarbital three times daily is added.
2. **Psychosis** may be secondary to either steroid therapy or SLE.
   a. **Steroid-induced psychosis** will improve with tapering of systemic corticosteroids. Major tranquilizers, such as 1 mg of haloperidol twice daily, initially will assist in control of psychotic manifestations.
   b. **Systemic lupus erythematosus-related psychosis.** The occurrence of SLE-related psychosis does not necessarily require an increase in steroid therapy. If adequate behavioral control is achieved with major tranquilizers and no organic signs are present on either physical examination or cerebrospinal fluid analysis, corticosteroids are not initiated or increased.
3. **Parenchymal central nervous system disease.** In the presence of new focal neurologic findings, 20 mg of prednisone is given three times daily until either improvement or toxicity is observed. Some neurologic lesions are not responsive to steroids. If no improvement is evident after about 3 to 4 weeks of high-dose therapy, prednisone is tapered to avoid complications. Dosages of prednisone above 60 to 80 mg daily rarely produce additional therapeutic benefit but markedly increase the risk for serious side effects. Any trial of very high-dose prednisone in severe disease should continue only for a predetermined, limited period of time. Pulse methylprednisolone therapy may be helpful for patients who do not respond to standard therapy. Cytotoxic agents such as IV cyclophosphamide have been used in steroid-unresponsive SLE patients with severe central nervous system disease.
4. **Peripheral nerve disease.** Peripheral neuropathy is common. Mononeuritis multiplex usually represents small-vessel vasculitis. If the patient is unresponsive to 60 mg of prednisone daily in three divided doses, then 1 to 3 mg of azathioprine per kilogram or 1 to 2 mg of cyclophosphamide per kilogram may be initiated.

I. **Renal disease.** For the initial management of active renal disease, as defined by active urinary sediment including red blood cells and red cell casts, proteinuria, and a decrease in creatinine clearance, the intensity of therapy is often defined by the severity of presentation and extra-renal manifestations of disease. Response to a chosen treatment is assessed by serial urinalyses, 24-hour urine testing, and determination of levels of serum complement and anti-DNA antibodies. Although renal biopsy is helpful in characterizing the type of renal lesion and extent of acute and chronic change, it is not mandatory. Patients with diffuse proliferative or membranoproliferative glomerulonephritis have the worst prognosis, but the natural history of clinically silent, diffuse proliferative disease with normal renal function has not been determined. Chronic changes of fibrosis and atrophy suggest little reversible disease and a poor prognosis. Any therapeutic regimen must consider both short-term and long-term effects encountered during the management of chronic nephritis.

Infection and drug-related causes of renal abnormalities must be sought and corrected. Vigorous control of blood pressure and avoidance of nephrotoxins is mandatory.

1. **Corticosteroid therapy** is the mainstay of treatment for active nephritis. The dosage, route of administration, and duration of therapy vary depending on the initial presentation, presence of comorbidities, and prior treatment modalities. Two approaches have been employed for the management of active nephritis.

   Prednisone (60 mg daily in divided doses) for 1 to 2 months: Resolution of signs of active disease commonly permits tapering of prednisone. A recurrence of active urinary sediment, increased proteinuria, and decreased kidney function may prompt an increase in steroid dosage, a switch to "pulse" steroids, or a decision to perform a kidney biopsy in preparation for consideration of cyclophosphamide therapy.

   High-dose, "pulse" methylprednisolone: This regimen is defined by courses of 1,000 mg/d for 3 days monthly for 6 months, with 0.5 mg of oral prednisone per kilogram between pulses, to control both renal and extrarenal manifestations. It is used as (a) initial therapy for active nephritis, (b) sole therapy to avoid cumulative side effects of long-term daily steroids, or (c) therapy for exacerbations of severe disease that do not respond to daily oral steroids.

   Although prednisone clearly helps to relieve acute exacerbations of disease, long-term corticosteroid therapy is associated with **serious side effects.**

   a. **Physical appearance** is altered by weight gain that produces truncal fat deposition (moon facies, buffalo hump), hirsutism, acne, easy bruising, and purple striae. Although individual patients differ in their susceptibility to these changes, reduction of the steroid dosage will eventually reduce the severity of these manifestations.
   b. **Infection** occurs with greater frequency in corticosteroid-treated patients. Corticosteroids may mask both local and systemic signs of infection. Minor infections have a greater potential to become systemic. Latent infections, especially mycobacterial varieties, may become activated, and opportunistic agents such as fungi, *Nocardia,* and *Pneumocystis carinii* may cause serious clinical problems. Skin testing for delayed hypersensitivity to *Mycobacterium tuberculosis* should be performed before the initiation of corticosteroid therapy. However, a negative reaction may reflect the altered immunity of active SLE rather than lack of previous exposure to *M. tuberculosis.*
   c. **Mental function** may be altered. Minor reactions include irritability, insomnia, euphoria, and inability to concentrate. Major reactions may include severe depression, mania, and paranoid psychoses.
   d. **Glucose intolerance** may be induced or exacerbated by corticosteroids. Insulin may be required to control hyperglycemia and should be adjusted as the corticosteroid dosage is changed.
   e. **Hypokalemia** may be caused by preparations with mineralocorticoid activity. Serum potassium should be checked frequently, especially if congestive heart failure, nephrosis, or peripheral edema producing secondary hyperaldosteronism is present.
   f. **Sodium retention, edema, and hypertension** may be induced by all corticosteroid drugs. When these effects become clinically signifi-

cant, agents with fewer salt-retaining properties can be used. Alternative steroid preparations are listed in Appendix E. Because steroids should be given only for major SLE manifestations, it is usually not feasible to control hypertension by a reduction in dosage; therefore, blood pressure must be controlled by appropriate antihypertensive therapy.

g. **Myopathy** may occur in patients receiving long-term, high-dose steroids. The muscles are not tender, and unlike inflammatory myositis, steroid-induced myopathy is usually not characterized by elevated serum muscle enzymes. Proximal weakness is the most common symptom. Weakness of the pelvic girdle is more common than shoulder-girdle symptoms. Biopsy may be useful in distinguishing inflammatory, SLE-related myositis from non-inflammatory, corticosteroid-induced myopathy. Drug-induced myopathy will gradually improve with a reduction of corticosteroid dosage.

h. **Skeletal abnormalities** include osteopenia and osteonecrosis. Corticosteroids may reduce gastrointestinal calcium absorption, induce secondary hyperparathyroidism, and also reduce collagen matrix synthesis by osteoblasts. Compression fractures in the vertebral spine represent a major secondary complication, especially in older patients. They occur in about 15% of steroid-treated patients. Prophylactic vitamin D_3 (400 U twice daily) and calcium (1,500 mg/d from dietary and supplemental sources) are recommended. Patients receiving long-term corticosteroid therapy (for more than 1 month) should undergo baseline and yearly bone density evaluations and treatment with suitable bisphosphonates if necessary (see Chapter 46). Osteonecrosis occurs most frequently in weight-bearing joints, especially the femoral heads. The mechanism is unknown (therapy is discussed in Chapter 45). Reduction in corticosteroid dosage is desirable whenever possible, although it is unlikely to affect established osteonecrosis.

i. **Hypoadrenalism** may occur during periods of physiologic stress in patients with suppression of the hypothalamic-pituitary-adrenal axis resulting from exogenous steroid administration. During episodes of surgery or major intercurrent illness, it is advisable to provide supplemental steroid therapy to patients who are receiving corticosteroid therapy or who have discontinued such therapy within the previous year. Hydrocortisone (300 mg/d or equivalent dosage in three divided doses) may be given IV or IM during the period of maximum stress and subsequently tapered during 5 days. The stress of major nonsurgical illness may be managed with an increase in daily steroid dosage to at least the equivalent of 30 mg of prednisone.

j. **Other side effects** of corticosteroids include increased intraocular pressure, which may precipitate glaucoma, and the occurrence of posterior subcapsular cataracts. Although dyspepsia may accompany the use of steroids, it usually responds to antacids or histamine_2 blockers and administration of medication with meals. Enhancement of peptic ulcer disease probably does not occur. Menstrual irregularities, night sweats, and pancreatitis have been associated with corticosteroid therapy. Pseudotumor cerebri, associated with rapid steroid dosage reduction, is a rare complication.

2. **Cytotoxic drugs** are used in either severe corticosteroid-resistant disease or in the context of unacceptable steroid side effects. In patients with diffuse proliferative glomerulonephritis, cyclophosphamide has shown to retard progression of scarring in the kidney and reduce the risk for end-stage renal failure. Monthly infusions of IV "pulse" cyclophosphamide (0.5 to 1.0 g/m^2 of body surface area) preserve renal function more effectively than do corticosteroids alone, but the rate of relapse following a 6-month course is high. Most patients require extended therapy. Potential toxicities are substantial: nausea and vomiting (often requiring treatment with antiemetic drugs); alopecia (reversible); ovarian failure (nearly

universal in patients more than 30 years old) or azoospermia; and hemorrhagic cystitis, bladder fibrosis, and bladder transitional cell or squamous carcinoma. Intermittent IV cyclophosphamide may decrease the incidence of bladder complications associated with daily oral therapy. Azathioprine (1 to 3 mg/kg daily) is a far less toxic drug that avoids the potential complications of alopecia, sterility, and hemorrhagic cystitis associated with cyclophosphamide, but it is considered less effective. Each agent requires careful monitoring of complete blood cell counts. Allopurinol should not be used with azathioprine because it inhibits azathioprine catabolism. The long-term toxicity of these agents may include both hematopoietic malignancy and solid tumors (lymphomas with azathioprine, bladder carcinoma with cyclophosphamide).

3. **Other regimens.** Controlled trials of plasmapheresis have not shown benefit in most cases. Currently, clinical experience is being gathered with methotrexate and mycophenolate mofetil, but no controlled studies are available. Clinical experience with cyclosporin A (3 to 6 mg/kg daily) suggests that it might be useful in membranous glomerulonephritis. Side effects, particularly hypertension and renal toxicity, appear to be infrequent.

J. Special management considerations

1. **Idiopathic drug reactions.** The possibility of an increase in allergic drug reactions in SLE patients is controversial. However, some observations suggest that sulfonamide and quinolone drugs may exacerbate SLE. Fever and meningeal irritation have been reported in SLE patients taking ibuprofen, sulindac, and tolmetin.
2. **Drug-induced lupus.** Medications associated with drug-induced lupus (see Table 30-2) have been used extensively and effectively in patients with idiopathic SLE. Although the risk for exacerbating the underlying disease is often discussed, such risk has not been established and does not contraindicate the use of an otherwise indicated medication.
3. **Pregnancy.** The effects of pregnancy on SLE are variable and are discussed in detail in Chapter 24.
4. **Contraception.** Because SLE is a disease of women of childbearing age, contraception is an important issue. Barrier protection condoms and a diaphragm are preferable because they have no adverse effects. However, the patient's willingness to use these methods effectively must be considered. Because hormonal manipulation might theoretically exacerbate SLE, oral contraceptives with progesterone only or with a combination containing the lowest estrogen dose are preferable.
5. **Hormone replacement.** The effects of estrogen replacement therapy on SLE disease activity remain unclear. Although it may prove useful as a means to reduce the risk for osteoporosis and atherosclerosis in women with SLE, estrogen replacement therapy in SLE patients is controversial and is the subject of a national collaborative study. It is clearly contraindicated in those with a history of thrombosis or anti-phospholipid antibodies.
6. **Hemodialysis.** SLE patients appear to tolerate long-term hemodialysis as well as any population with chronic renal failure. Clinical impressions suggest that SLE patients may have more quiescent disease once on dialysis, but they may still occasionally experience SLE disease activity.
7. **Transplantation.** SLE patients may undergo renal transplantation without any apparent increase in morbidity in comparison with other transplantation populations. Recurrences of lupus in transplanted allografts are rare.

VIII. Prognosis. The prognosis of SLE has improved, largely because milder forms of disease have been recognized, but also through the availability of potent antibiotics, the development of intensive care units, and probably the use of corticosteroids and immunosuppressive agents in the more severely ill patients. Prognosis depends on the pattern of organ involvement; patients with renal and central nervous system disease have the worst 5-year survival rates. Infection continues to be a major cause of death. Recent series show 5-year survival rates of about 90%.

A. **Drug-induced lupus.** Many drugs (see Table 30-2) have been implicated in the induction of a lupuslike syndrome, with manifestations ranging from an isolated positive ANA test result to a clinical lupus syndrome. Procainamide and hydralazine are the drugs most frequently reported to produce a lupus-like syndrome.
   1. **Clinical features.** Skin rash, arthritis, pleural and pericardial effusions, lymphadenopathy, splenomegaly, anemia, leukopenia, elevated erythrocyte sedimentation rate, and transient false-positive serologic tests for syphilis may all be included. Pleuropulmonary disease is prominent, and renal and central nervous system disease are characteristically absent. Most manifestations resolve after discontinuation of the drug.
   2. **Laboratory studies.** The laboratory profile of a patient with drug-induced lupus may help distinguish the syndrome from spontaneous SLE. Serum complement is rarely reduced in the drug-induced syndrome, and antibodies to native (or double-stranded) DNA are usually absent. However, antibodies to single-stranded DNA are often present, in addition to antibodies to histones and ribonucleoproteins.
   3. **Treatment** of drug-induced lupus involves discontinuation of the offending agent and symptomatic management of the clinical manifestations. Because most manifestations are reversible, therapy is usually of short duration. A positive ANA test result alone should prompt review of the indications for use of the inciting agent but does not *per se* require the addition of therapeutic agents.

B. **Discoid lupus erythematosus**
   1. **Clinical presentation.** Disease may be limited to the skin and assume the chronic discoid form, with scaling red plaques and follicular plugging. Healing of these lesions is associated with central scarring and atrophy. Although chronic discoid lupus erythematosus remains primarily cutaneous in the majority of patients, SLE will develop in a small percentage (about 5%). Conversely, patients with SLE may have discoid lesions among the cutaneous manifestations of their disease. Certain types of skin lesions, such as those of subacute cutaneous lupus erythematosus, may reflect a specific immunogenetic predisposition.
   2. **Therapy** follows the same principles as those outlined for skin disease in SLE: avoidance of sun and ultraviolet exposure and use of topical steroids and hydroxychloroquine (see Chapter 11 for more information regarding discoid lupus erythematosus).

Bibliography

Boumpas DT, et al. Systemic lupus erythematosus: emerging concepts. Part 1. *Ann Intern Med* 1995;122:190.

Boumpas DT, et al. Systemic lupus erythematosus: emerging concepts. Part 2. *Ann Intern Med* 1995;123:42.

Klippel JH, Dieppe PA, eds. *Rheumatology,* 2nd ed. London: Gower Medical Publishing, 1997.

Lahita RG, ed. *Systemic lupus erythematosus.* New York: Churchill Livingstone, 1992.

Ropes MW. *Systemic lupus erythematosus.* Cambridge, MA: Harvard University Press, 1976.

Wallace DJ, Hahn BH, eds. *Dubois' lupus erythematosus,* 5th ed. Baltimore: Williams & Wilkins, 1997.

31. SYSTEMIC SCLEROSIS AND RELATED SYNDROMES

Robert F. Spiera

Scleroderma is a systemic disorder characterized by microvascular injury and fibrosis in affected organs. It is a relatively uncommon disorder, with an estimated incidence of between 10 to 20 per million annually, affecting women more commonly than men and often beginning in the third or fourth decade of life. Environmental factors have been implicated in subsets of scleroderma patients, but in the majority of cases, the disease is idiopathic. There is at best a weak genetic contribution to disease susceptibility.

I. Pathogenesis. The etiology and pathogenesis of scleroderma are unknown. The principal pathologic processes in affected organs are microvascular injury and fibrosis with excess deposition of extracellular matrix, in particular, collagen. It is not clear whether the primary process is endothelial injury causing ischemia and secondary fibrotic changes, or alternatively whether the exuberant fibrosis results in vascular injury. Recently, the role of possible autonomic dysregulation in the pathogenesis of the disorder has gained attention. Inflammation seems to play a role early in the disease course, and inflammatory perivascular infiltrates primarily consisting of T cells are seen in the dermis, particularly at the border between the reticular dermis and subcutaneous fat. Inflammation similarly seems to play a role in early alveolar disease, and in some patients with muscle disease. Vascular lesions generally consist of luminal narrowing caused by intimal proliferation. There is evidence of endothelial cell injury and platelet activation. Cytokines, including transforming growth factor-beta, interleukin-1 (IL-1), IL-2, and platelet-derived growth factor, have been implicated in fibroblast dysregulation and excess collagen production. Locally acting vasoactive molecules, including endothelin (vasoconstricting) and nitrous oxide (vasodilating), may also play a role in the disease process and afford future avenues of potential therapeutic intervention.

Auto-antibodies can be found in up to 95% of patients with systemic sclerosis, although a pathogenetic role has not yet been identified; they may be an epiphenomenon of immune systemic activation and tissue injury. A role for cellular immunity is supported by the correlation of increased IL-2 and soluble IL-2 receptor levels with disease activity, and the clinical and pathologic similarities between scleroderma and graft-versus-host disease. In this regard, investigators have demonstrated cellular mosaicism in women with scleroderma, with retention of fetal cells in skin lesions, and in the peripheral blood of women with systemic sclerosis. This suggests that a graft-versus-host type of reaction, induced by retained fetal cells, might contribute to the pathogenesis of scleroderma in some patients.

II. Clinical features. Scleroderma is a heterogeneous disorder with great variation in its presentation and clinical course. The hallmark features are hardening of the skin and Raynaud's phenomena. The pattern of skin involvement, namely *limited* versus *diffuse,* can be used to distinguish subsets of the disease and has implications regarding the involvement of other organ systems and prognosis. Morbidity and overall prognosis are a function of the pattern and degree of internal organ involvement, and are variable among patients. The course of the illness is characterized either by inexorable progression or by initial progression and then remission in some cases. Some patients have intermittent flares. Constitutional symptoms, including weight loss and fatigue, are common, whereas fever is uncommon in the absence of infection. Specific organ system involvement is addressed below.

A. Vascular. Vascular disease is nearly universal in scleroderma. Microvascular injury is felt to play a major role in pathogenesis, and the distribution thereof largely determines what organ systems will be affected. The most clinically overt indication of vascular disease is the presence of Raynaud's phenomena, which occurs in 95% of patients with scleroderma. In fact, when the diagnosis of scleroderma is suspected, the absence of Raynaud's phenomena should caution the clinician to search for other possible etiologies of a sclerosing illness. Typical changes of Raynaud's phenomena are pallor, cyanosis, then erythema in response to cold stimuli, although other factors can stimulate these symptoms, such as stress or smoking. They can also occur spontaneously. As opposed to the spasm in the primary Raynaud's phenomena, patients with scleroderma have structural changes in the arteries secondary to intimal hyperplasia and adventitial fibrosis that lead to attenuation of the lumen. Vasoconstriction in these already compromised vessels can lead to significant ischemia distally and can result in digital infarction and progressive auto-amputation. Similar changes are felt to contribute to visceral disease in the lungs and kidneys. Studies have similarly suggested "visceral" Raynaud's phenomena in the heart and kidney. Nailfold capillary changes, including tortuosity of capillary loops and areas of loop dropout, can be readily observed by use of an ophthalmoscope at 40 power with oil immersion. Telangiectases, which develop later in the course of the disease and can involve the oral mucosa, face, lips, and hands, also represent microvascular change.

B. Skin. Thickened, tight skin is the hallmark feature of systemic sclerosis, and the term scleroderma itself in fact is derived from Greek roots meaning "hard skin." Although systemic sclerosis without skin involvement has been described ("scleroderma *sine* scleroderma"), skin involvement in general is a readily recognizable, universal feature. In the earliest, edematous phase, there may be puffy, painless swelling in the hands and fingers. As the disease progresses, the skin becomes thickened and bound down, with loss of normal appendicular structures. The appearance can initially be erythematous, and later hypopigmented or hyperpigmented. Pruritus is a common complaint, and skin breakdown, particularly over extensor surfaces of the small joints of the hands, can result in poorly healing ulcerations with infections. The changes generally begin distally in the hands and progress proximally, with involvement of the neck and face, typical thinning of the lips, and a pursed appearance of the mouth resulting from perioral involvement. Telangiectases are commonly seen in the distal upper extremities and face. Subcutaneous calcifications occur mostly in the hands and near bony eminences. Overlying skin can become painful and inflamed, and calcifications can also lead to poorly healing wounds.

The pattern of skin involvement is variable, but two distinct courses have been recognized, which allow stratification of patients into distinct subgroups with differing serologic associations, clinical courses, and patterns of organ involvement. In *limited scleroderma,* the cutaneous disease remains distal and does not extend proximally to the forearms, although the face and neck can be involved. There can be a spontaneous regression of skin involvement within 2 years of disease onset. The limited pattern has also been referred to as the CREST syndrome, an acronym for calcinosis, Raynaud's esophageal dysmotility, sclerodactyly, and telangiectases, which are typical features. Organ involvement tends to occur earlier in *diffuse scleroderma,* and renal crisis and interstitial fibrotic lung disease are major causes of morbidity and mortality. Early classification of the patient with systemic sclerosis is important in regard to both prognosis and identification of key organ systems at risk.

C. Pulmonary. Lung involvement is a major cause of mortality in systemic sclerosis. Interstitial disease often begins at the bases and can be progressive. Interstitial lung disease can occur early in the course of diffuse scleroderma, but it is a very late, indolent process when occurring in patients with the limited form. Symptoms generally include dyspnea and a nonproductive cough, and the examination can reveal the typical dry "velcro" rales of fibrotic lung disease. Chest radiographs can reveal increased interstitial markings, especially at the bases. High-resolution computed tomography (CT) has a greater sensitivity in terms of detecting early abnormalities, and pulmonary function testing can reveal diminished vital capacity, diffusion capacity, and compliance, even in patients without symptoms. Bronchoalveolar lavage in some patients is suggestive of alveolitis, and there is interest in identifying patients with an inflammatory component to their lung disease (i.e., lavage fluid containing primarily polys), who might be candidates for immunosuppressive therapy. Pulmonary hypertension can also occur, as a secondary phenomenon in the setting of interstitial lung disease or as a primary process independent of parenchymal lung involvement, particularly in patients with limited scleroderma. Echocardiography can estimate pulmonary arterial pressures noninvasively. Infection is also a major issue, particularly in patients with esophageal disease and dysphagia, who are often at risk for aspiration. The incidence of lung cancer in patients with scleroderma also seems to be increased.

D. Renal. Before the introduction of angiotensin-converting enzyme (ACE) inhibitors, hypertensive renal crisis was a major cause of mortality in patients with diffuse scleroderma. This syndrome is characterized by a hyperreninemic state with accelerated hypertension, rapidly progressive azotemia, microangiopathic hemolysis, and consumptive thrombocytopenia. Urinalysis reveals evidence of protein and red blood cells. In the absence of appropriate diagnosis and therapy, severe complications, including hypertensive retinopathy, encephalopathy, and renal failure, can ensue. In some patients, normotensive renal crisis can occur, and this may be associated with corticosteroid use. In a patient in whom scleroderma has been diagnosed, particularly a patient with rapidly progressive, diffuse disease, regular blood pressure monitoring is essential, and daily self-monitoring of blood pressure at home is advisable.

E. Gastrointestinal. Gastrointestinal involvement is common in scleroderma and is the cause of clinical symptoms in nearly 50% of patients. Any segment of the gastrointestinal tract can be involved. Early pathologic changes include vasculopathy and smooth-muscle atrophy and fibrosis, which eventually result in dysmotility. There is also evidence that neuropathic changes contribute to disordered myoelectric function, even before the development of atrophic or fibrotic changes.

Esophageal abnormalities are often the predominant complaint. Reflux is common and is related to lower esophageal sphincter incompetence and impaired esophageal motility. Erosive esophagitis and even strictures can develop. Dysphagia and odynophagia are common and can interfere with nutrition. Cineesophagography or manometric evaluations can help distinguish the pattern of esophageal involvement. Stomach involvement is less commonly symptomatic, but gastroparesis can contribute to dyspepsia and a sense of bloating. Gastric telangiectases occur but are uncommonly a cause of bleeding. Intestinal hypermotility can lead to bloating and cramps in addition to bacterial overgrowth, malabsorption, and diarrhea. Colonic manifestations often include constipation or pseudo-obstruction. Wide-mouthed colonic diverticula are common but are often not of clinical significance.

F. Cardiac. Myocardial fibrosis can occur in scleroderma and is a poor prognostic feature. The early lesion appears to be contraction band necrosis and is likely related to local microvascular disease and intermittent ischemia resulting from spasm. Fibrotic replacement of normal myocardium can cause arrhythmias, which indicate a poor prognosis. Effusive pericarditis can occur but is not a common feature. Pulmonary hypertension can occur in the setting of fibrotic lung disease or as a primary vascular problem in patients with limited scleroderma. Systemic hypertension can also contribute to myocardial dysfunction.

G. Musculoskeletal. Arthralgias and morning stiffness are common and are often related to involvement of periarticular structures rather than arthritis *per se.* Contractures, particularly of the hands but also in large joints such as the shoulders, can lead to major functional limitations and are related to fibrosis of tendon sheaths or to sclerodermatous involvement of the overlying skin. Tendon friction rubs about the hands and feet are a typical feature in patients with diffuse scleroderma. Radiographs can reveal acro-osteolysis of digital tufts, which is likely related to repeated digital ischemia. Subcutaneous calcinosis can be seen as well.

Myopathy can occur secondary to fibrotic disease and atrophy, and less commonly as a result of an inflammatory myositis or an obliterative endarteropathy.

H. Serologies and laboratory investigations. Antinuclear antibodies can be found in 90% of patients. Anti-centromere antibodies can be found in more than 50% of patients with limited scleroderma (CREST syndrome). Anti-topoisomerse-1 (SCL-70) antibodies are found in 30% of patients with diffuse disease. The diagnosis is made on a clinical basis, however, and should not rely on serologic confirmation. Serologies provide supportive but not diagnostic information.

Other laboratory investigations are helpful in defining organ system involvement (e.g., creatine phosphokinase and aldolase in patients with weakness and possible myositis, or urinalysis and serum creatinine to screen for renal involvement), or monitoring for toxicities of ongoing therapies.

III. Treatment. No drugs have been proved to have a disease-modifying role in scleroderma in terms of altering the progression of the underlying pathogenic process. D-Penicillamine has been of interest, given its ability to interfere with cross-linking of collagen, which would in theory retard progression of this fibrosing illness. Some retrospective studies have suggested an improvement in skin and lung disease and survival in comparison with historical controls. A recent trial, however, comparing very low-dose (62.5 mg daily) with high-dose (750 to 1,000 mg daily) penicillamine did not show benefit in the higher-dose group. Colchicine has been of interest also, owing to its antifibrotic properties *in vitro*. Other agents currently under investigation include high-dose methotrexate, cyclosporin A, interferon-τ, and recombinant human relaxin. Photophoresis is also being used in some centers, although it has not been approved by the Food and Drug Administration for use in scleroderma.

Although disease-modifying therapy has been elusive, major strides have recently been made in treating specific organ complications of systemic sclerosis.

A. Vascular. Avoidance of smoking and cold exposure is paramount. Systemic vasodilators, including calcium channel blockers (e.g., extended-release nifedipine started at 30 mg daily or diltiazem started at 120 mg daily) and alpha blockers (e.g., prazosin started at 1 mg twice daily), are helpful in reducing the severity and frequency of vasospastic episodes. Topical nitrates can be of use. Iloprost, a prostacyclin analog administered IV, has been of value in patients with ischemic ulcerations related to Raynaud's phenomena, but it is not presently available in the United States. Sympathetic blockade may be quite effective in controlling severe or persistent vasospasm. Surgical approaches, in particular digital sympathectomy, can be useful in salvaging digits at risk. Hygiene is critical, as is aggressive therapy of secondary superinfection and avoidance of trauma. Surgical amputation is generally avoided; autoamputation of distally infarcted digits may occur. Anti-platelet therapy, such as aspirin (81 to 325 mg daily), or even full-dose anticoagulation has been advocated to improve perfusion in those patients with a low-flow state in their digits.

B. Skin. D-Penicillamine has been used in patients with rapidly progressive skin disease, although results are not impressive. Colchicine, potassium *p*-aminobenzoate, dimethyl sulfoxide, and photophoresis have also been used but are of uncertain value and are not supported by clinical trial evidence. No therapy has been proved to relieve calcinosis, although small case series have recently suggested a possible role for diltiazem in that regard. Colchicine (0.6 mg twice daily) seems to be helpful in the setting of inflammatory ulcerating lesions. Surgical debulking of calcinosis is generally not pursued, as recurrence is common, but it can be of value in instances of recurrent infection or extreme pain.

C. Pulmonary. Pulmonary fibrosis is a major cause of mortality in systemic sclerosis. Unfortunately, established fibrotic disease is not amenable to therapy other than supportive modalities. Early stages, however, may be more treatable, and there are some data supporting a role for cyclophosphamide in patients with alveolitis, which may be the earliest lesion. Bronchoalveolar lavage may be useful in determining whether an inflammatory alveolitis that could warrant such aggressive therapy is present. Pulmonary hypertension has a dismal prognosis and traditionally has been refractory to therapy. Vasodilators, generally with high-dose calcium channel blockers, and anticoagulation afford symptomatic benefit. More recently, administration of prostacyclin and nitric oxide by continuous IV infusion pumps has been shown to improve function and survival in patients with primary pulmonary hypertension and is now also being used in patients with systemic sclerosis. There is little published experience in lung transplantation in scleroderma.

D. Renal. ACE inhibitors have had a profound impact on scleroderma renal crisis. Blood pressure should be monitored closely in patients with diffuse disease, and periodic assessment of renal function is important, as approximately 10% of patients experience normotensive renal crisis that is responsive to ACE inhibitors. Standard ACE inhibitors, such as enalapril started at 5 mg daily or captopril started at 25 mg three times daily, are employed, and the dose is aggressively titrated upward to achieve adequate blood pressure control. In a normotensive renal crisis, the dose is increased to the maximum tolerated by blood pressure or until the parameters of active disease are controlled (e.g., microangiopathy, progressive azotemia, urinary sediment abnormalities). In a minority of patients, IV enalapril started at 1.25 mg every 6 hours is necessary. Renal transplantation has been performed successfully in scleroderma patients.

E. Gastrointestinal. Proton pump inhibitors (20 mg of omeprazole daily or 30 mg of lansoprazole daily) represent a tremendous advance in the management of reflux and esophagitis, and they now are being used for long-term therapy in patients with systemic sclerosis. Prokinetic agents such as cisapride (started at 10 mg four times daily) can help with early satiety and in reflux as well. In some patients, endoscopic dilation of strictures helps to relieve symptoms of dysphagia. Octreotide and erythromycin may be of value in improving gastric and intestinal motility. Bacterial overgrowth causes bloating and diarrhea and may require periodic empiric courses of antibacterial agents; quinolones such as ciprofloxacin (500 mg daily for 2 weeks) or tetracycline (250 mg twice daily) have been useful.

F. Cardiac. Pericarditis is not a frequent cause of symptoms or cardiovascular compromise, but when necessary it can be treated with antiinflammatory drugs or corticosteroids (often first with 30 mg of prednisone daily). Asymptomatic effusions do not usually require therapy. Other cardiac complications, such as arrhythmias and congestive heart failure, are treated in standard medical fashion.

G. Musculoskeletal. Arthralgias or tendon friction rubs can be treated with nonsteroidal antiinflammatory drugs, although these must be used cautiously given the gastrointestinal and renal concerns in this patient population. Low-dose corticosteroids (7.5 mg or less of daily prednisone) are helpful, but there are some concerns regarding an association of prednisone therapy with the development of renal crisis in patients with diffuse disease. Physical therapy and occupational therapy should be a mainstay of management, with particular attention to maintaining range of motion, muscle strengthening, the use of paraffin baths, and splinting when appropriate. Surgical reconstruction can be helpful in selected patients with severe contractures causing functional limitation.

Inflammatory myositis is treated with substantial doses of corticosteroids (often first with 40 to 60 mg of prednisone daily) and other immunosuppressive therapies, such as methotrexate or azathioprine. Idiopathic myositis would be treated similarly.

IV. Related syndromes

A. Localized scleroderma. Morphea is characterized by plaques of asymmetric fibrotic dermal lesions that can be histologically indistinguishable from the lesions of scleroderma. It is not associated with visceral disease, and survival does not differ from that of the general population. The lesions often spontaneously regress within several years, although in rare patients morphea can become generalized. Linear scleroderma usually occurs in children, often as a linear, indurated patch of dermal fibrosis in a lower extremity. In some instances, facial hemiatrophy in the typical *coup de sabre* deformity can occur. No proven therapeutic interventions are available.

B. Eosinophilic fasciitis is characterized by thickening and inflammation of fascia, with puckering and tightness of the overlying skin. Pain, weakness, and contractures can occur. In many patients, there is an antecedent history of trauma. Diagnostic biopsy must be deep and include fascia, where eosinophilic and lymphocytic infiltrates can be identified. Laboratory findings often include eosinophilia and the presence of acute-phase reactants. The skin changes can resemble those of scleroderma, but the syndrome is not generally associated with Raynaud's phenomena or sclerodactyly. Also, visceral disease and antinuclear antibodies are much less common. The distinction is crucial, as eosinophilic fasciitis is often dramatically responsive to modest or high doses of corticosteroids and is often a self-limited illness.

C. Chemically induced symptoms. Scleroderma-like illnesses have been reported after exposure to bleomycin, vinyl chloride, and silica dust. An association between silicone gel-filled breast implants and the development of scleroderma has been suggested, but epidemiologic studies have not supported a causal relationship. A scleroderma-like illness appeared in Spain in 1981 and was ultimately linked to ingestion of a toxic rapeseed oil. Ingestion of contaminated tryptophan is felt to be the cause of the eosinophilia myalgia syndrome, characterized by myalgias, arthralgias, neuropathy, and skin changes resembling those of scleroderma, but with less prominent Raynaud's phenomena.

D. Mixed connective tissue disease. Patients with rheumatic diseases can often demonstrate overlapping features. Mixed connective tissue disease is an antibody-defined overlap connective tissue disease demonstrating features of lupus, systemic sclerosis, and myositis. Patients often present with puffy hands and arthralgias, and joint symptoms can be a prominent part of the clinical course. Raynaud's phenomena, esophageal dysmotility, and interstitial lung disease in addition to inflammatory myopathy can be seen. These patients have antinuclear antibodies that stain in a speckled pattern of immunofluorescence and detectable and often high titers of antibodies to ribonucleoproteins (anti-RNP). Patients with various features of rheumatoid arthritis, systemic sclerosis, lupus, polymyositis, and other rheumatic signs and symptoms but with nonspecific serologies are classified as having undifferentiated connective tissue disease. With observation, a classic disease may emerge. Therapy tends to be focused on the dominant disease manifestations.

Bibliography

Artlett CM, Smith JB, Jiminez SA. Identification of fetal DNA and cells in skin lesions from women with systemic sclerosis. *N Engl J Med* 1998;338:1186.

Chartash EK, et al. Tryptophan-induced eosinophilia-myalgia syndrome. *J Rheumatol* 1990;17:1527.

Clements PJ, Furst DE. *Systemic sclerosis.* Baltimore: Williams & Wilkins, 1996.

Clements PJ, et al. High-dose (HI-DPA) vs. low-dose (LO-DPA) penicillamine in early diffuse systemic sclerosis (SSc) trial: analysis of trial. *Arthritis Rheum* 1997;40[S173].

Mayes M. Epidemiology of systemic sclerosis and related diseases. *Curr Opin Rheumatol* 1997;9:557.

McLaughlin VD, et al. Reduction in pulmonary vascular resistance with long-term epoprostenol (prostacyclin) therapy in primary pulmonary hypertension. *N Engl J Med* 1998;338:273.

Seibold JR. Systemic sclerosis: clinical features. In: Klippel JH, Dieppe PA, eds. *Rheumatology.* London: Mosby–Yearbook Europe Limited, 1994.

Spiera RF, Gibofsky A, Spiera H. Silicone gel-filled implants and connective tissue disease: an overview. *J Rheumatol* 1994;21:239.

Steen VD. Systemic sclerosis: management. In: Klippel JH, Dieppe PA, eds. *Rheumatology.* London: Mosby–Yearbook Europe Limited, 1994.

Steen VD, et al. D-Penicillamine therapy in progressive systemic sclerosis. *Ann Intern Med* 1982;97:652.

Wigley FM. Management of severe Raynaud's phenomena. *J Clin Rheumatol* 1996; 2:103.

Wigley FM, et al. Intravenous iloprost infusion in patients with Raynaud's phenomena secondary to systemic sclerosis: a multicenter placebo-controlled, double-blind study. *Ann Intern Med* 1994;120:199.

32. VASCULITIS

Yusuf Yazici and Michael D. Lockshin

I. **Definition.** The vasculitides are a heterogeneous group of systemic inflammatory disorders that have as their common manifestation the inflammation of blood vessels with demonstrable structural injury to the vessel walls. The major ischemic manifestations are defined by the type and size of the involved blood vessels and the tissue and organ damage caused by vascular occlusion.

II. **Etiology and pathogenesis.** Although the specific cause of many of these disorders is not known, the inciting agents and disease mechanisms have been characterized in many. Infectious organisms, drugs, tumors, and allergic reactions are some of the defined triggers. Pathogenetic factors include immune complex disease, anti-neutrophil cytoplasmic antibodies, anti-endothelial cell antibodies, and cell-mediated immunity.

III. **Clinical manifestations common to the vasculitides.** Although each of the vasculitic disorders has its own clinical signature, they share specific clinical manifestations to one degree or another. When the physician deals with a patient who has a multisystem disorder, and once infection and neoplasm have been ruled out appropriately, a vasculitic disorder should be strongly considered if combinations of the following manifestations are prominent:

1. Constitutional symptoms, including fatigue, weight loss, fever, weakness, failure to thrive.
2. Skin rash.
3. Joint inflammation.
4. Neuropathy or central nervous system disjunction.
5. Pulmonary infiltrates or nodules.
6. Sinus or nasal inflammation.
7. Kidney inflammation or insufficiency.
8. Gastrointestinal or liver inflammation.
9. Laboratory abnormalities, including anemia, leukocytosis, thrombocytopenia, and elevated erythrocyte sedimentation rate (ESR) or C-reactive protein (CRP).

IV. **Historical perspective.** The first description of systemic vasculitis as a disease entity dates back to the nineteenth century. Although the first cases of Henoch-Schönlein purpura (HSP) and polyarteritis nodosa (PAN) were described in 1801 and 1866, respectively, most reports were published in the twentieth century. In 1908, Takayasu first noted the large-vessel vasculitis that carries his name, and Klinger recognized the syndrome later detailed by Wegener in 1936. Later, Behçet delineated the systemic disease bearing his name, and Churg and Strauss detailed a PAN-like syndrome with eosinophilia and pulmonary infiltrates in 1951.

V. **Classification.** As the number of vasculitic syndromes increased, the need for a system of classification became evident. Although many clinical overlap syndromes may exist, the following clinical parameters can be employed to diagnose the disorder, define its severity, and then construct the correct therapeutic plan.

A. **Vessel size.** The occlusion of blood vessels as a consequence of inflammation leads to different clinical manifestations, defined by the type and size of blood vessel involved and the tissue bed that is perfused by the vessel. Thus, the physician can employ the presenting patient findings as a diagnostic tool. For example, large-vessel involvement might cause blindness, stroke, or a myocardial infarction; medium-vessel disease can lead to renal or bowel dysfunction; and small-vessel disease can cause skin and other tissue lesions and ischemia (Table 32-1).

Table 32-1. Clinical manifestations of vasculitis according to vessel size

Vessel size	Disorder
Large vessels (aorta and its branches)	Giant cell arteritis Takayasu's arteritis Primary angiitis of the central nervous system
Medium-sized vessels (main visceral arteries)	Polyarteritis nodosa Kawasaki disease
Small vessels (venules, capillaries, arterioles, and small arteries)	Churg-Strauss syndrome Wegener's granulomatosis Henoch-Schönlein purpura Microscopic angiitis Mixed cryoglobulinemia

B. Pathology and type of inflammation. The types of inflammation involving blood vessels fall into two broad categories, necrotizing and granulomatous; however, overlaps can exist. In the necrotizing type, seen classically in PAN, inflammatory lesions are focal and segmental and consist of macrophages, CD4+ T lymphocytes, and polymorphonuclear leukocytes. Fibrinoid necrosis may or may not exist, but disruption of the internal elastic lamina is expected. The granulomatous lesion of Wegener's granulomatosis (WG) in the lung reveals focal necrotizing lesions with or without granulomatous inflammation or multinucleated giant cells.

C. Characteristic clinical patterns. WG—lung, sinus, kidney; PAN—aneurysms, neuropathy; HSP—rash, abdominal pain, joint problems.

D. Pathogenic mechanisms. Immune complex—PAN; anti-neutrophil cytoplasmic antibodies—WG.

E. Laboratory abnormalities.

F. Inciting agents. Hepatitis B virus—PAN; hepatitis C virus—mixed cryoglobulinemia; parvovirus—PAN, WG; human immunodeficiency virus—PAN.

VI. Clinical presentation. Most patients with vasculitis have nonspecific systemic symptoms, involvement of multiple organ systems, or both. They commonly present as diagnostic challenges. The diagnosis is based on a combination of clinical, serologic, histologic, and angiographic findings. A complete history and physical examination are mandatory, as most diagnoses are defined by clinical rather than laboratory findings. A history of asthma, atopy, and eosinophilia may suggest Churg-Strauss syndrome (CSS); jaw claudication and scalp tenderness could lead to a diagnosis of temporal arteritis; and involvement of the lung, kidney, and upper respiratory tract should suggest the possibility of WG.

VII. Supporting laboratory, imaging, and biopsy data. Although the diagnosis of the vasculitides is usually based on the clinical presentation, certain supporting data are employed in solidifying the diagnosis, defining the extent of the disease and the degree of tissue damage, and guiding therapeutic choices. However, it must be appreciated that if the clinical picture dictates immediate therapeutic action, awaiting the results of more sophisticated tests or biopsies may not be appropriate.

A. Routine laboratory tests. The level of inflammation can be defined by the presence of anemia, leukocytosis, thrombocytosis, and elevation of the Westergren ESR or CRP. All values may be abnormal on disease presentation and improve or normalize after therapy is instituted.

B. Organ-specific testing. Testing for organ involvement is often guided by the clinical manifestations and also includes routine blood testing and imaging.

1. Renal involvement can be best clarified with measurement of serum creatinine, urinalysis, and possibly a 24-hour urine collection for determination of creatinine clearance and protein. An elevated creatinine level and active urinary sediment with red blood cells, casts, and proteinuria commonly reflect active kidney inflammation.

2. **Muscle inflammation.** An elevated creatine kinase level could represent muscle damage resulting from inflammation or myocardial infarction resulting from coronary vasculitis.
3. **Lung involvement.** A posterolateral chest roentgenogram or computed tomography (CT) can be quite helpful in defining a pulmonary infiltrate or nodule or pleural involvement.
4. **Liver involvement.** Abnormal results of liver function tests may reflect liver inflammation or associated infectious hepatitis.
5. **Sinus involvement.** A routine sinus series roentgenogram or CT may help to define the presence and extent of mucosal inflammation.

C. Testing for type of vasculitis or its etiology. These tests are used in specific clinical circumstances, as guided by the disease presentation and the results of the above routine tests.

1. Consider an infectious trigger: hepatitis B or C, human immunodeficiency virus.
2. Consider an immune complex disorder: complement consumption with low C3 and C4 levels, presence of cryoglobulins (e.g., hepatitis C).
3. Consider an autoimmune disorder such as systemic lupus erythematosus (SLE): antinuclear antibody (ANA), anti-DNA testing.

D. Disease-specific testing

1. **Anti-neutrophil cytoplasmic antibody (ANCA) testing.** These antibodies are found in the serum of patients with specific types of vasculitis and are helpful as adjunctive diagnostic tools in the setting of a clinical picture consistent with WG, microscopic polyangiitis, and CSS. Two different indirect immunofluorescence staining patterns characterize these antibodies: cytoplasmic (c-ANCA, reflecting antibodies to serine proteinase) and perinuclear (p-ANCA, reacting with myeloperoxidase). A few points about ANCA are important: (a) Most patients with WG have c-ANCA positivity and most with microscopic polyangiitis or CSS have p-ANCA positivity; (b) the definite diagnosis of WG continues to be based on biopsy results, not ANCA positivity; (c) decisions regarding disease activity should be based on clinical signs, not the ANCA titer; (d) 10% of patients may be negative for ANCA in the setting of active vasculitis.
2. **Tissue biopsy.** Like any test, a tissue biopsy should be considered if it is needed to define a diagnosis, guide therapy, or clarify the prognosis. In general, the simplest and safest procedure with the highest yield should be chosen, as defined by the specific clinical setting. At times, the disease severity and comorbidities are such that one employs the clinical picture alone in guiding the treatment. Certain procedures are associated with both a high yield and low risk: skin biopsy in patients with dermatitis, temporal artery biopsy in giant cell arteritis (GCA), muscle biopsy in PAN. Others entail a higher risk with a high diagnostic yield: lung biopsy in WG, kidney biopsy in microscopic polyangiitis, sural nerve biopsy in PAN, and brain biopsy in primary angiitis of the brain.
3. **Imaging procedures**
   a. **Magnetic resonance imaging (MRI), computed transaxial tomography (CTT).** These procedures may be needed to define the presence of specific organ involvement or extent of disease. Examples include MRI of the brain to assess for infarcts or CTT of the chest to characterize lung disease.
   b. **Angiography.** In special circumstances, this procedure can add greatly to diagnostic accuracy and definition of the type and extent of vascular involvement. This is particularly true when diagnostic questions remain after the initial clinical evaluation of PAN and Takayasu's arteritis. MR angiogram can be employed as a noninvasive method of evaluating vessel involvement.

VIII. **Giant cell arteritis** is a disease of the elderly, usually starting after age 50. It affects primarily white people, and women are twice as likely to be affected. Common presenting symptoms are fatigue, headache, and tenderness of the scalp, particularly around the temporal and occipital area. Jaw claudication (pain when chewing) is seen in two-thirds of patients. Headache is the presenting symptom in two-thirds, and half have the proximal soreness and stiffness of polymyalgia rheumatica (PMR). Temporal arteries can be palpable, tender, and nodular, with reduced pulsation. In some series, visual disturbances have been reported in 20% of patients, but the frequency has declined over the years, probably because of earlier diagnosis and treatment. Transient ophthalmologic symptoms can lead to permanent blindness if not treated promptly.

A. **Laboratory findings.** The ESR is usually elevated, often over 100 mm/h. A normal ESR is unusual but does not rule out GCA. Anemia and thrombocytosis are common.

B. **Temporal artery biopsy.** Different rheumatologists have different approaches to temporal artery biopsy. Things to keep in mind are as follows: (a) Perform a biopsy when the diagnosis is in doubt; (b) do not delay treatment for the sake of the biopsy; and (c) remember that in a third of patients biopsy results are negative because the lesions can involve the artery in a skip fashion. Pathology shows granulomatous arteritis with giant cells and destruction of the internal elastic lamina. Color duplex ultrasonography can have a place in the diagnosis of GCA; the most specific finding is a dark halo around the artery, which may represent edema. The diagnosis of GCA should be considered in any patient over the age of 50 with recent onset of headache, loss of vision, myalgias, fever of unknown origin, a high ESR, or anemia. It should be remembered that PAN can also affect the temporal arteries.

C. **Polymyalgia rheumatica.** GCA can accompany PMR, a syndrome characterized by proximal muscle aches and stiffness that is usually bilateral and symmetric. The ESR is usually elevated, but a normal ESR does not rule out PMR. GCA may develop in some patients after years of PMR, or vice versa.

D. **Treatment** is with corticosteroids. Initially, prednisone or an equivalent should be given in a dose sufficient to control the disease and then continued at the lowest dose that controls symptoms and lowers the ESR. Biopsy for GCA is not mandatory and should not delay treatment if clinical suspicion is high, as blindness from arteritis can occur suddenly and at any time. Most rheumatologists use 10 to 20 mg of prednisone daily for **PMR** and 40 to 60 mg of prednisone daily for **GCA** because of the higher risk for arteritic complications in GCA. There is usually a dramatic response to steroids in PMR patients, seen within days. Corticosteroid tapering begins after a month; most patients are on 5 to 10 mg of prednisone at 6 months. Even though controversy exists over the length of treatment, patients will usually need to be on steroids about a year, and some for as long as 2 years. Relapses are most likely in the first 18 months and are managed by increasing the dose of steroids. Side effects of corticosteroids should be kept in mind and will occasionally necessitate the use of steroid-sparing agents such as methotrexate or azathioprine.

IX. **Takayasu's arteritis** is a chronic inflammatory disorder of unknown etiology affecting the aorta and its major branches. It predominantly affects women ages 15 to 25, with a female-to-male ratio of 9:1. It has two phases—an early systemic phase, characterized by malaise, fever, night sweats, weight loss, myalgias, and arthralgias, and a later occlusive phase, with symptoms of claudication, headaches, syncope, and visual disturbances. Physical examination can reveal arterial bruits over the involved vessels, and an absence of pulses is seen later in the disease. Hypertension is common but is often spuriously low in the arms, so that measurement of blood pressure in the legs is required.

A. The **diagnosis** of Takayasu's arteritis should be considered when symptoms of vascular insufficiency (claudication, transient visual disturbances, syncope) occur in the setting of bruits, weak pulses, and discrepancies of limb blood pressure in young women.

B. The **differential diagnosis** includes SLE, syphilitic aortitis, mycotic aneurysm, aortitis secondary to rheumatic fever, Behçet's syndrome, Crohn's disease, and ankylosing spondylitis, all of which can involve the large vessels (secondary Takayasu's arteritis). In addition, temporal arteritis, congenital coarctation, thrombotic or embolic disease (as in endocarditis), anti-phospholipid antibody syndrome, and myxoma can sometimes mimic Takayasu's arteritis.

C. Laboratory studies, except for a high ESR in the early phase, are nonspecific and usually not helpful. Chest radiography might show a widened aortic shadow, irregularity of the descending aorta, and cardiac enlargement with hilar fullness. Arteriography is most helpful. MRI may show a very thickened and altered aorta. Visualization of the whole aorta is needed because multiple parts may be involved. Suggestive findings include a segmental, smooth, tapered pattern of stenosis and complete occlusion of the large vessel.

D. Treatment is primarily with oral corticosteroids. Untreated disease has a significant mortality rate. Most patients respond to a dose of 1 mg/kg daily, but there is also evidence that a starting dose of 30 mg/d with a maintenance dose of 5 to 10 mg/d is effective therapy. Cytotoxic therapy has been used in patients failing steroid treatment. Surgery and percutaneous transluminal angioplasty also have been used in advanced disease with variable success. Tuberculosis is sometimes associated with Takayasu's arteritis, so a PPD (purified protein derivative) skin test should be performed and prophylactic tuberculosis therapy given to patients with positive test results.

X. Isolated angiitis of the central nervous system is a recently recognized vasculitic disorder primarily involving the central nervous system. Typical patients are in their forties or fifties. Onset is highly variable, usually with a prodrome of 6 months. The most common symptoms are headaches, which can spontaneously remit for long periods. Nonfocal neurologic deficits are characteristic, including a decrease in cognitive function. Any anatomic area can be involved with signs and symptoms, which range from transient ischemic attacks, strokes, paraparesis, and cranial neuropathies to seizures. Cerebrospinal fluid analysis findings are abnormal in more than 90% of patients and include modest pleocytosis, normal glucose levels, and increased protein. The cerebrospinal fluid should be cultured and infection ruled out. MRI and CT have made diagnosis easier; suggestive findings include multiple, bilateral supratentorial infarcts. Angiography has proved less useful. Histologic confirmation through **leptomeningeal biopsy** is the gold standard. Therapy is with corticosteroids and cyclophosphamide (CTX) and is usually continued for 6 to 12 months after remission.

XI. Polyarteritis nodosa is an acute necrotizing vasculitis of medium-sized and small arteries. Before the 1994 International Chapel Hill Consensus Conference, PAN also included microscopic polyangiitis. After this conference, microscopic polyangiitis was separated from PAN, with involvement of vessels smaller than arterioles indicating microscopic polyangiitis and not PAN. Most series, however, still consider renal involvement with a pattern of microscopic polyangiitis to be part of PAN.

A. Etiology. In most cases, the etiology of PAN is not known; some cases, however, are a consequence of hepatitis B viral infection. In France, hepatitis B-related PAN formerly accounted for about one-third of all cases of PAN, but there has been a decrease in the number of cases since the development of vaccines against hepatitis B. Other viruses (human immunodeficiency virus, cytomegalovirus, parvovirus B19, human T-lymphotrophic virus type 1, hepatitis C virus) are also implicated as etiologic agents.

B. The **pathologic lesion** that best defines PAN is a focal, segmental, necrotizing vasculitis of medium-sized and small vessels. The existence of uninvolved segments just next to the diseased areas is typical of PAN. The lesion may occur in any artery of the body, but involvement of the aorta and pulmonary arteries is rare. Arterial aneurysms and thromboses can occur at the site of the vascular lesion.

C. Clinical presentation. The majority of patients present with constitutional symptoms (malaise, fever, weight loss), peripheral neuropathy, and gastrointestinal or cutaneous involvement. Peripheral neuropathy is most commonly in the form of painful mononeuritis multiplex or multiple mononeuropathies. Cutaneous lesions are present in 27% to 60% of patients. Vascular purpura is typically papulopetechial. Inflammatory lesions are infrequent, but when present they are the ideal site for biopsy. Livedo reticularis is common. When possible, the biopsy specimen should include the dermis to detect medium-sized vessel involvement. Myalgias and arthralgias are also common. Kidney involvement is diverse and can be vascular or glomerular. According to the type of tissue involvement, it is possible to diagnose two different diseases: microscopic polyangiitis when glomerulonephritis is seen, and PAN when vascular nephropathy is observed. Gastrointestinal involvement can be severe and present with abdominal pain, bleeding, and bowel perforation. Orchitis and epididymitis are also seen in PAN. Although the spectrum of the clinical presentation may vary, most patients will have severe manifestations and appear acutely ill.

D. Laboratory studies. The ESR is usually high. Positivity for ANCA is rare in PAN. Hepatitis B surface antigen (HBsAg) should be sought in all cases. Angiography often shows microaneurysms and stenoses in medium-sized vessels. Although the diagnosis of PAN is clinical, it is useful to demonstrate vasculitis in biopsy specimens. Skin, skeletal muscle, sural nerve, and kidney are the usual sites. Biopsy specimens of apparently unaffected muscles may reveal vasculitis in a small fraction of patients.

E. Treatment. Initial management of PAN without hepatitis B is with high-dose corticosteroids (40 to 60 mg/d). CTX is added for severe cases. Traditionally, oral CTX has been used, but recent studies have shown that IV administration can be as effective as the oral with fewer side effects. In hepatitis B-related PAN, corticosteroids and CTX may allow the virus to persist, which can lead to chronic hepatitis and liver cirrhosis. Good results have been reported treating these patients with a combination of antiviral agents, plasma exchange, and corticosteroids. Relapses are rare in patients who achieve remission.

XII. Kawasaki disease is an acute febrile disease occurring most commonly in infants and children under the age of 5. The first case was described in Japan in 1961.

A. Clinical presentation. Vasculitis, especially of the coronary arteries, is the most serious and life-threatening complication. The onset is typically abrupt, with remitting or continuous high fever that generally lasts 1 to 2 weeks. Within 2 to 4 days of onset, bilateral conjunctival congestion occurs. Dryness, redness, and fissuring of the lips are observed within 2 to 5 days, and a "strawberry" tongue (as in scarlet fever) can be seen. Painful cervical lymphadenopathy appears shortly before or simultaneously with the fever. Exanthema of the trunk and reddening of the palms and soles with consequent desquamation are usual. Cardiovascular involvement can include carditis with heart murmurs and electrocardiographic changes. Coronary artery lesions with dilatation or aneurysms may be seen on echocardiography. Other symptoms include abdominal pain, vomiting, diarrhea, and arthritis. Kawasaki disease should be included in the differential diagnosis of all febrile illnesses associated with rash in children. The angiitis of Kawasaki disease usually lasts about 7 weeks and is most commonly seen in the medium-sized and large arteries, including the coronary and iliac arteries.

B. The **etiology** of Kawasaki disease is not known. Although many hypotheses involving an infectious cause have been proposed, none has been confirmed.

C. Treatment. Management is supportive in uncomplicated cases. Coronary artery involvement should assessed with two-dimensional echocardiography weekly for the first month. If changes are detected, high-dose IV gamma globulin as a single infusion of 2 g/kg is given. Low-dose aspirin (3 to 5 mg/kg daily) is used until the coronary artery changes regress. Long-term management should include coronary angiography and follow-up for coronary artherosclerosis.

XIII. Wegener's granulomatosis is a relatively rare disease (3 per 100,000 in the United States) with the classic triad of necrotizing granulomatous vasculitis of the upper and lower airways, systemic vasculitis, and focal necrotizing glomerulonephritis. A less aggressive, milder form of WG exists (limited WG), with involvement predominantly in the lungs and an absence of glomerulonephritis, that carries a better prognosis. WG affects male and female subjects at about the same rate, and about 80% to 90% of the patients are white.

A. Clinical presentation. The diagnosis is usually made within 6 months of initial symptoms, but unusual presentations of the mild form may elude diagnosis for years. It is important to distinguish WG from other pulmonary-renal syndromes, such as Goodpasture's syndrome and SLE. Most patients seek care because of upper and lower respiratory tract symptoms. Sinus pain, purulent sinus drainage, nasal mucosal ulceration, and otitis media are common; tracheal inflammation can lead to subglottic stenosis. At presentation, 80% of patients have no renal involvement and 50% have no overt lung disease; however, pulmonary problems, renal problems, or both eventually develop in more than 80% of patients. The glomerulonephritis is characterized by focal necrosis, crescent formation, and an absence or paucity of immunoglobulin deposits. Identical "pauci-immune" necrotizing glomerulonephritis occurs in CSS and microscopic polyangiitis, the other two ANCA-associated small-vessel vasculitides. Other WG manifestations include ocular inflammation, cutaneous purpura, peripheral neuropathy, arthritis, and diverse abdominal visceral involvement. Necrotizing granulomatous pulmonary inflammation produces radiographic densities, and the lesions may cavitate. Alveolar capillaritis can cause pulmonary hemorrhage with irregular infiltrates. Massive pulmonary hemorrhage is a life-threatening manifestation and requires aggressive immunosuppressive treatment.

B. Laboratory data. Patients usually have normochromic, normocytic anemia, leukocytosis, thrombocytosis, and an elevated ESR. WG, in contrast to the immune complex vasculitides, is associated with antineutrophil cytoplasmic antibody (ANCA), especially c-ANCA, which has a 98% specificity but a 30% to 99% sensitivity. Titers are usually associated with disease activity; consequently, only 30% to 40% of patients with limited WG or generalized WG in remission have c-ANCA positivity. A small minority (5%) can be positive for p-ANCA also. The limited form of the disease can be difficult to diagnose on clinical grounds, and the presence of c-ANCA may strongly influence the diagnosis. The strongest diagnostic evidence nonetheless comes from biopsy specimens of the involved tissues, which show granulomas. Lymphomatoid granulomatosis and necrotizing sarcoidosis may be confused with WG. The causative agent(s) leading to granuloma formation are unknown.

C. Treatment. Patients are initially given oral cyclophosphamide (2 mg/kg daily) and oral prednisone (1 mg/kg daily). The prednisone is changed to an alternate-day regimen in about 4 to 6 weeks, and then the dose is gradually tapered. Cyclophosphamide is continued for at least 1 year after complete clinical remission. Leukocyte count is a guide to cyclophosphamide dose adjustment, and one should aim to keep the neutrophil count above 3,000/mm^3. An increased risk for infection, especially with *Pneumocystis carinii,* and bladder cancer should be kept in mind at all times. When compared with oral cyclophosphamide and corticosteroids, pulse IV cyclophosphamide and corticosteroids are equally effective in achieving initial remission; however, in the long term, treatment with pulse cyclophosphamide does not maintain remission or prevent relapses to the degree that oral cyclophosphamide treatment does. Methotrexate and azathioprine are alternatives to cyclophosphamide in less severe forms of WG, and both have been used for maintenance after achievement of remission in generalized WG. Relapses are associated with respiratory tract infections and with chronic nasal carriage of *Staphylococcus aureus*. Some studies suggest that trimethoprim/sulfamethoxazole may be useful in inducing remission in the initial phases of WG or in preventing relapses.

XIV. Microscopic polyangiitis is a pauci-immune necrotizing vasculitis of the small vessels without evidence of granulomatous inflammation. *ANCA positivity is common.*

A. Clinical presentation. Pulmonary and renal involvement are commonly seen, with approximately 90% of patients having glomerulonephritis. Microscopic polyangiitis is the most common cause of pulmonary-renal syndrome. Alveolar hemorrhage can complicate the picture. The onset is usually insidious and the prognosis is more guarded than in classic PAN.

B. Laboratory studies. More than 80% of patients have ANCA, most often p-ANCA. This helps to distinguish microscopic polyangiitis from ANCA-negative small-vessel vasculitis but does not distinguish it from other ANCA-related vasculitides. Pathologically, microscopic polyangiitis can cause a necrotizing vasculitis identical to PAN. At the Chapel Hill Consensus Conference, microscopic polyangiitis and PAN were distinguished by the absence of vasculitis in vessels other than arteries in PAN and the presence of vasculitis in vessels smaller than arteries (arterioles, venules, and capillaries) in microscopic polyangiitis. By this definition, the presence of glomerulonephritis or pulmonary alveolar capillaritis would exclude a diagnosis of PAN.

C. Treatment of microscopic polyangiitis includes corticosteroids and cytotoxic agents; doses and duration of treatment are similar to those used for WG. High-dose IV steroids, followed by oral steroids and oral or IV cyclophosphamide in cases with major organ involvement, is a useful treatment strategy. About one-third of patients relapse and are treated with a repeated regimen similar to the induction therapy.

XV. Churg-Strauss syndrome is a rare disorder characterized by hypereosinophilia, systemic vasculitis, and necrotizing granulomatous inflammation that occurs in people with asthma and allergic rhinitis. Pulmonary infiltrates occur in up to 90% of patients, and a cutaneous eruption is seen in 70%. Cardiac manifestations (pericarditis, cardiomyopathy, and myocardial infarction) account for about half of deaths. Peripheral neuropathy is found in 70% of patients; its occurrence in susceptible patients is highly suggestive of CSS. Renal disease, seldom seen, is generally mild.

A. Laboratory findings. Approximately 70% of patients have ANCA, more commonly p-ANCA; virtually all have eosinophilia. Anemia and an elevated ESR are also found with active disease. The diagnosis of vasculitis should be substantiated by biopsy of one of the involved tissues.

B. The **differential diagnosis** of CSS includes WG, microscopic polyangiitis, PAN, chronic eosinophilic pneumonia, and the idiopathic hypereosinophilic syndrome. Neither asthma nor a history of allergies is a prominent feature of WG, in which eosinophilia is rarely found. Renal involvement is less severe in CSS, and the histopathologic features of the granulomatous lesions of CSS and WG are very different. The absence of vasculitis or granuloma formation in chronic eosinophilic pneumonia and in the idiopathic hypereosinophilic syndrome helps to differentiate these entities from CSS.

C. Treatment. Most cases of CSS respond well to corticosteroids. Initial management requires high doses of prednisone (1 mg/kg daily) or the equivalent; methylprednisolone pulses have also been used. Life-threatening complications call for cyclophosphamide in addition to steroids. Both oral and IV pulse cyclophosphamide has been used, with differing rates of success. Relapses are rare after complete remissions.

XVI. Henoch-Schönlein purpura is the most common vasculitis of childhood. Half of the time, it is preceded by an upper respiratory tract infection, but the etiology remains unknown. Boys and girls are affected equally. The median age of onset is 4 years. It follows a self-limiting course in most patients. HSP can accompany familial Mediterranean fever in those regions where the latter is endemic.

A. **Clinical presentation.** The classic triad is palpable purpura with a normal platelet count, colicky abdominal pain, and arthritis. Palpable purpura occurs in 100% of patients but is the presenting symptom in only half. Dependent areas are usually involved, and involvement of the buttocks is common. Arthritis is transient and usually involves the knees and ankles; there are no permanent sequelae. Up to one-third of patients may experience hemoptysis and half have occult gastrointestinal bleeding, but serious hemorrhage is rare. Ten percent to fifty percent have renal involvement, ranging from transient isolated microscopic hematuria to rapidly progressive glomerulonephritis. HSP and immunoglobulin A (IgA) nephropathy are similar, but the latter is confined to the kidney, whereas the former is a systemic disease.

B. The **diagnosis** is made on clinical grounds. Laboratory tests may indicate the organs involved and are mostly used to rule out other causes.

C. **Treatment** is largely supportive and includes hydration and monitoring. Nonsteroidal antiinflammatory drugs (NSAIDs) can be used for joint pain and will not aggravate the purpura. However, they should be avoided if renal insufficiency is present. Corticosteroids have been used in the management of abdominal pain, edema, and nephritis.

XVII. Cryoglobulinemic vasculitis. Cryoglobulins are circulating immunoglobulins that precipitate at low temperatures. They are grouped into three categories: type 1, composed of a single monoclonal immunoglobulin; type 2, characterized by polyclonal IgG; and type 3, which is monoclonal or polyclonal IgM. The IgM is an auto-antibody with rheumatoid factor activity. Mixed cryoglobulins lead to immune complex disease by depositing in the vessels, activating complement, and causing inflammation.

A. **Clinical presentation.** The most frequent manifestations are palpable purpura, arthralgias, and nephritis. Histologic section reveals leukocytoclastic vasculitis. Skin ulcers, Raynaud's phenomenon, hepatic abnormalities, and splenomegaly can also be seen. Hepatitis C virus has been detected in more than 90% of patients with mixed cryoglobulins in various population studies, but the exact pathogenic role of hepatitis C virus in this setting is still unclear. Mixed cryoglobulins and rheumatoid factor are typically detectable in the serum. For reliable detection, blood must be maintained at 37°C during transport and clotting. Serum must then be stored at 4°C for at least 7 days for cryoglobulins to be observed.

B. **Cryocrit,** a method for detecting and quantifying cryoglobulins, measures the percentage of packed cryoglobulins in graduated test tubes after cold incubation and centrifugation of the serum. The cryocrit is usually between 1% and 3% in type 3 and between 2% and 7% in type 2, and it may be up to 50% in type 1 cryoglobulinemia. There is, however, no correlation between the cryocrit and disease severity. Very low levels of C4 and normal or slightly low levels of C3 are common and aid in the diagnosis. The main cause of morbidity is renal involvement.

C. **Treatment.** Mild disease with purpura and arthralgias is usually treated with NSAIDs. Serious visceral involvement, such as glomerulonephritis, calls for treatment with corticosteroids and cytotoxic drugs such as CTX and azathioprine. Plasmapheresis has also been used with some success. Recently, interferon-alfa has been successfully used in patients with cryoglobulinemic vasculitis associated with hepatitis C infection. However, further studies are still needed.

XVIII. Pseudovasculitis. These are conditions that obstruct blood flow in vessels without an accompanying inflammation of the vessel wall. They need to be kept in the differential diagnosis of any suspected vasculitis. A useful mnemonic to recall the more frequently seen pseudovasculitic conditions is AMACEC (antiphospholipid antibody syndrome, myxoma, amyloidosis, cholesterol emboli, endocarditis, and calciphylaxis).

A. **Anti-phospholipid antibody syndrome** causes both large- and small-vessel occlusions, leading to gangrene, livedo, and skin ulcers. Signs of inflammation, including a raised ESR, are usually absent. It should be kept in mind that anti-phospholipid antibody syndrome may also be seen in the setting of true vasculitis, as in patients with SLE.

B. **Myxomas** are benign cardiac tumors, most commonly found in the left atrium. They can cause extracardiac symptoms of petechial skin rashes, Raynaud's phenomenon, glomerulonephritis, arthritis, myositis, pleurisy, and pericarditis, often accompanied by fever, increased ESR, leukocytosis, hypocomplementemia, positivity for ANA, and thrombocytopenia. Diagnosis is usually made with echocardiography.

C. **Amyloidosis** can also sometimes mimic vasculitis and be accompanied by PMR and GCA-type symptoms of scalp tenderness and claudication of the jaw. Histology shows amyloid deposits in the vessel walls.

D. **Cholesterol embolism** is caused by the shedding of cholesterol crystals from atheromatous plaques. It is most commonly seen in elderly men. It is usually seen in the setting of diffuse atherosclerosis, commonly after abdominal surgery or diagnostic angiography, during which emboli become dislodged. When emboli occlude small arteries, the symptoms are indistinguishable from those of true vasculitis. Livedo reticularis in the lower extremities is common. More serious complications are occlusion of intestinal or coronary arteries. Renal failure may develop. Myalgias with muscle tenderness are common. The key element in diagnosis is clinical suspicion. Histologic demonstration of cholesterol emboli may be diagnostic. Treatment is by excision of the atheromatous plaque. Steroids are not helpful, and anticoagulation should be avoided.

E. **Infective endocarditis** is associated with a true vasculitis and embolic phenomena. True vasculitic lesions can be caused by an immune complex vasculitis. Emboli occluding the vessel lumen are more common. Skin, brain, spleen, and kidney are the organs frequently involved. Patients can also have arthralgias, arthritis, and an increased acute-phase response and be positive for rheumatoid factor, which make diagnosis difficult; SLE may also be suggested, given that these patients commonly have valvular disease.

F. **Calciphylaxis** is a rare and potentially lethal syndrome, almost always associated with chronic renal failure. Even though calcifications develop in many patients with chronic renal failure, in some, a severe condition develops that is characterized by skin necrosis and gangrene of the extremities. Organ involvement can also occur. Calciphylaxis is thought to be a hypersensitivity reaction involving parathyroid hormone, vitamin D, and hypercalcemia. Treatment is aimed at local management of skin ulcers and at keeping the calcium/phosphate product low.

XIX. Miscellaneous vasculitides

A. **Relapsing polychondritis** is a rare disease characterized by inflammation of cartilage, mainly of the ears, nose, larynx, and joints.

1. **Clinical presentation.** The most common clinical manifestation is a destructive auricular chondritis with sparing of the ear lobule. Articular symptoms are second in frequency and are usually self-limited, with a nonerosive oligoarticular or polyarticular peripheral arthritis. Inflammatory eye disease may also occur. Leukocytoclastic vasculitis causing skin lesions and aneurysms of the thoracic-abdominal aorta and cerebral artery can occur. In 30% of cases, there is an association with rheumatoid arthritis, Sjögren's syndrome, WG, microscopic polyangiitis, and malignancies (including carcinoma of the lung, breast, and colon and myeloproliferative disorders). There are no specific laboratory tests for relapsing polychondritis, but biopsy of an affected area is diagnostic, showing loss of basophilic staining of the cartilage matrix accompanied by perichondral inflammation at the interface of cartilage and soft tissue and fibrocyte and capillary endothelial cell proliferation.
2. **Treatment.** Although NSAIDs can control mild episodes of inflammation, corticosteroids are the mainstay of treatment, initially in dosages of 0.75 to 1 mg/kg daily. Immunosuppressive drugs are used as steroid-sparing agents in patients requiring long-term steroid therapy.

B. Behçet's syndrome. First described by Hulusi Behçet of Istanbul, this syndrome is a systemic vasculitis involving both arteries and veins.

1. The **clinical presentation** is characterized by recurrent oral and genital aphthous ulceration, chronic relapsing uveitis, and a variety of skin manifestations, including the *pathergy reaction* (nonspecific hyperreactivity of the skin), erythema nodosum, and superficial thrombophlebitis. Uveitis can lead to blindness in up to 20% of patients with eye disease. Male and young patients have a more severe course than do female and older patients. Behçet's syndrome has been associated with HLA-B51 and is mainly observed in countries around the Mediterranean and in the Far East. The natural history of Behçet's syndrome is one of exacerbations and remissions. Disease manifestations as a rule usually become less severe with time.
2. **Treatment.** Mild oral and genital ulcers can be treated with local corticosteroids. Thalidomide has also been used successfully in treating mucocutaneous lesions. Colchicine, which has traditionally been used for every aspect of Behçet's syndrome, seems to be effective mainly for the treatment of mucocutaneous lesions in female patients. Immunosuppression is the mainstay of treatment for eye disease; azathioprine has been shown to maintain visual acuity and prevent new eye disease, and cyclosporin A is used for disease flares. The role of heparin or anticoagulants for thrombophlebitis is still being debated. Anti-platelet drugs are preferred for milder cases.

Bibliography

Ansell BM, et al., eds. *The vasculitides, science and practice.* London: Chapman and Hall, 1996.

Guillevin L, et al. A prospective, multicenter, randomized trial comparing steroids and pulse cyclophosphamide versus steroids and oral cyclophosphamide in the treatment of generalized Wegener's granulomatosis. *Arthritis Rheum* 1997;40:2187.

Hamuryudan V, et al. Azathioprine in Behcet's syndrome: effects on long-term prognosis. *Arthritis Rheum* 1997;40:769.

Hoffman GS. Classification of the systemic vasculitides: antineutrophil cytoplasmic antibodies, consensus and controversy. *Clin Exp Rheumatol* 1998;16:111.

Hunder G. Vasculitis: diagnosis and therapy. *Am J Med* 1996;100[Suppl 2A]:37.

Hunder GG, ed. Vasculitis. *Rheum Dis Clin North Am* 1995;21:4.

Jennette JC, Falk RJ. Small-vessel vasculitis. *N Eng J Med* 1997;337:1512.

Klippel JH, Dieppe PA, eds. *Rheumatology,* 2nd ed. London: Mosby, 1998.

Koldingsnes W, et al. Wegener's granulomatosis: long-term follow-up of patients treated with pulse cyclophosphamide. *Br J Rheumatol* 1998;37:659.

Lhote F, Cohen P, Guillevin L. Polyarteritis nodosa, microscopic polyangiitis and Churg-Strauss syndrome. *Lupus* 1998;7:238.

Schmidt WA, et al. Color duplex ultrasonography in the diagnosis of temporal arteritis. *N Engl J Med* 1997;337:1336.

Stegeman CA, et al. Trimethoprim-sulfamethoxazole (co-trimoxazole) for the prevention of relapses of Wegener's granulomatosis. *N Engl J Med* 1996;335:16.

Tervaert JWC, Kallenberg CGM. Cell adhesion molecules in vasculitis. *Curr Opin Rheumatol* 1997;9:16.

Trentham DE, Le CH. Relapsing polychondritis. *Ann Intern Med* 1998;129:114.

Yazici H, Husby G, eds. Vasculitis. *Baillieres Clin Rheumatol* 1997;11:2.

33. ANKYLOSING SPONDYLITIS

Eric S. Schned

Ankylosing spondylitis (AS) is an inflammatory disorder of unknown etiology that primarily affects the spine, axial skeleton, and large proximal joints of the body. A distinctive feature of the disease is the striking tendency toward fibrosis and secondary ossification and ankylosis of involved joints. The disease typically affects young men in the second through fourth decades, although women may also be affected. There is a spectrum of clinical severity, ranging from asymptomatic sacroiliitis to the classic form of immobilizing spinal encasement. AS is strongly associated with the HLA-B27 histocompatibility antigen. Recent investigations suggest that most spondyloarthropathy, including AS, is characterized by disease susceptibility genes that are triggered by environmental agents such as microorganisms.

Pathologic changes consistent with AS have been recognized in human skeletons 5,000 years old. The disease was long considered a form of rheumatoid arthritis (RA) and was variously called rheumatoid spondylitis, von Bechterew disease, and Marie-Strumpel disease until the 1930s, when it was classified as a distinct pathologic and clinical entity.

Diagnostic criteria have been developed for AS and recent modifications have been published (Table 33-1).

I. Prevalence and genetic aspects

A. Prevalence figures differ depending on the population studied and the methods used to detect and define disease. Because disease susceptibility is strongly associated with the HLA-B27 antigen, disease prevalence tends to parallel the frequency of the gene in different populations. This accounts for the low prevalence in Africans, African Americans, and Japanese, and the high prevalence in Native-American tribes. The overall prevalence of AS in the U.S. population was recently estimated to be 1.29 per 1,000 persons.

A positive family history of AS may be found in about 15% to 20% of cases. The risk for development of AS in an HLA-B27–positive relative of a case is approximately 20%. The risk for development of AS in a random population of HLA-B27–positive persons is only about 2%. These data suggest that although the HLA-B27 gene confers distinct genetic susceptibility on a person, other factors, presumably environmental, also play a crucial role (see below).

B. Genetic aspects. In 1973, Schlosstein and Brewerton independently reported a strong association of HLA-B27 with AS. Subsequent studies have shown the HLA-B27 histocompatibility antigen to be present in about 8% of the normal American white population, with equal sex distribution, whereas 90% to 95% of spondylitic patients bear the antigen. However, the overall prevalence of HLA-B27 antigen is lower among African Americans (<2%), and it appears that clinical AS is less common in this group than in white populations.

Molecular studies have identified at least nine different HLA-B27 subtypes (B*2701–B*2709). The HLA-B*2705 gene subtype is primordial and is the allele most frequently found in American white and African-American populations.

C. Sex distribution. AS is identified more commonly in male than in female subjects by a ratio of about 3 : 1. However, the diagnosis in women may be overlooked or missed for various reasons, such as attribution of symptoms to other causes or reluctance to perform a radiographic examination of the pelvis in young women.

II. Pathophysiology

A. Pathogenesis. In 1990, Hammer and colleagues introduced the human HLA-B27 gene into transgenic rats, in which a disease very similar to AS subsequently developed. In 1994, they showed that arthritis did not develop in

Table 33-1. Proposed clinical criteria for ankylosing spondylitis

Diagnosis
Clinical criteria
Low back pain and stiffness for more than 3 months, improved by exercise, unrelieved by rest
Limitation of lumbar spine motion in both sagittal and frontal planes
Limitation of chest expansion (corrected for age and sex)
Radiologic criterion: Sacroiliitis grade ≥ 2 bilaterally or grade 3–4 unilaterally
Grading: Define ankylosing spondylitis if radiologic criterion is associated with at least one clinical criterion.

From van der Linden S, et al. Evaluation of diagnostic criteria for ankylosing spondylitis. A proposal for modification of the New York criteria. *Arthritis Rheum* 1984;27:366.

germ-free HLA-B27–positive transgenic mice. These experiments lend strong evidence to (a) the direct participation of the HLA-B27 gene, and (b) the additional requirement for bacteria to cause the disease.

A search for triggering bacterial pathogens has centered on enteric bacteria. *Klebsiella pneumoniae,* a common gut pathogen, has been studied extensively. *Klebsiella* shares a homology of six amino acids with HLA-B27, which suggests a role for molecular mimicry. Perhaps the presence of the HLA-B27 gene confers a degree of immune tolerance to gram-negative bacteria, or, alternatively, results in an increased immunologic reaction. Occult bowel inflammation has been reported in a large number of people with AS, which strengthens the hypothesis of a role for gut pathogens and links the clinical entities of AS and inflammatory bowel arthropathy.

The demonstration of persisting bacterial organisms and possibly even live microorganisms in the peripheral joints of persons with reactive arthritis has led to speculation that similar antigens or microorganisms could exist in spondylitic joints, but so far no such studies have been reported.

B. Pathology

1. **Skeletal sites** of inflammatory involvement in AS are as follows:
    a. The **axial skeleton** (including sacroiliac joints, intervertebral disk spaces, and apophyseal and costovertebral joints).
    b. The **anterior central joints** (e.g., manubriosternal joint, sternoclavicular joint, and symphysis pubis).
    c. The **large proximal synovial joints** (hips, knees, shoulders).
2. **Extraskeletal sites** of inflammation and post-inflammatory fibrous tissue include the uveal tract, aortic root wall, apical lung parenchyma, and heart valves.
3. **Pathologic findings.** Fibrocartilage is the primary site of inflammation in articular tissues. Other areas of inflammation include subchondral bone (osteitis), the annulus fibrosis of intervertebral disks, perispinal ligaments, periarticular ligamentous-bony junctions (enthesitis), periosteum (periostitis), and occasionally synovial membranes (synovitis).

    In all these tissues, the initial cellular inflammatory changes are followed by fibrosis and often ossification, which lead ultimately to bony ankylosis.

III. Clinical presentation

A. The **classic presentation** occurs in a young man between 15 and 40 years old who experiences the insidious onset of intermittent or persistent low back pain and stiffness that is often *worse in the morning hours* and *after prolonged rest.* The pain is typically *relieved by physical activity.* It is usually centered in the lumbosacral spine but may also be present in the buttocks and hips and occasionally radiate into the thighs.

B. Chest pain. The patient may complain of thoracic spine, neck, or shoulder pain and stiffness. Thoracic involvement can lead to anterior chest pain that may mimic angina pectoris.

C. **Peripheral arthritis** occurs in one-half of patients during the course of AS. Involved joints are usually large and proximal, such as the hips and shoulders.
   1. **Hip** involvement is a major source of disability in AS.
   2. **Heel pain** may occur secondary to local enthesopathy of the calcaneus; Achilles tendinitis is also common.

D. **Subsets of ankylosing spondylitis**
   1. **Juvenile ankylosing spondylitis.** In childhood, AS usually presents in older boys as an asymmetric *oligoarticular arthritis* of the lower extremities, often predating back symptoms. *Heel pain* is a common complaint. However, with time, the child acquires more typical features of adult AS. Almost all children affected are positive for HLA-B27.
   2. **Asymptomatic sacroiliitis.** Among asymptomatic HLA-B27–positive relatives of probands with AS and among random asymptomatic persons who are HLA-B27–positive, 20% may be found to have radiographic sacroiliitis. Also, about one-fourth of HLA-B27–positive patients with acute anterior uveitis will have subtle clinical or radiographic evidence of sacroiliitis. Some of these patients may progress to overt clinical disease.

E. **Extraskeletal manifestations**
   1. **Aortic valve regurgitation** is present in 3% to 5% of patients. When present, it should be followed closely, as it often progresses to heart failure. Complete heart block may develop when fibrosis extends from the aortic root to the electrical conduction system.
   2. **Pulmonary involvement**
      a. **Restriction of the thoracic cage** during respiration, caused by fusion of costovertebral joints, can result in reduced lung volumes but rarely leads to impaired gas exchange.
      b. **Apical lobe fibrobullous disease** of unknown pathogenesis occurs in 1% of patients with advanced AS.
   3. **Acute iritis,** usually unilateral, will occur in 25% of patients at some time during the course of AS. Some patients experience recurrent episodes with scarring and secondary glaucoma. Studies have shown an independent association of idiopathic iritis with HLA-B27. Subtle clinical, radiographic, or bone scan changes of AS can be demonstrated in many of these patients.
   4. **Renal function** is normal in AS.

F. **Complications**
   1. Patients with ankylosed spines have an increased susceptibility to **vertebral fractures,** especially in the cervical region, after falls or even minimal trauma because of the rigidity of the spine.
   2. The **cauda equina syndrome,** which causes pain in the buttocks or lower extremities, bladder or bowel dysfunction, and variable sensory loss is sometimes seen in long-standing AS. It is a consequence of nerve root compression by abnormal bony growths.

IV. **Physical examination**

A. **Sacroiliac (SI) joints.** Early signs include local tenderness over the SI joints and tenderness with paraspinal muscle spasm at lumbosacral vertebral levels. SI joint involvement may be elicited by special maneuvers to stress the joint.
   1. **Lateral compression of the pelvis** with both the examiner's hands will elicit pain in the involved joint(s).
   2. **Gaenslen's sign.** The patient lies supine on the edge of the examining table with knees flexed and with one buttock over the edge. The patient lowers the unsupported leg off the table. This maneuver elicits pain in the SI joint on the same side as the lowered leg because the SI joint is stretched open, like the binding of a book.

B. **Spine.** Loss of spinal motion (lateral motion, flexion, and extension) occurs early in most cases, and several maneuvers can be employed to detect and then follow such changes. With progression of disease, there is typically loss of the normal lordosis, progressive kyphosis of the thoracic spine, fixed flexion of the neck, and ultimately a stooped posture with fixed flexion contractures of the hips and knees. In the **Schober test (spinal forward flexion),** the patient stands erect. The examiner makes marks at two points along the spine (the lumbosacral junction and a point 10 cm above). The distance between the marks is measured in maximum forward flexion. *Less than 5 cm of distraction* is abnormal.

C. **Costovertebral involvement** is reflected in decreased chest expansion, which can be measured at the fourth intercostal space in men or under the breast in women. *Less than 5 cm of chest expansion* during inspiration in the adult is considered reduced.

D. **Extraaxial joint involvement** is usually proximal and asymmetric, and it tends to cause early contractures.

E. **Other signs.** The signs associated with aortic regurgitation, acute iritis, and upper lobe fibrosis are not specific. Rheumatoid nodules are notably absent. Fever is seldom present, although it can occur transiently during acute flares of arthritis.

V. Laboratory studies

A. **HLA-B27** is present in 95% of white spondylitic patients.

B. The **erythrocyte sedimentation rate** is elevated in many cases but does not correlate well with disease activity.

C. **Hematologic tests.** A mild normocytic anemia is seen in severe cases. The white cell count is normal.

D. **Pulmonary function tests** in patients with thoracic involvement usually indicate a diminished vital capacity and total lung capacity and an increased residual volume and functional residual volume. Flow measurements are usually normal.

E. **Immunologic tests.** No specific abnormalities occur.

F. **Radiographs.** The radiographic appearance of advanced AS is characteristic.

1. **Sacroiliac joints.** The earliest radiographic changes often occur here.
   a. Punched-out **erosions.**
   b. **"Pseudo-widening"** of the joint.
   c. Adjacent sclerosis.
   d. Bony bridging of the joint with complete loss of joint space may develop.
2. **Spine**
   a. Vertebral chondritis and adjacent subchondral osteitis followed by fibrosis and ossification lead to bony bridging of adjacent vertebrae (**syndesmophytes**). The advanced radiographic appearance of the ossification process of AS is aptly named **bamboo spine.**
   b. The **Romanus sign** is an erosion surrounded by sclerosis at a vertebral body margin.
   c. Periostitis of the periphery of the vertebral body leads to early **"squaring"** of vertebral bodies.
3. **Peripheral joints.** Initially, the radiographic appearance of proximal joints in AS may resemble that of RA. However, there is a greater tendency in AS to central articular erosion, proliferative new bone formation in periarticular tissues, and bony ankylosis. Concentric joint space narrowing and lateral osteophytes are distinctive radiographic signs of hip disease in AS.
4. **Ligamentous-bony junctions.** Inflammation and secondary ossification at these junctions in areas such as the pelvis (sacrotuberous and sacrospinal ligament insertions), the greater trochanter of the femur, plantar fascia, and the Achilles tendon lead to proliferative bone margins and whiskery spicules.

G. **Nuclear scans.** Technetium stannous pyrophosphate bone scans can often detect areas of active inflammation in AS before standard radiographic changes are present.

H. **Computed tomography (CT)** and **magnetic resonance imaging (MRI).** These scans may identify erosions in sacroiliac joints before they appear on radiographs.

VI. Differential diagnosis

A. Distinguishing AS from the multitude of other causes of low back pain is challenging. Testing for HLA-B27 is impractical and expensive to perform in all patients complaining of back pain. It should be reserved for patients exhibiting signs and symptoms suggestive, but not diagnostic, of AS. The **clinical history,** however, may be a sensitive and specific tool in the differential diagnosis. If four or more of the following features are present, the diagnosis of AS should be strongly considered:

1. Age of onset less than 40 years.
2. Insidious onset.
3. Low back pain lasting longer than 3 months.
4. Association with morning stiffness.
5. Improvement with exercise.

B. Conditions that should be distinguished from AS are the following:

1. Lumbosacral disk disease and "lumbar strain." The clinical feature of pain intensifying with rest and improving on exercise in spondylitic patients may be useful. Although sciatica-like pain may occur in AS, accompanying neurologic signs of lumbar root compression are unusual.

2. Other seronegative spondyloarthropathies. In any of the other seronegative spondyloarthropathies, skeletal inflammation may develop that is essentially identical to that of classic AS. Usually, the extraarticular manifestations of these diseases allow clinical differentiation, but there is probably an overlapping spectrum of features. The spondylitis of **Reiter's syndrome** and **psoriatic arthropathy** is usually less severe than that of typical AS, and syndesmophytes tend to be asymmetric.

3. Degenerative joint disease of lumbosacral apophyseal and intervertebral joints. The older age of the patient and the presence of typical osteophytes on radiography usually facilitate differentiation. The SI joints can be affected by osteoarthritis, but radiographic involvement is limited to the lower part of the joints, whereas complete involvement is the rule in AS.

4. Diffuse idiopathic skeletal hyperostosis (Forestier disease) is an idiopathic enthesopathy seen in elderly persons that can mimic AS but lacks apophyseal and SI involvement.

5. Osteitis condensans ilii is an asymptomatic sclerosis of the iliac subchondral bone in parous women that may cause radiographic confusion with AS. Sclerosis is *only on the iliac side* of the joint in this condition.

VII. Treatment. The **aims of management** in AS are to control pain, maintain maximum skeletal mobility, and prevent deformities. There is no specific therapy or cure for AS. Management requires patient education and cooperation and consists of dedication to a program of posture control, exercises, and judicious use of medications and surgical intervention when appropriate.

A. Physical therapy. All patients should be enrolled in a physiotherapy program. Maintenance of erect posture is critical in all activities, including sitting, standing, and walking. The patient should sleep in a prone position or supine on a firm mattress with one small or no pillow. Walking and swimming are excellent ways to maintain joint mobility.

B. Drugs. The role of drugs is to relieve pain and inflammation so that posture can be preserved and an exercise program maintained.

1. Indomethacin (25 to 50 mg three to four times daily or one 75-mg slow-release capsule twice daily) is the most commonly prescribed drug.

2. Other nonsteroidal antiinflammatory drugs, such as naproxen (500 mg twice daily), sulindac (200 mg twice daily), piroxicam (20 mg daily), and tolmetin (400 mg three times daily), are reported to offer comparable pain relief.

3. Salicylates, for unknown reasons, seldom provide an adequate therapeutic response in AS.

4. Sulfasalazine (500 mg to 1 g twice daily with meals) relieves spinal symptoms and decreases acute-phase reactants. It is especially useful early in disease. Neutropenia occurs in 1% to 3% of patients, so monitoring of the white blood cell count and patient education about reporting of signs of infection are important. Gold and antimalarial agents are not beneficial. Immunosuppressive agents, such as methotrexate, cyclophosphamide, and azathioprine, may be helpful but have not been proved effective in controlled trials. Systemic steroids may be helpful to treat acute flares but should be used with extreme caution on a long-term basis because of serious side effects.

5. **Intraarticular corticosteroids** may occasionally be useful for acutely inflamed joints. Indications and dosages are discussed in Chapter 4.

C. **Surgery.** Surgical procedures are usually reserved for patients with far-advanced disease causing painful deformities or loss of function. Total hip replacement is the most commonly performed procedure. However, total knee replacements, cervical and lumbar osteotomies to relieve severe spinal kyphosis, and stabilization of atlanto-axial subluxation may be necessary. Unfortunately, ectopic ossification at the operative site may occur.

VIII. **Prognosis.** The course of AS varies. In some patients, the disease progresses relentlessly (often despite therapy), with fusion of axial and peripheral joints. In others, bony ankylosis may develop gradually with little pain or discomfort. In still others, skeletal involvement may be limited to only mild sacroiliitis and never progress to serious spondylitis or ankylosing disease.

Although AS is not curable, rehabilitation yields impressive achievements. Most patients who maintain disciplined exercise and posture programs and take antiinflammatory medication judiciously are able to lead relatively normal and active lives with minor adjustments in life-style. Relentlessly crippling disease develops in fewer than 10%. Most longitudinal studies of AS show survival curves approximating that of the general population.

Bibliography

Calin A, Fries JJ. Striking prevalence of ankylosing spondylitis in "healthy" W27-positive males and females. *N Engl J Med* 1975;293:835.

Hammer RE, et al. Spontaneous inflammatory disease in transgenic rats expressing HLA-B27 and human beta2m: an animal model of HLA-B27-associated human disorders. *Cell* 1990;63:1099.

Lawrence RC, et al. Estimates of the prevalence of arthritis and selected musculoskeletal disorders in the United States. *Arthritis Rheum* 1998;41:778.

Moll JMH, et al. Associations between AS, psoriatic arthritis, Reiter's disease, the intestinal arthropathies, and Behçet's syndrome. *Medicine* 1974;53:343.

Schlosstein L, et al. High association of an HL-A antigen, W27, with ankylosing spondylitis. *N Engl J Med* 1973;288:704.

Taurog JD, et al. The germ-free state prevents development of gut and joint inflammatory disease in HLA-B27 transgenic rats. *J Exp Med* 1994;180:2359.

34. ENTEROPATHIC ARTHRITIS

Kyriakos A. Kirou and Allan Gibofsky

Enteritis has been pathogenetically linked to arthritis in certain human (and experimental animal model) systemic inflammatory disorders, collectively comprising the enteropathic arthritides. Bacteria have been thought to play a significant role in these diseases, either when exposure to normal intestinal flora is increased (as in ulcerative colitis, in which intestinal permeability is increased), or when enteric infection with certain "arthritogenic" bacteria, such as *Shigella,* occurs (reactive arthritis). However, synovial fluid cultures are characteristically negative, and by definition, septic arthritides are excluded from the classification of enteropathic arthritides. Genetic factors are also implicated. In particular, inflammatory bowel disease-related arthritis and reactive arthritis belong to the clinically distinct group of spondyloarthritides, which are characterized by familial aggregation and a strong association with the class I major histocompatibility complex (MHC) allele HLA-B27 (see Chapter 6). Other common features of the spondyloarthritides, of which ankylosing spondylitis is the prototype, include sacroiliitis (with or without spondylitis), enthesitis, asymmetric oligoarthritis, uveitis, mucocutaneous inflammation, and seronegativity for rheumatoid factor. Notably, subclinical gut inflammation has been documented in all forms of spondyloarthritis.

Enteropathic arthritides that are *not associated with HLA-B27* include those occurring in the context of Whipple's disease and celiac disease and after intestinal bypass surgery. If the inclusion criteria for enteropathic arthritides were loosened to accept disorders that simply combine joint and abdominal symptoms, the list could be extended to include vasculitic syndromes, pancreatic disease, Behçet's disease, and familial Mediterranean fever.

I. **Inflammatory bowel disease.** Ulcerative colitis and Crohn's disease share similar extra-intestinal and rheumatic manifestations. Both peripheral and axial arthritis can occur.

A. **Epidemiologic and genetic considerations**

1. In whites, the prevalence of either ulcerative colitis or Crohn's disease is between 50 and 100 in 100,000.
2. **Peripheral arthritis** occurs in 10% to 25% of patients and is slightly more common in Crohn's disease. Men and women are equally affected, and the peak age of onset is between 25 and 44 years. There is no association with HLA-B27.
3. **Axial involvement** is more frequent in Crohn's disease (5% to 22%) than in ulcerative colitis (2% to 6%). There is no male predominance, as there is in ankylosing spondylitis, and only 50% to 70% of patients are positive for HLA-B27. In fact, the presence of ankylosing spondylitis in patients negative for HLA-B27 should predict inflammatory bowel disease or psoriatic arthritis.

B. **Clinical manifestations and diagnosis**

1. **Peripheral arthritis**

a. Usually acute, migratory, and transient. Recurrences are common.

b. Asymmetric and oligoarticular pattern, typically involving the large and small joints of the lower extremities. Dactylitis can occur.

c. Usually follows bowel symptoms. It tends to correlate with extent and activity of gut inflammation and often coincides with other bowel activity-related extra-intestinal manifestations (erythema nodosum, enthesitis, aphthous oral ulcerations, finger clubbing, and possibly also uveitis).

d. **Laboratory studies**

(1) Anemia and a high erythrocyte sedimentation rate are common with flares of arthritis.

(2) Results of synovial fluid analysis are consistent with inflammatory arthritis: 4,000 to 40,000 leukocytes per milliliter (70% to 90% polymorphonuclear leukocytes). Cultures are sterile.
(3) Joint radiographic findings are nonspecific, with soft-tissue swelling and juxtaarticular osteoporosis. Asymmetric metatarsophalangeal erosions and reactive bone formation can rarely be seen.

e. Differential diagnosis of inflammatory bowel disease peripheral arthritis

(1) Migratory arthritis should be distinguished from rheumatic fever.
(2) Acute monarthritis can closely resemble septic arthritis, gout, or pseudogout.

2. Axial involvement (sacroiliitis and spondylitis)

a. Clinically and radiographically indistinguishable from idiopathic ankylosing spondylitis.

b. Occurs independently of bowel disease activity and extent, and frequently precedes it by several years. In as many as 6% of patients with ankylosing spondylitis, Crohn's disease may evolve.

c. Differential diagnosis in cases in which intestinal symptoms are not present at presentation can be difficult. Other causes of low back pain should be considered (see Chapter 18).

C. Treatment

1. Therapy should be directed primarily at the intestinal inflammation, as it will usually control the acute peripheral arthritis also.
2. Sulfasalazine (1 g twice daily) is effective in ulcerative colitis (both treatment of active disease and prevention of relapses) but less so in Crohn's disease. Importantly, it has been recently shown to be useful and well tolerated in the management of peripheral arthritis in many forms of spondyloarthritis. However, it may be less effective in axial inflammation than a nonsteroidal inflammatory drug (NSAID), such as indomethacin.
3. NSAIDs in standard doses are effective in the treatment of peripheral arthritis and axial inflammatory symptoms. However, because they may induce flares of ulcerative colitis, they should be used with caution.
4. Intraarticular corticosteroid injections can be very helpful, especially in monarticular disease. Systemic corticosteroids should not be used for arthritis alone.
5. Colectomy cures peripheral arthritis in ulcerative colitis but does not alter the course of spondylitis.

D. Prognosis

1. Prognosis for **peripheral disease** is generally good. Chronic disease will develop in only 10% of patients.
2. Prognosis for **axial disease** is similar to that of ankylosing spondylitis.

II. Enteropathic reactive arthritis is a form of spondyloarthritis that typically occurs 1 to 3 weeks after an acute intestinal infection with certain arthritogenic bacteria (e.g., *Shigella flexneri, Campylobacter jejuni,* and some *Salmonella* and *Yersinia* species). It is usually seen in a patient positive for HLA-B27. Occasionally, diarrhea can be subclinical, making the diagnosis less obvious. The large joints of the lower extremities are usually affected, and full Reiter's syndrome can occur (see Chapter 36). Antibiotics have not been shown to alter the disease course.

III. Other spondyloarthritides. Less prominent intestinal symptoms may occur in other forms of spondyloarthritis. In fact, endoscopic studies of the colon and ileum have shown macroscopic inflammatory lesions in 18% to 50% of patients with spondyloarthritis. The prevalence of such lesions is even higher by histologic criteria. Acute inflammatory changes resemble those of bacterial enteritis, and chronic inflammatory lesions are similar to those seen in Crohn's disease. Chronic gut inflammation is associated with more severe and persistent arthritis or spondylitis, and the condition occasionally evolves into clinically apparent Crohn's disease.

IV. Whipple's disease. This rare multisystem disease has been recently shown to be caused by a gram-positive actinomycete (*Tropheryma whippelii*).

A. Clinical presentation. Whipple's disease affects men ages 35 to 60. It is characterized by the insidious onset of fever, arthritis, malabsorption, generalized lymphadenopathy, skin hyperpigmentation, uveitis, or progressive encephalopathy. The typically symmetric, transient, and nondeforming polyarthritis occurs in 80% of the patients and may precede enteritis by several years.

B. Diagnosis. Until recently, the diagnosis depended on duodenal biopsy and the demonstration of deposits in lamina propria macrophages that stained with periodic acid–Schiff (PAS). In other tissues, electron microscopic demonstration of characteristic rod-shaped bacilli was necessary. However, a specific diagnosis can now be made from tissue and even from peripheral blood, with use of the polymerase chain reaction to verify the presence of the causative microorganism.

C. Treatment. Antibiotic therapy is effective, but relapses can occur. Parenteral antibiotic therapy with penicillin G (1.2 million U/d) and streptomycin (1 g/d) is recommended for the first 2 weeks, followed by oral trimethoprim/sulfamethoxazole (160/800 mg twice daily) for 1 to 2 years. Agents that do not cross the blood–brain barrier should probably be avoided.

V. Intestinal bypass arthritis (arthritis-dermatitis syndrome). Jejunoileostomy or jejunocolostomy, performed for morbid obesity, often results (after 2 to 30 months) in the arthritis-dermatitis syndrome. A symmetric and migratory nondeforming polyarthritis of the large joints is observed in 20% to 80% of patients and may become chronic in 25%. Other features include erythema nodosum, macular and vesiculopustular skin lesions, Raynaud's phenomenon, serositis, glomerulonephritis, retinal vasculitis, and superficial thrombophlebitis. The syndrome has been attributed to bacterial overgrowth in the blind loop with alteration of bowel permeability and formation of bacterial antigen-containing immune complexes.

A. Laboratory studies, including evaluation of peripheral blood, synovial fluid, stool, and **joint radiography** are not diagnostically helpful.

B. Treatment. NSAIDs are effective against arthritis, but courses of oral antibiotics (e.g., with tetracycline, clindamycin, or metronidazole) may offer additional help. Nevertheless, only surgical re-anastomosis of the bypassed intestinal segment provides a cure. By 1985, bypass surgery for obesity was largely abandoned, so the clinician is unlikely to see further cases.

VI. Celiac disease, or gluten-induced enteropathy, is a rare disease characterized by mucosal abnormalities of the small intestine and malabsorption. Association with many autoimmune disorders has been noted, and arthritis occurs in fewer than 50% of patients.

A. Clinical presentation and diagnosis. Arthritis is usually polyarticular and often involves hand and wrist joints. Half of patients have no intestinal symptoms. In that clinical scenario, the presence of malaise, weight loss, and low serum folate levels can be very helpful in diagnosis. Bone pain resulting from osteomalacia may also occur.

B. Treatment. Arthritis usually responds well to a gluten-free diet.

VII. Pancreatic disease. Chronic pancreatitis or pancreatic cancer can sometimes be associated with nodular subcutaneous fat necrosis and arthritis. A history of alcoholism is common.

A. Laboratory studies. Serum pancreatic enzymes are usually elevated. Synovial fluid may contain calcified necrotic fat particles, which can be confused with negatively birefringent crystals on polarized microscopy.

B. Treatment. Prompt diagnosis is essential, and therapy should be focused on the underlying pancreatic disease.

VIII. Syndromes associated with vasculitis, such as Henoch-Schönlein purpura and systemic lupus erythematosus, can give rise to both abdominal pain (caused by involvement of mesenteric arteries) and arthritis. Diagnostic and treatment efforts are directed at the primary disease.

Bibliography

Calin A, Taurog JD. *The spondyloarthritides.* Oxford, UK: Oxford University Press, 1998.

Lowsky R, et al. Brief report: diagnosis of Whipple's disease by molecular analysis of peripheral blood. *N Engl J Med* 1994;331:1343.

Mielants H, Veys EM. Enteropathic arthritis. In: Koopman WJ, ed. *Arthritis and allied conditions.* Baltimore: Williams & Wilkins, 1997.

Singer R. Diagnosis and treatment of Whipple's disease. *Drugs* 1998;55:699.

35. PSORIATIC ARTHRITIS

Joseph A. Markenson

Psoriatic arthritis (PA) is an inflammatory arthropathy occurring in 5% to 7% of patients with psoriasis [excluding subjects who are positive for rheumatoid factor (RF) and presumably have coexisting psoriasis and rheumatoid arthritis (RA)]. Psoriasis is a common disease afflicting 1% to 2% of the general population. Dermal psoriasis usually appears in the second to third decades, but the onset of associated arthritis is usually delayed by two decades. The pathogenesis of PA is unknown, although a genetic component is evident. Concordance between monozygotic twins is higher (70%) than in RA (30%), yet the lack of complete concordance suggests that other (e.g., environmental) factors are involved. Because many lesions of psoriasis are colonized with staphylococci and streptococci, there is some thought that psoriatic arthritis may be a form of reactive arthritis in which microbial superantigens result in T cells that cross-react with human auto-antigens. Family studies suggest an extremely high (>50%) risk in first-degree relatives of patients with arthritis. The female-to-male ratio is 1:1, whereas in RA it is 3:1.

I. **Clinical presentations.** Five distinct patterns of PA are recognized.

A. Patients with **oligoarticular disease** constitute 70% of all cases of PA. It is characteristically asymmetric, affecting a large joint such as a knee and a few scattered distal interphalangeal (DIP), proximal interphalangeal (PIP), and metacarpophalangeal (MCP) joints, often in association with diffuse swelling of one or more fingers and toes ("sausage digits").

B. **Symmetric polyarthritis,** which resembles RA, is the next most common pattern. Patients are usually RF-negative and constitute about 15% of all cases of PA. Constitutional symptoms such as morning stiffness and fatigue are common and tend to parallel the activity of joint disease.

C. **Asymmetric involvement of distal interphalangeal joints** of the hands and feet is sometimes referred to as "classic" psoriatic arthropathy, but this pattern appears in no more than 10% of cases of psoriatic arthritis; digits affected often have characteristic psoriatic nail changes. This pattern may evolve into the oligoarticular pattern.

D. **Arthritis mutilans** is a particularly disabling form, occurring in fewer than 5% of all cases of PA. The deformity, most striking in the fingers and toes, is caused by osteolysis of the affected joints.

E. **Psoriatic spondyloarthritis** occurs in up to 5% of patients with PA and presents with clinical and radiographic features that may be indistinguishable from those of idiopathic sacroiliitis or ankylosing spondylitis. The histocompatibility antigen HLA-B27 is found in 40% of this group.

II. **History.** Symptoms are highly variable according to the anatomic patterns described above. Although interphalangeal (IP) joints of the fingers and toes are most commonly affected, larger joints such as the knee and ankle may be involved.

The extraarticular manifestations such as vasculitis, lung disease, and pericarditis seen in RA are generally not seen in PA. Inflammatory eye disease does occur in up to 30% of patients with PA. Constitutional symptoms such as malaise, morning stiffness, and fever are less common and are more often seen with the symmetric polyarticular pattern. Back pain may be indicative of psoriatic spondylitis or sacroiliitis. There is an increasing awareness of an association between temporomandibular joint disease and psoriatic arthritis.

III. **Physical examination** reveals cardinal signs of inflammation in affected joints. IP joint involvement is often associated with a sausage appearance of the digits (dactylitis). The most common form of PA has the characteristic asymmetric "skip-hit" pattern of digit involvement. Psoriasis may be obvious or may manifest only as an obscure patch in the scalp or umbilicus, or as nail pitting (onychodystrophy). Arthritis usually follows well-established cutaneous or nail lesions, although some patients exhibit characteristic patterns of PA in the absence of such. Nail changes alone may not be diagnostic, but the presence of more than 20 pits is suggestive and more than 60 diagnostic of PA. With all nail changes, especially those involving the toenails, fungal and bacterial infections, which may also cause hyperkeratosis and onycholysis, should be ruled out.

IV. Laboratory studies

A. Rheumatoid factor is seen in fewer than 10% of PA patients.

B. Polyclonal hypergammaglobulinemia is occasionally present.

C. Serum complement in patients with PA tends to be higher than normal; however, this finding is of no diagnostic significance. Theoretically, elevated synovial fluid complement levels might distinguish PA from RA. Such measurements are frequently subnormal in RA.

D. Serum uric acid. In 10% to 20% of patients with psoriasis, levels of uric acid may be elevated in relation to the severity of the skin disease.

E. The **erythrocyte sedimentation rate** and other acute-phase reactants are elevated and parallel the activity of the arthritis.

F. Test results for **antinuclear factors** are usually negative.

G. Radiographic features considered classic for PA are destructive lesions involving predominantly the DIP joints of fingers and the IP joints of the toes. Bony ankylosis of the DIP joints of the hand and toes, along with bony proliferation of the base of the distal phalanx, and resorption of the tufts of the distal phalanges of hands and feet are also commonly seen. Other classic features are fluffy periostitis of large joints, "pencil-in-cup" appearance of DIP joints, an asymmetric joint pattern, and gross destruction of isolated small joints. Changes in the spine and sacroiliac (SI) joints may be similar to those seen in ankylosing spondylitis, but SI joint changes in PA are often unilateral, and syndesmophytes can sometimes be distinguished from those of ankylosing spondylitis.

V. Differential diagnosis

A. Reiter's syndrome. The cutaneous lesions of Reiter's syndrome resemble pustular psoriasis. Reiter's syndrome usually affects large joints in an oligoarticular fashion and infrequently involves the DIP joints or produces sausage digits. Both illnesses may be associated with spondyloarthritis. The incidence of HLA-B27 is higher in Reiter's syndrome than in PA. Radiographically, Reiter's syndrome may demonstrate periostitis of the plantar surfaces of the calcaneus, metatarsal bones, or ankles. In PA, periostitis is usually limited to the long bones.

B. Gout. Acute psoriatic monarthritis can resemble but should be differentiated from gout by the absence of monosodium urate crystals in the synovial fluid. Hyperuricemia may occur in up to 20% of patients with skin psoriasis but is uncommon during acute flares of PA. In contrast to monarticular PA, acute gouty arthritis usually resolves completely in 1 to 2 weeks, even if untreated.

C. Rheumatoid arthritis is the most difficult entity to differentiate from PA. Distal and asymmetric IP joint involvement and the absence of RF support the diagnosis of PA. The presence of skin psoriasis and onychodystrophy helps distinguish PA from RA. (Patients with symmetric arthritis and psoriasis who are positive for RF are usually considered to have coexistent RA and psoriasis.) Subcutaneous nodules are absent in PA. The radiographic features (see section **IV.G**) may help differentiate PA from RA.

D. Human immunodeficiency virus (HIV) infection. PA is more aggressive in patients with HIV infection, which suggests a pathogenesis different from that of RA. (HIV depletes CD4+ T cells and RA is almost absent in HIV patients, unlike PA, which is a CD8+ T-cell disease). However, the incidence of skin disease (psoriasis) is not greater than in the normal population. HLA-associated antigens are similar and appear in the same frequency as in non–HIV-infected patients with PA (HLA-Bw38, -Bw39, and -Cw6). In contrast, in HIV-associated Reiter's disease, the frequency of HLA-B27 can be higher than 75%.

VI. **Treatment.** The management goals and therapeutic efforts applied to PA and RA have similar features. However, nonsteroidal antiinflammatory drugs (NSAIDs) are used as the base therapy in many PA patients, whereas combined disease-modifying antirheumatic drugs (DMARDs) are now used early in RA treatment.

A. **Physical therapy** is used as an adjunct to drug therapy to help preserve joint range of motion and minimize muscle weakness.

B. **Drug therapy** is aimed at decreasing inflammation of synovial tissue to allow maintenance of joint function. NSAIDs are the drugs of choice. Therapeutic options follow in order of use.

1. **Nonsteroidal antiinflammatory drugs.** The reader is referred to Appendix E for a more complete discussion of the agents listed below.

a. **Ibuprofen** (600 mg four times daily), **naproxen** (250 to 500 mg twice daily), **fenoprofen** (300 mg four times daily), **ketoprofen** (75 mg three times daily), and **flurbiprofen** (100 mg three times daily) are other propionic acid derivatives that are applicable to the treatment of PA.

b. **Indomethacin** (200 mg/d) in divided doses is usually an effective antiinflammatory agent for both spondyloarthritis and peripheral arthritis.

c. **Sulindac** (200 mg twice daily), an NSAID much like indomethacin, requires less frequent dosing and may be associated with less gastrointestinal intolerance.

d. **Piroxicam** is a long-acting NSAID given in a single daily dose of 20 mg.

e. **Diclofenac** (75 mg twice daily) is effective but requires monitoring with liver function tests.

f. **Nabumetone** (1,000 to 2,000 mg/d) is well tolerated and may be associated with fewer gastric ulcers, although the same degree of gastric intolerance is noted as with the above-mentioned NSAIDs.

g. **Arthrotec** (50 to 75 mg twice daily), a combination tablet of diclofenac and misoprostol, may be used for patients at high risk for gastrointestinal side effects.

2. **Disease-modifying antirheumatic drug therapy and combination therapies**

a. **Gold salts.** A course of aurothiomalate is indicated for the treatment of progressive, severe PA, especially when the disease resembles RA. A full course usually starts with sequential weekly IM injections of 10, 25, and then 50 mg until a total dose of 1,000 mg has been achieved. If successful, monthly maintenance injections of 50 mg are given indefinitely. The efficacy of auranofin (20 mg/d PO) in RA approaches that of injectable gold preparations. It has not been systematically evaluated as treatment for PA; however, this author has had moderate success with it in treating patients with PA. (The toxicity of gold preparations and relevant laboratory surveillance are discussed in Chapter 28.)

b. **Antimalarial therapy** has been associated with exfoliative skin reaction in persons with psoriasis; however, recent studies have concluded that such drugs can be used safely and that they have the potential for inducing remission of PA. Hydroxychloroquine (200 mg/d for 1 month followed by 400 mg/d) is recommended. Hydroxychloroquine therapy probably should be considered when PA fails to respond to NSAIDs or gold.

c. **Sulfasalazine** has been used in the treatment of RA (see Chapter 28), and trials of PA are in progress. It is effective as a second-line drug with an onset of action later than that of NSAIDs and before that of gold. Side effects are mainly gastrointestinal intolerance and skin rash.

d. **Immunosuppressive drugs.** Oral or parenteral **methotrexate** is an extremely effective therapy for both the arthritic and skin manifestation of psoriasis. Evidence now exists in RA that liver biopsy is not necessary, and an algorithm has been developed to follow toxicity. Opinions are divided regarding whether toxicity to methotrexate is different in PA, and a biopsy must still be performed. This author, however, is following the American College of Rheumatology recommendations for monitoring liver toxicity in RA. A dosage of 7.5 to 25.0 mg/wk (maximum dosage, 50 mg/wk) is usually successful in suppressing cutaneous and articular manifestations of psoriasis. A commonly employed oral regimen consists of a series of three doses (2.5 to 10.0 mg each) administered at 12-hour intervals during a 36-hour period each week. The drug is hepatotoxic, and authorities recommend a liver biopsy at a cumulative dose of 1,500 mg. Careful monitoring of liver function tests, complete blood counts to detect bone marrow suppression, and chest radiographs to detect methotrexate-induced pulmonary infiltrates are mandatory.

e. **Corticosteroid therapy** has limited application in the management of PA. For patients with oligoarticular disease, in which disability results from involvement of one or a few joints, intraarticular steroid therapy may be preferred to systemic use of antiinflammatory drugs. Topical corticosteroids are useful for psoriatic skin disease. Oral corticosteroids should be avoided if possible because of increased relapses and flares, particularly skin disease, when doses are adjusted.

f. **Preliminary open trials with retinoid (etretinate)** suggest that it is beneficial at a mean daily maintenance dose of 30 mg. Results are seen usually between 6 weeks and 3 months. The mechanism of action is unknown. Etretinate cannot be used in women of childbearing age. Side effects include mucocutaneous lesions, proximal arthralgias and myalgias, and extraspinal calcifications.

g. **Cyclosporin A** has been used with efficacy in patients with severe PA refractory to other treatments. Careful observation of serum creatinine levels and blood pressure monitoring are mandatory.

h. **Photochemotherapy** with methoxypsoralen and long-wave ultraviolet A light (PUVA) will benefit a group of nonspondylitic patients with synchronous joint and skin flares.

i. **Reconstructive surgery** is of value in patients with end-stage joint destruction. Procedures employed and indications are similar to those for RA (see Chapters 28 and 54).

VII. Prognosis. The prognosis for patients with PA varies according to the anatomic pattern. The severity of arthritis tends to parallel the severity of skin disease. Most patients have mild episodic disease affecting only a few joints. For these, the prognosis is generally favorable. In approximately 5% of patients, severe disabling and deforming arthritis develops. The axial spondyloarthropathy of PA is associated with many of the same extraarticular manifestations seen in idiopathic ankylosing spondylitis (uveitis, cardiac disease, conduction defects, aortitis), and these features may significantly contribute to morbidity. Complications of therapy, especially oral corticosteroids, have been the largest contributing factor to mortality in several large series.

Bibliography

Arnett FC, et al. Psoriasis and psoriatic arthritis: association with human immunodeficiency virus infection. *Rheum Dis Clin North Am* 1991;17:59.

Green L, et al. Arthritis in psoriasis. *Ann Rheum Dis* 1981;40:366.

Grekin RC, et al. Retinoids in the treatment of psoriasis: monotherapy and combinations. *Dermatol Clin* 1984;2:439.

Kammer G, et al. Psoriatic arthritis: a clinical, immunologic and HLA study of 100 patients. *Semin Arthritis Rheum* 1979;9:75.

Moll JMH, Wright V. Psoriatic arthritis seminar. *Arthritis Rheum* 1978;3:55.
Perlman GG, et al. Photochemotherapy and psoriatic arthritis. *Ann Intern Med* 1979;91:717.
Wright V. Psoriatic arthritis: a comparative study of rheumatoid arthritis and arthritis associated with psoriasis. *Ann Rheum Dis* 1961;20:123.

36. REITER'S SYNDROME AND REACTIVE ARTHRITIS

Robert D. Inman

In 1916, Hans Reiter reported the case of a Prussian lieutenant in whom diarrhea developed; shortly thereafter, he experienced arthritis, conjunctivitis, and urethritis. Ironically, Reiter attributed this symptom complex to a spirochetal infection, but the association of the syndrome with his name has persisted. Although the early descriptions of Reiter's syndrome (RS) define a clinical triad of arthritis, conjunctivitis, and urethritis, most authors now accept the presence of a seronegative asymmetric arthritis plus one characteristic extraarticular feature (described below) as sufficient for the diagnosis. An antecedent infection of the gastrointestinal or genitourinary tract can often be identified, but not invariably. The pathogens implicated in such infections are *Yersinia, Salmonella, Shigella, Campylobacter* (gastrointestinal infections), and *Chlamydia* (genitourinary infections). It is not clear whether a wider range of "arthritogenic" organisms should be included in this list, but the evidence for other organisms playing a triggering role in RS has remained circumstantial.

Although RS occurs in children and the elderly, it is usually seen in young adults, with a significant male predominance. It may be that RS is underrecognized in female patients, as some clinical features (e.g., cervicitis) may be less symptomatic than the extraarticular features in male patients (e.g., balanitis). However, serious, even refractory, RS does occur in women, and the clinician should be alert to a typical constellation of symptoms in either sex. Despite the strong immunogenetic influence on the disease, a positive family history for RS is uncommon. It has been observed that if there is a positive family history, it tends to be for RS, whereas patients with ankylosing spondylitis are more likely to have relatives with that disease than with RS. At present, there are no predictive features that discriminate systemic target organ involvement from disease limited to the joints, or that discriminate a benign, self-limited course (averaging 3 to 4 months) from a more chronic course. Retrospective studies have noted that a sustained antibody response against the triggering pathogen is characteristic of those patients in whom a more chronic course of RS develops.

I. Pathogenesis. Despite the strong association with the HLA-B27 antigen, the mechanism whereby this HLA gene might confer disease susceptibility to RS remains unknown. There are three hypothetical routes by which HLA might interact with a triggering infectious agent. The first is molecular mimicry, whereby an autoimmune response develops after the infection because of cross-reactivity of host and microbial antigens. The clinical significance of cross-reacting antibodies in such studies remains undefined. The second is an altered cellular immune response to the pathogen; proponents argue that unique determinants in the antigen-binding groove of the HLA-B27 molecule specifically present "arthritogenic" peptides to the responding CD8+ T-cell population. The idenficiation of such pathogenic T cells has proved problematic in both clinical and experimental systems, although CD8+ T cells recognizing microbial peptides have been isolated. The third possibility is an altered microbial-host cell interaction, by which certain HLA alleles modulate host response to arthritogenic organisms. This might implicate altered invasion, intracellular killing pathways, or cytokine production. Whatever the mechanism, it is likely that the synovitis that ensues is related to local deposition and persistence of microbial antigens, but definitive proof is lacking to resolve the issue.

II. Diagnosis

A. History. A careful history should be taken to address any recent exposure to an enteric pathogen (a diarrheal illness after travel) or a sexually transmitted pathogen (a new sexual partner). The typical interval between the triggering infection and RS is 1 to 4 weeks, but exceptions earlier or later have been described. A prior history of low back pain or recurrent tendinitis is not uncommon. A history of recent antibiotic therapy is relevant to interpretation of any culture results. Prior episodes of uveitis may not be mentioned by the patient unless specifically sought.

B. **Constitutional symptoms.** Fatigue may not be present in the acute phase but can become significant in chronic RS.

C. **Physical findings**

1. **Fever** is usually low-grade (<38°C) in most patients. Significant or sustained fever should suggest that the original infection may still be active.
2. **Arthritis.** The cardinal feature is an asymmetric arthritis, typically oligoarticular and predominantly in the lower extremities. Most common are knees, ankles, and metatarsophalangeal joints, but involvement of an upper extremity can be seen. Acute sacroiliitis may present as a diffuse low back pain that is difficult to localize but may be felt in the deep gluteal area.
3. **Enthesitis.** Plantar fasciitis and Achilles tendinitis are quite specific for RS and should be sought carefully. Any tendinous insertion into bone can be involved, and tendinitis of hip adductors may be misdiagnosed as arthritis of the hip joint.
4. **Genitourinary symptoms.** Urethritis can be manifested by dysuria and by urethral discharge in male patients. Cervicitis in female patients is usually asymptomatic. Prostatitis and hemorrhagic cystitis may also occur.
5. **Ocular symptoms.** Conjunctivitis may be mildly or markedly symptomatic, with a burning sensation and local crusting around the eye. Uveitis is generally associated with pain and photophobia and sometimes loss of visual acuity.
6. **Gastrointestinal symptoms.** Antecedent diarrhea has generally resolved by the onset of arthritis but may persist at a low level for prolonged periods.
7. **Mucocutaneous symptoms**
   a. **Circinate balanitis** appears as coalescing, superficial genital ulcers.
   b. **Keratoderma blennorrhagicum** is characterized by the appearance of keratotic skin lesions on the palms and soles.
   c. **Mucosal ulcers** can appear on the tongue or buccal mucosa and are generally painless, but not invariably so.
8. **Cardiac and neurologic features** are rare.
   a. Heart block, pericarditis, aortic insufficiency.
   b. Myelopathy, cranial nerve lesions.

III. **Laboratory studies**

A. **Hematologic findings.** An elevated erythrocyte sedimentation rate is usually present in an acute episode. The anemia of chronic disease usually accompanies a more prolonged course.

B. **Urinary findings.** Pyuria is common, hematuria less common. Urethral discharge contains abundant neutrophils.

C. **Synovial fluid.** An elevated white blood cell count (10,000 to 50,000), with a predominance of neutrophils, is usually seen in active disease. Synovial fluid glucose and complement levels are generally normal, and determinations are not routinely ordered. Results of a Gram's stain are carefully examined, and a synovial fluid specimen is sent for culture.

D. **Culture.** In general, a careful search for persistent pathogens should be undertaken. The arthritogenic organisms listed above (e.g., *Salmonella*) may on occasion be associated with a true septic arthritis, so that appropriate cultures of synovial fluid should always be performed. Urethral discharge or persistent diarrhea should also occasion appropriate cultures (for chlamydial infection and gonorrhea in the former, for gram-negative enteric pathogens in the latter). Immunofluorescence studies of urethral swabs are increasingly being used for assessing chlamydial urethritis. Polymerase chain reaction to identify pathogens in synovial fluid is a valuable research tool, but its use has not yet been established in routine clinical practice.

E. **Tissue typing.** The HLA-B27 antigen is present in 70% to 80% of patients with RS but is of diagnostic value only in the appropriate clinical setting (i.e., high pretest probability). A negative test result does not exclude the diagnosis but may alert the clinician to the possibility of alternative diagnoses.

F. Radiographs. Generally, radiographic findings are normal in the acute disease, but reactive new bone at entheses may accompany chronic disease. Radiographic sacroiliitis may occur in the course of RS and is *classically asymmetric.* Clinical suspicion of sacroiliac disease with normal radiographic findings is an indication for bone scan confirmation of sacroiliitis. Evaluation of sacroiliac joints by computed tomography (CT) or magnetic resonance imaging (MRI) has been shown to increase the sensitivity of imaging, but the specificity of these techniques is not clearly defined. CT can demonstrate sacroiliac erosions, as can a properly taken Ferguson view of the sacroiliac joints that is interpreted by an experienced bone radiologist.

IV. Differential diagnosis

A. Septic arthritis. Appropriate cultures of synovial fluid, and of all potential portals of entry, should be performed to exclude septic arthritis. The most common diagnosis to exclude in a young patient is gonococcal arthritis. RS and disseminated gonococcal infection may both involve tenosynovitis, urethritis, conjunctivitis, and dermatitis.

B. Colitic arthropathy. Arthritis following diarrhea may represent the rheumatic complication of either Crohn's disease or ulcerative colitis, and gastrointestinal endoscopy and radiology may be required to exclude this possibility. Arthritis may be the presenting manifestation of inflammatory bowel disease and may precede bowel complaints for some period of time.

C. Psoriatic arthritis. Skin rash coincident with arthritis may represent psoriatic arthritis rather than RS, and indeed the histopathologic findings of psoriasis and keratoderma are similar. Coexisting urethritis and conjunctivitis, or antecedent diarrhea, would favor a diagnosis of RS. Pitting of the nails occurs in both conditions, but the nail dystrophy of psoriatic arthritis is generally more severe.

D. Rheumatoid arthritis. If chronic polyarthritis suggests rheumatoid arthritis, the presence of asymmetry and sacroiliitis and negativity for rheumatoid factor would favor RS. The extraarticular features of rheumatoid arthritis are distinct from those of RS.

E. Human immunodeficiency virus (HIV) infection. There are indications from some series that RS may occur with higher frequency and severity in patients with HIV infection. The frequency of this clinical overlap is not known. Patients in a high-risk category should be screened for HIV serology. There may be a unique arthropathy associated with HIV, but this is not fully resolved. In some patients, the episode of RS occurs long before clinically overt acquired immune deficiency syndrome (AIDS). This is an important consideration when any immunosuppressive therapy is being considered.

V. Treatment

A. Antibiotics. It has generally been held that antibiotics do not influence the course of RS, but recent evidence suggests that tetracycline compounds (e.g., doxycycline) may shorten the course of post-chlamydial RS. In any event, it is reasonable to institute appropriate antibiotic therapy if any culture results indicate a persisting infection (e.g., chlamydial urethritis). There is no evidence that antibiotic therapy alters the natural course of post-dysenteric RS.

B. Arthritis therapy

1. **Antiinflammatory drugs.** In general, the new nonsteroidal antiinflammatory drugs are superior to aspirin for controlling synovitis. Indomethacin (50 mg three times daily) and diclofenac (50 mg three times daily) are generally well tolerated in the young patients who represent the majority of patients. Recent evidence from a 36-week trial suggests that sulfasalazine is superior to placebo in improving the peripheral arthritis of RS. It is used at a dose of 500 mg to 1 g twice daily, and the granulocyte count is carefully monitored.
2. **Immunosuppressive therapy.** There has been favorable experience with methotrexate (5 to 15 mg/wk) and azathioprine (50 to 150 mg/d) in cases of chronic disease refractory to other measures. These agents are generally reserved for severe disease. As is the case in rheumatoid arthritis, clinicians

are more commonly using methotrexate earlier, when the response to nonsteroidal antiinflammatory drug therapy is unsatisfactory.

3. **Steroid therapy.** Intraarticular steroid injections may be of benefit, but oral steroids are rarely, if ever, indicated. Local steroid injection in the sacroiliac joint under fluoroscopic guidance has a role, particularly when this is the dominant symptomatic joint.

C. **Ocular disease.** Uveitis should be managed jointly by an ophthalmologist and a rheumatologist. Generally, local steroid drops will suffice, but oral steroids may be required in severe cases. Refractory uveitis can be the indication for intervention with methotrexate or azathioprine therapy.

VI. **Prognosis.** In most patients, significant improvement with antiinflammatory therapy occurs during a 3- to 4-month period. However, a recent 5-year follow-up study of patients with post-*Salmonella* RS reported that two-thirds of the patients continued to have subjective complaints at this interval, and that more than a third demonstrated objective changes in the joints. Long-term functional disability occurs in only a minority of patients. This variability in clinical course should be mentioned in discussions with the patient.

Bibliography

Careless D, Inman RD. Etiopathogenesis of reactive arthritis and ankylosing spondylitis. *Curr Opin Rheumatol* 1995;7:290.

Clegg DO, et al. Comparison of sulfasalazine and placebo in the treatment of reactive arthritis (Reiter's syndrome). *Arthritis Rheum* 1996;39:2021.

Cremers MCW, et al. Second-line treatment in seronegative spondyloarthropathies. *Semin Arthritis Rheum* 1994;24:71.

Inman RD. Treatment of seronegative spondyloarthropathies. In: Klippel J, Weyand CM, eds. *Primer on the rheumatic diseases.* Atlanta: Arthritis Foundation, 1997:193.

Thomson GT, et al. Post-*Salmonella* reactive arthritis: late clinical sequelae in a point source cohort. *Am J Med* 1995;98:13.

37. GOUT

Theodore R. Fields and Nicholas P. Scarpa

The first clinical description of a syndrome called podagra, a classic pattern of gout, was in the fifth century B.C. Despite its early recognition, gout continued to plague humankind until the middle of the twentieth century, when practical and effective therapy emerged. The introduction of allopurinol and nonsteroidal antiinflammatory drugs (NSAIDs) has made it possible to alter the course of the disease dramatically.

Gout is a heterogeneous disorder with primary and secondary forms characterized by hyperuricemia and urate crystal-induced arthritis.

I. **Epidemiology.** In the United States, approximately 12% of family members of gout patients are affected. Ninety percent of primary gout patients are men. The peak age for the first attack of gout is during the fifth decade. Primary gout is thought to be a polygenic disease.

II. **Disease classification**

A. **Primary gout.** In primary gout, hyperuricemia results from a disorder of purine metabolism or from abnormal excretion of uric acid. Most patients with primary gout fall into an idiopathic category because no precise genetic or metabolic defect can be identified. In approximately 1% of the primary gout group, specific enzyme defects have been found. Deficiency of hypoxanthine guanine phosphoribosyltransferase (HGPRT) and increased activity of phosphoribosylpyrophosphate (PRPP) synthetase are the best-characterized forms.

B. **Secondary gout** constitutes about 10% of all gout cases. It can result from a variety of disorders that cause hyperuricemia as a result of overproduction or impaired excretion of uric acid (Table 37-1).

III. **Acute gout**

A. **Clinical presentation**

1. The **intense articular inflammation** associated with the presence of intracellular monosodium urate crystals in synovial fluid is usually the first and most characteristic manifestation of an acute gouty arthritis. Classically, acute gout presents as a monarthritis (approximately 70% of cases); however, a polyarticular arthritis occurs in a significant percentage of patients. The onset of pain is sudden; within hours it may become excruciating to the point that the weight of bed sheets is intolerable. Weight bearing, even wearing footwear, may become impossible. The intense inflammation and erythema over the affected joint resemble tenosynovitis or cellulitis. Some patients also experience chills and fever with the acute onset.
2. Acute gouty arthritis occurs most commonly in men (95% of cases), with the initial attack occurring in the fourth or fifth decade. Gouty arthritis rarely develops in women before the onset of menopause.
3. Important **predisposing factors** of an acute gouty attack include diuretic use, recent surgery, alcohol abuse, chronic renal disease, rapid weight reduction, and infection. A positive family history of gout is helpful in supporting a diagnosis of primary gout. In patients taking cyclosporine, an especially rapidly progressing form of gout can develop, often with tophi.
4. The **joints most commonly affected** include the first metatarsophalangeal joints (podagra), the dorsum of the foot, the ankle, the knee, and occasionally the joints of the upper extremity. Gouty involvement is also seen in Heberden's and Bouchard's nodes, especially in elderly women on diuretics.

B. **Laboratory studies**

1. **Synovial fluid examination.** The most important procedure in establishing the diagnosis of acute gouty arthritis is the examination of the synovial fluid by compensated polarized microscopy.

Table 37-1. Classification of hyperuricemia

Overproduction of uric acid
Primary gout
Myeloproliferative disorders
Lymphoma
Hemoglobinopathies
Hemolytic anemia
Psoriasis
Cancer chemotherapy
Underexcretion of uric acid
Chronic renal failure
Lead nephropathy (saturnine gout)
Drugs: diuretics (except spironolactone), ethambutol, low-dose aspirin, cyclosporine
Lactic acidosis (alcoholism, preeclampsia)
Ketosis (diabetic, starvation)
Hyperparathyroidism
Hypertension
Overproduction and underexcretion
Glycogen storage disease, type 1
Mechanism unknown
Sarcoidosis
Obesity
Hypoparathyroidism
Paget's disease
Down syndrome

a. **Principles of polarizing microscopy.** The polarizing microscope consists of the usual optics with added polarizer and analyzer lenses that orient white light into a single plane. When a birefringent crystal is examined and rotated into the proper position, it will appear as a bright object against a dark field. When a first-order red compensator is added to the system, the specimen background appears rose (first-order red). Crystals examined with a compensator have characteristic colors that change when they are rotated 90 degrees as a result of the optical properties of the crystals and the compensator's deceleration of a characteristic frequency of light. The complex physics underlying this phenomenon are clearly described elsewhere.

b. **Crystal identification.** If carefully sought, urate crystals can be found in the synovial fluids of 85% of acute gout patients. Urate crystals can also often be found in asymptomatic knee and first metatarsophalangeal joints in patients with gout. Urate crystals are slender and needle-shaped and have strong negative birefringence under polarized light. (Calcium pyrophosphate crystals are pleomorphic, are predominantly rhomboid-shaped, and have weakly positive birefringence.) In most joint fluids, urate crystals can be found inside neutrophils; however, in chronic gout, crystals may also be found free in the synovial fluid. Under polarized light, urate crystals appear yellow when parallel to the axis of the red compensator and blue when perpendicular to the axis. (An axis reference line is etched on the housing of the compensator.) The calcium pyrophosphate crystals of pseudogout have the opposite orientation.

2. **Biochemical findings.** Serum uric acid levels are usually elevated but are normal in about 10% of patients with acute gout. The creatinine and urea nitrogen levels will be elevated if secondary gout attributable to renal failure is responsible for the acute attack. Lead poisoning, which can also cause nephropathy, can be detected by measuring an elevated level of copropor-

phyrin III or lead in the urine. If one of the genetic enzyme deficiencies of primary gout is suspected, erythrocyte enzymes can be assessed in a few specialized laboratories.

3. **Radiographs** usually show only soft-tissue swelling in the first attack of gout. With recurrent or chronic disease, tophi and periarticular erosions with overhanging edges can be seen in the affected joints. On rare occasions, magnetic resonance imaging (MRI) can be useful in distinguishing tophi from other soft-tissue lesions.

C. **Differential diagnosis.** Of paramount importance in the differential diagnosis of acute monarthritis is septic arthritis. Infection can be excluded only by Gram's stain and appropriate culture of the aspirated synovial fluid. The remainder of the differential diagnosis includes trauma, pseudogout, and atypical rheumatoid arthritis (RA). Although identification of calcium pyrophosphate crystals supports the diagnosis of pseudogout, both gout and pseudogout may coexist. The diagnosis of atypical RA often requires a prolonged period of observation before a clinical pattern of disease consistent with RA emerges.

D. **Treatment.** In the eighteenth and nineteenth centuries, physicians were frustrated by the myriad of impotent remedies proposed to cure gout. Today, however, physicians have a choice of treatment remedies that can dramatically alter the courses of acute and gouty arthritis. Detailed information on individual drugs appears in Appendix E. Regardless of the drug regimen chosen, resting the involved joint is an important adjunctive therapy.

1. **Indomethacin** is better tolerated than oral colchicine. The dosage of indomethacin is 50 mg three times daily until the attack has almost completely resolved, then 50 mg twice daily until the patient is asymptomatic. A therapeutic effect is usually seen in 8 hours. A suppository form of indomethacin has been approved for use in those patients unable to tolerate the oral form.
2. **Other NSAIDs** have also been used in treating acute gouty arthritis as alternative regimens.
   a. **Sulindac.** The dosage is 400 mg initially, then 200 mg twice daily, with gradual tapering during 5 days as inflammation subsides.
   b. **Naproxen.** The dosage is 500 mg initially, then 250 mg q8h, with gradual tapering during 5 days.
   c. **Ibuprofen.** The dosage is 800 mg initially, then 400 mg q6h, with gradual tapering during 5 days.
3. **Colchicine.** A therapeutic response to colchicine in the past has been considered diagnostic of acute gout, but it is now recognized to be nonspecific.
   a. **Oral colchicine** may cause nausea and diarrhea at the doses needed for control of an acute attack and is rarely recommended as first-time therapy. Occasional patients can tolerate five to six 0.6-mg doses PO hourly and may use this regimen. However, side effects usually outweigh therapeutic benefits.
   b. **Intravenous colchicine** is used infrequently in current practice. It should be avoided if possible in patients with severe renal or hepatic disease. Patients who have received a full IV dose of colchicine should receive no further colchicine (by any route) for 7 days. IV colchicine should not be used in patients with significant leukopenia or decreased marrow reserves, and it should be avoided if the patient is already taking oral colchicine. It should also be avoided in patients on hemodialysis. Some clinicians have stopped using IV colchicine in view of its potential toxicity. Consult current product labeling for dosage and clinical safety information.
4. **Allopurinol** or **probenecid** should **not** be started during an acute gout episode because reduction of the serum uric acid level may be associated with prolongation of the attack.
5. **Corticosteroids.** Although not the treatment of choice in patients without concomitant medical problems, the side effect profile of steroids makes this class of drugs appropriate in some of the more complex gout cases.

Prednisone (20 to 40 mg daily for up to 3 days, with subsequent rapid taper) can be successful. Local steroid injection is an additional therapeutic option.

IV. Asymptomatic hyperuricemia is arbitrarily defined as serum uric acid values that exceed the mean plus two standard deviations in an asymptomatic population. Therefore, by definition, 2.5% of the population will be affected. It should be stressed that most patients with hyperuricemia are asymptomatic and do not acquire renal or articular disease.

A. Diagnosis. Many clinical laboratories use an auto-analyzer colorimetric technique based on the ability of urate to reduce phosphotungstic acid. For men, the upper limit of a normal uric acid level is 8.0 mg/dL, and for women, it is 6.5 mg/dL. Several common substances, such as caffeine, vitamin C, and acetaminophen, produce spurious uric acid elevations with the colorimetric technique. The true serum uric acid level as measured by the uricase method is approximately 1 mg lower per deciliter than the value measured by the automated technique. Evaluation of the patient with asymptomatic hyperuricemia includes exclusion of drug effects or other conditions listed in Table 37-1. Diuretic therapy is a particularly common cause of uric acid elevation, which usually does not require treatment.

B. Treatment of asymptomatic hyperuricemia is a subject of controversy. No strong evidence has been offered that asymptomatic hyperuricemia results in chronic renal disease or joint deformity. Factors in the evaluation of the patient that might lead one to consider individualized therapy to lower serum uric acid include a family history of renal stones and the degree of hyperuricemia. Patients with repeated uric acid elevations above 10 mg/dL have an increased risk for development of gout or urolithiasis; probenecid or allopurinol therapy may be warranted. There is no established treatment protocol for lesser degrees of hyperuricemia, but the cost and possible toxicity of long-term allopurinol or uricosuric therapy argue against their routine use in patients with asymptomatic hyperuricemia and uric acid levels below 10 mg/dL. The risk for urolithiasis is less than 1% of patients per year. Although it is proposed that hyperuricemia may be a risk factor for the development of arterial hypertension and other cardiovascular abnormalities, the data are not sufficiently compelling to warrant treatment.

V. Interval gout is characterized by asymptomatic periods between acute gout attacks. Some patients never experience a second attack. In most patients, a second attack occurs within 6 months to 2 years (75% to 80%). Because the second attack or subsequent attacks cannot be predicted, most physicians take a conservative approach initially. Many patients will not need treatment. Factors that influence a decision to treat with uric acid-lowering agents include a history of renal calculi or uric acid excretion greater than 1,000 mg daily (see section **IV** for a complete discussion).

VI. Chronic gout is characterized by recurrent episodes of oligoarthritis and polyarticular arthritis, joint deformity, tophi, or urolithiasis. With the variety of medications available today for the treatment of hyperuricemia and acute gout attacks, the incidence of tophaceous gout is diminishing steadily.

A. Physical examination. Joint examination may reveal an asymmetric polyarthritis that can be very deforming and sometimes difficult to distinguish from RA. Tophi occur in approximately 15% of patients. The more common locations of tophi include the olecranon bursae, finger joints, and helix of the ear. To distinguish possible tophi on the helix of the ear from other entities, one may compress a microscope slide against the lesion, and if the lesion appears white in color, it is a tophus. If the lesion appears yellow in color, this usually signifies a sebaceous cyst, and finally, if the color is the same as the surrounding tissue, this represents normal cartilage. Material scraped or aspirated from tophi can be definitively identified with a polarizing microscope as discussed in section **III.B.1.** Destruction of cartilage by tophi may lead to secondary degenerative joint disease. Other rare locations of tophi that have been described include the vocal cords, heart valves, and spinal column in addition to the conduction system of the heart.

B. Laboratory studies

1. Serum studies

a. Uric acid. Elevated uric acid values occur in about 90% of gout patients.

b. Creatinine. Elevated levels may reflect gout-related nephropathy or primary renal disease.

2. Urine studies. Patients with primary gout can be subdivided into **over-excreters** of uric acid (15% of patients) and **normal excreters** based on quantitative urinary excretion of urate. On a regular diet, normal persons will excrete 300 to 800 mg of uric acid daily. The patient should be instructed to avoid alcohol or aspirin ingestion and to eat no more than one moderate serving of meat daily during the 3 days preceding the urine collection. Foods with a very high purine content, such as organ meats (liver and kidney) and anchovies, should also be avoided before the collection. A uric acid collection obtained during an acute gout attack is unreliable as a result of fluctuating serum acid levels not usually seen in the basal state.

3. Radiographs. Soft-tissue swelling and osteopenia may occur as nonspecific early changes on radiographs. As the disease progresses, soft-tissue tophi may be seen as well as punched-out, sharply marginated areas of bony destruction. Pure urate stones are radiolucent, and imaging studies must take this into account.

C. The **differential diagnosis** includes RA, osteoarthritis, and pseudogout. At times, it can be exceedingly difficult to distinguish rheumatoid nodules from tophi without the aid of a biopsy specimen or aspirate. The absence of crystals in the synovial fluid distinguishes chronic gout from osteoarthritis. The demonstration of calcium pyrophosphate crystals in synovial fluid as well as chondrocalcinosis on radiography may help to distinguish chronic gouty arthritis from pseudogout.

D. Complications. Pure urate stones are found in approximately 80% to 90% of all gout patients in whom urolithiasis develops, in comparison with 10% of the general population. Any patient with gout in whom urolithiasis develops should have recovered stones analyzed chemically, and a 24-hour urine specimen should be obtained for determination of uric acid, calcium, and phosphate excretion. Other diseases associated with stone formation include hyperparathyroidism, cystinuria, and renal tubular acidosis, all of which require appropriate serum and urine studies to elucidate the etiology of urolithiasis. The treatment of choice in nephrolithiasis of gout is allopurinol, which lowers both serum and urinary uric acid values. Patients should be encouraged to maintain high urine volumes, and particularly in large "over-producers" of uric acid, alkalinization of the urine is warranted.

E. Treatment

1. Patient education. It is important that the patient realize that gout is a chronic disease and that certain life-style modifications, such as maintenance of an ideal weight and moderation of alcohol intake, are important. A purine-restricted diet may be of benefit in some patients, but only small changes in serum uric acid can be attained. Other factors worth emphasizing are ingestion of at least 2 L of fluids daily to help prevent renal stones and avoidance of alcohol and low-dose aspirin, which aggravate hyperuricemia.

2. Drug therapy. The goals of therapy are to prevent renal parenchymal damage and nephrolithiasis and to suppress articular flares. Drug strategy in chronic gout is determined by the pattern of 24-hour urate excretion and the severity of disease.

a. Colchicine prophylaxis. Colchicine (0.6 mg daily or twice daily) is effective in diminishing the frequency and severity of spontaneous gout flares and flares induced by initial allopurinol and probenecid therapy. Colchicine may be discontinued after a 6-month symptom-free interval if allopurinol or probenecid has been started. Otherwise, it is continued indefinitely. In the elderly and those with impaired renal function, the dose is 0.6 mg daily. In dialysis patients, oral colchicine is generally best avoided. Some clinicians have abandoned long-term colchicine prophylaxis for several reasons. First, colchicine does not lower urate levels or prevent tophi. Second, acute attacks can be handled as described in section **III.D,** and oral colchicine at times can cause toxicity, including bone marrow suppression and myopathy. Third, no randomized controlled studies are available to demonstrate the benefit of colchicine alone as a preventive agent in interval gout.

b. Recurrent gout attacks are treated as described earlier (see section **III.D**). The patient may be given a supply of indomethacin (the drug of choice for acute attacks) with instructions to take 50 mg q6h at the first sign of a gout prodrome and to call the physician. When indomethacin is self-administered in this manner, a gout attack may be aborted with only two to three doses.

c. Uricosurics. The goal is to lower urate to approximately 6.0 mg/dL (auto-analyzer measurement). Most commonly, these drugs are used in patients less than 50 years of age.

(1) Indications (all must be present)

(a) Normal urate excreter (<800 mg/24 h).

(b) Normal renal function.

(c) Absence of tophi.

(d) No history of renal calculi.

(2) Administration. Prophylactic colchicine (0.6 mg twice daily) should begin 3 days before therapy. **Probenecid** is the uricosuric drug of choice. The initial dosage is 250 mg twice daily for 1 week. The dosage is increased to 500 mg two to three times daily depending on serum uric acid response. Adequate hydration must be maintained to prevent uric acid precipitation in renal tubules.

d. Allopurinol. The goal is to lower urate to approximately 6.0 mg/dL.

(1) Indications (only one need be present)

(a) Hyperexcretion of urate (>800 mg/24 h).

(b) History of renal calculi.

(c) Tophi.

(d) Renal insufficiency and gout.

(e) There is another indication for lowering urate, and uricosuric drugs are ineffective, not tolerated, or contraindicated.

(f) Before cytotoxic therapy for neoplasia.

(g) Continued attacks of gout despite colchicine prophylaxis, uricosuric drugs, or both. The severity of the gout attacks and the presence of radiographic joint damage are taken into consideration in the individual case.

(2) Administration. Prophylactic colchicine (0.6 mg twice daily) can be started 3 days before initiation of allopurinol therapy. Some clinicians avoid oral colchicine in this setting and treat any flares of gout with NSAIDs or corticosteroids. Colchicine is appropriate for patients in whom prevention of gouty attacks during the initiation of the allopurinol therapy is felt to be especially important. When colchicine prophylaxis is used in this setting, it is generally continued for 6 months. The initial allopurinol dosage is 100 mg daily, which is increased weekly until the maintenance dosage of 300 mg daily is reached. Dosages as high as 600 to 800 mg/d may be needed in a few patients to achieve clinical control. If the creatinine clearance is less than 20 mL/min, the toxicity (skin rash, vasculitis, agranulocytosis) of allopurinol increases. The dosage of allopurinol is decreased according to decreased renal function. For a glomerular filtration rate of 20 to 30 mL/min, the dose of allopurinol should be reduced to 100 mg/d.

(3) Allopurinol allergy. Oxypurinol (an active metabolite of allopurinol) has been shown to be as effective as allopurinol and can be used (by special release from the manufacturer) in patients with allopurinol allergy. However, cross-reactive allergy has occurred in as many as 50% of cases. IV and oral desensitization regimens for allopurinol have been published.

e. **Joint aspiration and intraarticular injection of corticosteroid** preparations may be indicated for patients with persisting chronic synovitis. The technique and dosage regimen are described in Chapter 4.

f. **Prevention of nephrolithiasis.** In patients with renal stones, the following measures may be used.

(1) **Urine alkalinization.** A urine pH greater than 6.0 can be achieved with one of the following:

(a) Sodium or potassium citrate (Polycitra) (20 mL four times daily). However, compliance with a regimen of dosing four times daily is difficult.

(b) Acetazolamide (500 mg at bedtime).

(2) **Large urine volume.** The patient should be instructed to drink adequate fluids to produce at least 2 L of urine daily.

g. **Surgical therapy.** Surgical removal of large tophi is indicated if they become infected or interfere with joint function.

VII. The **prognosis** of properly managed gout is excellent, and most patients have a normal life span. Chronic deforming arthritis and periarthritis can occur in long-standing untreated cases. In rare patients with severe tophaceous renal disease, chronic renal failure may develop.

Bibliography

Bomalaski J, Schumacher R. Podagra is more than gout. *Bull Rheum Dis* 1984;34:6.

Fam AG. "Problem" gout: clinical challenges, effective solutions. *J Musculoskeletal Med* 1997;14:63.

Kelley WM, Harris ED. *Textbook of rheumatology.* Philadelphia: WB Saunders, 1997.

38. PSEUDOGOUT (CALCIUM PYROPHOSPHATE DIHYDRATE CRYSTAL ARTHROPATHY)

Theodore R. Fields and Nicholas P. Scarpa

Pseudogout is an inflammatory arthropathy, with acute and chronic forms, caused by the deposition of calcium pyrophosphate dihydrate (CPPD) crystals in synovial structures. Chondrocalcinosis (calcified cartilage seen on radiographs), found in the majority of pseudogout patients, was first recognized in 1957 by Zitnan and Sitaj. McCarty in 1962 defined the relationship of intrasynovial CPPD crystals to chondrocalcinosis. The prevalence of pseudogout is not known. However, 8% of all people older than 60 years have radiographic evidence of chondrocalcinosis. The prevalence of chondrocalcinosis increases with age to involve as many as 28% of the population in the ninth decade. The mode of inheritance of CPPD is unsettled. However, an autosomal dominant pattern has been described in some populations in which disease begins in early adulthood, progresses rapidly, and is polyarticular.

I. **Pathogenesis.** Aging, osteoarthritis, genetic defects, and certain metabolic disorders are thought to induce abnormalities in cartilage that enhance deposition of CPPD crystals. Crystals are shed into the joint and undergo phagocytosis by leukocytes. The release lysosomal enzymes results in an acute inflammatory response. If inflammation persists, the cellular infiltrate of the synovium changes to a mononuclear pattern with fibroblastic proliferation in the chronic form of the disease.

Diseases associated with CPPD include hyperparathyroidism, hemochromatosis, hypophosphatasia, hypomagnesemia, gout, neuropathic arthropathy, and osteoarthritis. The association of CPPD with hypothyroidism is controversial. Diabetes has been shown *not* to be linked with pseudogout.

Osteoarthritis and chondrocalcinosis are both common disorders, and their exact relationship has not been established. It is possible that chrondrocalcinosis is a disease marker for certain cartilage changes in osteoarthritis.

II. **History.** CPPD deposition syndromes occur in the following clinical patterns:

A. **Acute pseudogout.** Acute monarthritis occurs in nearly 25% of patients with CPPD. Elderly women are afflicted more often then men. The knee is the most commonly involved joint. Ankle, wrist, and shoulder involvement is also common, and acromioclavicular pseudogout has been described. Attacks are usually self-limited, lasting several days to several weeks. Surgical procedures, especially parathyroidectomy, and severe medical illness may precipitate acute pseudogout attacks.

B. **Chronic pseudogout**

1. **Pseudo-rheumatoid arthritis.** This chronic polyarticular inflammation occurs in up to 5% of patients with CPPD deposition. In some patients, prominent symptoms of fatigue, malaise, and morning stiffness may also develop, making the distinction from rheumatoid arthritis difficult.
2. **Atypical osteoarthritis,** the most common pattern of CPDD arthropathy, tends to be distinguished from true osteoarthritis by the involvement of the wrists and metacarpophalangeal joints. Flexion contractures and periarticular tendinous involvement also occur in this subgroup of patients. Formation of osteophytes occurs, but it is not as exuberant as that seen with true osteoarthritis.

C. **Asymptomatic chondrocalcinosis** refers to the radiographic finding of calcified cartilage in patients without joint complaints. It is very common in the eighth decade and later.

D. **Pseudoneuropathic joints.** The deposition of CPPD crystals in the presence of destructive arthropathy, as seen in Charcot's joints, has been described.

This is usually a chronic relapsing arthropathy with a female predominance of 14:1 and associated with tendon ruptures, especially at the shoulder joints.

III. Physical examination

A. Articular features. Signs of inflammation are prominent, particularly in the knees, hips, and wrists. Involvement of the small joints of the hands and feet is less common.

B. Extraarticular features. Signs of other diseases associated with CPPD arthropathy may be present, such as skin pigmentation and the hepatomegaly of hemochromatosis or the band keratopathy and muscle weakness of hyperparathyroidism.

IV. Laboratory studies

A. Biochemical. There are no known specific biochemical abnormalities of pseudogout itself. The chemical abnormalities noted in other diseases associated with the development of pseudogout may, however, be present. These values include low serum levels of magnesium and phosphate in addition to elevated levels of calcium, ferritin, and uric acid. Low thyroxine levels are not any longer believed to be related to pseudogout.

B. Synovial fluid. Study of aspirated joint fluid is required to confirm the diagnosis. The white blood cell count ranges from 3,000 to 50,000, with 70% or more neutrophils. No organisms are present on Gram's stain. Results of cultures are negative. CPPD crystals can be identified with compensated polarized microscopy. CPPD crystals are rhomboid-shaped and exhibit weakly positive birefringence. These crystals can also be seen on light microscopy with use of alizarin red S stain.

C. Radiographs. Chondrocalcinosis can be demonstrated in approximately 75% of pseudogout patients. Fibrocartilage sites that are most likely to demonstrate chondrocalcinosis include knee menisci, the symphysis pubis, and the triangular cartilage of the wrist. Chondrocalcinosis appears as linear or punctate radiographic densities within cartilage. Subchondral bone cysts and hooklike osteophytes of metacarpophalangeal joints may also be observed.

V. Differential diagnosis

A. Disorders resembling acute pseudogout

1. **Gout.** The only absolute method of distinction is the characterization of crystals in synovial fluid. However, the simultaneous existence of both gout (monosodium urate crystals) and pseudogout (CPPD) can occur.
2. **Septic arthritis.** The finding of prominent systemic signs of infection, when present, may offer a clue to the diagnosis; aspiration of synovial fluid with Gram's stain and appropriate cultures are essential.
3. **Hydroxyapatite crystal deposition disease** may produce synovitis or tendinitis. Crystals may be seen with electron microscopy but not with routine polarizing microscopy. Therefore, the diagnosis must be made clinically. This disorder tends to develop in patients with calcifications of the shoulder area and patients on hemodialysis. In young, premenopausal women, goutlike inflammation of the first metatarsophalangeal joint, or pseudopodagra, may be caused by CPPD crystals.
4. **Other causes of monarthritis, including osteoarthritis and neuropathic arthropathy,** are reviewed in Chapter 9.

B. Metabolic disorders associated with syndromes of calcium pyrophosphate dihydrate deposition include hyperparathyroidism, hemochromatosis, ochronosis, gout, hypomagnesemia, Wilson's disease, and hypophosphatasia. Other associations include aging, osteoarthritis, neuropathic joints, trauma, and septic arthritis.

VI. Treatment. In the acute attacks of pseudogout, a combination of joint aspiration and drug therapy is very beneficial. The affected joint should be mobilized quickly so that patients do not suffer complications from prolonged joint inactivity.

A. Joint aspiration alone removes a significant quantity of inciting crystals and chemical mediators, thereby often allowing the synovitis to subside. In those with protracted courses, intraarticular injection of a long-acting corticosteroid preparation is usually beneficial.

B. Antiinflammatory drugs

1. **Indomethacin** (50 mg every 8 hours with tapering doses during 5 days) is usually effective.
2. **Other nonsteroidal antiinflammatory drugs (NSAIDs),** such as naproxen and sulindac, have efficacy similar to that of indomethacin and are often better tolerated in the elderly than is indomethacin.

C. Chronic pseudogout can be managed with NSAIDs and periodic intra-articular corticosteroid injections. Any associated diseases such as hemochromatosis and hyperparathyroidism should be managed appropriately, but treatment of the underlying disease may not prevent the recurrent attacks of arthropathy.

VII. Prophylaxis. Some evidence favors long-term prophylaxis with oral colchicine (0.6 mg PO twice daily) for patients with recurrent acute attacks. Several "letters to the editor" suggest a benefit of hydroxychloroquine, in doses similar to those used for rheumatoid arthritis, in preventing pseudogout flares.

VIII. Prognosis. Pseudogout itself has no known effect on life expectancy; associated diseases carry their own prognoses. Joint symptoms can be controlled by the treatment regimens outlined in section **VI.** Patients with associated osteoarthritis may eventually require prosthetic joints if symptoms and disability become chronic and severe.

Bibliography

Chaisson CE, et al. Lack of association between thyroid status and chondrocalcinosis or osteoarthritis: the Framingham osteoarthritis study. *J Rheumatol* 1996;23:711.

Ellman MH, Brown NL, Porat AP. Laboratory investigations in pseudogout patients and controls. *J Rheumatol* 1980;7:77.

McCarty DJ, ed. Conference on pseudogout and pyrophosphate metabolism. *Arthritis Rheum* 1976;19:275.

Utsinger PD, Zvaifler NJ, Resnick D. Calcium pyrophosphate dihydrate deposition disease without chondrocalcinosis. *J Rheumatol* 1975;2:258.

39. RHEUMATIC DISEASE IN PATIENTS INFECTED WITH THE HUMAN IMMUNODEFICIENCY VIRUS (AIDS)

Edward J. Parrish

It is not surprising that a number of musculoskeletal complaints and inflammatory phenomena develop in persons infected with the human immunodeficiency virus (HIV), given the fact that they are subject to a vast array of pathogens and have marked degrees of immune dysregulation, cytokine production, cell growth abnormalities, and a propensity to anaplasia. Although a clear picture of the epidemiology of rheumatic disease is not available, studies in small populations and anecdotal evidence persuade us not only that the occurrence of some of the following diseases is increased, but also that their manifestations (and therapies) may be altered by the presence of HIV and intercurrent HIV-related processes. Table 39-1 provides an overview of the range of rheumatic diseases reported in this population. What we cannot predict is the effect that aggressive antiretroviral therapy will have on these manifestations. At present, combination therapies are able to reduce dramatically the viral load in a sizable proportion of infected persons and to restore some immune capabilities in others. The rate of AIDS-related deaths and hospitalizations has declined throughout the United States, giving much hope. However, viral strains resistant to present drugs are emerging and spreading through the population. Further, impoverished countries lack the resources to provide effective therapies.

I. General approach to the HIV-infected patient with rheumatic complaints. The principles of sound medical practice apply as much in the diagnosis and therapeutics of the HIV-infected population as in uninfected persons. However, a few important features are worth emphasizing with this patient group.

- **A. Approach to diagnosis.** More often than not, the complaints of many patients are periarticular, enthesopathic, and "myofascial" rather than articular. The inability to define adequately the anatomic structures involved often frustrates the diagnostician. Therefore, a descriptive and generic approach to diagnosis is more helpful than are definitive classification systems until we learn more about the nature of these syndromes.
- **B. Suspicion of infection or neoplasia** should be paramount. Many phenomena are the direct result of these two underlying processes or will be unmasked by their presence. The clinical expression of infectious agents can be decidedly different in the immunosuppressed patient.
- **C. Complicating factors.** The incidence and array of neuropathies in particular are high. Neuropathy may coexist with or mimic a number of rheumatic diseases. Depression mimics and complicates rheumatic and neuropathic disease. Current drug regimens used to treat HIV-infected persons contain an impressive list of medications that cause both rheumatic and neurologic complaints. Likewise, the use of alcohol and illicit drugs notoriously produces a confounding range of pathology and should be thoroughly reviewed with all patients. Additionally, the use of "alternative" pharmaceuticals, megavitamins, herbs, and "health foods" by people with HIV is extensive. Like any ingested chemical, a number of these may cause or potentiate disease.
- **D. Interpretation of laboratory tests.** The frequency of auto-antibodies is increased in this population, reflecting the presence of chronic infections, immune dysregulation, and medication use. The physician should be particularly discriminating in the use and interpretation of laboratory tests, therefore, to avoid complicating rather than clarifying a diagnostic dilemma.
- **E.** The social problems faced by HIV-infected persons are often more debilitating than their physical problems. Ostracism from family and friends and loss of living quarters and jobs may make access to and compliance with medical care difficult. Even after all these years, prejudice and fear significantly challenge the medical community globally and personally.

Table 39-1. Rheumatologic disease in HIV-infected persons

Arthralgias
Painful articular syndromes
Osteonecrosis
Enthesopathy/periosteal syndromes
Hypertrophic osteoarthropathy
Arthritis
Reactive
Associated with HLA-B27
Not associated with HLA-B27
Psoriatic
Associated with AIDS
Septic
Myopathy
Vasculitis
Necrotizing
Eosinophilic
Leukocytoclastic
Angiitis of the central nervous system
Sicca syndrome
Diffuse infiltrative lymphocytosis syndrome
Autoimmune phenomena
Lupuslike syndromes

II. Musculoskeletal disorders in human immunodeficiency virus infection

A. Myopathy

1. **Clinical spectrum.** The occurrence of myopathy is one of the most striking features of HIV disease. It is likely the most common rheumatologic problem encountered, yet it is often overlooked because of its highly variable expression. The majority of cases are silent and found incidentally as transient increases in muscle enzymes. Typically, symptoms and findings will wax and wane with little persistent clinical consequence. Pain is often absent, or the patient will complain of "achiness." Rarely, the pain may be debilitating. Although the distribution is usually proximal, as in idiopathic polymyositis, it can be distal and in this form is frequently confused with neuropathy. Indeed, superimposed neurogenic complaints and findings are common. Sometimes, atrophy will gradually develop in the muscle groups involved. Dysfunction may lead to falling or inability to ambulate.
2. **Prevalence.** Myalgia has been reported in 10% to 35% of patients, and the incidence of muscle atrophy was 6% in one cohort.
3. **Pathology.** The range of histologic findings in muscle from HIV-infected patients is broad. Of note, most biopsy specimens have features indistinguishable from those of idiopathic autoimmune polymyositis—that is, variation in fiber size, often with an inflammatory mononuclear cell infiltrate. Frank necrosis may be present and associated with polymorphonuclear cell infiltration. Nemaline rods may be present, usually without inflammation. Red ragged fibers were found only in patients treated with azidothymidine (AZT). These have been seen in other diseases also, especially thyroid-associated myopathy, and are therefore not specific for drug-induced disease. Pyomyositis, a disorder often caused by *Staphylococcus aureus* and previously limited to the tropics, is increased in the HIV population. Nonpyogenic infectious agents may infiltrate muscle locally or diffusely. Neoplastic infiltration, especially with lymphoma, is not uncommon.
4. **Etiology.** The waxing and waning nature of the complaints and findings of muscle disease in the HIV-infected population suggests that underlying low-grade myopathy may be quite common but of little consequence. This implies

that for clinically significant disease to develop, additional insults are likely. Inciting factors may include drugs, intercurrent infection, or fever.

a. **Drug toxicity**
   (1) **Azidothymidine** has been shown to cause an inflammatory myositis in humans. The defect appears at the mitochondrial level and is manifested by the appearance of red ragged fibers and loss of specific mitochondrial peptides.
   (2) **Other therapeutic agents.** Sulfonamides, penicillin, rifampin, phenytoin, cimetidine, and chloroquine are just a few of the medications that have been associated with myopathy. Although these drugs rarely cause muscle disease, they should be considered especially when significant muscle impairment develops with a temporal relationship to the use of new medications.
   (3) **Alcohol and illicit drugs.** In the rush to look for other causes of myopathy, one must remember that the use of recreational drugs is common in many persons infected with HIV. Besides ethanol, the most common offenders are cocaine, crack, and mixtures of heroin. The extent to which these drugs, even in small quantities, contribute to significant myopathy is not fully appreciated.

b. **Infectious causes.** Besides HIV itself, a number of infectious agents appear frequently in HIV-infected persons, in particular mycobacteria, Microsporidia, *Toxoplasma,* hepatitis B virus, hepatitis C virus, and human T-cell lymphotropic virus type I (HTLV-I).

5. **Differential diagnosis.** It is important to differentiate myopathic processes from a number of conditions that may mimic or exacerbate their manifestations. Above all, consider infection. Although the incidence of direct infection is not common, it is sufficient to require diligence. Most importantly, neuropathy may cause concomitant atrophy and weakness in addition to associated pain; these findings can be virtually indistinguishable on clinical grounds from those of a primary myopathic process. Enthesopathy and periostitis, especially in the distal femur, can produce a confusing picture. Bursitis and arthritis, especially of the shoulder and pelvic girdle, can mimic muscle disease. Rarely, soft-tissue processes such as erythema nodosum or phlegmon may lead some to consider a localized infectious myositis. Underlying osteomyelitis could be difficult to distinguish from primary muscle disease. Adrenal insufficiency is common in HIV-infected persons. Although it does not cause muscle disease itself, one of the most common complaints of the steroid-deficient person is myalgia.

6. **History and physical examination.** The clinician will most often be rewarded by focusing on the temporal relationship between the onset of muscle disease and the introduction of new medications or other clinical changes. When this is not fruitful and especially when the onset is abrupt, a strong suspicion for occult infection or malignancy should be pursued, whether or not fever is present. Virtually any such process can be local or diffuse. Tenderness is more indicative of an inflammatory process, although hyperesthesia from a neuropathy can occur.

7. **Laboratory studies**
   a. **Electrolyte abnormalities.** Weakness or frank myonecrosis can occur from alterations in potassium, phosphorus, calcium, or magnesium levels. Patients with metabolic abnormalities or those with nutritional deficiencies may demonstrate such findings.
   b. **Muscle enzymes.** Creatine kinase (CK) and aldolase are the most common and sensitive indicators of muscle damage. Either may be elevated exclusively. In general, the CK level should be checked first and aldolase measured as needed if the CK level is not elevated and clinical suspicion is high. In the face of intercurrent infection, trauma, fever, or use of cocaine or alcohol, the CK level may become dramatically elevated. Typically, after the insult has been eliminated, CK will return to the normal range within a few days.

c. **Biopsy and imaging.** Biopsy should be considered whenever infection is suspected or when clinical deterioration continues in the face of therapy. Additionally, muscle biopsy should be considered before the patient is committed to long-term immunosuppressive medications. As in idiopathic autoimmune polymyositis, biopsy may miss the areas of involvement. The probability of a diagnostic biopsy may be enhanced by the use of imaging techniques. Magnetic resonance imaging (MRI) has been shown to be particularly sensitive in the definition of inflammatory and infiltrative muscle disease. Additionally, ultrasonography and radionuclide techniques with gallium or technetium pyrophosphate can be helpful.

8. **Treatment**

a. **What to treat.** Because of the multiplicity of causes and the waxing and waning nature of muscle disease in this population, the fortuitous finding of myopathy by laboratory criteria does not in itself require intervention. CK elevations in particular often do not correlate with complaints or physical findings and may persist at even high levels without clinical significance. Pain and weakness are the main reasons for initiating therapy.

b. **Modalities**

(1) The patient should **discontinue any offending agents,** particularly alcohol, illicit drugs, and any medications that are not absolutely necessary.

(2) **Treatment of infection.** Any direct infection of muscle or any intercurrent infection should be treated.

(3) **Antiretroviral therapy** is indicated for those patients with HIV-related myositis who are not presently on a medication regimen.

(4) **Pain relief.** Symptomatic relief of pain is often required. This is particularly true in muscle disease, in which pain leads to disuse and disuse leads to atrophy. Mild analgesics may be sufficient, but often nonsteroidal antiinflammatory drugs (NSAIDs) are necessary to resolve the symptoms.

(5) **Physical and occupational therapy** should be started early to prevent wasting and contractures.

(6) **Intravenous immune globulin** works quickly and may be administered at necessary intervals, with months between treatments often possible in some patients.

(7) **Steroid therapy.** When the above measures have failed or when complaints and dysfunction progressively worsen, steroid therapy at low dose appears to have dramatic results and is well tolerated. Prednisone (30 mg daily tapered to 10 mg daily during a 10-day period) is satisfactory for most patients. One may then switch to an alternate-day therapeutic schedule with further tapering as the patient can tolerate. The toxicity of low-level steroid maintenance therapy for several months is not yet known. Within days of initiation of steroid therapy, however, exacerbation of mucocutaneous candidiasis and reactivation of herpes simplex are seen. Usually, these abate with steroid taper and antifungal or antiherpes regimens, respectively. There is presently no role for cytotoxic drug therapy.

c. **When to stop azidothymidine.** AZT is being used less and less in antiretroviral cocktails. However, in those who presently have good retroviral suppression on AZT, discontinuation of the drug must be weighed against the benefit it confers. Cessation for even brief periods has been shown to lead to overgrowth of resistant virus that cannot be suppressed by reinstitution of AZT. Discontinuing AZT is helpful in resolving myopathy in only 50% of the cases in which it is suspected of being a factor. AZT-induced cardiomyopathy is the most serious consequence and demands discontinuation of the drug.

B. **Human immunodeficiency virus-associated painful articular syndromes**

1. **Definition and differentiation.** These syndromes are unique to HIV-infected persons. They are among the most common musculoskeletal mani-

festations but because of the paucity of anatomic findings are the most difficult to delineate. It is convenient to distinguish them arbitrarily from HIV-associated arthropathy by the absence of joint effusions. The clinical presentations require differentiation from enthesopathy, periostitis, myositis, and neuropathy, although these may coexist. One may discern two types on clinical grounds:

a. **Acute.** The acute painful articular syndrome is dramatic. Typically, the patient is carried by friends into the emergency department and complains of the rapid onset of pain in the knees or ankles. It is frequently symmetric. The physical findings are unimpressive except that the patient may not be able to stand. Response to NSAIDs is poor. Often, narcotics are required for pain control. The symptoms abate within 2 to 24 hours, although they may last for a few days. The recovery is with minimal residuum.

b. **Subacute.** Typically, this syndrome has a gradual onset during a period of a few weeks. It too has a predilection for knees and ankles. At times, it appears as a classic patellofemoral syndrome and may be accompanied by some degree of quadriceps femoris atrophy. Often, direct palpation in the area of complaint will elicit diffuse tenderness of muscle, tendons, and bone, suggesting myositis, enthesitis, or periostitis. Most cases gradually resolve during weeks or months and require minimal intervention. Some are progressive and lead to significant debility.

2. **Pathology.** Little is known about the etiology of these syndromes, but recurrent ischemia may be an underlying factor. This is supported by the following evidence:

a. The acute form is most reminiscent of the musculoskeletal pain of a sickle cell crisis in its rapidity of onset and resolution, and in the poor correlation between the severity of complaints and the physical findings.

b. Necropsy specimens of knee synovium show effacement consistent with recurrent ischemic insult.

c. Some have suggested a predilection toward osteonecrosis in HIV-infected patients. Although no studies have been performed to support this claim, anecdotes of extensive aseptic necrosis in persons without other known predisposing factors tend to support this possibility.

3. **Treatment**

a. **Acute.** Response to NSAIDs is poor as a rule, although the use of IM ketorolac may hold promise. Otherwise, narcotic analgesia usually suffices until the episode abates.

b. **Subacute.** NSAIDS are variably helpful; usually indomethacin is required for sufficient control. At times, the level of disability is so severe that a trial of systemic steroid is warranted. Usually, this produces dramatic relief. Steroids often may be tapered rapidly to minimal dosage and discontinued during 1 week.

C. Human immunodeficiency virus-associated arthropathy

1. **Clinical presentation.** This resembles the subacute form of the painful articular syndrome, but joint effusion is present. Indeed, it may likely be a continuum of the same process. Symptoms develop during a period of weeks and abate, usually within a month. There is a predilection for the lower extremities, and the pain may be quite severe, with direct distal femur tenderness. The joint fluid is typically not inflammatory ($<10^3$ cells per milliliter), although the patient may respond dramatically to intraarticular steroid. As an important distinction from classic presentations of reactive arthritis, these patients do not possess the HLA-B27 major histocompatibility complex (MHC) class I phenotype and do not demonstrate the extraarticular manifestations of Reiter's syndrome (i.e., conjunctivitis, urethritis).

2. **Pathology.** Although the joint fluid is not inflammatory, synovial biopsy in these patients usually shows some degree of mononuclear and plasma cell infiltrate. This is usually mild and seldom of the severity seen in other forms of inflammatory arthropathy. Periosteal reaction may be found on

radiographs, and these patients may have hypertrophic osteoarthropathy. For this reason, it is prudent to exclude intercurrent infection, especially of a pulmonic source, in these patients. It is tempting to view this syndrome as part of a continuum of periarticular ischemia that produces the acute painful articular syndromes.

D. Reactive arthropathy

1. **Clinical syndromes.** Since the first description by Winchester and coworkers in 1987, no group of rheumatic syndromes has been the topic of so much discussion as the reactive arthritides in patients infected with HIV. The central issue has been whether HIV contributes to reactive arthritis. The arguments obviously hinge on the question of whether there is indeed an increased incidence of reactive arthritis in the HIV-infected population. The difficulty of comparing equivalent populations, the lack of adequate diagnostic criteria for some disease states, and the incomplete manifestation of some syndromes have hampered the resolution of this question. The best study, which prospectively evaluated all patients in an infectious disease clinic, concluded that incomplete Reiter's syndrome and enthesopathy were increased in frequency in HIV-infected patients. This does not, however, imply a direct causal role for HIV in the arthropathy. The advent of highly effective antiretroviral therapies has not resolved the question. One might explain an increased incidence on the basis of exposure to or persistence of the same pathogens (*Chlamydia* and enteric pathogens) known to elicit reactive arthritis in non–HIV-infected persons.

   The spectrum of reactive arthropathy or spondyloarthropathy is impressive. Findings range from frank synovitis to enthesitis and axial skeleton involvement. Extraarticular manifestations include dermal (psoriasiform, keratoderma blennorrhagicum, circinate balanitis), ocular (conjunctivitis, uveitis), mucosal (palatine and buccal ulcerations), genital (urethritis, cervicitis, prostatitis), and intestinal involvement. Any combination of findings may coexist. In the HIV-infected patient, two categories are frequently found—the post-infectious and psoriasis-related reactive type of arthritides.

   a. **Post-infectious**

      (1) **Enteric pathogens.** Infection with an array of enteric pathogens is common in HIV disease. Chronic or recurrent diarrhea is virtually the norm, and the causes are legion. There appears to be an increased frequency of salmonellosis. Small-bowel biopsy in some patients reveals lesions similar to those found in Whipple's disease, raising the question of whether other bowel flora such as mycobacteria may result in systemic disease.

      (2) **Venereal infection.** The high incidence of sexually transmitted diseases in the HIV-infected population is mirrored in the increased frequency of gonococcal and chlamydial infection. There is evidence that gonococcal and chlamydial products may persist in joint fluids in persons with arthritis. Some have suggested that inadequate therapy and other host factors lead to incomplete eradication. It is unclear whether HIV infection is associated with persistence of these agents or their products.

   b. **Psoriatic.** There is an increase in both the frequency and severity of all forms of psoriasis in HIV-infected patients. This includes the vulgaris, pustular, and erythroderma forms. There is also an increase in the extra-dermatologic manifestations of the disease, including arthritis. Interestingly, the extra-dermatologic disease tends to follow patterns more commonly associated with variants of Reiter's syndrome, including an increased incidence of conjunctivitis, urethritis, and enthesopathy. No excess of HLA antigens associated with classic psoriasis has been found in this group; indeed there was an increase in HLA-B27. Thus, the line between psoriatic and reactive arthropathy is indistinct in the HIV-infected population.

2. **Treatment**
   a. **Nonsteroidal antiinflammatory drugs** are often sufficient to control both joint and extraarticular manifestations of the disease. Long-term use is usually required. Many cases will respond only to indomethacin, as has been found in non–HIV-infected persons with similar complaints. Cyclooxygenase-2 (COX-2) inhibitors may show promise in this population.
   b. **Sulfasalazine,** increasingly used to treat Reiter's syndrome in the non-HIV population, has been shown anecdotally to be helpful in achieving disease control in patients unresponsive to NSAID therapy alone. Dosages of 1 to 2 g/d are often adequate.
   c. **Etretinate.** This medication was incidentally found to relieve joint symptoms in patients with psoriasis. It appears to be helpful in those without overt skin disease but with enthesopathy. Its use must be weighed against possible hepatic and hematologic toxicity.
   d. **Gold.** Parenteral gold was reported to be effective in one patient with Reiter's arthropathy and another with the psoriatic form. Although studies have suggested its utility in psoriatic arthropathy in non–HIV-infected persons, it does not appear to have a role in Reiter's syndrome.
   e. **Immunosuppressive and cytotoxic therapy.** Anecdotes reporting the onset of AIDS, opportunistic infection, Kaposi's sarcoma, and death in some patients soon after the institution of methotrexate or azathioprine has led to the widespread notion that these agents are contraindicated in HIV-infected patients. Prudence would require exhaustion of other modalities and the presence of significant debility before a course of therapy with either agent was undertaken.
   f. **Antibiotics.** Recent studies suggest that efforts to eradicate gonococci and *Chlamydia* with long-term (3 months) antibiotic therapy appear to resolve or relieve reactive arthritis. Most studies have chosen tetracycline derivatives, which incidentally have antiphlogistic properties. It would be reasonable, after thorough culture and use of DNA probes, to consider doxycycline in persons with persistent joint disease. Doxycycline is known to inhibit certain matrix metallo protease (MMP) enzyme systems.

E. **Sicca syndrome**

1. **Clinical presentation.** Xerostomia and xerophthalmia are common in HIV-infected patients and can be quite severe. This can further compromise their otherwise tenuous nutritional state by causing a decrease in caloric intake. Often, the causes are multifactorial, including an array of medications (neuroleptic agents, NSAIDs, antibiotics) and infection (*Candida*). In a number of HIV-infected patients, however, features consistent with Sjögren's syndrome develop, including parotitis with an inflammatory cell infiltrate within salivary glands. The infiltrating mononuclear cells are CD8+ lymphocytes rather than the CD4+ cells of classic autoimmune Sjögren's syndrome. Further, there is a notable absence of the auto-antibodies (anti-Ro, anti-La) classically found in the idiopathic syndrome. A subset of patients manifests far more extensive visceral involvement by CD8+ lymphocytes, especially of the lungs, gastrointestinal system, and central nervous system. This has been designated **diffuse infiltrative lymphocytosis syndrome.**
2. **Treatment.** Avoidance of medications that exacerbate xerostomia and xerophthalmia is important. In particular, the physician should find substitutes for, or eliminate, antihistamines, decongestants, NSAIDs, antihypertensives, tricyclic antidepressants, and other anticholinergic agents. Aggressive treatment of candidiasis is important. Instructing the patient to use dietetic gelatin lozenges and increase fluid intake with meals may help. Use of topical methylcellulose lacrimal substitutes will often prevent corneal abrasion.

F. **Autoimmune phenomena.** Much interest has been generated by the finding of auto-antibodies and immune complexes in patients with HIV. Antinuclear antibodies, rheumatoid factor, anti-platelet antibodies, and direct anti-globulin (Coombs') antibodies are examples. A few have clinical significance, including those associated with the development of anemia and thrombocytopenia. Anti-phospholipid antibodies occur in 85% of HIV-infected persons; however, they do not appear to be associated with as high a frequency of thrombotic events as in non–HIV-infected patients with the anti-phospholipid syndrome.

G. **Lupuslike syndrome.** The plethora of autoimmune laboratory findings coupled with an array of cutaneous, articular, central nervous system, and visceral inflammatory disease has, at times, produced some diagnostic uncertainty. Often, particularly when HIV infects young women, the clinical and laboratory manifestations may be virtually indistinguishable from those of systemic lupus erythematosus. Fortunately, in the majority of HIV-infected persons who are positive for antinuclear antibodies, they are present in very low titers, and rarely, if ever, is anti–ds-DNA antibody demonstrated. Patients with collagen vascular disease often have cross-reacting antibodies against constituents of the HIV or cells infected with HIV, which leads to false-positive results of assays for HIV antibodies. Typically, however, they demonstrate antibodies to only one or two proteins of HIV on Western blot, not to products of all three major retroviral genes (gag, pol, and env) simultaneously. Therefore, in patients in whom such a question arises, it is important to inform the laboratory technologist and define the actual Western blot pattern.

H. **Vasculitis.** Vasculitides of various sorts have been documented in patients with HIV. The presence of necrotizing vasculitides such as polyarteritis nodosa is often a harbinger of rapid demise. Leukocytoclastic angiitis and eosinophilic vasculitides of small and medium vessels are seen more frequently. Isolated angiitis of the central nervous system may play a role in the development of stroke or dementia in these patients. Hepatitis B and C viruses have been implicated in the development of necrotizing and cryoglobulinemic vasculitides, respectively. Modalities directed at control of viral replication in both of these entities have met with disappointing results to date.

III. **Additional observations**

A. **Cytomegalovirus** produces a vasculitis by direct infection and necrosis of the vascular endothelium. This may mimic noninfectious vasculitis.

B. **Endocarditis** is well-known for its array of immune clinical syndromes, including arthritis, leukocytoclastic vasculitis, stroke, and glomerulonephritis. Certainly, in the population using IV drugs, it remains a common cause of morbidity and mortality.

C. **Syphilis** continues to live up to its "accolade" as the great imitator. In the presence of HIV, reactivation can occur and the clinical presentation may be quite atypical. Lues, especially in the secondary stages, may have an associated arthropathy.

D. The use of **interferon-alfa** appears to predispose to autoimmune disease and serologic phenomena, particularly thyroid abnormalities. With its use in the treatment of Kaposi's sarcoma and as an antiretroviral agent, we might expect an increase in these features as patients live longer.

E. **Lymphoma** often takes atypical forms in patients with HIV infection. In particular, destructive bony or joint lesions often mimic infectious or inflammatory lesions. Localized infiltration of muscle may cause a mass lesion, pain, or weakness. Paraneoplastic syndromes include arthropathy, myopathy, vasculitis, and neuropathy.

F. **Erythema nodosum** may be confused with a phlegmon, infiltrative mass lesions, or arthritis, depending on its location and appearance. Post-infectious, intercurrent mycobacterial or paraneoplastic stimuli for erythema nodosum are common in the HIV-infected population.

G. **Parvovirus infection** is associated with a rheumatoid-like polyarticular arthritis in non–HIV-infected adults. Some observers feel that it may play a role in bone marrow suppression during HIV infection.

H. **Mycobacteria, tuberculous and atypical forms,** may cause joint infection by direct extension or hematogenous spread. Atypical forms may be isolated from blood or joint fluid. Tubercle bacilli are somewhat more difficult to isolate; if they are strongly suspected, synovial membrane biopsy with tissue culture and histologic assessment may be required. Unlike the clinical picture in persons not infected with HIV, osteomyelitis caused by atypical mycobacteria may proceed with rapid destruction of bone.

I. Lipodystrophy syndromes increasingly reported with the use of protease inhibitor therapy can give the appearance of muscle wasting.

Bibliography

Berman A, et al. Rheumatic manifestations in populations at risk for HIV infection: the added effect of HIV. *J Rheumatol* 1991;18:1564.

Cuellar ML. HIV infection-associated inflammatory musculoskeletal disorders. *Rheum Dis Clin North Am* 1998;24:403.

Espinoza LR, et al. Rheumatic manifestations associated with human immunodeficiency virus infection. *Arthritis Rheum* 1989;32:1615.

Itescu S, et al. A diffuse infiltrative CD8 lymphocytosis syndrome in human immunodeficiency virus (HIV) infection: a host immune response associated with HLA-DR5. *Ann Intern Med* 1990;112:3.

Rynes RI, et al. Acquired immunodeficiency syndrome-associated arthritis. *Am J Med* 1988;84:810.

Winchester R, et al. The co-occurrence of Reiter syndrome and acquired immunodeficiency. *Ann Intern Med* 1987;106:19.

40. INFECTIOUS ARTHRITIS

Barry D. Brause

I. Diagnosis and therapy
The clinical presentation, course, and prognosis in patients with septic arthritis are determined by the interaction of specific pathogens and host inflammatory responses with the involved synovial tissue, cartilage, and bone. Early recognition of the pathologic process along with timely, appropriate medical and surgical intervention can neutralize the destruction and provide a favorable functional outcome.

II. Pathogenesis. Invasion of the synovial membrane by microorganisms is the initial event in all pyogenic arthritides involving native (nonprosthetic) articulations. Subsequently, infection extends into the joint space, where a paucity of phagocytes, antibodies, and complement permits a closed-space infection to be established. As the pathologic process continues, the avascular cartilage is degraded by bacterial and leukocyte enzymes. The infection progresses at a rate determined by the virulence of the pathogen, the nature and extent of the inflammatory reaction, and the vulnerability of the underlying host tissue. Polymorphonuclear leukocytes, recruited by microbial chemotactic factors, appear to be essential for the evolution of tissue destruction. Inflamed hypertrophic synovium becomes an aggressive form of granulation tissue (pannus), which expands throughout the entire articulation. Irreversible loss of joint function is related to the extent of cartilaginous dissolution and subsequent overgrowth of adjacent osseous tissue.

III. Routes of infection. Microbial arthritis can arise by three routes of infection: hematogenous seeding, extension from sepsis in adjacent tissue, and implantation. Infections of the skin and soft tissues, genitourinary tract, respiratory tract, and gastrointestinal tract can spread to the synovial membrane through the bloodstream. Local septic processes in tissue contiguous to the joint, such as cellulitis, infected skin ulcerations, paronychia, infected synovial cysts, and osteomyelitis, can invade synovial membranes by direct extension. Microorganisms can be introduced into articular tissue through traumatic injury, arthrocentesis, intraarticular injections, and orthopedic surgery.

IV. Predisposing factors include the following (approximate frequencies appear in parentheses):

A. Extraarticular infection (25% to 50%).

B. Previous damage to joint resulting from rheumatoid arthritis, degenerative joint disease, crystal-induced arthritis, systemic lupus erythematosus, neuropathic arthropathy, trauma, or surgery (27%).

C. Serious underlying chronic illness, usually associated with impaired immunologic defenses, including malignancy, diabetes mellitus, hepatic cirrhosis, and parenteral drug abuse (19%).

D. Immunosuppressive or corticosteroid therapy (50%).

V. Clinical presentation

A. Articular. The acute onset of joint pain is the most characteristic symptom, with increasing severity on flexion, extension, or weight bearing. Articular pain is induced by even minimal degrees of joint motion. Arthralgia produced only by extreme flexion or extreme extension is suggestive of periarticular inflammation, as seen in septic bursitis. Local soft-tissue swelling, tenderness, erythema, and warmth accompany a restricted range of motion in the involved articulation. Fever is an almost constant feature of pyarthrosis (90% of cases), and systemic sepsis with septic shock can occur with particularly virulent pathogens in vulnerable patients. Synovial effusions are present in 90% of cases. Bacterial arthritis usually affects only one joint; however, polyarticular infection is seen in 10% of patients and frequently reflects concomitant bacteremia. Knees and hips are the most commonly infected joints, but septic arthritis in parenteral drug abusers often affects the sternoclavicular, sacroiliac, or shoulder articulations. Sepsis within the hip joint can be difficult to diagnose, as focal symptoms may be minimal and effusions undemonstrable. Viral arthritides commonly involve multiple joints, particularly in the hands and wrists. Mycobacterial and fungal arthritides generally have a subacute or chronic clinical presentation.

B. Dermatitis-arthritis syndromes. Certain pyarthroses are accompanied by dermatologic manifestations along with articular involvement. This presentation is most commonly recognized with *Neisseria gonorrhoeae* and *Haemophilus influenzae.* Gonococcal arthritis often is associated with prodromal or concomitant tenosynovitis and erythematous papular, vesiculopustular, or petechial skin rashes characteristic of the disseminated stage of gonococcemia. *H. influenzae* pyarthrosis can be associated with tenosynovitis and erysipeloid, pustular, or petechial rashes. Similar presentations have been described for bacterial arthritis associated with *Neisseria meningitidis* and *Streptobacillus moniliformis* (rat bite fever). The pathognomonic appearance of erythema chronicum migrans can be essential for the diagnosis of early *Borrelia burgdorferi* arthritis (Lyme disease), which is discussed in Chapter 41. Exanthems are important features in the presentation of viral arthritis associated with rubella and hepatitis B.

VI. Laboratory studies

A. The peripheral blood white blood cell (WBC) count is normal in 30% of patients.

B. Culture all possible foci of infection (sputum, urine, skin lesions, oropharynx, urethra, uterine cervix, rectum), and obtain at least two blood cultures. Specific culture media for gonococci (Thayer-Martin or chocolate agars) should be employed in addition to routine media for specimens from mucosal surfaces and skin lesions. In 49% of cases, the same organism is cultured from an extra-articular site and the joint.

C. Radiographs of the joint should be obtained to document the extent of previous damage, observe for evidence of osteomyelitis, and provide a baseline for follow-up studies. The earliest radiographic sign of joint infection is periarticular soft-tissue swelling with displacement of the adjacent fat pads by synovial edema or an articular effusion during the first week of pyarthrosis. After this period, periarticular osteopenia (subchondral bone rarefaction) develops as a result of local hyperemia in addition to bone atrophy secondary to relative immobility. With more fulminant infection, uniform joint space narrowing becomes visible by radiography as a consequence of articular cartilage dissolution. Subsequently, osseous erosions, induced by pannus, can be seen in subchondral sites or in peripheral areas between the joint capsule insertion and the joint cartilage, where the synovium is in direct contact with bone. Eventually, fibrous or bony ankylosis may develop in chronic infections. Radiologic evaluation of the infected joint is helpful but not diagnostic, as these anatomic changes are not specific for septic processes.

D. Radioisotope bone scans may be of value in diagnostic problems involving deep-seated joints such as hip, shoulder, or spine. However, the findings are not specific, and the scan usually has little role in the initial evaluation of acute infectious arthritis.

VII. Arthrocentesis.

Aspiration of synovial fluid is mandatory for any joint inflammation in which infection is a possibility. Initial aspiration is by closed-needle technique, with a needle large enough (16- to 18-gauge) to permit recovery of thick, purulent material (see Chapter 4 for details of joint aspiration). Hip joint sepsis represents an exception to this approach. In this situation, a radiographically guided aspiration may be more appropriate, and assessment should include an orthopedic surgical evaluation because arthroscopic or open surgical drainage may be necessary.

Synovial fluid analysis is the basis for initiation of therapy and confirmation of the specific microbiologic diagnosis (Table 40-1). The following studies are

Table 40-1. Synovial fluid analysis

	Normal	Inflammation	Bacterial infection
Color	Colorless, pale yellow	Yellow	Yellow
Turbidity	Slight	Turbid	Turbid, purulent
Leukocyte count	200–1,000	1,000–10,000	10,000– >100,000
Cell type	Mononuclear	Neutrophils	Neutrophils
Synovial fluid/blood			
Glucose	0.8–1.0	0.5–0.8	<0.5
Gram's stain	Negative	Negative	Positive (65%)
Culture	Negative	Negative	Positive

ranked in order of importance; if the size of the synovial fluid sample is small, culture and Gram's stain receive priority.

A. Culture. Optimally, fluid should be inoculated onto media promptly at the bedside, or the sample should be promptly delivered to the laboratory for immediate incubation. Media should be selected for gram-positive and gram-negative aerobes (blood agar and MacConkey agar), *N. gonorrhoeae* and *H. influenzae* (chocolate agar or Thayer-Martin agar), anaerobes (thioglycolate broth), and, if indicated, fungi and mycobacteria. Cultures of synovial fluid confirm the specific etiologic microorganism in all bacterial arthritides except in gonococcal infection, in which only 50% positivity is found, and the diagnosis is then made on the basis of urethral, cervical, pharyngeal, and rectal cultures or the presence of tenosynovitis and the characteristic skin lesions of disseminated gonococcemia. The age-related incidence of bacterial agents in septic arthritis is seen in Table 40-2.

B. Gram's stain. Pending the results of cultures, the Gram's stain is the cornerstone of initial antibiotic selection (see section **VII. A**).

C. Cell count and differential. Synovial fluid leukocytosis with predominance of neutrophils is common, but the range of WBC counts is wide (6,800 to 250,000 cells). The probability of infection increases with higher WBC counts; 40% of patients with bacterial arthritis have synovial fluid WBC counts greater than 100,000, whereas rheumatoid arthritis and crystal-induced arthritis rarely produce these counts.

Note: Gout and pseudogout crystals can be found in the synovial fluids of patients with septic arthritis.

D. Synovial fluid glucose. In septic joints, this value is usually less than 50% of simultaneous serum levels; however, this relationship holds only for fasting specimens because postprandial blood glucose may not equilibrate promptly with synovial fluid. The synovial fluid glucose level is reduced in only 50% of infected patients, and reductions can be seen in uninfected, inflamed joints in patients with rheumatoid arthritis.

Table 40-2. Age-related bacteriology of septic arthritis

Microorganism	<2 y	2–15 y	16–50 y	>50 y
Staphylococcus aureus	40%	50%	15%	70%
Streptococci	25%	30%	5%	15%
Haemophilus	30%[a]	9%[a]	—	—
Neisseria gonorrhoeae	—	5%	75%	—
Gram-negative bacilli	3%	5%	5%	8%

[a] *Haemophilus* no longer seen with high frequency in children vaccinated with *Haemophilus influenzae,* type b vaccine.

E. **Countercurrent immunoelectrophoresis** can rapidly detect antigens from pneumococci, meningococci, and *H. influenzae* in joint fluid (and urine) and is helpful in establishing the microbiologic diagnosis. Countercurrent immunoelectrophoresis can be diagnostic when prior antibiotic therapy interferes with routine cultures.

VIII. Initial treatment

A. **Antibiotic therapy,** empirically based on Gram's stain results, is summarized in Table 40-3. Administration should be initiated promptly and parenterally to ensure reliable serum levels. Most antimicrobial agents achieve effective synovial fluid levels with parenteral dosing; therefore, intraarticular instillation or irrigation is not indicated and may be hazardous. Antibiotics injected directly into the joint space can cause a chemical synovitis and can be absorbed systemically, resulting in potentially toxic serum levels.

B. **Joint immobilization** (usually in extension) should be employed only initially when joint pain is incapacitating. As soon as possible, range of motion exercises should be started (without weight bearing), as this technique may enhance nutritional diffusion to cartilage and assist in restoring natural cartilage repair mechanisms inhibited by immobilization. Such exercises should also prevent the development of contractures. Weight bearing should be avoided until joint inflammation has resolved substantially to reduce the risk for damage to articular cartilage.

C. **Analgesics** that do not affect fever should be used, such as codeine (30 mg q4h). Antiinflammatory drugs (e.g., aspirin, indomethacin) should not be used initially so that the response to treatment can be assessed. (In addition, these agents are antipyretics.)

IX. Subsequent treatment

A. **General measures.** The daily assessment of patient status includes temperature, strength and appetite, change in range of motion in the joint, peripheral blood WBC count, and resolution of any extraarticular foci of infection.

B. **Selection of definitive antibiotic therapy** occurs as culture results become available. Antibiotic guidelines for specific pathogens are set forth in Table 40-4.

C. **Duration of antibiotic therapy** varies with different types of bacterial arthritis. Gonococcal arthritis can be treated with 7 days of parenteral therapy, whereas other bacterial pathogens require 2 to 4 weeks of antibiotic therapy, depending on the microorganism, response to therapy, and condition of

Table 40-3. Initial antibiotic therapy for pyogenic arthritis, based on Gram's stain of synovial fluid

Gram's stain finding	Initial antibiotic therapy	Alternative antibiotic therapy
Gram-positive cocci	Nafcillin[a]	Vancomycin
Gram-negative cocci	Ceftriaxone, cefotaxime, or ceftizoxime[b]	Spectinomycin[b] or ciprofloxacin (additional coverage needed if *Neisseria meningitidis* suspected)
Gram-negative bacilli	Gentamicin	Ceftazidime[c]
Septic clinical picture—no organism seen	Ampicillin/sulbactam[a] plus gentamicin	Vancomycin plus ceftizoxime[a]

[a] Vancomycin should be used if methicillin-resistant *Staphylococcus aureus* is prevalent.
[b] Ceftizoxime and spectinomycin should not be used if *Neisseria meningitidis* is a possible pathogen.
[c] Gentamicin should be used if patient is a compromised host (e.g., hepatic cirrhosis, diabetes mellitus, intravenous drug abuse, neoplastic disease, or immunosuppression).

Table 40-4. Antibiotic therapy based on culture identification of organism

Organism	Antibiotic	Alternative agent
Staphylococcus aureus	Nafcillin	Vancomycin
Methicillin-resistant *S. aureus*	Vancomycin	
Streptococci (non-enterococcal)	Penicillin	Cefazolin or vancomycin
Enterococci	Penicillin plus aminoglycoside[a]	Vancomycin plus aminoglycoside[a]
Neisseria gonorrhoeae	Third-generation cephalosporin[b]	Spectinomycin or ciprofloxacin (if patient not pregnant)
Enterobacteriaceae	Third-generation cephalosporin	Aminoglycoside,[a] ciprofloxacin, or aztreonam
Haemophilus influenzae	Third-generation cephalosporin	Trimethoprim/sulfamethoxazole or chloramphenicol
Pseudomonas	Aminoglycoside[a]	Ceftazidime

[a] Gentamicin, tobramycin, or amikacin.
[b] Ceftriaxone, ceftizoxime, or cefotaxime.

the underlying articular tissues. Treatment of infections in prosthetic total joint arthroplasty is discussed in section **X.H.**

D. Serial joint aspiration. Because septic arthritis is a closed-space infection, drainage procedures are essential to decrease intraarticular pressure and reduce leukocyte enzyme activity. Simple arthrocentesis is commonly adequate to accomplish this aspect of therapy, and serial aspirations are necessary as prompted by reaccumulations of inflammatory effusions, often on a daily basis and occasionally twice daily. The response to therapy can be monitored by serial synovial fluid leukocyte counts. After 5 to 7 days of effective treatment, the joint fluid WBC count should decline by 50% to 75%. Failure to achieve such a reduction should be viewed as an indication of inadequate therapy, and surgical drainage should be considered.

E. Surgical drainage, often with synovectomy, is indicated in the treatment of hip infections (particularly with *Staphylococcus aureus* or gram-negative bacilli) because of the mechanical difficulty encountered in percutaneous needle aspiration of this deep articulation. Operative debridement is essential when pyarthrosis is inadequately responsive to arthrocentesis as a consequence of loculation of infection by intraarticular adhesions or underlying joint disease. Arthroscopic techniques have often been employed instead of open arthrotomy for debridement in these situations, especially when the knee is involved. Arthroscopy provides for more complete visualization of the tissue (by magnification and access to posterior compartments), decreases morbidity (lower complication rate), increases joint mobility (earlier postoperative motion because of decreased incision size and associated pain), and is more economical (shorter hospitalization period). The indications for open surgical drainage include the following:

1. Hip infection.
2. Failure of needle aspiration to drain the joint adequately (widely varying WBC counts in repeated aspirates suggest loculated pockets of purulence).
3. Lack of local or systemic response to therapy (e.g., joint fluid cultures remain positive, patient remains febrile after 72 to 96 hours of antibiotic therapy). A low threshold for early exploratory arthrotomy or arthroscopy should be maintained in the compromised host with gram-negative bacillary arthritis.

4. Recrudescent or recurrent infection should prompt consideration of surgical drainage and debridement with histopathologic examination of synovial tissue and cultures for fastidious bacteria, mycobacteria, and fungi if appropriate.

X. Specific entities and problems

A. Gonococcal arthritis

1. Diagnostic features

a. **Polyarthritis and monarthritis** occur in approximately equal proportions at presentation.

b. **Pustulovesicular skin lesions,** often with central necrosis, occur in 44% of cases.

c. **Tenosynovitis** occurs in 68% of cases.

d. **Positive cultures** are obtained from urethra (81%), synovial fluid (60%), blood (24%), pharynx (17%), and rectum (13%).

2. Treatment

a. **Drug therapy** (as recommended by the Centers for Disease Control and Prevention)

(1) Ceftriaxone (1 g IM or IV q24h), ceftizoxime (1 g IV q8h), or cefotaxime (1 g IV q8h for 7 days).

(2) For persons allergic to β-lactam drugs, ciprofloxacin (400 mg IV q12h), ofloxacin (400 mg IV q12h), or spectinomycin (2 g IM q12h) should be employed. Quinolones should not be used during pregnancy or in patients likely to have acquired infection in Asia, where resistance has been demonstrated. In certain geographic areas (e.g., Cleveland, Ohio), where strains with decreased susceptibility to quinolones are endemic, quinolones should not be used to treat gonorrhea. Reliable patients with uncomplicated disease in whom all symptoms resolve within 24 to 48 hours may complete therapy (for a total of 7 days of treatment) with either oral cefixime (400 mg twice daily); if not pregnant, with oral ciprofloxacin (500 mg twice daily); or oral ofloxacin (400 mg twice daily).

(3) Indications for hospitalization include inability of patient to follow or tolerate an outpatient regimen, uncertain diagnosis, and presence of a purulent joint effusion.

B. Tuberculous arthritis

1. **Diagnostic features.** Presentation is typically a chronic monarthritis or spondylitis. Skeletal tuberculosis is usually a combined osteomyelitis and arthritis, as infective lesions in epiphyseal bone invade the adjacent joint. The chest radiographic findings are often normal, and constitutional symptoms may not be present. The tuberculin skin test result is almost always positive. Synovial fluid analysis reveals an elevated WBC count (usually 10,000 to 20,000/μL) with neutrophil predominance (80% of cases). Acid-fast stains of joint effusions are positive in only 27%, and although joint fluid culture is positive in 83%, cultivation requires 4 to 6 weeks of incubation. Synovial biopsy is the procedure of choice for immediate diagnosis; histopathology demonstrates granuloma formation in 95%, caseation in 55%, and the tubercle bacillus in 10% of cases.

2. **Treatment** consists of isoniazid (300 mg/d) and rifampin (300 mg twice daily) for at least 12 months, with pyrazinamide (25 mg/kg daily; maximum of 2.5 g/d) for the initial 2 months.

C. Atypical mycobacterial arthritis

1. **Diagnostic features.** *Mycobacterium marinum* is the most common cause of atypical tuberculous arthritis. Presentation is usually a subacute or chronic interphalangeal or metacarpophalangeal monarthritis. Symptoms commonly develop several weeks after local traumatic contact with marine life (fish, fishing equipment, fish tanks). Diagnosis is assisted by synovial biopsy revealing granulomas or acid-fast bacilli. Mycobacterial cultures of synovial tissue are diagnostic; however, the microbiology laboratory should be alerted to incubate specimens at 30°C for optimal results.

2. **Treatment** consists of rifampin (300 mg twice daily) and ethambutol (15 mg/kg daily for 6 weeks) or minocycline (100 mg twice daily) for 16 weeks.

D. **Fungal arthritis**

1. **Diagnostic features.** Fungal arthritis usually presents as a chronic monarticular infection, but acute polyarticular disease with or without erythema nodosum can be seen. Diagnosis depends on synovial tissue histopathology and mycotic cultures. Key features of specific types of fungal arthritis follow:
   a. **Blastomycosis** primarily involves the lungs, with spread to skin and bone; knee, ankle, and elbow are the most commonly affected joints. Synovial fluid culture is positive for the organism in 90% of cases.
   b. **Candidiasis** causes hematogenous septic arthritis in immunosuppressed hosts. Two-thirds of patients present acutely, 40% have multiple joint involvement, and 65% have evidence of osteomyelitis.
   c. **Coccidioidomycosis and histoplasmosis** both exhibit an acute, self-limited, hypersensitivity-type polyarthritis with erythema nodosum. Subsequently, a chronic granulomatous infectious synovitis may develop.
   d. **Sporotrichosis** affects joints rarely by extension of infection from the usual cutaneous and lymphatic or osseous sites of involvement. More frequently, a slowly progressive polyarticular infection develops as a result of hematogenous seeding of the synovium.
2. **Treatment** of blastomycosis, coccidioidomycosis, histoplasmosis, and sporotrichosis can be successful with oral imidazoles. Candidiasis is treated with IV amphotericin B. Surgical debridement is often necessary to eradicate fungal infection.

E. **Viral arthritis.** Rubella virus, hepatitis B virus, and parvovirus are the most common identifiable viral pathogens, although arthritis can be a manifestation of mumps, infectious mononucleosis (Epstein-Barr virus), herpes simplex, or infection with arbovirus, enterovirus, varicella-zoster, or adenovirus.

1. **Diagnostic features.** Rubella is accompanied by a polyarthritis after appearance of the exanthem and usually resolves within 2 weeks. Polyarthritis also may develop following rubella vaccination. Prodromal hepatitis B is associated with polyarthritis and skin eruptions such as urticaria, maculopapular rashes, petechiae, purpura, and angioneurotic edema. Joint symptoms usually resolve after 1 to 3 weeks coincident with the onset of jaundice. Recurrent arthritis can be seen with chronic active hepatitis or persistent antigenemia.
2. **Treatment** consists of nonsteroidal antiinflammatory drugs.

F. **Lyme disease** is discussed in Chapter 41.

G. **Septic bursitis**

1. **Diagnostic features.** Because of their superficial location, the prepatellar and olecranon bursae are most frequently infected, usually following trauma. Patients present with the acute (2 days) or subacute (12 days) onset of local pain and inflammation, with cellulitis in 75% and regional lymphadenopathy in 25% of cases. Pain is evident on palpation of the bursa and on extreme flexion and extreme extension of the adjacent joint but not on limited motion, as seen in septic arthritis. Infection of the prepatellar or olecranon bursa does not imply involvement of the deeper joints, as there is normally no communication between the two spaces. However, infection of a synovial cyst (e.g., Baker's cyst) does imply the presence of septic arthritis. Bursal fluid analysis reveals abnormalities similar to those of infected joint fluid. The etiologic pathogen is *S. aureus* in more than 90% of cases.
2. **Treatment** involves drainage by percutaneous aspiration and antibiotic therapy. Clinically mild infections can be treated with oral antibiotics for 3 to 4 weeks. If such patients worsen or fail to improve within 1 to 2 days, parenteral therapy should be instituted as for more severe infections, with IV treatment for 2 weeks followed by 2 weeks of oral therapy. Serial

needle aspirations are necessary for reaccumulations of bursal fluid, and surgical drainage with bursectomy is indicated for persistent infection or chronic inflammation.

H. Prosthetic joint infection

1. **Diagnostic features.** Total joint replacement infections can present as acute, fulminant illness with fever, joint pain, local swelling, and erythema when caused by relatively virulent organisms (e.g., *S. aureus*). Subacute presentations with gradually progressive joint pain and no fever suggest indolent infection with a relatively avirulent organism (e.g., *Staphylococcus epidermidis*). A painful prosthetic joint can be caused by both infection and noninfectious, mechanical loosening. Radiography, bone scan, leukocyte scans, WBC counts, and sedimentation rate are not diagnostic for infection. Therefore, the diagnosis of prosthetic joint infection rests on isolation of the pathogen by arthrocentesis or, occasionally, by exploratory arthrotomy. Staphylococci are the predominant organisms (*S. epidermidis,* 22%; *S. aureus,* 22%), with streptococci in 21%, gram-negative bacilli in 25%, and anaerobes in 10% of cases.
2. **Treatment.** Eradication of the pathogen in prosthetic joint infection requires removal of the prosthesis. Metallic joint excision followed by 6 weeks of bactericidal parenteral antimicrobial therapy and subsequent reimplantation is successful in 90% to 97% of cases. Prosthetic joint removal with reimplantation in a one-stage procedure employing antibiotic-impregnated cement is successful in 70% to 80% of patients. Occasionally, protracted oral antibiotic therapy is given to suppress prosthetic joint infection when the prosthesis cannot be removed, the pathogen is relatively avirulent, or the prosthesis is not loose.
3. **Prevention.** Because prosthetic joint infection is a catastrophic event for the patient, prevention is of considerable importance. The hematogenous route is responsible for 20% to 40% of these infections. The use of prophylactic antibiotics in patients with prosthetic joints for events or procedures associated with anticipated bacteremia is controversial at the present time, and the adequacy and cost effectiveness of such measures have not been determined. The American Dental Association and the American Academy of Orthopedic Surgeons have jointly advised that prophylactic antibiotics be given to selected patients undergoing dental procedures associated with significant bleeding (including periodontal scaling). The selected patient populations include persons with inflammatory arthropathies (including rheumatoid arthritis and systemic lupus erythematosis), immunosuppression, diabetes mellitus, malnutrition, hemophilia, previous prosthetic joint infection, and all those who have undergone joint replacement within the past 2 years. Clinical decisions regarding prophylactic antibiotics for expected bacteremias in patients with prosthetic joints should be made on an individual basis. The following schedules are for consideration by physicians who wish to employ prophylactic antibiotics in some settings for certain patients.
   a. **Dental procedures** (associated with gingival hemorrhage)
      (1) **Amoxicillin, cephalexin, or cephradine** (2 g PO 1 hour before procedure), or
      (2) **Clindamycin** (600 mg PO 1 hour before procedure).
   b. **Certain genitourinary and gastrointestinal procedures**
      (1) **Amoxicillin** (2 g PO) or **vancomycin** (1 g IV; 1-hour infusion), plus
      (2) **Ciprofloxacin** (750 mg PO), plus
      (3) **Metronidazole** (500 mg PO 1 hour before procedure; omit metronidazole for urinary tract procedures).

Bibliography

American Dental Association, American Academy of Orthopaedic Surgeons. Advisory statement: antibiotic prophylaxis for dental patients with total joint replacements. *J Am Dent Assoc* 1997;128:1004.

Brause BD. Infections with prostheses in bones and joints. In: Mandell GL, Bennett JE, Dolin R, eds. *Principles and practice of infectious diseases,* 4th ed. New York: Churchill Livingstone, 1994:1051.
Broy SB, Stuhlberg SD, Schmid FR. The role of arthroscopy in the diagnosis and management of the septic joint. *Clin Rheum Dis* 1986;12:489.
Cuellar ML, Silveira LH, Espinoza LR. Fungal arthritis. *Ann Rheum Dis* 1992;51:690.
Garrido G, et al. A review of peripheral tuberculous arthritis. *Semin Arthritis Rheum* 1988;18:142.
Goldenberg DL, Reed JI. Bacterial arthritis. *N Engl J Med* 1985;312:764.
Hannsen AD, Rand JA. Evaluation and treatment of infection at the site of a total hip or knee arthroplasty. *J Bone Joint Surg* 1998;80A:910.
Ho G Jr, Mikolich DJ. Bacterial infection of the superficial subcutaneous bursae. *Clin Rheum Dis* 1986;12:437.
Mikhail IS, Alarcon GS. Nongonococcal bacterial arthritis. *Rheum Dis Clin North Am* 1993;19:311.
Scopelitis E, Martinez-Osuna P. Gonococcal arthritis. *Rheum Dis Clin North Am* 1993;19:363.
U.S. Department of Health and Human Services, Centers for Disease Control and Prevention. 1998 Guidelines for treatment of sexually transmitted diseases. *MMWR Morb Mortal Wkly Rep* 1998;47[RR-1]:63.

41. LYME DISEASE

Steven K. Magid

Lyme disease has become an increasingly common cause of arthritis and disability. Although it is most prevalent on the East Coast, the disease is also common in Wisconsin and Minnesota, and in fact may be found throughout the continental United States.

I. **History.** Lyme disease was first described in the United States by Steere et al. (1977) when clusters of an illness first thought to be juvenile rheumatoid arthritis were noted in three small Connecticut communities. These cases were associated with a rash, already known in Europe as erythema chronicum migrans and now referred to as erythema migrans (EM). In Europe, EM was thought to be transmitted by the sheep tick. Spirochetes were noted in the skin lesions, and antibiotics were successfully used to treat the rash. It was soon appreciated that a proportion of the Connecticut patients remembered a tick bite at the site of their rash. In addition, there was a 30-fold higher incidence of EM and Lyme disease in areas inhabited by the *Ixodes dammini* tick (later renamed *Ixodes scapularis*). Eventually, spirochetes were isolated from blood, cerebrospinal fluid, and EM lesions of patients with what was soon appreciated to be a systemic disorder—Lyme disease.

II. **Microbiology.** In 1982, *I. dammini* (*scapularis*) ticks collected in the locale of EM patients were found to contain spirochetes in their midgut. These organisms were eventually grown on selective media. They led to the development of the EM rash and an antibody response in exposed laboratory animals. These spirochetes were of the genus *Borrelia,* belonging (along with genera *Leptospira* and *Treponema*) to the order Spirochaetales; they were named *Borrelia burgdorferi* (*Bb*). Genetic differences have been reported between the Bb genospecies seen in the United States and those seen in Europe and elsewhere. The strain that infects humans in the United States is called *Bb sensu stricto.* The two most important genospecies in Europe are *Bb garinii* and *Bb afzelii.* The differences in genospecies may account for some of the differences between the clinical presentation of Lyme disease in Europe and in the United States. *Bb* isolated from ticks will grow easily in culture medium. This is not the case with clinical specimens, from which the organism is difficult to isolate and grow.

More than 30 *Bb* proteins have been identified by immunoblot techniques. There are three major outer surface proteins (Osp): Osp A (30 kd), Osp B (34 kd), and Osp C (23 kd). There is also a 41-kd flagellar antigen that is shared by other spirochetes. In addition, the 18-, 28-, 35-, 37-, 39-, 45-, 58-, 66-, and 93-kd antigens evoke important immune responses.

III. **Vectors.** *Bb* is transmitted from the tick by inoculation of saliva and the regurgitation of midgut contents into the bite site. Lyme disease is not thought to be transmitted by sexual contact or by breast milk. Although *Bb* may survive in banked blood, as of 1994, transfusion-associated Lyme disease had not been reported. The life cycle of *I. dammini* spans 2 years and includes three stages of development: larva, nymph, and adult. If infected, ticks may spread Lyme disease during each stage. However, ticks at the nymphal stage are the most important vector. Nymphs are most active during the spring and summer, when many people are outdoors in shorts and short sleeves. And nymphs are so small, they are easily overlooked. This probably accounts for the peak onset of Lyme disease during these months. The preferred host of the *I. dammini* tick is the white-footed mouse. Adult ticks feed on deer and other rodents, but it is the deer that most often serves as the mating ground of the adult tick (hence the name deer tick). Humans, birds, and many other animals also serve as vectors. In the endemic areas of the northeast, 30% to 50% of nymphal and adult ticks may be infected with *Bb* (in some areas, the rate of infection may be even higher). In the north central United States, rates of 10% to 20% are reported, in contrast to the Pacific Coast, where the rate of tick infection is approximately 1% to 2%.

A number of different members of the *I. ricinus* complex of ticks are involved in the dissemination of Lyme disease. On the East Coast, *I. scapularis* is the most important vector. In the Western United States, *I. pacificus,* the Western black-legged tick, is responsible. *I. ricinus* is the main vector in western and central Europe; and *I. persulcatus* is found in eastern Russia, China, and Japan.

IV. Epidemiology. According to the Centers for Disease Control and Prevention, Lyme disease is the most common vector-borne disease in the United States. Since 1982, more than 95,000 cases have been reported in the United States. This is almost certainly a vast underestimate, as many cases are thought not to be reported. In the United States, Lyme disease causes 95% of all vector-borne diseases. The overall incidence in the United States is about 5 in 100,000. However, in endemic areas, it may be as high as 1 to 3 in 100 per year! Through 1995, cases have been reported in all states except Montana. In 1995, the eight states (Connecticut, Rhode Island, New York, New Jersey, Pennsylvania, Maryland, Wisconsin, and Minnesota) with the highest reported rate of Lyme disease accounted for 91% (10,613) of the 11,700 cases reported. New York State reported 38% (4,438) of all cases. Cases have been reported from most European countries, the (former) U.S.S.R., China, Japan, and Australia. Lyme disease may occur in all age groups. There is a peak in children and in persons ages 30 through 49. The earliest cases of Lyme disease were thought to have occurred 25 years ago on Cape Cod and in Connecticut. However, the spirochete has been identified in ticks collected more than 50 years ago! There has obviously been a rapid spread of Lyme disease since that time.

V. Clinical presentation. Steere has outlined a useful clinical classification for Lyme disease. In this scheme, Lyme disease is divided into early localized (stage 1), early disseminated (stage 2), and late disseminated (stage 3) infection (Table 41-1).

A. Early localized (stage 1). Lyme disease is initiated by the injection of the *Bb* spirochete into the skin by an infected tick. After local spread, the characteristic rash of EM develops 3 to 32 days later (mean, 7 days) in approximately 70% of patients. Only one-third of patients may remember the actual tick bite. EM may be seen anywhere, but it frequently occurs on the thigh, groin, and axilla. In children, the earlobe crease is a common site. The size may be from 3 cm to 70 cm (mean, 15 cm). A hallmark of the rash is its gradual expansion in size—up to 1 to 2 cm a day. As it expands, bright red outer borders develop. Typically, there is a central clearing, and the rash takes on a ringlike appearance. However, the rash may also be vesicular, necrotic, or targetlike. The skin may be burning, painful, and pruritic. If antibiotics are not given, the lesions usually clear within a month (range, 1 day to 14 months). If antibiotics are used, the lesions clear in several days. During the early localized stage, there may be minor constitutional symptoms and regional lymphadenopathy.

B. Early disseminated (stage 2). Within days to weeks of the tick bite, the spirochete spreads systemically via blood or lymph. At this time, blood culture results may be positive. There are many possible manifestations of Lyme disease, but often a characteristic syndrome develops. Early on, there may be excruciating headaches and a stiff neck. These episodes typically occur in short, hour-long attacks. There are frequently migrating, intense pains in joints, bursae, tendons, muscles, and bones. The patient may appear ill and complain of debilitating malaise and fatigue. These symptoms appear during the phase of hematogenous spread. Later, in stage 2, the spirochetes seem to establish themselves preferentially in certain sites, including the nervous system, heart, and musculoskeletal system. The spirochete may be found in pathologic specimens from the heart, retina, muscle, bone, synovium, spleen, liver, meninges, and brain. Secondary EM occurs in approximately 50% of patients who note primary EM. These lesions resemble primary EM but are smaller and tend to migrate less. They are frequently multiple and annular, with merging borders.

Table 41-1. Manifestations of Lyme disease by stage[a]

	Early infection		
System[b]	Localized (stage 1)	Disseminated (stage 2)	Late infection—persistent (stage 3)
Skin	Erythema migrans	Secondary annular lesions, malar rash, diffuse erythema or urticaria, evanescent lesions, lymphocytoma	Acrodermatitis chronica atrophicans, localized scleroderma-like lesions
Musculoskeletal system		Migratory pain in joints, tendons, bursae, muscle, bone; brief arthritis attacks; myositis[c]; osteomyelitis[c]; panniculitis[c]	Prolonged arthritis attacks, chronic arthritis, peripheral enthesopathy, periostitis or joint subluxations below lesions of acrodermatitis
Neurologic system		Meningitis, cranial neuritis, Bell's palsy, motor or sensory radiculoneuritis, subtle encephalitis, mononeuritis multiplex, myelitis,[c] chorea,[c] cerebellar ataxia[c]	Chronic encephalomyelitis, spastic parapareses, ataxic gait, subtle mental disorders, chronic axonal polyradiculopathy, dimentia[c]
Lymphatic system	Regional lymphadenopathy	Regional or generalized lymphadenopathy, splenomegaly	
Heart		Atrioventricular nodal block, myopericarditis, pancarditis	
Eyes		Conjunctivitis, iritis,[c] choroiditis,[c] retinal hemorrhage or detachment,[c] panophthalmitis[c]	Keratitis
Liver		Mild or recurrent hepatitis	
Respiratory system		Nonexudative sore throat, nonproductive cough, adult respiratory distress syndrome[c]	
Kidney		Microscopic hematuria or proteinuria	
Genitourinary system		Orchitis[c]	
Constitutional symptoms	Minor	Severe malaise and fatigue	Fatigue

[a] The classification by stages provides a guideline for the expected timing of the manifestations, but this may vary from case to case.
[b] Systems are listed from the most to the least commonly affected.
[c] The inclusion of this manifestation is based on one or a few cases.

1. **Neurologic manifestations**
   a. **Cranial nerves.** Weeks to months after the onset of Lyme disease, neurologic symptoms develop in 15% to 20% of patients. Bell's palsy is particularly common. It is usually unilateral but may be sequential or bilateral. Other cranial neuropathies are less common and may occur with or without Bell's palsy. Involvement of cranial nerves III, IV, and VI may cause extraocular palsy. If the fifth cranial nerve is involved, facial dysesthesia may occur. Dizziness, otalgia, sore throat, and deafness may occur with cranial nerve VIII involvement. Optic atrophy and Argyll-Robertson pupils may occur if the optic nerve is involved.
   b. **Peripheral nerves. Neuropathies** are sometimes seen and frequently involve the median nerve.
   c. **Radiculopathy** may be unilateral, often in the dermatome of the tick bite. It commonly involves T-5 and T-8 through T-12. The radiculopathy may be sequential and bilateral.
   d. **Aseptic meningitis.** Recurrent attacks of prostrating headaches may occur and are often associated with stiff neck, photophobia, nausea, and vomiting. Patients are frequently afebrile. Such severe attacks may last weeks and alternate with periods of milder headache. Spinal fluid shows a lymphocytic pleocytosis with increased production of immunoglobulin G (IgG). Evidence of local antibody to *Bb* may be found. Oligoclonal banding may also be seen.
   e. **Encephalitis** may begin in stage 2. It is manifested by lethargy, fatigue, dementia, poor concentration and memory, and emotional lability.

      It has not been established whether peripheral and cranial neuropathies are always associated with central nervous system infection. It is also not known whether resolution of neurologic signs and symptoms without treatment are indicative of resolution of infection, or if infection persists in a latent state.
2. **Cardiac manifestations.** Several weeks after the EM rash, cardiac involvement may develop in 4% to 8% of patients. Atrioventricular block in fluctuating degrees is the most common finding. The duration is usually brief (3 days to 6 weeks). Complete heart block rarely occurs and, when present, usually does not last more than a week. A permanent pacemaker is usually not needed. Ventricular tachycardia has been reported. Other manifestations may include acute myopericarditis, mild left ventricular dysfunction, cardiographic abnormalities, and rarely pancarditis. The latter may be fatal. Valvular lesions are not seen.
3. **Joint manifestations.** Arthritis is usually considered a late manifestation of disease, but acute attacks may begin in the early disseminated phase. They may appear as early as a few weeks after disease onset. At a mean of 6 months after the onset of Lyme disease (range, 2 weeks to 2 years), attacks of arthritis will develop in 60% of patients. It is usually asymmetric and oligoarticular (involving four or fewer joints). Large joints are preferentially involved, especially the knee. Initially, these attacks are brief and may last days or weeks and then remit without antibiotic therapy. Although some patients have continuous inflammation, most do not. The leukocyte counts in specimens of Lyme disease effusions obtained by arthrocentesis range from 500 to 110,000/mm^3; polymorphonuclear leukocytes predominate. As demonstrated by polymerase chain reaction (PCR), culture, and staining, the involved joints are usually directly infected with *Bb*.

C. Late persistent infection (stage 3)

1. **Arthritis**
   a. **Clinical presentation.** In one study, 55 patients with untreated EM were followed. Eleven patients had EM as the only manifestation of Lyme disease, with no joint involvement at all. Ten patients had EM with arthralgias, 28 had EM with intermittent arthritis, and only 6 had EM with chronic arthritis. The most common pattern was an asymmetric oligoarthritis or monarthritis of large joints. Most patients had knee

involvement at some point in their illness. Characteristically, the knees became very swollen (sometimes massively). They appeared warm but not "hot." Pain was moderate but not severe. In three patients, Baker's cysts developed with early rupture. Arthritis of the ankle, wrist, and occasionally elbow and hand has also been seen. Temporomandibular joint involvement is also frequent. It is rare for more than five joints to be involved. Although it is unusual for small joints to be involved, a rheumatoid arthritis-like picture has been reported. Nodules are unusual but have been described in atypical locations.

b. **Chronic arthritis.** Arthritis dominates stage 3. With time, the above-mentioned episodic attacks may last for months rather than weeks. Eventually, chronic arthritis (defined as arthritis lasting more than a year), may develop. This occurs in fewer than 10% of Lyme disease patients, and it has been suggested that the presence of the HLA-DR4 haplotype, in addition to a lack of response to antibiotics, places a person at greater risk for the development of chronic arthritis. The transition from episodic attacks to chronic arthritis has been associated with the development of antibodies to Osp A. To explain the fact that in some patients with chronic arthritis the PCR does not show *Bb* sequences, many theories have been advanced. It appears that some cases of chronic Lyme arthritis may not be caused by persistent *Bb* infection, but rather by a "reactive" or immune process. It is interesting to note that chronic arthritis may spontaneously resolve, even after years.

2. **Neurologic manifestations.** Chronic or late Lyme neuroborreliosis may have manifestations in both the peripheral and central nervous systems.

a. **Chronic radiculoneuropathy** presents mainly with sensory symptoms, especially radicular pain or distal paresthesias. They usually affect the limbs, rather than the trunk, in a "stocking-glove" distribution.

b. Patients with **encephalopathy** usually complain of difficulty with memory and concentration. Hypersomnolence, depression, irritability, and marked memory loss are noted.

c. **Leukencephalitis and encephalomyelitis** are rare in the United States. Optic neuropathy, spastic paraparesis, bladder dysfunction, ataxia, dysarthria, and encephalopathy may also be seen.

VI. Diagnosis. The diagnosis of Lyme disease is a *clinical* one. Laboratory data are used solely as a means of confirmation. Supporting clinical evidence includes epidemiologic data, characteristic clinical presentations, and the exclusion of other disorders in which joint, cardiac, and neurologic phenomena occur. Serologic testing remains the best way to confirm a clinical diagnosis in a patient with suspected Lyme disease.

A. The **immunofluorescence assay (IFA)** was the first to be developed. An indirect immunofluorescence technique involving the whole *Bb* organism is used. Antibodies detected by this technique are seen within weeks of the onset of the disease.

B. Enzyme-linked immunosorbent assay (ELISA) is usually considered to be the preferred screening method. The sensitivity, specificity, and reproducibility are considered better than those of the IFA. Sonicated, whole-*Bb* extracts are used as the antigens. IgM antibodies appear 2 to 4 weeks after the EM rash. They peak after 8 weeks and usually normalize by 4 to 6 months. Continued or late appearance of IgM antibodies may be indicative of ongoing or recurrent infection. IgG antibodies occur within 6 to 8 weeks after the EM rash, peak after 4 to 6 months, and may remain elevated indefinitely.

C. Western blot. This technique separates the major *Bb* proteins on an agar gel by molecular weight. By overlaying a patient's sera, it is possible to determine which *Bb* proteins (if any) are the targets of an antibody response. Some of the more important *Borrelia* antigens identified by Western blot include 31-kd Osp A; 34-kd Osp B; 21- to 24-kd Osp C (varies with the strain of *Bb* used); Bmp A (p39), which appears to be highly specific for Lyme disease; 41-kd flagellin (a motility component with strong cross-reactivity to flagellins of other organisms); and 58-, 60-, 66-, and 72-kd heat shock proteins (which are widely conserved in all cells and have strong homology with other organisms).

Characteristic patterns of antibody formation after infection with *Bb* have been used by the Centers for Disease Control and Prevention to develop criteria for a "positive" Western blot. IgM2 of three positive bands: 24 (Osp:C), 39 (Bmp A), and 41 (Fla) kd. IgG5 of 10 bands: 18, 21 (= 24), 28, 30, 39, 41, 45, 58 (not GroEL), 66, and 93 kd.

D. The **polymerase chain reaction** is a technique that "amplifies" a single copy of *Bb* DNA into many millions of copies, allowing the detection of even a single *Bb* genome. It is most useful in testing inflammatory fluids such as cerebrospinal and joint fluid rather than blood. The PCR technique is limited by the fact it cannot distinguish between the DNA from living *Borrelia* and the DNA from nonviable organisms. In addition, special laboratory techniques are required to avoid false-positive results in this highly sensitive test.

E. Cellular immunity testing. T cells reactive against *Bb* have been found in the blood, synovial fluid, and cerebrospinal fluid of Lyme disease patients. The interest in this test stems from the occasional Lyme disease patient with a positive T-cell proliferation test result in the absence of a positive serologic test result. However, this circumstance is decidedly rare. The utility of the T-cell proliferation test is limited by the fact that it is difficult to perform and interpret. Fresh T cells are required, the results depend on the way the *Bb* organisms are prepared, and there are many interlaboratory variations in reported results. Although considerable discussion and debate about the utility of clinical T-cell testing are ongoing, at present it cannot be routinely recommended.

F. Urinary antigen testing is based on the ability to detect Osp that has been shed and filtered by the glomerulus. It currently has no clinical role.

G. False-negative results of immunofluorescence assay or enzyme-linked immunosorbent assay may be caused by the following:

1. Testing during the first weeks of infection, before antibody development. It is important to recognize that in tertiary neuroborreliosis and in Lyme arthritis, results of serologic testing are almost universally positive.
2. Laboratory variation or error. Studies have demonstrated marked interlaboratory variations in test results.
3. Early use of antibiotics, which may abort a humoral immune response.
4. T-cell suppression of antibody production early in the course of the disease.
5. Immune complex sequestration of antibodies.

   Lyme disease patients with negative IFA or ELISA serologies may occasionally be positive for cerebrospinal fluid antibodies or, as mentioned above, demonstrate a T-cell proliferation response to *Bb*.

H. False-positive results of immunofluorescence assay or enzyme-linked immunosorbent assay are common. They may be caused by the following:

1. Cross-reactivity with other spirochetes
   - **a.** Nonpathogenic oral spirochetes and those that cause gingivitis.
   - **b.** *Treponema pallidum* (and *Treponema* organisms that cause yaws and pinta).
   - **c.** Cross-reactivity with homologous non-*Bb* proteins (heat shock proteins or flagellin).
2. Polyclonal B-cell activation, particularly in patients whose serum contains rheumatoid factor, antinuclear antibodies, or anti-thyroid antibodies, and in patients with malaria, Epstein-Barr virus infection, and Rocky Mountain spotted fever.
3. Prior, possibly asymptomatic *Bb* infection. If another type of illness occurs in these patients, it may be wrongly attributed to Lyme disease. This is exemplified by a report of four patients who were initially thought to have Lyme disease but were shown to have endocarditis. This highlights the care with which a diagnosis of Lyme disease must be made.

VII. Treatment

A. Protection from ticks may be the most important method of combating Lyme disease. This is accomplished by the following:

1. Wearing protective, light-colored clothing tucked in at the ankles and wrists.

2. Using insect repellent on clothing.
3. Inspecting for ticks. It probably takes more than 24 hours for transmission of *Bb* after tick attachment.
4. Proper tick removal.
5. Modifying residential landscapes (clear leaf litter, brush, tall grass; remove stone walls, wood piles; erect deer barriers).
6. Area application of acaricides. This is effective but raises safety concerns.

B. Facts about tick bites

1. **Tick removal.** Proper removal minimizes the risk for inoculation of tick gut contents. Use tweezers to grasp the tick behind its head, pull slowly and gently.
2. The **risk** for acquiring Lyme disease varies and depends on the local *Bb* infection rate of ticks (which may range from 1% to 50%). It is likely that most tick bites (cited as >95%) do not result in the transmission of Lyme disease. Transmission rates also vary with the duration of tick attachment; it is thought that transmission of Lyme disease rarely occurs earlier than 48 hours after attachment.
3. **Use of prophylactic antibiotics.** Studies have not been able to prove the efficacy of prophylactic antibiotic treatment after a tick bite. In addition, it has been stated that the risk for acquiring Lyme disease after an observed tick bite is equal to the risk for an adverse drug effect, including anaphylaxis and photosensitivity (especially with doxycycline).

C. Recommended strategy for possible infection. After a tick bite has been sustained, one approach is to observe the area of the bite to see if EM develops. If it does, antibiotics should be given. Similarly, if a flulike illness or fever develops, antibiotics should also be given. More controversial is whether antibiotics should be given for a worried patient or a worried doctor! Much of this depends on an evaluation of the risk for Lyme disease, the prevalence of *Bb*-infected ticks in the area, and whether or not the tick was engorged. An exception to this would be a pregnant patient, to whom a 10-day course of oral amoxicillin might be offered.

D. Recommended approach to seropositive patients

1. **Without signs or symptoms.** Most experts do *not* advocate treatment in this group of patients, especially if the Western blot does not confirm the diagnosis. However, patients with a positive Western blot result and no symptoms may be offered a lumbar puncture, with treatment based on the results. Alternatively, an empiric course of oral antibiotics may be given. In clinical practice, the latter may be the easiest route to follow.
2. **With nonspecific symptoms.** This is the most difficult group to evaluate. In general, most patients with Lyme disease will have objective evidence of the disease on history, physical examination, and laboratory testing. The pitfalls of treating ELISA-positive patients with nonspecific symptoms but without Western blot confirmation of Lyme disease should be appreciated.

E. Treatment of confirmed Lyme disease. The treatment protocols currently recommended are summarized in Table 41-2.

1. **Early localized (stage 1).** Antibiotic treatment of EM is felt to shorten the course of the rash and decrease the chance of disease progression. *Bb* is sensitive, in animal studies and *in vitro,* to tetracycline, ampicillin, ceftriaxone, imipenem, and erythromycin. The advantages of doxycycline over tetracycline are better gastrointestinal absorption and central nervous system penetration and twice-daily dosing. However, neither should be used in pregnant women or in children. It is important to be aware of the possibility of photosensitivity reactions. Cefuroxime axetil (Ceftin) seems to be as effective as doxycycline. Azithromycin may be less effective than amoxicillin. The greater the number of extra-cutaneous manifestations, the slower the antibiotic response and the greater the risk for late disease. A higher dose and longer duration of antibiotic treatment may be required in this setting. If treatment is given early in Lyme disease, the antibody response may disappear. In this setting, recurrent infections have been reported.

Table 41-2. Recommendations for antibiotic treatment[a]

Early Lyme disease[b]
Doxycycline, 100 mg bid for 10–21 days
Amoxicillin, 500 mg bid for 10–21 days
Erythromycin, 250 mg qid for 10–21 days (less effective than doxycycline or amoxicillin)
Lyme carditis
Ceftriaxone, 2 g qd IV for 14 days
Penicillin G, 20 million units IV for 14 days
Doxycycline, 100 mg PO bid for 14–21 days, may suffice[b]
Amoxicillin, 500 mg PO tid for 14–21 days, may suffice[b]
Neurologic manifestations—facial nerve paralysis
For an isolated finding, oral regimens for early disease, used for at least 21 days, may suffice
For a finding associated with other neurologic manifestations, intravenous therapy (see below)
Lyme meningitis[c]
Ceftriaxone, 2 mg qd by single dose for 14–21 days
Penicillin G, 20 million units qd in divided doses for 10–21 days
Possible alternatives for Lyme meningitis
Doxycycline, 100 mg PO or IV for 14–21 days
Chloramphenicol, 1 g IV for q6h for 10–21 days
Lyme arthritis
Doxycycline, 100 mg PO bid for 30 days
Amoxicillin and probenecid, 500 mg each PO qid for 30 days
Penicillin G, 20 million units IV in divided doses daily for 14–21 days
Ceftriaxone, 2 g IV qd for 14–21 days
In pregnant women
For localized early Lyme disease, amoxicillin, 500 mg tid for 21 days
For disseminated early Lyme disease or any manifestation of late disease, penicillin G, 20 million units qd for 14–21 days
For asymptomatic seropositivity, no treatment necessary

[a] These guidelines are to be modified by new findings and should always be applied with close attention to the clinical course of individual patients.
[b] Shorter courses are reserved for disease that is limited to a single skin lesion.
[c] Regimens for radiculoneuropathy, peripheral neuropathy, and encephalitis are the same as those for meningitis.

2. **Early disseminated (stage 2).** Oral antibiotics are generally effective during early stage 2 disease. They are effective for secondary EM, migratory musculoskeletal pain, severe malaise, isolated Bell's palsy, and possibly acute arthritis. Longer courses may be required for persistent symptoms. However, IV antibiotics are generally needed for any neurologic sign other than Bell's palsy and for abnormal lumbar puncture findings. Some specialists advocate a lumbar puncture for all patients with neurologic signs or symptoms, including Bell's palsy, because abnormal findings would suggest that IV therapy should be given. The antibiotics standard for high-degree atrioventricular block or cardiomegaly are ceftriaxone and penicillin G. A temporary pacer and an intensive care unit setting are also indicated.
3. **Arthritis.** The optimal treatment regimen for arthritis has still not been completely defined. Early on in the course of the disease, bouts of arthritis may be self-limited and resolve without antibiotics. Although arthritis has been treated with both oral and parenteral antibiotics, some patients prefer initial oral treatment. It may take many months for a clinical response to occur. Those who fail an initial oral antibiotic course should be treated

with IV antibiotics. Some physicians may opt to treat IV from the start, particularly if neuroborreliosis has not been ruled out. A fibromyalgia picture with nonspecific complaints has been described. Antibiotics are not effective in treating this malady. Intraarticular steroids should be avoided before the institution of antibiotic therapy because they have been associated with an increased risk for antibiotic failure. Arthroscopic synovectomy of the knee has also been reported to be beneficial in treating chronic Lyme arthritis refractory to other modalities.

4. **Pregnancy.** There have been case reports of *Bb* causing prematurity, stillbirth, central nervous system infection, and cardiac malformations in the fetus. However, follow-up studies do not directly implicate Lyme disease as a cause of the congenital malformations. Seropositivity in an otherwise asymptomatic pregnant patient or a prior history of Lyme disease in a patient who is currently pregnant does not confer an increased risk to the fetus. Nonetheless, most physicians believe that active Lyme disease in a pregnant patient warrants aggressive and usually IV treatment.

VIII. Vaccines. Recombinant Osp A vaccine has been shown to protect against Lyme disease in a mouse model. A chemically inactivated whole-cell vaccine has been approved for use in dogs. In humans, recombinant Osp A vaccination is being studied. A phase II randomized, double-blind, placebo-controlled study of 350 residents of an island highly endemic for Lyme disease showed high efficacy and no significant side effects (participants had no prior infection). Another study done in subjects with prior Lyme disease showed good tolerance. Two double-blind phase III trials of recombinant Osp A have been completed. Both studies demonstrate safety and efficacy. It has been postulated that the vaccine may work by causing antibody-mediated death of spirochetes in the tick midgut, before the spirochetes can be transmitted to the vaccinated host.

Bibliography

Abramowicz M, ed. Treatment of lyme disease. *Med Lett Drugs Ther* 1997;39:47.

Burgdorfer W, et al. Lyme disease: a tick-borne spirochetosis? *Science* 1982;216:1317.

Centers for Disease Control and Prevention. Lyme disease—United States, 1987 and 1988. *JAMA* 1989;262:2209.

Dattwyler RJ, et al. Seronegative Lyme disease: dissociation of specific T- and B-lymphocyte responses to *Borrelia burgdorferi*. *N Engl J Med* 1988;319:1441.

Kaell AT, et al. Positive Lyme serology in subacute bacterial endocarditis: a study of four patients. *JAMA* 1990;264:2916.

Logigian EL, Kaplan RF, Steere AC. Chronic neurologic manifestations of Lyme disease. *N Engl J Med* 1990;323:1438.

Rahn DW, Evans J, eds. Lyme disease. American College of Physicians, Philadelphia, 1998.

Rahn DW, Malawista SE. Lyme disease: recommendations for diagnosis and treatment. *Ann Intern Med* 1991;114:472.

Sigal LH, et al. A vaccine consisting of recombinant *Borrelia burgdorferi* outer surface protein A to prevent Lyme disease. *N Engl J Med* 1998;339:216.

Steere AC. Lyme disease. *N Engl J Med* 1989;321:586.

Steere AC, et al. Lyme arthritis: an epidemic of oligoarticular arthritis in children and adults in three Connecticut communities. *Arthritis Rheum* 1977;20:7.

Steere AC, et al. Vaccination against Lyme disease with recombinant *Borrelia burgdorferi* outer surface lipoprotein A with adjuvant. *N Engl J Med* 1998;339:209.

Steere AC, Schoen RT, Taylor E. The clinical evolution of Lyme arthritis. *Ann Intern Med* 1987;107:725.

42. OSTEOMYELITIS

Barry D. Brause

Although the distinction made between the acute and chronic forms of osteomyelitis has some value in therapy and prognosis, no abrupt shift from one category to the other occurs in most cases. A more useful classification, based on the pathogenetic route of infection, divides cases into three types: (a) hematogenous osteomyelitis; (b) introduced infection, which results from contamination accompanying surgical and nonsurgical trauma; and (c) contiguous infection, which results from the spread of microorganisms from adjacent infected tissue and includes osteomyelitis associated with peripheral vascular disease.

I. **Etiology, epidemiology, and pathogenesis.** Osteomyelitis represents the invasion of microorganisms into bone, and virtually all microbes can infect bone. Bacteria are the usual pathogens, and staphylococci are the most common etiologic agents in all three types of osseous infection. *Staphylococcus aureus* causes approximately 60% of cases of hematogenous and introduced osteomyelitis and is the most prominent pathogen when osseous infection develops from sepsis in contiguous tissue. *Staphylococcus epidermidis* and the other coagulase-negative staphylococci have become the major pathogens in bone infections associated with indwelling prosthetic materials and foreign bodies, such as joint replacement implants and fracture fixation devices, which are responsible for 30% of these cases. Streptococci, gram-negative bacilli, anaerobes, mycobacteria, and fungi are causative agents in a variety of clinical situations (Table 42-1).

A. **Hematogenous osteomyelitis.** The anatomic osseous site of involvement in hematogenous infection is age-dependent. From birth through puberty, the metaphyseal regions in the long bones of the extremities (tibia, femur, humerus) are most frequently involved owing to their large blood flow during these developmental years. In adults, blood-borne pathogens preferentially infect the spine (lumbosacral, thoracic) because vertebrae receive relatively more blood flow with maturation. In bacteremia, the more vascular anterior end plates are seeded, and osteomyelitis commonly involves two adjacent vertebral bodies and the intervertebral disk space. The septic process compromises the nutrient supply to the intervertebral disk, resulting in disk necrosis and disk space narrowing, which is often the earliest radiographic sign of vertebral osteomyelitis. The etiologic pathogens in hematogenous osteomyelitis reflect the microorganisms associated with bacteremia in specific patient populations (see Table 42-1).

B. **Introduced osteomyelitis.** Patients are at risk for the introduced form of osteomyelitis whenever the skin and soft tissues overlying and protecting bone are breached by trauma or surgery. Approximately 70% of compound fractures are contaminated by skin and soil microflora, but thanks to effective debridement and perioperative antibiotic therapy, infection develops in only 2% to 9%. Prophylactic antibiotics and extensive antiseptic operative techniques allow large foreign bodies to be inserted into bones during reparative and reconstructive orthopedic surgery with infection rates below 2%. Indwelling foreign bodies decrease the magnitude of a bacterial inoculum necessary to establish infection in bone, and they permit pathogens to persist on the surface of avascular material, often within host- or microbe-derived biofilms, sequestered from circulating immune factors and systemic antibiotics.

C. **Osteomyelitis by contiguous spread (including vascular insufficiency).** Osteomyelitis develops by contiguous spread in one-third to two-thirds of diabetic patients with long-standing foot ulcers, and more hospital days are utilized to treat foot infections than any other complication of diabetes mellitus. Osseous involvement reflects unsuccessful reversal of or compensation for underlying severe neuropathy and vascular insufficiency, which prevent a skin ulcer from healing, so that progressively deeper microbial invasion culminates in spread

Table 42-1. Predispositions, anatomic sites, and prominent pathogens in forms of osteomyelitis

Form of osteomyelitis	Predisposing condition	Site	Prominent pathogens
Hematogenous	None	Long bones	*S. aureus*
Childhood	Sickle cell hemoglobinopathy	Multiple	Streptococci *Haemophilus* *Salmonella* *Staphylococcus aureus*
Adult	Urinary tract infection or instrumentation	Vertebrae	GNB Streptococci
	Skin infection	Vertebrae	*S. aureus* Streptococci
	Respiratory infection	Vertebrae	Streptococci *Mycobacterium tuberculosis*
	IV drug abuse, or vascular catheters	Vertebrae	GNB Staphylococci *Candida*
	AIDS	Multiple	Fungi
	Endocarditis	Vertebrae	*Mycobacterium* Streptococci Staphylococci
Introduced type	Fractures	Fracture site	*S. aureus* *S. epidermidis* GNB
	Prosthetic joint	Prosthesis	*Staphylococcus epidermidis* *S. aureus*
Contiguous spread	Skin ulcer	Foot, leg	Polymicrobial Staphylococci Streptococci GNB Anaerobes
	Sinusitis	Skull	Streptococci Anaerobes
	Dental abscess	Mandible Maxilla	Streptococci Anaerobes
	Human or animal bites	Hand	Streptococci Anaerobes *Pasteurella*
	Felon	Finger	*S. aureus*
	Gardening	Hand	*Sporothrix*

GNB, gram-negative bacilli.
From Brause BD. Osteomyelitis. In: Bennett JC, Plum F. *Cecil-Loeb Textbook of Medicine,* 20th ed. Philadelphia: WB Saunders, 1996:1625.

to contiguous bone. This clinical scenario is also seen in patients with chronic skin ulcerations resulting from other conditions associated with severe sensory neuropathy (e.g., meningomyelocele) or vascular insufficiency (e.g., decubitus ulcers, vasculitis, atherosclerosis, and arteriosclerosis). The most common pathogens are staphylococci, streptococci, gram-negative bacilli, and anaerobes. Multiple organisms are isolated in more than 60% of cases.

In all three forms of osteomyelitis, the microorganisms induce local metabolic changes and inflammatory reactions that produce osseous edema. As infection spreads within the bone, local thrombophlebitis develops, increasing edema and intraosseous pressure, which can result in ischemic necrosis of large areas of bone, called sequestra. If the osseous cortex is breached, subperiosteal abscesses can develop, with periosteal inflammation and periosteal formation of new bone in adjacent soft tissue, called an involucrum.

D. **Chronic osteomyelitis.** Unsuccessful therapy of acute osteomyelitis results in relapsing or chronic infection. Microorganisms persist in foci of gross or microscopic necrotic bone (sequestra) and intermittently invade surrounding tissues, causing the acute exacerbations of chronic osteomyelitis. Because of the avascular nature of sequestra, persistent pathogens are not eradicated by systemic antibiotics; however, local immune responses may control or eliminate the septic process. Recrudescent infection usually involves only local tissue but may spread through the overlying soft tissue to produce a drainage tract or sinus that eventually reaches the skin surface, creating a cutaneous draining sinus orifice. The sinus commonly drains sporadically from an osseous origin (often at a site of necrotic bone, or sequestrum) and reflects the degree of active infection and inflammation in the bone. Rare complications of chronic osteomyelitis include squamous cell carcinoma in overlying draining sinus tracts and secondary amyloidosis.

II. **Clinical features and presentation**

A. **Acute hematogenous osteomyelitis in childhood.** The majority of children with acute hematogenous osteomyelitis show evidence of systemic illness—fever, chills, malaise, leukocytosis, elevated erythrocyte sedimentation rate—along with local symptoms. Focal bone pain is a characteristic feature, with overlying erythema, warmth, and swelling variably seen. Limb motion may be limited by local pain (pseudoparalysis) when the infection is near an articulation. Adjacent joint effusions can occur but are usually sterile when the epiphyseal cartilage is intact.

B. **Adult hematogenous osteomyelitis (including vertebral osteomyelitis).** Vertebral osteomyelitis most often presents subacutely with prominent back pain and spine tenderness following urinary tract instrumentation or infection (30%), skin infection (13%), or respiratory infection (11%). In one-third of cases, the source of the bacteremia is unidentifiable. Fever is present in fewer than 50% of patients and is commonly low-grade. The infection can extend beyond the vertebral column and produce suppuration at the particular spinal level of involvement, such as a retropharyngeal abscess, mediastinitis, empyema, or subdiaphragmatic and iliopsoas abscesses, in addition to meningitis. If paresis, sensory deficits, or bowel or bladder dysfunction develop, spinal epidural abscess, the most feared complication of vertebral osteomyelitis, should be considered and evaluated immediately. Tuberculous infection should be considered in relatively indolent infections of the spine, hip, and knee.

C. **Introduced osteomyelitis.** Osteomyelitis following trauma or bone surgery commonly presents with persistent or recurrent fever, increasing pain at the operative site, and poor wound healing. Incisional healing difficulties include protracted drainage, cellulitis, suture abscesses, wound hematomas or seromas, and dehiscence. Bone infection should also be considered in cases of fracture non-union and failed arthrodesis. Prosthetic joint infection is associated with joint pain (95%), fever (43%), or cutaneous sinus drainage (32%).

D. **Osteomyelitis by contiguous spread.** Osseous involvement by spread of infection from an overlying chronic ischemic or neuropathic foot ulcer typically presents in patients with long-standing insulin-dependent diabetes mellitus or other vascular or neuropathic disease and involves the metatarsals (44%) or the proximal phalanges (32%). It is characterized by erythema (86%), swelling (75%), cellulitis, and necrosis, but pain is variable because of the frequent presence of sensory neuropathy (94%). Features correlated with the development of osteomyelitis in patients with such ulcers include the duration of unhealed ulceration (mean, 4 months), size of the ulcer (area ≥ 2 cm^2

and depth >3mm), and the presence of exposed bone. Additional presentations of osteomyelitis caused by contiguous spread of infection are listed in Table 42-1.

E. Chronic osteomyelitis. Acute exacerbations of chronic osteomyelitis present with local bone pain and tenderness in the area of previous osseous involvement. Fever with focal swelling, erythema, and increased warmth may also occur. Purulent drainage through an old or new cutaneous sinus frequently develops and usually is accompanied by defervescence as the inflammatory process is decompressed.

III. Diagnosis. The diagnosis of osteomyelitis is based on the compilation of clinical observations (history and physical examination) and findings from well-chosen imaging studies, and on the exercise of sound clinical judgment to give appropriate weight to the data collected. It is essential to be mindful of the pathogenesis attributed to the specific clinical situation being evaluated. Establishing the presence of osteomyelitis includes both confirming the site of bone involvement and identifying the causative microorganism(s). Osseous infection should be differentiated from septic arthritis and bursitis, cellulitis, soft-tissue abscesses, bone fractures, and neoplasms, and from bone infarcts seen with sickle cell hemoglobinopathy and Gaucher's disease. Anatomic delineation of bone infection depends substantially on imaging techniques.

A. Radiology. The earliest osseous roentgenographic changes in hematogenous infection are medullary areas of lucency, which require 30% to 50% decalcification to be seen and take 2 to 4 weeks to develop. As sepsis progresses, periosteal elevation, thickening, and new bone formation may be seen, with sequestra and sclerosis occurring in chronic cases. Vertebral osteomyelitis appears initially as disk space narrowing with subsequent cortical degradation at the adjacent end plates. With the introduced form of osteomyelitis, bone resorption is evident at the site of the fracture, fixation device, or bone-cement interface of a joint prosthesis. When bone infection develops by spread from contiguous tissue, subperiosteal bone lucencies and cortical erosions are demonstrable and followed by lytic medullary lesions. Periosteal reaction is commonly seen in patients with chronic, deep ulcerations overlying bone but is not diagnostic of osteomyelitis. There is commonly a delay in radiographic improvement during the healing phase of bone infection, and 30% of patients have worsening roentgenographic findings while they are improving clinically on therapy. **Computed tomography (CT)** can be useful in demonstrating small osseous changes, sequestra, and extraosseous extension of infection. Roentgenography is the most specific and least expensive imaging technique for diagnosing osteomyelitis. In patients with very acute, fulminant infection (such as childhood hematogenous osteomyelitis), roentgenograms may not be sufficiently sensitive to reveal diagnostic abnormalities at the time of presentation, and additional studies are needed. However, most cases of bone infection present subacutely, with adequate duration of infection for demineralization to occur, and can be well evaluated by radiologic techniques.

B. Radionuclide scans. Technetium diphosphonate bone scans, gallium citrate scans, and indium-labeled leukocyte scintigraphy are much more sensitive than roentgenography and usually demonstrate increased radionuclide uptake at the onset of symptoms. However, these imaging methods are plagued by inadequate specificity and spatial resolution, so they cannot be relied on to be definitively diagnostic.

Inflammatory and degenerative processes in surrounding soft tissues, areas recently subjected to orthopedic surgery or trauma, bone fractures, and neoplasms produce abnormal findings on nuclide scans in the absence of osteomyelitis. Table 42-2 lists the approximate sensitivity and specificity of various imaging techniques in clinical situations in which the diagnosis is ambiguous because of the presence of a pathologic process in adjacent tissues (e.g., cellulitis, edema) or a comorbid state in the osseous tissue (e.g., diabetic osteoarthropathy, bone infarction, recent trauma).

Table 42-2. Estimated relative value of different imaging techniques for the diagnosis of osteomyelitis in complicated cases

Imaging technique	Sensitivity (%)	Specificity (%)
Roentgenography	69	82
Technetium bone scan	77	36
Gallium scan	95	38
Indium-labeled WBC scan	74	69
Sequential indium and technetium scans	86	72
Magnetic resonance imaging (MRI)	83	75

Complicated cases include patients with diabetes, neuropathic osteoarthropathy, cellulitis, and recent trauma (orthopedic surgery, fractures).
WBC, white blood cell.

C. **Magnetic resonance imaging (MRI)** can detect osteomyelitis earlier and with a sensitivity equal to or greater than that of roentgenography, and its spatial resolution is much better than that of scintigraphy. Negative MRI findings are strong evidence against the presence of osteomyelitis. However, this technique is too nonspecific to be the optimal determinant for the presence of bone infection. An increased MRI signal represents small increases in tissue water content. Gadolinium is deposited in the extracellular fluid compartment in areas of increased vascular permeability and thereby increases the sensitivity of MRI for inflammation of all etiologies. MRI detects the bone edema of osteomyelitis; however, differentiation of nonspecific reactive marrow edema from adjacent foci of infection or other causes of soft-tissue edema is often not possible. The specificity of MRI for osteomyelitis is significantly diminished because of false-positives related to sterile inflammation, edema in tissues adjacent to bone, bone infarction, recent trauma, diabetic osteoarthropathy, heterotopic bone formation, neoplasm, and local radiation therapy (see Table 42-2). A recently developed technique that uses fat suppression with MRI scans has increased the specificity, but not yet to the level needed for confidence.

D. **Microbiologic studies.** The specific etiologic pathogen in osteomyelitis should be delineated because the microbe is never sufficiently predictable to allow routine presumptive therapy (see Table 42-1). Moreover, knowledge of the antimicrobial sensitivity of the isolated causative bacterium is essential to design optimal therapy. Blood cultures are positive in 25% to 50% of children with acute hematogenous osteomyelitis but in fewer than 10% of the other forms of bone infection. If septic arthritis or soft-tissue abscess accompanies the osseous infection, arthrocentesis or abscess aspiration cultures can be diagnostic. However, superficial cultures of open wounds, wound drainage, or skin ulcerations and cultures of cutaneous sinus tracts do not delineate the true bone pathogen(s). Sinus tract and sinus drainage cultures often reflect colonizing flora and cannot be relied on to identify the actual cause of the deep osseous infection. In patients with deep, chronic skin ulcers by which infection has spread to bone, curettage cultures from the base of the ulcer have a 75% correlation with osseous tissue cultures. Bone aspirate cultures are positive in 50% to 60% of patients, whereas bone biopsy cultures are positive in 70% to 93% of cases and should be sought (percutaneously or by operative debridement) when there is no overlying skin ulcer and the microbiologic etiology has not been otherwise determined. Specific cultures for mycobacteria, fungi, and anaerobes should be considered when routine bacterial cultures are negative.

E. **Guidelines for diagnosing osteomyelitis (based on pathogenesis)**

1. **Childhood acute hematogenous osteomyelitis**

   a. Plain roentgenograms of the suspect bone. CT if additional detail is needed.

   b. Technetium bone scan, if the roentgenograms are not diagnostic.
   c. MRI with gadolinium if roentgenograms and technetium bone scan are not diagnostic but clinical suspicion is strong.
   d. Blood cultures.
   e. Bone biopsy for cultures and histopathology.

2. **Adult acute hematogenous osteomyelitis (vertebral osteomyelitis)**
   a. Plain roentgenograms of the suspect bones. CT if additional detail is needed.
   b. MRI with gadolinium if roentgenograms are not diagnostic.
   c. Blood cultures.
   d. Bone biopsy for cultures and histopathology.

3. **Introduced form of osteomyelitis**
   a. Plain roentgenograms of the suspect bones. CT if additional detail is needed. Serial roentgenography or CT at intervals during a 4-week period to observe any meaningful osseous changes.
   b. Arthrocentesis (if a prosthetic joint is present) for cultures.
   c. Bone biopsy, usually with debridement surgery, for cultures.

4. **Osteomyelitis caused by contiguous spread of infection**
   a. Plain roentgenograms of the suspect bones. CT if additional detail is needed. Serial roentgenography or CT at intervals during a 4-week period to observe any meaningful osseous changes.
   b. Indium-labeled leukocyte scan (or sequential indium or technetium scan), if suspicion is not strong, for the negative predictive value of a negative scan result. (A positive scan result would not be as diagnostic as meaningful osseous changes on serial roentgenograms.)
   c. MRI with gadolinium and fat suppression if clinical suspicion is strong.
   d. Culture base of soft-tissue ulcer before starting antibiotic therapy. Prepare ulcer base with iodine, then alcohol (allow alcohol to evaporate). Abrade ulcer base with a culture swab.
   e. Avoid percutaneous bone biopsy, if possible, because (a) this trauma may induce bone necrosis and infection, (b) the histopathology of neuropathic osteopathy may resemble that of osteomyelitis, and (c) the bone biopsy specimen can be contaminated with organisms from the contiguous infected soft tissue.
   f. If soft-tissue infection is present, treat with antibiotics and obtain serial roentgenograms with the patient off antibiotic therapy at intervals during a 4-week period to determine subsequently the presence or absence of osteomyelitis.

5. **Chronic osteomyelitis**
   a. Plain roentgenograms of the suspect bone.
   b. CT or MRI to delineate sequestra.
   c. Sinogram (roentgenogram with dye inserted into a cutaneous sinus tract) to demonstrate the osseous site of sinus tract origin, which often is the site of sequestrum.
   d. Bone biopsy (percutaneously or at debridement surgery) for cultures and histopathology.

      Note: Sinus tract cultures are not reliable for delineating the true etiologic pathogen.

IV. Treatment

A. Antibiotics. Acute osteomyelitis is curable with adequate antimicrobial therapy accompanied by surgical debridement when necessary. IV antibiotics are commonly used, but oral agents are also effective when the quantitative susceptibility of the pathogen is sufficient and when gastrointestinal absorption and compliance are ensured. The exact potency and duration of treatment necessary to eradicate bone infections are not known. Antimicrobial agents that produce trough serum bactericidal activity at a 1:2 titer have been associated with highly successful outcomes. Therapy should be administered for at least 4 to 6 weeks. Designing a therapeutic regimen for osteomyelitis depends substantially on the sensitivity of the isolated pathogen to specific antimicrobial agents, which underscores the essential importance of delineating the pathogen in these infections.

Chronic osteomyelitis is treatable but not curable with systemic antibiotics. Acute exacerbations of these persistent infections can be suppressed successfully by debridement of identifiable sequestra followed by protracted courses of parenteral or oral antimicrobial agents. Theoretically, depot administration of appropriate antibiotics to the site of infected, avascular bone via antibiotic-loaded polymethylmethacrylate beads could eradicate the persistent bacteria unreachable by systemic (blood vessel-dependent) therapy.

B. Surgery. When acute osteomyelitis is complicated by abscess formation or extensive necrosis, surgical debridement is an important adjunct to antibiotics. In cases associated with prosthetic joints or internal fixation devices, the foreign body usually needs to be removed to effect a cure. In chronic osteomyelitis, surgery is often the primary therapeutic treatment. Necrotic tissue and sequestra should be removed when possible, and dead spaces should be eliminated with packing, bone grafts, muscle pedicles, or skin grafts. Surgery is also important when neurologic structures are threatened (e.g., cord compression in vertebral osteomyelitis). In osteomyelitis associated with peripheral vascular disease, amputation of the affected area is frequently required if the infection does not respond to parenteral antibiotics.

Bibliography

Brause BD. Infections with prostheses in bones and joints. In: Mandell GL, Bennett JE, Dolin R, eds. *Principles and practice of infectious diseases.* New York: Churchill Livingstone, 1994:1051.

Crim JR, Seeger LL. Imaging evaluation of osteomyelitis. *Crit Rev Diagn Imaging* 1994;35:201.

Haas DW, McAndrew MP. Bacterial osteomyelitis in adults: evolving considerations in diagnosis and treatment. *Am J Med* 1996;101:550.

Lew DP, Waldvogel FA. Osteomyelitis. *N Engl J Med* 1997;336:999.

Lipsky BA. Osteomyelitis of the foot in diabetic patients. *Clin Infect Dis* 1997;25:1318.

Morrison WB, et al. Osteomyelitis in feet of diabetics: clinical accuracy, surgical utility, and cost-effectiveness of MR imaging. *Radiology* 1995;196:557.

Sapico FL, et al. The infected foot of the diabetic patient: quantitative microbiology and analysis of clinical features. *Rev Infect Dis* 1984;6:S171.

Torda AJ, Gottlieb T, Bradbury R. Pyogenic vertebral osteomyelitis: analysis of 20 cases and review. *Clin Infect Dis* 1995;20:320.

Weinstein M, et al. Multicenter collaborative evaluation of a standardized serum bactericidal test as a predictor of therapeutic efficacy in acute and chronic osteomyelitis. *Am J Med* 1987;83:218.

43. RHEUMATIC FEVER

Allan Gibofsky and John B. Zabriskie

Acute rheumatic fever (ARF) is the term used to describe a systemic rheumatic disease manifested clinically by a constellation of symptoms following pharyngeal streptococcal infection.

I. Etiology and pathogenesis. The disease occurs as a sequela of streptococcal pharyngitis, and the latent period from infection to onset of disease varies from 2 to 6 weeks or longer. ARF is almost exclusively associated with group A strains causing pharyngitis, and rarely if ever follows infections causing impetigo or kidney disease.

The available evidence suggests that the host's abnormal immune response, at both a cellular and humoral level, to streptococcal antigens cross-reactive with target mammalian antigens is responsible for the pathologic damage. These cross-reactive antigens include the hyaluronic capsule of the streptococcus and a number of streptococcal antigens, including M proteins, that share antigenic determinants with cardiac tropomyosin and myosin. Other antigenic determinants include renal, central nervous system, and skin antigens. A genetic basis for the disease has been suggested for more than 100 years, and family studies indicate that gene inheritance is either autosomal recessive or dominant with limited penetrance. Whether susceptibility to rheumatic fever is associated with certain major histocompatibility complex (MHC) alleles is controversial, although associations with HLA-DR4 and HLA-DR2 have been reported. Non-MHC markers have been described, and a monoclonal antibody called D8/17 identifies an antigen present on the B cells of 100% of rheumatic fever patients tested.

II. Prevalence. Both the prevalence and severity of rheumatic fever have declined dramatically during the last six decades in the United States and other developed countries; however, a resurgence in new and recurrent cases deserves renewed attention. Changes in living conditions, nutrition, and virulence of the organism, in addition to antibiotic therapy of streptococcal pharyngitis, have all been suggested as reasons for the decreased incidence. The overall incidence of rheumatic fever in the United States is currently estimated to be less than 1 in 100,000 children of school age per year, but groups with poor standards of living have a much higher incidence. In some developing nations, the incidence of rheumatic fever remains high, 60 in 100,000 children (5 to 14 years old) per year or more. Rheumatic heart disease, a chronic sequela of rheumatic fever, is the most common cause of heart disease in persons under age 40 in these countries. Rheumatic fever thus represents a significant worldwide health problem.

III. Clinical presentation

A. Antecedent streptococcal pharyngitis most commonly occurs 2 to 3 weeks before the onset of the symptoms of rheumatic fever. It may be mild, however, and a history of fever and sore throat cannot be elicited in all patients.

B. Fever, which has no specific pattern, is almost always present at the onset of an acute attack and fades away in days to weeks without antiinflammatory treatment. Fever resolves promptly with salicylate therapy.

C. Arthritis with fever is the most common manifestation of ARF, occurring in 50% to 75% of cases. It usually involves the large peripheral joints, especially the knees and ankles, but any joint may be affected. The arthritis, which occurs within 5 weeks of the streptococcal infection, when anti-streptococcal antibody titers are usually high, subsides without treatment in a few weeks and very rarely causes joint deformity. Carditis occurs less frequently in cases with severe arthritis.

D. Arthralgia without objective evidence of joint inflammation may precede the development of synovitis. Severe arthralgia, especially if migratory, is an important diagnostic feature.

E. **Carditis** is the most important manifestation of ARF because it frequently leads to chronic valvular damage. In rare cases, it is a cause of death from cardiac failure or arrhythmias associated with myocarditis during an acute episode. Carditis occurs in 40% to 50% of attacks of ARF in some series, but this incidence seems to be decreasing.

1. **Chest pain or dyspnea** may occur with ARF, but these complaints are often not specific to cardiac involvement.
2. **Major signs**
   a. **Significant new or changing murmurs,** described below, are characteristic of acute valvulitis and differ from the murmurs of valvular stenosis or regurgitation that may be heard later. They often disappear with resolution of acute inflammation.
      (1) **Mitral valvulitis murmur** is blowing, high-pitched, holosystolic, and apical and transmits to the axilla. It must be distinguished from the click/murmur of the mitral valve prolapse syndrome, which has a mid-systolic click and late systolic murmur.
      (2) **Carey Coombs murmur** is mid-diastolic, low-pitched, and apical and often associated with the mitral valvulitis. It is best heard with the patient in the left lateral recumbent position and should be distinguished from the murmur of mitral stenosis.
      (3) **Aortic valvulitis** murmur is a soft, high-pitched, decrescendo blow, heard immediately after the second heart sound along the left sternal border with the patient leaning forward. It must be distinguished from the murmur of a congenital bicuspid aortic valve.
   b. **Cardiomegaly** should be carefully monitored by physical examination and serial chest roentgenograms.
   c. **Congestive heart failure** occurs more commonly in children under 6 years of age and in patients without severe arthritis.
   d. **Pericarditis,** when present, usually occurs in association with other features of rheumatic carditis. Pericarditis may be manifested by chest pain, friction rub, effusions, and electrocardiographic changes. Large effusions are rare.
   e. **Other cardiac findings** may include tachycardia at rest (out of proportion to fever) and a soft, dull, variable first heart sound secondary to a prolonged PR interval. Atrioventricular block is commonly seen in cases of ARF without other evidence of carditis or subsequent rheumatic heart disease. It is thought to be a toxic manifestation of ARF and is not specifically indicative of carditis.

F. **Erythema marginatum,** a rare manifestation of ARF, is a nonpruritic rash that begins as a pink macule and spreads outward in a sharp ring with central clearing or as serpiginous coalescing lines. The rash is evanescent and rarely raised, blanches with pressure, is brought out by application of heat, and is distributed over the trunk and proximal extremities, never on the face, and rarely on the distal extremities. The rash may appear at any time in the course of ARF. Its appearance and resolution are unrelated to the course of other manifestations or to treatment. Rash secondary to drug reaction or systemic juvenile rheumatoid arthritis can usually be differentiated by the characteristics just mentioned and other associated clinical manifestations.

G. **Subcutaneous nodules** are firm, nontender, nonpruritic, freely movable swellings located in crops of variable numbers over bony prominences and tendons without overlying skin discoloration. They are smaller and less persistent than those of rheumatoid arthritis. Nodules are a late and infrequent manifestation associated with severe carditis.

H. **Sydenham's chorea** is a late manifestation of ARF and may follow other manifestations of ARF or may appear alone. It is characterized by involuntary, purposeless, abrupt, and nonrepetitive movements, muscular weakness, and emotional lability. The abnormal movements subside during sleep. When subtle, chorea is demonstrated when (a) squeezing the examiner's hand reveals an erratic "milkmaid's grip," (b) raising the hand straight ahead causes pronation of one or both arms, (c) extending the hands straight ahead causes spooning of the hand with wrist flexion and extension of fingers, and (d) protruding the tongue produces snakelike darting movements. Because the latent period from streptococcal infection to chorea is 1 to 6 months, anti-streptolysin O (ASO) titers and levels of acute-phase reactants may be normal. Investigation of other streptococcal antigens usually will reveal one or more with rising titers in all but those patients with isolated chorea. The duration of chorea ranges from 1 week to 1 year, with an average of 3 months. Some patients with Sydenham's chorea have an antibody that reacts with basal ganglia and cross-reacts with streptococcal cell membranes. Sydenham's chorea must be distinguished from other neurologic entities, including Huntington's chorea, central nervous system lupus, Wilson's disease, and toxic drug reactions (especially to the phenothiazines).

IV. Laboratory studies

A. Evidence of preceding streptococcal infection may be obtained by throat cultures (in about 25% of cases), and it is recommended that *three* successive cultures be taken before antibiotic treatment is begun. ASO antibodies are elevated in approximately 80% of cases, and serial serum samples should be drawn during the acute stage and 2 weeks later. Testing for anti-hyaluronidase, deoxyribonuclease B, and streptozyme titers increases the documentation of a preceding streptococcal infection to 97%.

B. Acute-phase reactants, such as C-reactive protein, and the erythrocyte sedimentation rate reflect ongoing inflammation and are useful in monitoring response to therapy.

C. Anti-heart antibodies that cross-react with streptococcal cell membranes are found in sera of ARF patients, but the test has not been standardized for routine use.

D. Serial chest roentgenograms are important to reveal cardiomegaly as a sign of carditis.

E. Serial electrocardiograms may reveal the nonspecific atrioventricular block discussed in section **III.E.2.e** or changes of myocarditis and pericarditis.

F. Echocardiography is useful in differentiating patients with bicuspid aortic valves or mitral prolapse syndrome from those with rheumatic heart disease. It may also be used to evaluate pericardial effusion and myocardial function.

V. The **revised Jones criteria** (Table 43-1) indicate a high probability of ARF when evidence of a preceding streptococcal infection is found simultaneously with the presence of two major criteria; a diagnosis of ARF based on the presence of

Table 43-1. Jones criteria (revised) for guidance in the diagnosis of rheumatic fever

Major criteria	Minor criteria
Carditis	Clinical
Polyarthritis	Fever
Chorea	Arthralgia
Erythema marginatum	Previous rheumatic fever
Subcutaneous nodules	Previous rheumatic fever or heart disease
	Laboratory
	Increased ESR or CRP
	Prolonged PR interval

PLUS: Supporting evidence of preceding streptococcal infection: increased ASO or other streptococcal antibodies, positive throat culture for group A streptococci, or recent scarlet fever.

ESR, erythrocyte sedimentation rate; CRP, C-reactive protein; ASO, anti-streptolysin O.
From special report: Jones criteria (revised) for guidance in the diagnosis of rheumatic fever. *Circulation* 1984;69:204A.

one major criterion and two minor criteria is less definitive. The Jones criteria were developed to provide uniformity and to minimize the overdiagnosis of ARF.

VI. Differential diagnosis

A. Bacterial infections, including septic arthritis, osteomyelitis, and subacute bacterial endocarditis, should be ruled out by appropriate culture. Lyme disease should be considered, especially in areas where it is endemic.

B. Viral infections, particularly rubella arthritis, arthritis associated with hepatitis B infection, and infectious mononucleosis, should be considered.

C. Collagen vascular disease, rheumatoid arthritis, systemic lupus erythematosus, and vasculitis such as Henoch-Schönlein purpura may be differentiated on clinical and laboratory grounds.

D. Immune complex disease induced by an allergic reaction to drugs may be suggested by history and by clinical features such as pruritic or urticarial rash.

E. Sickle cell hemoglobinopathies may superficially resemble ARF but are not difficult to differentiate.

F. Malignancies, especially leukemias and lymphomas, can present with fever and acute polyarthritis.

G. Mucocutaneous lymph node syndrome (Kawasaki disease) may initially resemble ARF, but the desquamating rash and absence of rising ASO titers should make differentiation possible.

VII. Treatment

A. Antibiotic treatment with penicillin, or erythromycin in case of penicillin allergy, is recommended for all patients in a standard 10-day course for streptococcal pharyngitis to eradicate residual organisms. There is, however, no evidence that such therapy significantly alters the acute or chronic phase of the disease. Penicillin prophylaxis (see section **VII.B.5**) is begun after the 10-day course of treatment to reduce the risk for recurrence of disease.

B. Antiinflammatory treatment provides symptomatic relief but does not appear to alter the duration of the attack or cardiac sequelae.

1. **General measures** that are helpful include the following:
   a. **Analgesics** for the management of joint pains, especially while diagnostic evaluation is in progress and before antiinflammatory treatment is started.
   b. **Sodium restriction, digitalis, and diuretics** for heart failure. Digitalis should be used with caution, as myocarditis is almost invariably present.
2. **Salicylates** are highly effective in controlling fever and arthritis but should not be used before an adequate period of observation allows a firm diagnosis to be established. A dosage of about 80 mg/kg daily in four divided doses, with a resultant blood level of 20 to 30 mg/dL, is usually effective in controlling fever, arthritis, and mild carditis when given for 2 weeks, followed by a dosage of about 60 mg/kg daily for 6 subsequent weeks.
3. **Corticosteroids** have not been shown to be more effective than aspirin in reducing long-term cardiac damage. Nevertheless, they are often used to treat carditis, especially when congestive failure is present. Prednisone (1 to 2 mg/kg daily in divided doses) is used for 2 to 4 weeks. Salicylates are often added for an additional 4 to 8 weeks.
4. **Treatment of chorea** includes keeping the patient in a quiet, protective environment and sedation with phenobarbital, diazepam, or chlorpromazine as needed. Valproic acid and haloperidol appear to be useful in reducing the severity of choreiform movements.
5. **Prophylaxis** with penicillin G (250,000 U PO twice daily) or benzathine penicillin (1.2 million U IM every 4 weeks) clearly reduces the chance of recurrent rheumatic fever and progressive cardiac damage. In areas where high exposure to streptococci is expected and in all cases of valvular damage, the injections should be given every 3 weeks. Alternatively, the injection is given every 4 weeks with supplemental oral penicillin dosing during the last 10 days of each month. With penicillin VK (250 mg PO twice daily) in place of penicillin G, absorption from the intestinal tract is improved and more

reliable. Benzathine penicillin prophylaxis has the advantage of ensured compliance, but cases of recurrent rheumatic fever have occasionally been reported, probably a consequence of individual differences in the pharmacokinetics of the drug. The penicillin-allergic patient may be treated with 250 mg of erythromycin twice daily. The minimum recommended duration of prophylaxis is 5 years from the last recurrence because recurrences are most common during this period. Recurrent attacks in adulthood have been reported, however, and as long-term prophylaxis appears to be benign, it is advisable to continue prophylaxis indefinitely. All patients with evidence of chronic rheumatic heart disease, regardless of age, should be on continuous prophylaxis because recurrent disease usually includes carditis.

Bibliography

Gibofsky A, Zabriskie JB. Rheumatic fever. In: Espinoza L, ed. *Infections in the rheumatic diseases.* New York: Grune & Stratton, 1988;367–373.

Gibofsky A, Kerwar S, Zabriskie J. Rheumatic fever: the relationships between host, microbe, and genetics. *Rheum Dis Clin North Am* 1998;24:237.

Human DG, Hill ID, Fraser CB. Treatment choice in acute rheumatic carditis. *Arch Dis Child* 1984;59:410.

Land HA, Bisno AL. Acute rheumatic fever: a vanishing disease in suburbia. *JAMA* 1983;249:895.

Markowitz M. Observations on the epidemiology and preventability of rheumatic fever in developing countries. *Clin Ther* 1981;4:240.

Patarrayo ME, et al. Association of a B-cell alloantigen with susceptibility to rheumatic fever. *Nature* 1979;278:173.

Schwartz RH, Hepner SI, Ziai M. Incidence of acute rheumatic fever: a suburban community hospital experience during the 1970s. *Clin Pediatr* 1983;22:798.

Special report: Jones criteria (revised) for guidance in the diagnosis of rheumatic fever. *Circulation* 1984;69:204A.

Zabriskie JB. Rheumatic fever: a streptococcal-induced autoimmune disease. *Pediatr Ann* 1982;11:383.

Zabriskie JB, Kerwar S, Gibofsky A. The arthritogenic properties of microbial antigens: their implications in disease states. *Rheum Dis Clin North Am* 1998;24:211.

44. OSTEOARTHRITIS

John F. Beary, III and Michael E. Luggen

Osteoarthritis (OA) is the most common musculoskeletal problem in people over age 50. It is characterized by *focal degeneration* of joint cartilage and *new bone formation* at the base of the cartilage lesion (subchondral bone) and at the joint margins (osteophytes). During the past two decades, OA has come to be viewed as a disease involving the *entire joint organ* (bone, cartilage, and supporting elements) rather than as primarily a cartilage problem.

A 1994 National Institutes of Health Conference created the following *comprehensive definition: Osteoarthritis* is the result of both mechanical and biologic events that destabilize the normal coupling of degradation and synthesis of articular cartilage and subchondral bone. Although it may be initiated by multiple factors, including genetic, developmental, metabolic, and traumatic causes, OA involves all tissues of the diarthrodial joint. Ultimately, OA is manifested by morphologic, biochemical, molecular, and biomechanical changes of both cells and matrix that lead to a softening, fibrillation, ulceration, and loss of articular cartilage; sclerosis and eburnation of subchondral bone; and the formation of osteophytes and subchondral cysts. When clinically evident, OA is characterized by joint pain, tenderness, limitation of movement, crepitus, occasional effusion, and variable degrees of local inflammation.

OA occurs in all mammalian species and is the earliest documented human disease. Human skeletons from 2 million years ago show evidence of the effect of OA, at the time that bipedality occurred in the evolutionary change from hominids to humans. The bipedal posture promotes OA changes in joints such as the aging lumbar spine and knees.

A. E. Garrod described OA as a clinical entity in 1907 and differentiated it from rheumatoid arthritis (RA). RA was noted to be inflammatory and erosive, whereas OA was a degenerative process with hypertrophic bone features.

I. Disease classification

A. Primary

1. **Localized osteoarthritis.** Heberden's nodes without other joint involvement represent the most common form of primary OA. Family studies reveal that genetic factors are important in the development of Heberden's nodes. These nodes are ten times more common in women than in men.
2. **Generalized osteoarthritis** was named by Moore in 1952. Generalized OA is defined by involvement of three or more joints or joint groups [e.g., the distal interphalangeal (DIP) joints are counted as one group]. By definition, conditions that are known to produce secondary generalized OA, such as ochronosis, are excluded. The DIP, proximal interphalangeal (PIP), first carpometacarpal (CMC), spine, knee, and hip joints are commonly involved. Other features of generalized OA include a predilection for postmenopausal women and episodic joint inflammation. A familial pattern, associated with Heberden's nodes, has been reported in a subset of generalized OA patients.
3. **Erosive osteoarthritis,** also known as inflammatory OA, may be a distinct disease. However, there is also a possibility that erosive OA merely represents the end of the OA spectrum characterized by severe disease. DIP and PIP joints of the hands are affected. Results of the test for rheumatoid factor (RF) are negative. Joint radiographs reveal both osteophytes and erosions. In one series, 15% of patients with erosive OA subsequently fulfilled criteria for a diagnosis of RA.

B. Secondary. See section **III.B** for causes.

II. Epidemiology. Primary OA is the most common form of arthritis in North America and Western Europe and affects 21 million Americans. The natural history of the disease takes about 20 years to be expressed; therefore, the majority of patients are over the age of 60. OA results in 68 million lost work days per year and 4 million hospitalizations per year. About 100,000 patients in the United States are unable to walk from bed to bathroom because of OA. OA of the knee is the second leading cause of disability in the elderly, following heart disease.

An interesting epidemiologic clue from the work of Nevitt et al. suggests that women who are long-term users of estrogen replacement therapy have decreased rates of OA of the hip, which adds support to the role of bone in the expression of this disease. This line of evidence is also consistent with findings of regional abnormalities of bone density and vascularity in periarticular densitometry studies and scintigraphy studies. Finally, epidemiologic studies suggest that low levels of vitamin D may be related to the progression of OA of the knee.

Radiographic surveys reveal that the majority of subjects over age 55 have radiographically confirmed disease. It is further estimated that 90% of people over age 70 have radiographic evidence of OA in at least one joint. Above age 55, women are affected more than men. Between the ages of 40 and 55, there is little difference in male versus female prevalence. Studies of ethnic groups in the United States reveal that African-American women are more likely to get knee OA than are Caucasians.

III. Pathogenesis

A. Primary osteoarthritis. The forces exerted on the normal joint by motion and weight bearing are dissipated by joint cartilage, subchondral bone, and surrounding structures (joint capsule and muscle). Joint cartilage has unique properties of compressibility and elasticity, attributable to the presence of an intertwined mesh of both collagen and proteoglycan (PG). Cartilage collagen is type 2 collagen and forms a three-dimensional network of cross-linked fibers that create the structural framework for cartilage. PGs are large molecules that individually consist of a protein core with negatively charged glycosaminoglycan side chains composed of keratan sulfate and chondroitin sulfate. PGs exist mostly as aggregates and are attached as side chains by a link protein to a core of hyaluronic acid. The PGs bind large amounts of water molecules, which are released when the cartilage is compressed and recaptured when compression is removed. The primary PG of articular cartilage is termed aggrecan and gives cartilage the ability to undergo reversible deformations.

Primary OA is a multifactorial disease process that involves the joint constituents (chondrocytes, collagen, PGs, subchondral bone, and synovial membrane) in various ways. Although a precise pathogenesis has not been elucidated, the following factors are germane to the development of primary OA:

1. **Aging.** The ability of articular cartilage to withstand fatigue testing diminishes progressively with age. However, no specific biochemical defect of aging cartilage has yet been identified. It is also of interest that in human cartilage, chondrocytes remain normal in number and metabolic activity as the tissue ages.
2. **Mechanical factors (wear and tear).** Accumulated microtrauma causes changes in subchondral bone that likely affect the ability of a joint to absorb the force of impulse loading, thus leading to degeneration of cartilage. This factor may account for occupational OA, such as that seen in the metacarpophalangeal (MCP) and shoulder joints of boxers, elbows of jackhammer operators, knees of basketball players, ankles of ballet dancers, and spines of coal miners.
3. **Genetic factors.** It is known that factors such as the collagen content of cartilage and the ability of chondrocytes to synthesize PGs are genetically determined. Primary OA in the form of Heberden's nodes also points to the importance of a genetic factor in pathogenesis. Polymorphisms of the type 2 collagen gene have recently been identified in a family with premature OA.
4. **Biochemical factors.** The principal early change in OA cartilage is a decreased content of PGs. (Collagen content remains normal.) The loss of PGs causes biomechanical problems, such as a loss of compressive stiff-

ness in the cartilage, decreased elasticity, and an increase in hydraulic permeability. Later, collagen unravels and is lost because of increased matrix metalloproteinase activity.

B. Secondary osteoarthritis. Disorders that damage joint surfaces and cause cartilage changes characteristic of OA are as follows:

1. **Mechanical incongruity of the joint**
   a. **Congenital and developmental disorders,** such as hip dysplasia, slipped femoral capital epiphysis, and multiple epiphyseal dysplasia.
   b. Prior joint **trauma.**
   c. Prior joint **surgery,** such as meniscectomy.
2. Prior **inflammatory** joint disease, such as RA or infectious arthritis.
3. Prior **bone disease,** such as Paget's disease or osteonecrosis.
4. **Bleeding dyscrasias.** Hemarthrosis affects 90% of patients with hemophilia, most commonly in the knee, ankle, and elbow. With recurrent hemarthrosis, a proliferative synovitis occurs, which promotes development of secondary OA. Large cystic areas and evidence of osteonecrosis may be seen on radiographs.
5. **Neuropathic joint disease.** Loss of pain or proprioception leads to decreased joint protection and subsequent secondary OA. Examples of diseases responsible for the development of neuropathic arthropathy include diabetes, syphilis, pernicious anemia, spinal cord trauma, and peripheral nerve injury. Radiographic findings reveal severe OA changes with loss of cartilage, exuberant osteophyte formation, bizarre bony overgrowth, fragmentation of subchondral bone with pathologic fractures, and eventually disintegration of the joint structure.
6. **Excessive intraarticular steroid injections** may be associated with OA. Two mechanisms are postulated:
   a. Intraarticular injection relieves pain and thereby allows overuse of an already damaged joint, and
   b. Cartilage may be directly damaged by injected steroids.
7. **Endocrinopathies and metabolic disorders** (see also Chapter 48).
   a. **Acromegaly.**
   b. **Cushing's disease** and long-term corticosteroid therapy via the mechanism of osteonecrosis. Corticosteroids inhibit osteoblast function and cause a secondary hyperparathyroidism, which activates osteoclasts and so accelerates subchondral bone damage.
   c. **Crystal arthropathies.** Calcium pyrophosphate dihydrate deposition (CPPD) disease is strongly associated with OA. Basic calcium phosphate crystals play a key role in the destructive arthropathy of large joints known as Milwaukee shoulder syndrome.
   d. **Gout.**
   e. **Ochronosis.** These patients lack homogentisic acid oxidase, which results in increased urinary excretion of homogentisic acid and increased binding of homogentisic acid to connective tissue. The latter presumably is responsible for the secondary OA seen in this disorder. The pigment is deposited in cartilage, skin, and sclera. Degenerative disease of the spine with calcification of the intervertebral disks is characteristic.
   f. **Wilson's disease.** Premature OA, pseudogout, and chondromalacia patellae are articular manifestations of this disorder of copper metabolism.
   g. **Hemochromatosis.** Hemosiderin granules are deposited in cartilage. CPPD crystals are also associated with this disease. The arthropathy of hemochromatosis characteristically involves the second and third MCP joints.

IV. Pathology. Various features are seen in cartilage and bone as the disease progresses.

A. Structural breakdown of cartilage. In order of progression, this process consists of the following:

1. Fibrillation and fissuring.
2. Focal and diffuse erosions of the cartilage surface.
3. Thinning and complete denudation of cartilage.

B. Changes in subchondral bone

1. Subchondral bony sclerosis.
2. Cyst formation.
3. Bone thickening with eburnation.
4. Reactive proliferation of new bone and cartilage at the joint periphery to produce osteophytes. Buckland-Wright has shown that bony changes of subchondral cortical sclerosis and osteophytosis precede changes in articular cartilage, measured radiographically as a loss in joint space width.

C. Other changes. Some mild degree of synovitis can be expected, perhaps a consequence of attempts to remove degenerative bone and cartilage debris from the synovial space. Additional changes include degeneration of menisci and periarticular muscle atrophy.

V. General clinical presentation

A. History

1. Symptoms

a. Symptomatic patients are usually **over the age of 40.** It should be noted that radiographic OA without clinical symptoms is quite common.

b. Patients complain of **pain** of insidious onset in **one or a few joints.** The pain is aching and poorly localized.

c. Pain first occurs after normal joint use and can be **relieved by rest.** As the disease progresses, pain during rest develops. Morning joint stiffness lasts less than half an hour.

d. Systemic symptoms are absent.

2. The most common **sites of involvement** are the DIP and first CMC joints of the hand and the first metatarsophalangeal (MTP) joint in the foot; hips; knees; and the lumbar and cervical spine. OA rarely involves the MCP joints, wrists, elbows, and shoulders or ankles, unless secondary OA is present. In general, correlation between joint symptoms and radiographic changes in early OA is poor. However, as the disease presses, pain is more common as a result of pathology in bone, which is richly innervated. Later-stage disease is characterized by osteophytes and radiographic joint space narrowing, particularly in large, weight-bearing joints such as the knee and hip.

B. Physical examination

1. Joints may be tender, especially if swelling and warmth (synovitis) are present. However, tenderness may be present without signs of inflammation. Pain with weight bearing may be present without pain on passive range of motion. Joint enlargement may result from the presence of effusion, synovial hyperplasia, or osteophytes.
2. In later disease stages, there may be **crepitus,** gross deformity, and subluxation (caused by cartilage loss, collapse of subchondral bone, bone cysts, and gross bony overgrowth).
3. **Limitation of motion** increases as disease progresses, perhaps caused by joint surface incongruity, muscle spasms and contracture, capsule contracture, or mechanical blockage by osteophytes or loose bodies.

C. Radiographic findings. Radiographs are not needed in the majority of clinical situations and can be reserved for situations of persistent unexplained joint symptoms. However, when a radiographic film is obtained, one must be aware that OA is very common and not overlook other arthritides or fractures when evaluating a painful joint. Special views may be needed to evaluate the extent of involvement of a particular joint.

1. **Radiographic criteria** for OA are as follows:

a. **Joint space narrowing** secondary to degeneration and disappearance of articular cartilage. Precise measurement of joint space narrowing is not available for routine clinical use but is currently used in research studies directed at testing disease-modifying therapies in knee OA.

b. **Osteophyte formation** at joint margins or sites of ligamentous attachment.
c. **Subchondral bone sclerosis.**
d. **Subchondral bone cysts.**
e. **Altered shape of a bone end caused by bone remodeling.**

D. **Other imaging modalities.** Scintigraphy has been shown to predict the progression of OA in some studies but is rarely used in routine practice. It is difficult to view the bone component of the joint organ with magnetic resonance imaging (MRI), but MRI can help to define ligament or meniscus abnormalities.

E. **Laboratory studies**

1. No specific or diagnostic abnormalities are seen in **primary OA.** No cartilage or bone markers of disease progress have been validated.
2. **Blood and urine.** Because of the localized nature of OA and the absence of systemic manifestations, clinical laboratory testing is usually not necessary to manage the patient. Values for the erythrocyte sedimentation rate, complete blood cell count, RF, chemistry studies, and urinalysis are generally normal. They are helpful in evaluating associated conditions and causes of secondary OA and in excluding other causes of arthritis. It should be kept in mind that low titers of RF are a common false-positive finding in the elderly.
3. **Synovial fluid,** when present, is usually noninflammatory, with fewer than 2,000 (mainly mononuclear) white blood cells per microliter.

VI. **Specific patterns of joint disease**

A. **Hands**

1. **History.** DIP joints are the most frequent site of hand involvement in OA, and PIP joints are also affected. The first CMC joint may be involved and be quite symptomatic, especially in patients whose occupations require repetitive use of this joint.
2. **Physical examination.** In patients with Heberden's (DIP) or Bouchard's (PIP) nodes, swellings over the joint are present, and the range of motion is decreased. The nodes are usually not tender. In some patients, small gelatinous cysts occur on the dorsal aspect of the DIP joints; they seem to be attached to tendon sheaths, resemble ganglia, and usually precede the development of Heberden's nodes. When the first CMC joint is affected, range of motion becomes limited, and a tender prominence develops at the base of the first metacarpal bone, which may lead to a "squared-off" appearance of the hand.
3. **Radiographs.** Because the physical signs of hand OA are so characteristic, hand radiographs are rarely needed. Patients with mild radiographic changes usually have no symptoms. Images of Heberden's nodes show joint space narrowing, subchondral sclerosis, cysts, and spurs. Although nodes may feel hard and bonelike, they may not be radiodense. When the first CMC joint is involved, subluxation of the base of the first metacarpal bone may be noted.

B. **Hips**

1. **History.** As a result of the key role of the hip in locomotion, patients with OA of the hip may be significantly disabled. Patients are usually older than those with hand involvement. Men are more often affected than women. In 20% of patients with unilateral disease, contralateral disease will develop within 8 years. Patients often complain of pain that increases with motion and weight bearing and decreases with rest. They may also complain of stiffness and a limp.

   Hip pain is usually felt on the outer aspect of the groin or inner thigh. Pain that originates in the hip may sometimes be perceived as originating in the medial knee or distal thigh (20% of patients), buttocks, or sciatic region. Patients may walk with an antalgic (pain-avoiding) gait, which may alter the gait pattern and cause pain in other joints of the lower extremities or the back. Sitting or rising may be especially difficult for these patients. It is important to distinguish true hip pain from pain caused by a lumbar radiculopathy, femoral hernia, or vascular insufficiency.

2. **Physical examination.** Decreased range of motion and pain on motion are the primary findings. Internal rotation is affected first. As deterioration progresses, there is further loss of rotation and loss of extension, abduction, and flexion. Joint contractures may develop. In the early stages of OA, flexion may not cause pain; however, extension and rotation will. In cases in which the radiation of the pain is atypical (to the knee), symptoms attributed to the hip can be reproduced by moving the hip through the extremes of motion while fixing all motion of the knee. Shortening of the limb caused by contracture or progressive lateral and upward subluxation of the femoral head may be observed. Compensatory lordosis of spine may also be observed secondary to flexion contracture of the hip.
3. **Radiographs.** Compared with OA symptoms in other joints, hip symptoms correlate better with radiographic findings. Virtually all patients with severe radiographic findings will have complaints attributable to the hip. Anteroposterior views of the **pelvis** should be obtained routinely when OA of the hips is suspected; these will provide information about the hips, sacroiliac joints, and pelvic bones. Advanced cases of hip OA may show protrusion acetabuli.
4. **Associated and predisposing conditions.** Some authors feel that OA of the hip is usually secondary to a developmental abnormality.
   a. **Congenital dysplasia of the hip** may account for 25% of OA cases in older Caucasian patients. The **acetabulum** does not develop properly and is shallow, which often results in femoral head subluxation and secondary degenerative changes. Patients may present with a limp in childhood or with premature OA in adulthood.
   b. **Slipped capital femoral epiphysis.** Just before the femoral epiphysis closes (between ages 16 and 19), the **femoral head** may be displaced posteromedially. These patients may present with a painful limp in adolescence or early adulthood.
   c. **Legg-Calvé-Perthes disease** is idiopathic osteonecrosis of the proximal femoral capital epiphysis, which occurs in young (3 to 8 years old) boys. The osteonecrosis often results in an abnormally large, flat femoral head with a wide, short neck.

C. Knees

1. **History.** The knee is frequently affected by OA. Even with normal walking, about four times the body weight is transmitted through the knee joint. Patients complain of trouble with kneeling, climbing stairs, and getting in and out of chairs. Locking of the knee may result from loose joint bodies. Morning stiffness is common but usually lasts less than 30 minutes.
2. **Physical examination.** Tenderness may be present along the joint line. Osteophytes may be palpated as irregular bony masses. Crepitus may be felt with the examiner's hand held over the patella during knee motion. Quadriceps atrophy may be present.
   a. **Medial and lateral compartment disease.** The medial compartment is the most frequently affected of the three knee compartments. Genu varus commonly occurs with medial compartment disease. Genu valgus, although less common, may occur when the lateral compartment is involved.

      The joint may be unstable as a result of cartilage loss and secondary lengthening of the collateral ligaments. It is important to compare the degrees of varus valgus deformity (of the extended knee) with and without weight bearing. If a change into varus alignment or an increase in the degree of deformity occurs with weight bearing, it is evidence of cartilage loss and compartment deformity rather than of ligamentous laxity alone.
   b. **Patellofemoral disease.** With patellofemoral OA, the patella loses side-to-side mobility, which results in a loss of about 10% of extension

and flexion. Pain and tenderness are most marked anteriorly. Pain may be elicited if the patella is held firmly against the femur and the quadriceps is isometrically contracted. Patellofemoral disease may occur alone without medial or lateral compartment disease.

3. **Radiographs**
   a. **Standard views** are the anteroposterior and lateral for most clinical situations. It is important to obtain these films during weight bearing to assess amounts of varus-valgus deformity and joint space narrowing. **Standing** films, with about 6 degrees of knee flexion, show the femoral cartilage and tibial plateau cartilage in direct contact and demonstrate joint space narrowing more reliably than non–weight-bearing films. Osteophytes and subchondral bone sclerosis and cyst formation are observed as OA progresses.
   b. **A tunnel view** is obtained with the knee in slight flexion to expose the intercondylar notch. This view allows evaluation of loose bodies, intraarticular spurs, and changes in the tibial intracondylar spines.
   c. The orientation of a **sunrise view** is tangential to the flexed knee; this view allows evaluation of the patellofemoral articulation.
4. **Associated and predisposing conditions**
   a. Fractures of the tibial plateau or femoral condyles with mechanical incongruence.
   b. Ligamentous injuries causing instability.
   c. Chronic patellar dislocation.
   d. Severe varus and valgus deformities.
   e. Internal derangement. Torn menisci predispose to OA, as do absent menisci after meniscectomy.
   f. Osteonecrosis (see Chapter 45).
   g. **Chondromalacia patellae** is a degeneration of the patellar cartilage most prominent in the age group of 15 to 30 years. There is pain during activity, especially *descending stairs.* Pain is elicited when the patella is pressed into the femoral groove as the patient tightens the quadriceps muscle.

D. **Spine.** Degenerative disease of the spine may be categorized as **osteoarthritis** or **spondylosis.** Because the posterior apophyseal joints are true diarthrodial joints, they may undergo the usual changes of OA, including joint space narrowing, sclerosis, and spur formation. The degenerative changes that affect the disks and vertebral bodies are properly referred to as spondylosis. Disks may herniate and compress the spinal cord or nerve roots. Degenerative changes of the vertebral bodies result in osteophytes that may cause mechanical compression of vital structures (spinal cord, nerve root, and, rarely, vessels).

1. **History**
   a. **Local pain and stiffness** may be caused by paraspinal ligament involvement or paraspinal muscle spasm.
   b. **Radicular symptoms** occur at all spinal levels, but are more common in the lumbar area and in the C5–6 and C6–7 roots.
      (1) Involvement of the **cervical spine** is usually seen at a neural foramen, secondary to impingement by osteophytes. Radicular symptoms tend to occur in the cervical spine because neural foramina and the spinal canal are relatively small in this area. Symptoms include neck pain that often radiates to the shoulder, upper back, and more distal aspects of the upper extremity. Weakness and paresthesias of the hand and arm may also occur.
      (2) **Lumbar spine.** Patients complain of low back pain that often radiates down the buttocks and may even extend into the legs and feet. The pain may increase with coughing and straining. With severe lesions, motor and sensory abnormalities may be present. A cauda equina syndrome with sphincter dysfunction can also develop (see Chapter 18.)

c. **Cord compression** by intervertebral ridges at cervical and thoracic levels may result in progressive myelopathy with minimal or no radicular pain.

d. **Mechanical compression of vital structures** also occurs mostly at the level of the cervical spine. Large anterior spurs may cause **dysphagia,** hoarseness, or cough. Compression of vertebral arteries may produce symptoms of **vertebrobasilar insufficiency** with vertigo, double vision, scotomas, headache, or ataxia. These symptoms often vary with head and neck position. Compression of the anterior spinal artery may produce a central cord syndrome.

2. **Physical examination.** The spinal examination may reveal decreased range of motion and local tenderness. A careful neurologic evaluation to detect absent reflexes, long-tract signs, and a radicular pattern of weakness and sensory abnormalities is important.

3. **Radiographs.** Severe degenerative changes may be present on radiographs with few symptoms. In contrast, a small spur that is critically placed may cause significant morbidity. **Oblique films** must be ordered to evaluate neural foramina. Standard anteroposterior and lateral views will not demonstrate impingement by a bone spur or a subluxation of an apophyseal joint. Osteophytes usually arise from the anterior and anterolateral aspects of vertebral bodies and are best seen on lateral films. A decrease in the intervertebral disk space secondary to disk degeneration is seen most often in the lower cervical and lumbar spine. A **vacuum phenomenon** indicative of disintegration of the nucleus pulposus of the disk may also be present. Anterior vertebral wedging may be seen. Specialized imaging methods such as computed tomography (CT) and MRI are useful for further selective investigations. CT may be of value in defining a bony cause of neurologic compression symptoms. MRI is useful to study soft-tissue structures of the neck, such as disks, when clinical examination and plain radiographs do not yield the diagnosis.

   In summary, advanced imaging techniques are best reserved for those clinical situations in which standard initial therapy has failed, or in which neurologic signs or symptoms are progressive.

E. **Feet**

1. **History.** The first MTP joint is one of the most common sites of OA involvement. Acute swelling and pain may be caused by bursal inflammation at the medial side of the metatarsal head (bunion). Patients often have a history of using improper footwear. In contrast, OA of the ankle or tarsal joints is rare and, when present, is usually secondary to trauma or to a systemic disease such as hemochromatosis.

2. **Physical examination** may reveal tenderness over the first MTP joint and hallux valgus deformity. The great toe is unable to bear weight normally, and added stress is placed on the metatarsal heads.

3. **Radiographs.** Typical changes of OA, such as sclerosis, joint space narrowing, and osteophyte formation, may be seen at the first MTP joint. Subluxation of the great toe with hallux valgus deformity may be noted. Radiographic changes in the midtarsal joints are common; however, they are infrequently associated with symptoms.

F. **Temporomandibular joint.** Crepitus, tenderness, and pain (often referred to the ear) are common problems that are sometimes attributed to dental malocclusion. Radiographic characterization of this joint is difficult. MRI can be utilized when more extensive imaging is indicated.

VII. **Differential diagnosis.** Primary OA can be confused with other forms of arthritis because it may occasionally present as an inflammatory polyarthritis of the hands or as monarticular arthritis. In addition, radiographic evidence of OA is so common that its presence may be unrelated to the true etiology of the patient's complaints. (See Chapters 14 through 21, which discuss diseases in specific anatomic regions.)

A. **Rheumatoid arthritis**
   1. **Monarticular rheumatoid arthritis.** When RA presents as monarticular arthritis of a large joint, differentiation from OA may be difficult and is based on the following:
      a. **Synovial fluid analysis.** RA fluid contains more white blood cells (>5,000) with a higher percentage of neutrophils, and has poorer viscosity than OA fluid.
      b. **Radiographs** in patients with RA usually show erosions and juxta-articular osteoporosis, although the findings are often normal in early RA. Osteophytes, subchondral bone cysts, and sclerosis suggest OA. However, Heberden's nodes and other degenerative abnormalities may coexist with RA.
      c. **Blood studies.** The erythrocyte sedimentation rate is often elevated, and RF is usually present in RA.
      d. **Follow-up observations** may eventually reveal a pattern of erosive joint destruction typical of RA. It may take as long as 2 years before the clinical picture is clear.
   2. **Polyarticular rheumatoid arthritis**
      a. **Distribution of joint involvement** is important when differentiating RA from inflammatory erosive OA.
         (1) **Rheumatoid arthritis.** MCP and PIP and wrist involvement.
         (2) **Osteoarthritis.** DIP and PIP and first CMC joints characteristically affected.
      b. **Radiographic features.** See section **V.C.**
      c. **Distinguishing clinical features of rheumatoid arthritis**
         (1) More inflammation with greater loss of joint function.
         (2) Involvement of a greater number of joints and in a symmetric fashion.
         (3) Quicker progression.
         (4) Less knee involvement.
         (5) More hand involvement.
         (6) Morning stiffness lasting longer than 30 minutes.
         (7) Significant systemic symptoms.

B. **Seronegative spondyloarthropathies.** These inflammatory diseases frequently involve the interphalangeal joints, single large joints, and the spine. Differentiating features are the following:
   1. **Psoriasis.** Skin and nail lesions and typical patterns of psoriatic arthropathy affecting interphalangeal joints (see Chapters 11 and 35).
   2. **Reiter's syndrome.** Presence of conjunctivitis, urethritis, and characteristic skin lesions (see Chapter 36).
   3. **Inflammatory bowel disease.** Complaints referable to large or small intestine (see Chapter 34).
   4. **Ankylosing spondylitis.** Sacroiliitis and fine, symmetric, marginal syndesmophytes (see Chapter 33).

C. **Crystal-induced arthritis**
   1. **Gout** affects primarily the first MTP joint in addition to other joints of the foot and lower extremity. Tophaceous deposits over the small joints of the hand may be confused with osteophytes. The diagnosis of gout is confirmed by the identification of urate crystals in the joint fluid (see Chapter 37).
   2. **Calcium pyrophosphate dihydrate arthritis (pseudogout)** may coexist with OA. The wrist, shoulder, knee, and ankle joints are commonly involved. Radiographs reveal chondrocalcinosis in most pseudogout patients. The diagnosis is confirmed by identifying birefringent, rhomboidal CPPD crystals in the joint fluid (see Chapter 38). Another type of crystal, basic calcium phosphate, is implicated in the pathogenesis of the destructive OA variant known as Milwaukee shoulder syndrome.

D. **Other disorders** that may coexist with OA but are important to identify and treat include the following:

1. **Infectious arthritis.**
2. **Neoplastic synovitis.** Lymphoma or leukemia may sometimes be identified by synovial fluid cytology.
3. **Pigmented villonodular synovitis.** The joint effusion is usually bloody. Diagnosis is confirmed by synovial biopsy.
4. **Neoplastic metastasis to juxtaarticular bone.** Bone scan is a useful diagnostic measure.
5. **Periarticular tendinitis or bursitis.**

VIII. Treatment. The American College of Rheumatology has published guidelines for the management of hip and knee OA; these are listed in the references. Therapy directed at other joints follows similar principles.

A. Nonpharmacologic therapy. Correction of predisposing factors should optimally take place before anatomic changes occur. Weight reduction in the obese patient is a particularly important intervention. Valgus-varus knee deformity and eversion-inversion ankle deformity may require surgical correction.

1. **Patient education** and self-management programs. Participation in Arthritis Foundation (1-800-283-7800) activities provides patients with a reliable flow of practical information.
2. **Joint rest.** Excessive use of an involved joint may increase symptoms and accelerate degenerative changes. It is important to protect joints. Weight-bearing joints may be unloaded by use of a cane (held in the hand opposite to the involved extremity and extended in tandem with it), crutches, or a walker. A neck collar may be useful for cervical OA. A first CMC joint splint can be quite helpful in a flare of CMC joint pain.
3. **Physical therapy** helps to relieve pain and stiffness, recover and maintain joint mobility, and strengthen supporting muscles. It is particularly helpful in patients with hip, knee, low back, and neck disease.
   a. **Therapeutic exercise.** See Chapter 56. The goal is to preserve range of motion and muscle strength.
   b. **Heat therapy** generally relieves pain and muscle spasm. Many methods are available, including diathermy and ultrasound (for deep pain), infrared, hot packs, warm bath or shower, and paraffin bath (for hands). See Chapter 56 for regimens.
4. **Occupational therapy** helps patients to adapt to their disabilities and helps minimize the stress placed on involved joints during activities of daily living (see Chapter 57).

B. Pharmacologic therapy

1. **Analgesics.**
   a. **Oral.** Acetaminophen is a standard baseline therapy. If sufficient analgesic effect is obtained, it avoids the gastric side effects of nonsteroidal antiinflammatory drugs (NSAIDs). The dosage of acetaminophen is 500 to 1,000 mg every 6 hours as required. Concurrent alcohol use should be avoided, and liver disease is a contraindication to use.
   b. **Topical.** Capsaicin cream (available in 0.025% and 0.075% strengths) is derived from the pepper plant and relieves pain via local reductions of substance P. It is applied three or four times per day to the affected area. Care must be taken to avoid contact with the eyes. It may take 2 weeks to obtain a therapeutic effect, so it is customary to use an oral medication during this period. The analgesic effects of acetaminophen and topical capsaicin are synergistic, and this is a particularly useful combination in the elderly.
2. **Nonsteroidal antiinflammatory drugs.** The choice of an NSAID should take into account such factors as efficacy, cost, adverse reactions, compliance, comorbidities, and past treatment. If NSAIDs are indicated after failure of the treatment modalities described above, they should be first used at low doses and on an as-needed basis if possible to minimize adverse reactions, especially in the elderly. The elderly are especially prone to peptic ulceration and unpredictable bleeding; these are clinically more serious than in young patients, who tend to have more physiologic reserve and are

less likely to suffer from multiple diseases and be taking multiple medications that can further exacerbate a gastrointestinal insult. In addition, the aging process leads to a slow decrease in renal function that in turn makes elderly patients more susceptible to the renal adverse actions of NSAIDs, as detailed below.

a. **Adverse reactions** to the NSAIDs include peptic ulcer in about 2%, rash in 2%, central nervous system effects such as tinnitus, and idiosyncratic hepatitis (rare). Dyspepsia is a frequent reason for NSAID discontinuation. Renal reactions, listed in order of decreasing frequency, are edema, transient acute renal insufficiency, tubulointerstitial nephropathy, hyperkalemia, and renal papillary necrosis.

b. **Choice of nonsteroidal antiinflammatory drug.** There is no evidence that one NSAID class is superior in efficacy to other classes. However, the first cyclooxygenase-2 (COX-2) inhibitor drug, which entered the U.S. market in February 1999, causes less gastrointestinal injury than do standard NSAIDs. It is reasonable to try a drug for 3 to 4 weeks, stop it if there is no therapeutic benefit, and then select another NSAID from a different structural class. Prescribing information for each drug listed below can be found in Appendix E.

   (1) **Cyclooxygenase-2 inhibitors.** Celecoxib, the first drug in this new class of NSAIDs, selectively inhibits the isoenzyme COX-2. This results in suppression of inflammation without disruption of the gastrointestinal protective effect of the COX-1 isoenzyme. In addition, celecoxib has no effect on platelet aggregation or bleeding time. The dose for osteoarthritis is 200 mg daily or 100 mg twice daily without regard to food. A second COX-2 medication, rofecoxib, was also approved by regulatory authorities in 1999. The dosage for OA is 12.5 to 25 mg once daily. The full safety picture for new drugs is typically clearer after they have been on the market for 2 to 3 years and used in larger populations. At that time, rarer adverse reactions have been detected and additional postmarketing studies have been completed.

   (2) **Acetic acids.** Sulindac is reputed to be associated with a lower rate of renal adverse reactions than other NSAIDs. It is supplied as 150-mg and 200-mg tablets. The dosage is 150 to 200 mg twice daily. Other members of this chemical family are indomethacin and tolmetin. Indomethacin is a potent analgesic but is not indicated for OA because it is poorly tolerated in the elderly.

   (3) **Propionic acids.** Members of this family include ibuprofen and naproxen. Specific information on these drugs is found in Appendix E. The dose of naproxen is 250 to 500 mg twice daily.

   (4) **Oxicam.** Piroxicam has the advantage of being taken in one daily dose, which assists with compliance. It is supplied as 10-mg and 20-mg capsules. The usual dosage is 20 mg once daily.

   (5) **Salicylates.** Aspirin products are less frequently used because of tolerance problems (gastrointestinal tract and central nervous system), particularly in the elderly. Enteric-coated aspirin (Ecotrin) is supplied as 325-mg or 500-mg tablets. The initial dosage is 500 mg four times daily. It should be taken after meals to minimize dyspepsia. Plain aspirin is not recommended for long-term use because it causes more occult blood loss than does Ecotrin. **Salsalate** is a non-acetylated salicylate that is associated with *minimal gastrointestinal toxicity* and does not affect platelet function. (Other drugs in this family are choline salicylate, choline magnesium trisalicylate, and diflunisal.) These non-acetylated drugs can be useful in arthritis secondary to bleeding dyscrasias because they have little effect on platelet function. Salsalate is supplied as 500-mg and 750-mg tablets. The usual dosage is 750 to 1,000 mg two to three times daily.

3. **Corticosteroids**
   a. **Systemic.** Oral corticosteroids have no role in the treatment of OA.
   b. **Intraarticular injections** may be of benefit if used judiciously in patients with one or two persistently inflamed joints. A joint should not be injected more than three times a year. Intraarticular corticosteroids can have an adverse effect on local cartilage metabolism; thus, excessive use of this treatment may aggravate OA rather than relieve it. Dosages for specific joints and precautions are listed in Chapter 4.
   c. **Intraarticular hyaluronic acid** is now available and can provide symptomatic relief lasting for several months when given as a series of injections. It is indicated for OA of the knee. These drugs (Synvisc and Hyalgan) are useful in patients who cannot tolerate NSAIDs or in whom NSAIDs have failed. Synvisc can be given in a series of three injections 1 week apart, versus five injections for Hyalgan.
4. **Experimental therapy.** At present, there are no therapies that reverse or halt the structural abnormalities of cartilage or bone in OA. Clinical trials are under way directed at cartilage targets and employing agents such as doxycycline and selective matrix metalloproteinase inhibitors. Biologic agents directed at targets such as interleukin-1ra are also being designed.

   In addition, one can expect to see clinical trials directed at bone targets in the future in accord with the "joint organ" concept.

IX. **Surgical treatment.** In addition to traditional surgical procedures and prosthetic joint replacement, a relatively recent advance is transplantation of cartilage in situations in which a focal defect is suitable for repair. Although it is not a routine procedure and is quite costly, cartilage transplantation adds to the tools available to preserve joint function.

A. **Indications**
   1. Relief of pain or severe disability after failure of conservative measures to halt or alleviate the pathologic process.
   2. Correction of a mechanical derangement that may lead to OA.

B. **Contraindications**
   1. Infection.
   2. Poor vascular supply.
   3. Emotional instability or occupational factors that make surgical rehabilitation unlikely to succeed.
   4. Obesity (relative contraindication).
   5. Serious medical illness (relative contraindication).
   6. Movement disorders, such as Parkinson's disease, and other neurologic diseases, such as Charcot's joint.

C. **Knee and hip procedures.** See Chapters 54 and 55 for a discussion of surgical therapy, including prosthetic joint replacement. Experienced surgeons obtain excellent functional results with hip and knee replacement surgery. Prostheses can be expected to last 15 years or so.

   Arthroscopic examination and removal of loose articular and meniscal debris can relieve pain and improve function. Simple joint irrigation can provide substantial clinical benefit in knees affected by OA.

X. The **prognosis of osteoarthritis** is highly variable. With DIP involvement of the hand, there is moderate pain and stiffness but little limitation of overall function. Disease of weight-bearing joints is more likely to cause disability. The time between the onset of hip pain and the development of serious disability averages 8 years. OA of the knee carries a worse prognosis than OA of the hip. Varus knee deformity and early onset of pain are poor prognostic signs.

Bibliography

Altman R, et al., and the OARS Task Force (Osteoarthritis Research Society). Design and conduct of clinical trials in patients with osteoarthritis. *Osteoarthritis Cartilage* 1996;4:217.

Buckland-Wright JC. Quantitative microfocal radiographic assessment of osteoarthritis of the knee from weight bearing tunnel and semiflexed standing views. *J Rheumatol* 1994;21:1734.

Buckland-Wright JC, et al. Accuracy and precision of joint space width measurements in standard and macroradiographs of osteoarthritic knees. *Ann Rheum Dis* 1995;54:872.

Dieppe PA, et al. Bone scintigraphy predicts the progression of joint space narrowing in osteoarthritis of the knees. *Ann Rheum Dis* 1993;52:557.

Hochberg MD, et al. Guidelines for the medical management of osteoarthritis. Part I. Osteoarthritis of the hip. Part II. Osteoarthritis of the knee. *Arthritis Rheum* 1995;38:1535,1541.

Lawrence RC, et al. Estimates of the prevalence of arthritis and selected musculoskeletal disorders in the United States. *Arthritis Rheum* 1998;41:778.

McAlindon TE, et al. Relation of dietary intake and serum levels of vitamin D to progression of osteoarthritis of the knee among participants in the Framingham study. *Ann Intern Med* 1996;125:353.

Nevitt MC, et al. Association of estrogen replacement therapy with the risk of osteoarthritis of the hip in elderly white women. *Arch Intern Med* 1996;156:2073.

Radin EL, Paul IL. Does cartilage compliance reduce skeletal impact loads? The relative force-attenuating properties of articular cartilage, synovial fluid, periarticular soft tissues and bone. *Arthritis Rheum* 1970;13:139.

Towheed TE, Hochberg MC. A systematic review of randomized controlled trials of pharmacologic therapy in osteoarthritis of the knee. *Semin Arthritis Rheum* 1997;26:755.

Westacott CI, et al. Alteration of cartilage metabolism by cells from osteoarthritic bone. *Arthritis Rheum* 1997;40:1282.

45. OSTEONECROSIS

Theresa Colosi and John H. Healey

I. Definition

Osteonecrosis (ON) is defined as the death *in situ* of a segment of bone from lack of circulation. Dead bone refers to dead cells, which include osteocytes in addition to the hematopoietic and fatty marrow cells within bone. Circulatory injury that compromises cell viability can secondarily jeopardize the structural integrity of bone. Bone has a rich blood supply, but it varies widely depending on the site. Certain locations are more susceptible to ON. The most common location for ON is the femoral head. Other relatively common locations include the distal femur, proximal humerus, and talus. ON usually affects adults less than 50 years old. This discussion pertains essentially to primary ON of the femoral head. Secondary ON also occurs. Areas of ON complicate osteoarthritis of the hip in 25% of cases.

II. Etiology

A. Four mechanisms of circulatory compromise of bone are recognized and one or more may play a significant role in a given patient:

1. **Mechanical disruption** (e.g., traumatic fracture/dislocation or stress fracture).
2. **Arterial occlusion** (e.g., embolism, sickle cells, invasion by Gaucher cells or fat, or nitrogen bubbles—"caisson disease").
3. **Injury** to or pressure on an intact artery (e.g., vasculitis, radiation injury, vasospasm).
4. **Venous outflow occlusion** (e.g., when venous pressure exceeds arterial pressure by any mechanism). This mechanism may, in fact, be the final common pathway of the other three mechanisms. ON may have a traumatic or an atraumatic cause. Traumatic ON occurs after injury to a bone with a vulnerable blood supply—for example, femoral head ON after hip dislocation or proximal humerus ON after proximal humerus fracture. Most cases of atraumatic ON are idiopathic or are associated with corticosteroid administration or ethanol abuse. The exact cause is unclear, although fat embolism and local clotting are probable mechanisms (Fig. 45-1).

B. Corticosteroid administration is a significant cause of ON because of its widespread use in a variety of diseases, including systemic lupus erythematosus, rheumatoid arthritis, inflammatory bowel disease, nephrotic syndrome, lymphoma and other myelogenous diseases, respiratory disease, and central nervous system disorders. In systemic lupus erythematosus, a high average daily dose (over 16.6 mg) and pulse therapy are considered important predictors for the development of ON.

C. Ethanol abuse also presents a clear dose-response relationship: consumption of more than 400 cc weekly results in a 10-fold greater risk for ON. Fat emboli from alcohol-induced fatty liver, increased blood cortisol levels, and altered lipid metabolism are all proposed mechanisms of ON in alcoholics.

D. Smoking is also a risk factor; smokers have a fourfold to fivefold greater risk for ON.

E. Atraumatic causes of ON are:

1. **Dysbaria** (decompression sickness or "caisson disease"), radiation therapy, and pregnancy. Decompression may precipitate ON if nitrogen bubbles, which may come out of solution subsequent to a rapid drop in barometric pressure, occlude arterioles.
2. **Radiation.** Radiation therapy may cause ON as a result of capillary injury and vasculitis. Theories on the mechanism of ON in pregnancy include venous congestion and the well-known phenomenon of hypercoagulability of pregnancy.
3. **Hypercoagulability.** A high incidence of coagulopathy exists in patients with ON. In a recent study, 26 patients with newly diagnosed ON of the

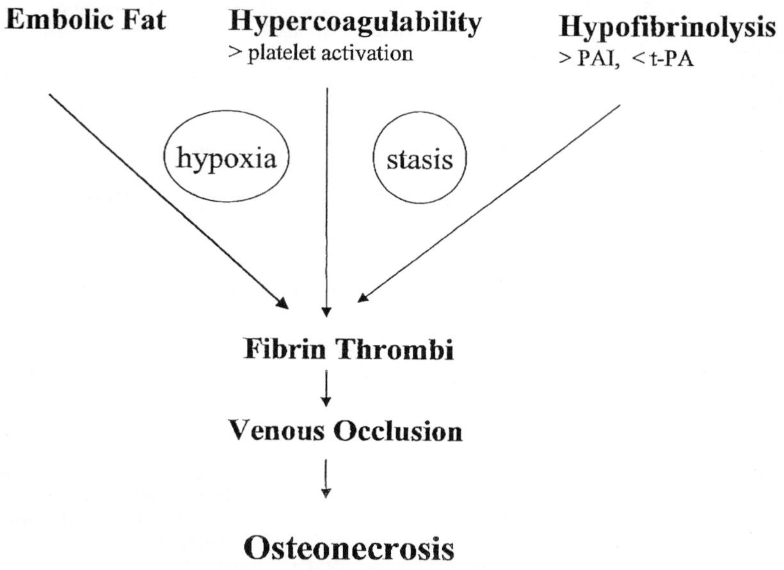

FIG. 45-1. Mechanisms of ischemic necrosis of bone.

femoral head underwent evaluation with a detailed coagulopathy profile. The proteins involved in thrombophilia and hypofibrinolysis—both of which may result in an increased incidence of thrombi—were studied. Eighty-three percent of these patients had a defined coagulopathy. Significant findings included high plasminogen activator inhibitor activity, low stimulated plasminogen activator activity, and high anti-cardiolipin immunoglobulin G.

4. **Association** with osteoporosis. In addition to coagulopathy, high-turnover osteoporosis or even osteomalacia may coexist with ON. In a histomorphometry study of transiliac bone specimens from 77 patients, investigators found a common profile: reduction in trabecular bone volume and osteoid seam thickness, in calcification rate, and in tetracycline-labeled surfaces. Total resorption surfaces were increased. These changes suggest a significant decrease in osteoblastic appositional rate and bone formation rate at the cell and tissue level. This decrease in appositional rate could explain a defect in healing of microfractures, which would facilitate the formation of subchondral fractures.

III. Diagnosis. One makes the diagnosis of ON on the basis of history, physical examination, and radiologic studies.

- **A.** A careful **history** should seek out the risk factors discussed previously.
- **B. Physical examination** findings may range from subtle (groin pain only) to significant (reduction in range of motion and pronounced antalgic gait).
- **C. Appropriate radiologic studies** include plain radiographs, bone scan, and magnetic resonance images (MRI). Results of these studies subsequently allow staging of the disease and provide guidelines to treatment. A currently used staging system is that of the University of Pennsylvania (Table 45-1). The importance of the system is that it incorporates the type and extent of radiologic and pathologic changes. The Japanese Investigation Committee for Avascular Necrosis of the Femoral Head also recently developed a classification system; it is based on plain anteroposterior radiographic findings and is used to predict prognosis and, thus, choose treatment.

Table 45-1. Steinberg-University of Pennsylvania staging system of osteonecrosis of the hip

Stage	0	Normal or nondiagnostic radiograph, bone scan, and MRI
Stage	1	Normal radiograph; abnormal bone scan, MRI A - Mild B - Moderate C - Severe
Stage	2	Lucent and sclerotic changes in femoral head A - Mild B - Moderate C - Severe
Stage	3	Subchondral collapse (crescent sign) without flattening A - Mild B - Moderate C - Severe
Stage	4	Flattening of femoral head A - Mild B - Moderate C - Severe
Stage	5	Joint narrowing, acetabular changes A - Mild (average of femoral head involvement) B - Moderate as determined in stage 4 and estimated C - Severe (acetabular involvement)
Stage	6	Advanced degenerative changes

Mild: <15% of the surface of femoral head or <2-mm depression; moderate: 15–30%; 2 to 4-mm depression; severe: >30% >4-mm depression.

D. Histology continues to be the standard for the definitive diagnosis of ON. Initially after vascular compromise, no histologic changes occur. Then examination of the marrow reveals death of hematopoietic cells, capillary endothelial cells, and lipocytes. Osteocytes shrink to produce the empty lacunae that are characteristic of dead bone. These early necrotic changes are associated with increased interstitial water, which produces a marrow abnormality detectable on MRI.

E. Osseous repair processes represent an integral part of the **pathology** of ON. Initially, reactive hyperemia and fibrous repair occur in the adjacent bone. New vessels from the adjacent fibrous repair tissue revascularize the leading edge of necrotic bone. Primitive mesenchymal cells, which subsequently differentiate into osteoblasts and osteoclasts, coexist with the new vessels. Appositional bone is deposited on existing dead trabeculae, which creates an osteosclerotic area radiographically. Creeping substitution subsequently removes the necrotic tissue. The histologic appearance in cortical bone is described as "cutting cones."

F. The **features** of ON are a composite of both necrotizing and reparative processes. When resorption progresses faster than formation of new bone, the bone becomes weak. Standard mechanical forces can then fracture the vulnerable bone. On radiographs, the subchondral radiolucent line representing collapsed cancellous trabeculae beneath an intact articular surface is known as the crescent sign. Subsequent segmental collapse of the articular surface, femoral head deformity, and joint incongruity lead to the development of secondary osteoarthritis.

IV. Treatment. The treatment of ON depends on the etiology, stage, and extent of the lesion. In the appropriate patient, avoidance of inciting factors such as steroid therapy, alchohol, and trauma is recommended. For patients with very early disease whose evaluation suggests synovitis, treatment consists of nonsteroidal anti-inflammatory medications and resting the affected hip by allowing only toe-touch weight bearing. Osteoporosis may respond to calcium, vitamin D, or antiresorptive therapy (e.g., bisphosphonates or calcitonin). For patients in an early stage of disease (i.e., before subchondral collapse has occurred), **core decompression** represents the best option for pain relief and prevention of progression to collapse and then to total hip arthroplasty. Core decompression is a surgical procedure in which the surgeon uses a cannulated device or drill to remove a core of bone from the femoral head and neck. Core decompression can help delay total hip arthroplasty significantly—on average, almost 10 years for patients with symptoms and normal radiographic findings, almost 5 years for patients with early radiographic changes (cystic and sclerotic lesions), and even 3 years for patients with structural failure of the femoral head (subchondral radiolucency with fracture or deformity of the femoral head). For patients who have progressed to an advanced stage of ON, total hip arthroplasty is the standard treatment.

V. Summary. ON is bone death secondary to circulatory compromise. The exact etiology is unclear, although several theories exist. ON may progress to a loss of bone structural integrity and thus damage the adjacent joint. The diagnosis is based on history and determination of important risk factors, physical examination findings, and radiologic studies, including plain radiographs and MRI. The treatment is based on the stage and extent of disease.

Bibliography

Arlot ME, et al. Bone histology in adults with aseptic necrosis. *J Bone Joint Surg* 1983;65-A:1319.

Favus MJ, ed. *Primer on the metabolic diseases and disorders of mineral metabolism,* 3rd ed. Washington, D.C.: American Society for Bone and Mineral Research, 1996.

Jones LC, et al. Coagulopathies associated with osteonecrosis of the femoral head. Presented at the 44th Annual Meeting of the Orthopedic Research Society, March 16–19, 1998, New Orleans, LA.

Ohzono K, et al. The fate of nontraumatic avascular necrosis of the femoral head: a radiologic classification to formulate prognosis. *Clin Orthop* 1992;277:73.

Simon SR, ed. *Orthopedic basic science.* Rosemont, IL: American Academy of Orthopedic Surgery, 1994;279.

Steinberg ME, Hayken GD, Steinberg DR. A quantitative system for staging avascular necrosis. *J Bone Joint Surg* 1995;77-B:34.

Urbaniak JR, Jones JP, eds. *Osteonecrosis: etiology, diagnosis, and treatment.* Rosemont, IL: American Academy of Orthopedic Surgery, 1997.

46. OSTEOPOROSIS

Joseph M. Lane and John H. Healey

Osteoporosis (OP) is a condition in which bone mass is below normal for an person's age, sex, and race. OP implies low quantities of mineralized bone, unmineralized matrix, microarchitectural defects, and susceptibility to low-energy, "fragility" fractures. A fracture is the result of a combination of bone mass, bone geometry, and the level and vector of trauma. **Osteomalacia (OM)** refers to an increase in unmineralized matrix, independent of the amount of bone mass. In practice, some patients have a mixture of OP and OM. **Osteopenia** refers to the radiographic finding of decreased bone density, which may be found in OP, OM, or other conditions.

Reduced bone mass is the most significant factor contributing to fractures. Normal, age-dependent bone loss is accelerated at menopause. Cancellous bone (also called trabecular bone) is lost more rapidly than cortical bone. Fractures usually occur earlier in principally cancellous bones (vertebrae) than in cortical bones (femoral neck). OP is the most common metabolic bone disease, contributing to fractures in 25% of women and 17% of men over age 70. It is important to appreciate the fact that we now have available excellent measurement and treatment tools which, in combination, can prevent or retard the development of OP.

I. Pathogenesis. Low initial levels of adult bone mass or an acceleration in bone loss can reduce bone mass and strength to below the fracture threshold (the bone mass below which the propensity to fracture is increased). Inadequate calcium intake and postmenopausal estrogen deficiency account for 90% of OP cases. Factors affecting primary and secondary OP are the following:

A. Nutritional abnormalities and social practices

1. Inadequate calcium intake.
2. Malabsorption.
3. Alcoholism.
4. Smoking.
5. Vitamin D deficiency.
6. Vitamin C deficiency.

B. Endocrine conditions

1. Menopause.
2. Hyperthyroidism.
3. Hyperparathyroidism.
4. Cushing's disease.
5. Diabetes mellitus.

C. Immobilization

1. Illness.
2. Weightlessness.

D. Iatrogenic causes

1. Corticosteroid therapy.
2. Long-term heparin therapy.
3. Long-term phenytoin (Dilantin) therapy.
4. Castration (oophorectomy, radiation, chemotherapy).
5. Excessive thyroid therapy.

E. Risk factors

1. Female sex. (Female maximal bone mass is lower than male maximal bone mass.)
2. White race. (Blacks have a greater bone mass; that of other races is probably intermediate but not as well-defined.)
3. Northwest European extraction. Other ethnic groups are less susceptible.
4. Lactation contributes to a cumulative negative calcium balance if calcium supplementation is inadequate.
5. Smoking.

6. Scoliosis.
7. Ectomorphic habitus.
8. Sedentary life-style.
9. Amenorrhea (marathon runners, ballerinas).
10. Family history (one-third have strong inheritance).
11. Collagen disorders: osteogenesis imperfecta, Ehlers-Danlos syndrome, Marfan syndrome.
12. History of low-energy fracture.
13. Systemic inflammatory disorders, such as rheumatoid arthritis and ankylosing spondylitis.

II. Clinical presentation. Back pain and fractures are the most characteristic presenting symptoms. Loss of height is a cardinal sign of vertebral OP. More than 60% of vertebral fractures are not symptomatic. Compression fractures are often multiple and most commonly occur in the T-11 to L-2 distribution. Fractures of the wrist (Colles' fracture), hip (femoral neck and intertrochanteric), and pelvis may be the first manifestation of OP. **High-turnover OP** results from increased bone resorption and occurs at the onset of menopause. **Low-turnover OP** is caused by decreased osteoblastic bone formation as a consequence of genetics, senility, and antimetabolites.

A. History. Multiple risk factors and at least one other pathologic factor are usually present.

B. Physical examination findings. Thin appearance, kyphosis, scoliosis, height loss, and percussion tenderness of spine.

C. Laboratory studies. Serum levels of calcium, phosphorus, and alkaline phosphatase are normal. Urinary calcium may be high in early postmenopausal period but is normal or low in chronic OP. Collagen breakdown products (N-telopeptide, pyridinoline cross-links) are elevated in high-turnover osteoporosis.

D. Radiographs

1. Osteopenia, loss of horizontal vertebral trabeculation.
2. Compression fractures: wedge, crush, or biconcave. Intact posterior elements.
3. Pedicles preserved. No lytic or blastic lesions.

E. Bone densitometry. Bone mass can be measured by noninvasive means (spinal and femoral dual-energy x-ray densitometry, radial single-photon densitometry, quantitative spinal computed tomography or ultrasound). Bone mass measurements correlate well with fracture risk. Values (called the T score) between 1 and 2.5 standard deviations (SD) below those for young, normal, peak bone mass indicate diminished bone mass or osteopenia, and values of 2.5 SD below normal represent full osteoporosis. Severe osteoporosis is defined as values of 2.5 SD below normal in the setting of a fragility fracture (World Health Organization). Serial measurements of bone density may identify patients losing bone rapidly and help monitor therapy.

F. Bone biopsy. Iliac crest biopsy reveals reduced bone mass and excludes concomitant OM, excessive osteoclastic bone resorption, and marrow disorders such as malignancies. This is the only method to assess bone quality and gives the most precise measure of bone turnover. It is not, however, a routine test.

III. Differential diagnosis. Treatable causes of secondary OP should be identified.

A. Multiple myeloma. An elevated erythrocyte sedimentation rate, proteinuria, monoclonal gammopathy, and radiographic lytic lesions suggest the diagnosis.

B. Metastatic malignancy may be associated with increased alkaline phosphatase, hypercalcemia, blastic bone lesions, and radiographic evidence of destructive lesions of a vertebral pedicle.

C. Osteomalacia. Low serum calcium and phosphorus levels, high levels of alkaline phosphatase, low levels of 25(OH)-vitamin D, and radiographic pseudofractures. Biopsy shows wide osteoid seams and delayed mineralization.

D. Hyperthyroidism is suggested by weight loss, heat intolerance, palpitations, elevated serum thyroxine, low level of thyroid-stimulating hormone, and elevated urinary calcium and hydroxyproline.

E. Hyperparathyroidism. Elevated calcium, low or normal phosphorus, and elevated serum parathormone level. Radiographic evidence of endosteal and periosteal resorption. Biopsy shows osteitis fibrosa cystica and tunneling resorption.

F. Renal osteodystrophy. Uremia, elevated phosphorus, low calcium, and ectopic calcification are diagnostic clues.

G. Gastrointestinal disease. Symptoms of malabsorption or a history of previous gastrointestinal surgery suggests a cause for OP or OM.

IV. Treatment

A. Orthopedic

1. **Limb fractures.** Routine fracture care, followed by bone mass assessment and appropriate treatment.
2. **Spine fractures.** Back pain from vertebral fractures often lasts between 4 and 6 weeks. It can be associated with ileus, pneumonia, skin decubitus ulcers, and thromboembolic complications. Bed rest and analgesics are recommended until the patient is comfortable (e.g., 1 week). Mobilize and ambulate as tolerated (pool therapy may help). Avoid long-term use of back braces, which ultimately weaken spinal muscles. Calcitonin for treatment of OP and pain. The development of such fractures should prompt an assessment of bone mass and treatment of OP.
3. **Physical therapy.** Daily walking; lumbar flexion and thoracic extension exercises. Sit-ups should be avoided.

B. Medical (in the presence of defined osteopenia or osteoporosis)

1. **Calcium carbonate** (1,500 mg elemental daily) or **calcium citrate** (1,200 mg daily).
2. **Vitamin D_3** (400 to 800 IU/d PO).
3. **Estrogen (hormone replacement therapy).** Consider strongly at menopause but beneficial at all postmenopausal ages. Increases bone mass and decreases fracture risk by 50%. Progesterone cyclically or in low doses continuously is required to prevent endometrial cancer. Improvement in bone mass and cardiovascular protection outweighs possible increased risk for breast cancer in many clinical situations.
4. **Calcitonin** in nasal form (i.e., 200 U of Miacalcin daily) increases spinal bone mass and decreases vertebral fracture risk by 37% but does not protect the hip. It may provide analgesia in the settings of vertebral fractures. Its complication rate is low (nasal irritation in 2% of cases).
5. **Bisphosphonates (alendronate).** Alendronate (10 mg daily) increases spine and bone mass and decreases the risk for fracture by 50%, a rate equal to that of hormone replacement therapy. Esophagitis is the main potential complication but can be eliminated by slow buildup of dosage and appropriate administration. Etidronate, at a dose of 400 mg orally/d for two weeks every three months is an alternative.
6. **Selective estrogen receptor modifiers.** Raloxifene (60 mg daily) is an anti-estrogen that inhibits bone resorption. It increases bone mass and affords fracture prevention for the spine. It increases postmenopausal symptoms and leg cramps (8%) but does not appear to be associated with uterine cancer at this time. One study suggests a 60% diminution in the risk for breast cancer. Tamoxifen, a breast cancer therapeutic agent, also limits bone resorption but is not approved for OP.
7. **Combination therapy.** If bone mass does not increase or fragility fractures continue to occur, combinations such as estrogen replacement therapy and bisphosphonate appear to be synergistic (15% enhancement over single agents).
8. **Exercise** (see below).

C. Prevention

1. **Calcium supplementation with vitamin D_3.** Doses of calcium should be increased with increasing age, to a maximum of 1,500 mg in postmenopausal women. The total daily calcium regimen can be taken as a combination of food and calcium pills (i.e., calcium carbonate or citrate). In a postmenopausal woman, three units of calcium are required daily. One unit is equivalent to a 500-mg calcium tablet, two pieces of cheese, one jar of yogurt, or one 8-oz glass of milk. The dosage of vitamin D_3 is 400 to 800 IU daily.

2. **Exercise.** Impact, stretching, strengthening, balance training. Tai-chi decreases the number of falls by 47%. Walking 20 minutes per day 3 times per week is helpful and is practical for most patients.
3. **Estrogen.** Consider low doses in patients with natural or premature menopause or other risk factors.
4. **Selective estrogen receptor modifiers.** Because it increases postmenopausal symptoms, raloxifene should be given at least 5 years after menopause (see above).
5. **Bisphosphonates.** Alendronate (5 mg daily or 10 mg thrice weekly) is effective in preventing bone loss.

D. Steroid-induced osteoporosis. Corticosteroids, especially when taken on a long-term basis, have a significant negative impact on bone mass. They increase bone resorption, decrease bone formation, and lead to secondary hyperparathyroidism. To counter these adverse actions, the following regimen is recommended for all patients treated with steroids for more than 1 month:

1. Bone mass measurement at baseline and yearly thereafter. These results will guide future therapeutic decisions.
2. Daily intake of 1,500 mg of calcium and 800 U of vitamin D_3.
3. Estrogen replacement therapy in postmenopausal women.
4. Assessment of testosterone levels in men with decreased bone mass and replacement treatment if appropriate.
5. Use of bisphosphonates or calcitonin in patients with persistently low bone mass or the development of new fragility fractures despite nutritional supplements and estrogen replacement therapy.

V. Prognosis

A. By maximizing peak bone mass and reducing the rate of bone loss, bone mass can be maintained above the fracture threshold.

B. Reduced bone mass is permissive of fractures. Fractures heal, but morbidity and mortality are high. Twenty percent of women die within 1 year of fracturing their hip.

C. Presently, bone mass can be augmented only by exercise and the use of antiresorptive agents in patients with high-turnover OP.

D. Experimental treatments may be beneficial for low-turnover OP.

1. Continuous 1,25- $(OH)_2$-vitamin D.
2. Third-generation bisphosphonates.
3. Sodium fluoride.
4. Intermittent parathyroid hormone.

Bibliography

Black DM, et al. Randomized trial of effect of alendronate on risk of fracture in women with existing vertebral fractures. *Lancet* 1996;348:1535.

Dawson-Hughes B. Osteoporosis treatment and the calcium requirement. *Am J Clin Nutr* 1998;67:5.

Delmas PD, et al. Effects of raloxifene on bone mineral density, serum cholesterol concentrations, and uterine endometrium in postmenopausal women. *N Engl J Med* 1997;337:1641.

Eastell R. Treatment of postmenopausal osteoporosis. *N Engl J Med* 1998;338:736.

Ettinger B. Overview of estrogen replacement therapy: historical prospective. *Proc Soc Exp Biol Med* 1998;217:2.

Lane JM: Osteoporosis. *Spine* 1997;22[24S]:32.

Marshall D, Johnell D, Wedel H. Meta-analyses of how well measures of bone mineral density predict occurrence of osteoporotic fractures. *Br Med J* 1996;312:1254.

Uusi-Rasi K, et al. Associations of physical activity and calcium intake with bone mass and size in healthy women at different ages. *J Bone Miner Res* 1998;13:133.

47. PAGET'S DISEASE OF BONE

John H. Healey

Sir James Paget, in 1877, described a condition he termed *osteitis deformans,* a disease of bone characterized by metabolic overactivity of affected bone and bony deformity. Paget's disease of bone is an age-related, localized disorder of bone metabolism in which increased bone resorption is followed by excessive production of woven bone. The result is enlarged and weakened bones. The disease may be monostotic or polyostotic (asymmetric).

I. **Epidemiology.** The disease is present radiographically in 3% of the population. Symptomatic Paget's disease is much less common. Persons of English extraction are most commonly affected, but no clear genetic pattern has been identified. There is a slight male predominance. Paget's disease is rare in patients less than 40 years old.

II. **Pathogenesis**

A. **Etiology.** The etiology is unknown. Evidence is accumulating, however, that Paget's disease of bone may be a "slow-virus" infection since the first report in 1974.

B. **Histology.** Increased bone turnover is evident. Osteoclast resorption may dominate. New bone is woven and has a mosaic pattern. Cement lines (reversal lines) are conspicuous.

C. **Genetics.** There is probably a significant genetic component. The disease is rare in Scandinavia and Japan.

D. **Radiology.** Paget's disease begins at one epiphysis and progresses to the other epiphysis of bone. Resorptive lytic flame is seen early at the leading edge of the lesion. Reactive bone formation enlarges the overall bone dimensions and leaves coarsened trabeculae and sclerosis.

III. **Clinical presentation.** Most patients with Paget's disease are asymptomatic. The disease is usually recognized fortuitously when a roentgenogram is obtained for another purpose or a lone elevated alkaline phosphatase is assessed. Symptomatic patients present with pain, deformity, or pathologic fracture. Clinically important degenerative arthritis, neural compression, changes in skin temperature, high-output heart failure, and bone sarcoma can occur in an area of Paget's disease (Table 47-1).

A. **Sites of involvement**

1. Sacrum (56%).
2. Spine (50%), lumbar most frequently.
3. Right femur (31%).
4. Cranium (28%).
5. Sternum (23%).
6. Pelvis (21%).
7. Left femur (21%).

B. **Associated conditions**

1. Hyperparathyroidism.
2. Hyperuricemia (40%).
3. Heart disease—congestive failure or valvular disease in most extensive cases.
4. Hearing loss.
5. Hypercalcemia in severe untreated cases, immobilized patients, or patients with fracture.
6. Osteoporosis resulting both from disuse and concomitant hyperparathyroidism.

IV. **Laboratory studies**

A. **Elevated serum alkaline phosphatase** indicates increased bone formation.

Table 47-1. Radiographic and clinical manifestations of Paget's disease of bone

Location	Radiographic findings	Clinical symptoms
Skull	Osteoporosis circumscripta	None
	Cranial enlargement	Occasionally painful
	Basilar invagination	Occipital neuralgia; lower cranial nerve impingement; medullary compression; ventricular obstruction and increased intracranial pressure; vertebral basilar artery insufficiency
	Temporal bone involvement	Hearing loss
	Auditory ossicle involvement	Hearing loss
Face, jawbones	Unilateral changes	Proptosis; trigeminal neuralgia; displacement of teeth
Spine	"Window frame" vertebra(e)	Nerve root compression; spinal stenosis
Pelvis, hip	Acetabular and femoral head disease with degenerative arthritis; protrusio acetabuli; sacroiliac joint ankylosis	Pain; end-stage arthritis
Knee joint	Bone and joint deformity	Pain; arthritis; fracture
Tibia, femur, humerus	Bowing, with or without fracture	Pain; arthritis; fracture

- **B. Elevated collagen breakdown products:** N- and C-terminal telopeptides, *N*-pyridinolines, hydroxyproline (less sensitive and slower to respond to therapy).
- **C.** Results of other chemistry and hematologic tests, [calcium, phosphorus] are usually normal.
- **D. Radiographs**
  - **1. Workup.** Anteroposterior and lateral views of entire involved bone and bone scan (to identify other sites of involvement) are necessary.
  - **2. Diagnostic features.** See section **II.D.**
  - **3. Associated findings**
    - **a.** Degenerative arthritis.
    - **b.** Bowing of long bones.
    - **c.** Spinal stenosis.
    - **d.** Paget's sarcoma, suggested by the appearance of lytic areas within sclerotic pagetic bone.

V. Differential diagnosis

- **A. Metastatic carcinoma.** Prostate and breast carcinoma in bone may resemble Paget's disease, but bony expansion is lacking and cortical destruction is more frequent. In any site, if destruction of bone, extracortical extension, or a possible soft-tissue mass is present, neoplasia must be ruled out, especially if pain is increasing.
- **B. Hemangioma of bone** (especially of vertebrae) may be sclerotic and resemble monostotic Paget's disease.
- **C. Caffey's disease.** Infantile cortical hyperostosis affects a young age group, may be more widespread, and predominantly affects cortical bone, although radiographic and histologic findings closely resemble those of juvenile Paget's disease.
- **D. Hyperparathyroidism.** Histology may be similar, and the conditions can coexist (7% to 14%). Biochemical and radiographic findings differ, however.

VI. Medical treatment

- **A. Asymptomatic patients** should be treated if a major joint, nerve, or weight-bearing bone is affected.

B. Symptomatic patients. Symptoms usually respond to treatment in 1 to 3 months, and improvement in biochemical parameters usually parallels improvement in symptoms. All agents now used inhibit osteoclast activity and block the initial resorptive phase of Paget's disease.

1. **Bisphosphonates** block osteoclast function and recruitment. However, they inhibit mineralization and osteoblast function to a variable degree.
   a. **Dosage**
      (1) Alendronate: 10 to 40 mg daily PO.
      (2) Pamidronate: 30 to 90 mg every week to month IV.
      (3) Etidronate: 5 to 20 mg/kg daily PO for 3 to 6 months. Lower dosages are preferred except in severe cases. A 6-month interval should elapse before a course is repeated.
      (4) Risedronate: 30 mg daily for 2 months.
   b. **Response.** Rapid improvement in symptoms and biochemical parameters is usually seen. A paradoxical increase in pain is observed in 15% of patients.
   c. **Side effects.** Increased pain, diarrhea, osteomalacic fractures, and delayed fracture healing.
2. **Calcitonin** is a polypeptide hormone with receptors in osteoclasts that decreases bone resorption.
   a. **Dosage.** Salmon calcitonin is the preferred agent because of its high activity and low antigenicity and cost. Initial dosages of 50 to 150 U daily SC for 1 to 3 months may be used, then tapered to a maintenance dosage of 50 U three times weekly for 3 to 6 months.
   b. **Response.** In two-thirds of patients, symptomatic relief and biochemical improvement may last 6 to 12 months after a therapeutic course is completed. Antibody formation does not preclude a good response but may require a switch to human calcitonin.
   c. **Side effects** include nausea, flushing, local reactions at injection sites, and urticaria; these respond to anti-emetics and antihistamines.
3. **Combination calcitonin and bisphosphonates** (low dose) may produce a faster, longer-lasting response and be more cost-effective.
4. **Gallium nitrate** blocks osteoclasts and may promote activity of osteoblasts. It is also a very effective treatment for hypercalcemia.
5. **Mithramycin,** a DNA inhibitor, has been successful in treating hypercalcemia of malignancy. Toxicity restricts its use to cases of acute neurologic compression syndromes in Paget's disease.

VII. Orthopedic treatment

A. Surgery may be successful, but deformity, poor bone quality, and soft-tissue hyperemia make surgery difficult. Calcitonin treatment for at least 6 weeks before procedures is recommended. Bisphosphonates should be avoided if an osteotomy is to be performed.

B. Fractures

1. Pseudofractures may persist for 6 to 12 months and should not be overtreated once symptoms subside.
2. Completed fractures usually heal with closed methods, but healing may be delayed.
3. Bisphosphonates should not be used.
4. Biopsy occasionally is necessary to exclude sarcoma.

C. Immobilization. Gallium nitrate, calcitonin, and occasionally mithramycin (now called plica mycin) will be necessary to treat hypercalcemia.

VIII. Prognosis. Bone sarcomas occur in fewer than 1% of patients and are almost always fatal. Benign giant cell tumors also occur and may respond to corticosteroid therapy. Multiple myeloma and metastases are also seen.

Uncomplicated Paget's disease generally responds to medical management and becomes quiescent. Degenerative arthritis and deformity usually require surgery. Medical management may prevent disease progression and is usually warranted.

Bibliography

Blumsohn A, et al. Different responses of biochemical markers of bone resorption to bisphosphonate therapy in Paget's disease. *Clin Chem* 1992;41:1592.

Mirra JM. Pathogenesis of Paget's disease based on viral etiology. *Clin Orthop* 1987; 217:162.

Reginster JY, Lecart MP. Efficacy and safety of drugs for Paget's disease of bone. *Bone* 1995;17 [Suppl 5]:485S.

Smidt WR, et al. An algorithmic approach to the treatment of Paget's disease of the spine. *Orthop Rev* 1994;23:715.

48. ENDOCRINE ARTHROPATHIES

Michael D. Lockshin

I. Pathogenesis and clinical manifestations. The musculoskeletal manifestations of endocrine diseases are highly variable. They include muscle dysfunction, disorders of bone metabolism, and cartilage deformation. Tendons, ligaments, and tendon attachment sites are regularly symptomatic. Crystal arthropathies and calcific tendinitis may be symptoms of endocrine disease. Table 48-1 lists the rheumatic manifestations of common endocrinopathies.

II. Diagnosis. Endocrinopathic musculoskeletal disease tends to be diffuse and poorly described. Except for crystal arthritis, it is more often periarticular than articular. The most important diagnostic step is to consider the possibility of endocrinopathy, then to evaluate whether the patient's symptoms might be explained by that abnormality. History, physical examination, and often radiology define the rheumatologic problem, and directed laboratory studies define the associated endocrinopathy.

- **A. Myalgias, proximal myopathies, and, on occasion, high levels of creatine kinase** suggest thyroid disorders. Less commonly, acromegaly and disorders causing hyperkalemia or hypokalemia will suggest primary muscle weakness. **Carpal tunnel syndrome** occurs in hypothyroidism, acromegaly, and diabetes. **Scleredema** of the upper back is characteristic of diabetes.
- **B.** Parathyroid disorders, acromegaly, most heritable disorders (Marfan syndrome, pseudo-hypoparathyroidism, ochronosis), and advanced diabetes show typical **radiologic abnormalities.**
- **C. Osteopenia** is characteristic of hyperparathyroidism and hyperadrenalism, but it also occurs in patients with thyroid and pituitary dysfunction.
- **D. Characteristic syndromes** may be diagnostic; the **cheiropathy** of advanced diabetes and **thyroid acropathy** in Graves' disease are examples. **Chondrocalcinosis** and characteristic metacarpophalangeal disease are diagnostic of hemochromatosis.

III. Laboratory studies. Radiographs often first suggest the possibility of an endocrinopathy. Routine clinical laboratory tests are usually not helpful. It is necessary to confirm the suspected endocrinopathy with appropriately directed tests.

IV. Differential diagnosis. Rheumatoid arthritis and osteoarthritis, gout, pseudogout, lupus, dermatomyositis, and scleroderma may each be suggested by some manifestation of an endocrinopathy. Normal levels of antinuclear antibody, rheumatoid factor, and muscle enzymes, and a normal erythrocyte sedimentation rate exclude these diagnoses, but abnormal test results do not positively confirm them. A noninflammatory **synovial fluid analysis** (except in pseudogout associated with diabetes, hyperparathyroidism, or hemochromatosis) is most characteristic of endocrinopathy. In myxedema, synovial fluid is often very viscous and colorless.

V. Treatment and prognosis

- **A. Treatment of the underlying endocrinopathy** relieves myalgia, myopathy, tendinitis, and, to some extent, osteopenia and skin manifestations, but it will not reverse established bone and cartilage deformity. The **rate of remission** varies with the endocrinopathy.
  1. In **thyroid** disease, myalgias remit within weeks to months, myopathy within months, and acropachy in years, if at all.
  2. In **parathyroid** disease, bone pain abates in months, and bone remineralization occurs within years. Normal bone structure may not be completely restored, particularly if bone trabeculae have become discontinuous.
  3. **Adrenal** myopathy improves in months.
  4. The skeletal changes of **pituitary, gonadal, and congenital** endocrinopathies usually do not regress. Estrogen replacement retards bone loss, but remineralization of osteoporotic bone requires calcium, calcitonin, and bisphosphonate therapy.

Table 48-1. Rheumatic manifestations and pathogenesis of common endocrinopathies

Endocrine abnormality	Rheumatic manifestation	Putative pathogenesis
Thyroid—hyper	Proximal myopathy	Muscle/protein metabolism
	Thyroid acropathy	Growth hormone
	Myalgia (during changing thyroid states)	Unknown
Thyroid—hypo	High creatine kinase	Muscle membrane abnormality
	Bland joint effusion	Abnormal cartilage metabolism
	Chondrocalcinosis	Unknown
	Hyperuricemia	Renal tubular dysfunction
	Myalgia (during changing thyroid states)	Unknown
Parathyroid—hyper	Osteopenia, bone resorption, fractures, cysts, myopathy, pseudogout	Increased osteoclast activity
Parathyroid—hypo	Osteopenia	Decreased osteoblast activity
Parathyroid—hypo (congenital)	Short stature, short metacarpals	Unknown
Pituitary—hyper	Increased cartilage, accelerated osteoarthritis, osteopenia	Growth hormone excess, abnormal joint mechnics
Pituitary—hypo	Short stature, osteopenia	Lack of growth hormone
Adrenal—hyper	Osteopenia	Effect on calcium metabolism and osteoblasts and osteoclasts
	Proximal myopathy	Muscle protein catabolism, hypokalemia
Gonads—hyper	Short stature	Premature closure of epiphyses
Gonads—hypo	Osteopenia	Unopposed osteoclast activity
Pancreas (diabetes)	Charcot's joints	Neuropathy
	Dupuytren's contracture	Unknown
	Palmar fasciitis	Unknown
	Carpal tunnel syndrome	Unknown
	Scleredema	Unknown
Other—hemochromatosis	Pyrophosphate arthropathy	Iron deposition in cartilage
	Hooks on metacarpophalangeal joints	Unknown
Other—miscellaneous (congenital)	Skeletal deformities	Varies with cause

5. The skeletal and soft-tissue abnormalities of **diabetes and hemochromatosis** do not improve.

B. **Medical treatment** (other than treatment of the endocrinopathy) is nonspecific and symptomatic. Nonsteroidal antiinflammatory drugs and analgesics are commonly used. There is no role for corticosteroid preparations, antimalarial agents, disease-modifying antirheumatic drugs (DMARDs), or immunosuppressive drugs. The following **specific precautions** are necessary:
   1. Patients with **hyperthyroidism** metabolize drugs rapidly; standard doses may be ineffective.
   2. Patients with **hypothyroidism** metabolize drugs slowly; standard doses may be toxic.
   3. In **diabetes and hyperparathyroidism,** renal dysfunction should be anticipated.
   4. In **hemochromatosis,** hepatic dysfunction should be anticipated.

C. **Surgical treatment** is useful for **carpal tunnel syndrome** and, on occasion, for orthopedic repair, but specific concerns are as follows:
   1. Osteopenic bones heal and hold prostheses poorly.
   2. Charcot's joints heal poorly and refracture. Fusions may be indicated.
   3. Diabetic cheiropathy responds very poorly to attempts at surgical correction.

Bibliography

Askari AD, et al. Arthritis of hemochromatosis. *Am J Med* 1983;75:957.

Benedetti A, et al. Joint lesions in diabetes. *N Engl J Med* 1975;282:1033.

Clouse ME, et al. Diabetic osteoarthropathy: clinical and roentgenographic observations in 90 cases. *Am J Roentgenol Radiat Ther* 1974;121:22.

Fatomechi V, et al. Dermopathy of Graves' disease (pretibial myxedema). Review of 150 cases. *Medicine (Baltimore)* 1994;73:1.

Grigic A, et al. Joint contracture in childhood diabetes. *N Engl J Med* 1975;292:371.

Lieberman S, et al. Rheumatologic and skeletal changes in acromegaly. *Endocrinol Metab Clin North Am* 1992;21:615.

McLean RM, et al. Bone and joint manifestations of hypothyroidism. *Semin Arthritis Rheum* 1995;24:282.

Poa HL, et al. Thyroid-induced osteoporosis. *Curr Opin Orthop* 1995;6:39.

Rosenbloom AL, et al. Limited joint mobility in childhood diabetes mellitus indicates increased risk for microvascular disease. *N Engl J Med* 1983;305:191.

Ross DS. Hyperthyroidism, thyroid hormone and bone. *Thyroid* 1994;4:319.

49. FIBROMYALGIA

Daniel J. Clauw and John F. Beary, III

Fibromyalgia (FM) is a painful, noninflammatory condition characterized by a history of widespread pain and diffuse tenderness on examination. Although FM is defined on the basis of pain and tenderness, most persons with FM also display a number of non-defining symptoms, including fatigue, sleep disturbances, headaches, and memory difficulties. In fact, it has become increasingly clear that considerable overlap exists between FM and "systemic" conditions (e.g., chronic fatigue syndrome) as well as "organ-specific" syndromes (e.g., migraine headache, tension headaches, irritable bowel syndrome, temporomandibular disorders, and mitral valve prolapse syndrome).

I. **Definition.** In 1990, FM was redefined by a subcommittee of the American College of Rheumatology. The new definition requires a history of chronic widespread pain (lasting longer than 3 months **in all four quadrants of the body** plus the axial skeleton) and the finding of tenderness in 11 or more of 18 points on examination. Tender points are discrete regions of the body. If a patient experiences pain when 4 kg of pressure is applied with digital palpation to any one of these points, it is considered a "positive" tender point. Patients whose chronic pain and tender points are confined to one quadrant of the body are diagnosed as having **regional myofascial disorder**.

Even when this definition was originally adopted, it was stated that these criteria were not meant to be strictly applied in clinical practice. Only about half of the patients seen in clinical practice who clearly have FM meet these strict criteria; **in many cases, pain is more limited in distribution,** or fewer than 11 tender points are noted. The usefulness of "tender points" is presently being debated because it is now clear that the primary problem in FM is a *generalized* disturbance in pain processing. Patients with FM exhibit more tenderness throughout the entire body, even in control areas such as the thumbnail or forehead. The tenderness is diffuse rather than regional and is not confined to certain types of tissues (i.e., muscle). Tender points merely represent regions of the body, such as the lateral epicondylar area, that are normally more tender. When a patient with FM is stimulated, the pain is likely to be amplified compared with that in a control subject.

Another problem with tender points is that in population-based studies, the number of tender points displayed by a patient is highly correlated with various measures of distress. In contrast, other methods of assessing tenderness, such as the use of a pressure gauge, are much less influenced by psychologic factors.

II. **Etiology and pathogenesis.** The precise cause for FM remains unclear. Numerous studies suggest a strong familial aggregation of FM, although none has established whether heredity or shared environmental influences are the cause. It is also clear that a number of environmental "stressors," including physical trauma, infection, autoimmune disorders, endocrine conditions, and emotional stress, seem to be capable of "triggering" the development of FM.

Several types of physiologic abnormalities have been identified in persons with FM and related conditions that may help explain the basis of symptoms. The hallmark of FM appears to be a central disturbance in pain processing that is largely unexplained by psychological factors. The evidence for this comes from numerous studies employing various types of experimental paradigms for pain testing. Abnormalities of neurotransmitters (e.g., substance P) in the cerebrospinal fluid of FM patients, and of cerebral areas involved in pain processing, such as the thalamus (seen on single-photon emission tomography), provide further, objective evidence. A number of abnormalities in both neuroendocrine and autonomic function have also been identified in subgroups of FM patients.

Although the dualistic notion that any illness is either "organic" or "functional" should be abandoned, because of the realization that all illnesses are likely to have a biologic basis, this debate continues with respect to FM. It is likely that this illness usually begins as a primarily physiologic problem, and it never progresses past this point in some cases because of appropriate treatment, good coping skills, and adequate support systems. In other cases with chronic symptoms, however, concurrent psychological, psychiatric, and behavioral factors become more prominent. Examples of such factors, which portend a worse prognosis, include maladaptive illness behaviors, secondary gain issues (e.g., litigation, compensation), and concurrent mood disorders.

III. Epidemiologic characteristics. Approximately 2% to 4% of the population in industrialized countries (e.g., the United States, Canada, Israel, and Germany) suffers from FM, as defined by the American College of Rheumatology criteria. However, these population-based studies suggest that it may be better to consider FM as the "end of a spectrum" rather than as a discrete, unique illness. For example, both the pain and tenderness domains are continuously distributed across a wide range in the population. Approximately 10% of the U.S. population suffers from chronic widespread pain, and 20% from chronic regional pain; both symptoms occur approximately 1.5 times more commonly in female patients. A wide continuum of tenderness can be noted within the population, so that some patients are very tender and others quite nontender. Women are more sensitive to cutaneous pressure than are men, and in fact are 10 times more likely to have 11 tender points than men. Because the American College of Rheumatology definition uses an arbitrary cutoff of 11 tender points to define the subset of patients with chronic widespread pain who meet FM criteria, FM is diagnosed predominantly in women.

Other studies have demonstrated that FM frequently coexists with other conditions. Approximately 25% of patients with rheumatoid arthritis, lupus, ankylosing spondylitis, osteoarthritis, hepatitis C, and a number of other conditions display concurrent FM.

These data suggest that it may be better to consider FM as a construct that helps explain chronic pain in the absence of a peripheral inflammatory or mechanical stimulus. This central or "non-nociceptive" pain occurs commonly throughout the entire body (in FM), in a single region of the body (e.g., temporomandibular syndrome, myofascial pain syndrome), or concurrently with other medical conditions (especially those characterized by chronic pain).

IV. Physical findings. The physical examination findings in FM are classically normal except for the presence of diffuse tenderness. Occasionally, patients will also display mild muscle weakness, perhaps because of pain or disuse.

V. Symptoms. The character of the pain in FM is different from that in most other musculoskeletal conditions. Although most persons with FM have a few areas where they always experience pain, this condition is characterized by wide variation in the location and intensity of pain. Patients frequently report a worsening of pain in response to activity, weather changes, menstrual status, and stressors. Subjective weakness, morning stiffness, swelling (especially of the hands and feet), and nondermatomal dysesthesias or paresthesias frequently accompany the pain. Fatigue and difficulties with short term-memory and concentration are also often present.

VI. Diagnostic testing. FM is a diagnosis of exclusion because there are no predictably abnormal findings on laboratory or imaging studies in this entity. Initial testing in a patient suspected of having FM should include routine hematology and chemistry panels, thyroid function tests, and a determination of sedimentation rate or C-reactive protein. Unless specific signs and symptoms suggest the presence of illnesses such as rheumatoid arthritis (e.g., synovitis on examination) or systemic lupus, tests for antinuclear antibodies and rheumatoid factor have a very low predictive value and should be avoided. For example, it has been estimated that for every antinuclear antibody test ordered for a patient with the nonspecific complaints of myalgias, arthralgias, and fatigue, there will be at least 20 false-positive results for every true-positive result (i.e., a patient with an autoimmune disorder). Certain laboratory abnormalities occur more commonly in persons with this spectrum of illness than in the general population, such as elevated antibody titers to certain viruses (e.g., Epstein-Barr virus), positivity for antinuclear antibodies, and lipid abnormalities. However, these tests are neither sensitive nor specific for FM.

VII. Treatment. Three types of treatment have been best demonstrated in randomized, controlled trials to be of benefit within this spectrum of illness: symptom-based pharmacotherapy, aerobic exercise, and cognitive behavioral therapy. Perhaps the most important role of the physician is to educate the patient that FM is a chronic condition wherein pain occurs even though there is no damage to the body, and that no pill or "magic herb" is available to "cure" their illness. Patients with this condition rarely improve significantly unless they accept the fact that they need to play an active role in their own treatment, which should include daily exercise and appropriate life-style modifications.

A. Pharmacotherapy. The class of drugs with established efficacy in FM is the tricyclic compounds; cyclobenzaprine (Flexeril) and amitriptyline (Elavil) are the best studied. These medications are tolerated best if they are taken *several hours before bedtime* (to help prevent the "hung-over" feeling that patients often report). They must be started at low doses (e.g., half of a 10-mg tablet) and slowly escalated by 5 to 10 mg every 1 to 2 weeks until efficacy is established or a dose of 50 mg daily is reached. Because FM is not an inflammatory condition, "antiinflammatory" doses of nonsteroidal antiinflammatory drugs (NSAIDs) are neither necessary nor of much benefit. In addition to tricyclics, analgesics (e.g., low doses of NSAIDs, acetaminophen, or tramadol) may be helpful. In some instances, other classes of antidepressants, such as those acting on the adrenergic or dopaminergic systems (venlafaxine, bupropion) or on serotonin receptors may be effective.

B. Aerobic exercise therapy can be extremely beneficial in FM and related conditions. Mildly affected persons can sometimes be adequately managed with these modalities alone. A graded, low-impact, aerobic exercise program is extremely beneficial. Patients should be instructed to begin with 5 to 10 minutes of low-impact exercise (e.g., water exercise, stationary bike, treadmill, walking) three to four times weekly and to increase this by 1 to 2 minutes a week. Beginning at high levels of exercise or escalating more rapidly is poorly tolerated and frequently will make the patient feel worse. The eventual goal should be 20 to 30 minutes of aerobic exercise four to five times weekly.

C. Cognitive behavioral therapy is an education-based program that has been successfully used to treat a number of chronic medical conditions, including chronic pain states, FM, and chronic fatigue syndrome. These programs, which can be undertaken in an individual or group setting, focus on teaching techniques that reduce symptoms (e.g., biofeedback, relaxation exercises). Maladaptive illness behaviors that the patient (usually unknowingly) displays and that make the illness worse are identified and explained. An example is the tendency for patients to "overdo it" on "good days," which will lead to several "bad days."

VIII. Prognosis. Although FM is typically a chronic illness lasting for several years, life expectancy is not affected. Most afflicted persons can expect to lead a relatively normal life with appropriate management.

Bibliography

Bennett RM, et al. Group treatment of fibromyalgia: a 6-month outpatient program. *J Rheumatol* 1996;23:521.

Clauw DJ. Fibromyalgia: more than just a musculoskeletal disease. *Am Fam Physician* 1995;52:843.

Clauw DJ, Chrousos GP. Chronic pain and fatigue syndromes: overlapping clinical and neuroendocrine features and potential pathogenic mechanisms. *Neuroimmunomodulation* 1997;4:134.

Goldenberg DL, Felson DT, Dinerman H. A randomized controlled trial of amitriptyline and naproxen in the treatment of patients with fibromyalgia. *Arthritis Rheum* 1986; 29:1371.

50. HYPERTROPHIC OSTEOARTHROPATHY AND OTHER RHEUMATIC MANIFESTATIONS OF NEOPLASIA

Alan T. Kaell

If a close temporal relationship exists between the discovery of a malignancy and the onset of a rheumatic syndrome, an association is often presumed. In many cases, the association may be coincidental. In other cases, the response of the rheumatic syndrome to successful management of the malignancy suggests an interrelationship of the two problems. Similarly, the recurrence of a rheumatic syndrome that heralds or follows the relapse of a malignancy is an even stronger indication of a pathogenetic linkage.

The pathogenesis of a rheumatic syndrome may be known in a patient with metastatic joint involvement or gout. For most other conditions, such as **hypertrophic (pulmonary) osteoarthropathy,** the pathogenesis remains speculative. Humoral, cellular, neural, and vascular mechanisms have been suggested.

The relationship between various rheumatic syndromes and malignant neoplasms takes any one of several forms:

1. Rheumatic syndrome as a manifestation of an established or occult malignancy.
2. Malignancy occurring in the setting of an established rheumatic syndrome.
3. Malignancy as a complication of antirheumatic therapy.
4. Rheumatic syndrome as a complication of antineoplastic therapy.

I. Rheumatic syndrome as a manifestation of neoplasia

A. Primary bone and joint neoplasms. Primary bone tumors such as chondrosarcoma, giant cell tumor, and osteogenic sarcoma may present as monarticular pain. They can either directly invade the joint capsule and synovium or induce a synovial reaction by involving juxtaarticular bone.

B. Tenosynovial sarcomas are rare and usually present as a painless soft-tissue mass near a joint of the lower extremity. Extension directly into the joint is uncommon. Three subtypes of sarcoma and their typical locations include synovial (lower limb, distal upper limb), clear cell (heel, toes, ankles), and epithelioid (hand, wrist, forearm). Radiographic findings are nonspecific, and diagnosis is by biopsy. These tumors are probably of mesenchymal and not synovial cell origin.

C. Lymphoproliferative disorders

1. Leukemia. Leukemic cells may directly infiltrate articular tissues. Polyarthritis occurs more often with hematologic malignancies than with solid neoplasms. In childhood, the metaphyseal portion of bones is occupied by red marrow. Acute lymphocytic leukemia can present as a migratory or symmetric polyarthritis by infiltrating the periosteum, joint capsule, or metaphysis. It may even mimic rheumatic fever or juvenile rheumatoid arthritis (JRA). The ankle or knee is usually involved. Characteristically, the joint pain is quite severe and disproportionate to any physical findings. The erythrocyte sedimentation rate may be normal. Articular manifestations may develop before the appearance of leukemic cells in the peripheral blood. An elevated serum lactate dehydrogenase or mild leukopenia may help distinguish children with malignant neoplasms who present with musculoskeletal complaints from those who ultimately have JRA. In some cases, immunocytologic analysis can identify leukemic cells in synovial fluid.

2. Vasculitis seen in leukemia is usually limited to cutaneous involvement (except for hairy-cell leukemia). Recurrent leukemic infiltrations into muscles may mimic localized, tender swelling of polyarteritis. Hairy-cell leukemia has been associated with polyarteritis nodosa. Rheumatic manifestations can precede or follow the clinical onset of leukemic symptoms and diagnosis. Rarely, temporal arteritis and polyarthritis, including rheumatoid arthritis (RA) and adult Still's disease, occur. Pathogenesis involves either leukemic infiltration or immune-driven inflammation.

3. **Lymphoma.** Monarticular or polyarticular symptoms may be related to lymphomatous involvement of juxtaarticular bone. Both Hodgkin's and non-Hodgkin's lymphoma may present with musculoskeletal symptoms. This is attributed to either induction of a synovial reaction by adjacent osseous lymphoma or direct invasion of the joint capsule or synovium. In patients with T-cell lymphomas, a chronic polyarthritis may also develop.

   Vasculitis associated with lymphoma is usually limited to cutaneous involvement, presumably on an immune basis. In rare patients with **intravascular lymphoma,** multiorgan involvement may mimic vasculitis and symmetric polyarthritis.

4. **Angioimmunoblastic lymphadenopathy** can be associated with rash, polyarthritis, polyclonal hypergammaglobulinemia, and Coombs'-positive hemolytic anemia. This condition may mimic systemic lupus erythematosus (SLE).

5. **Myelodysplastic disorders** have also been associated with a variety of musculoskeletal symptoms and signs, including polyarthritis, lupuslike conditions, polychondritis, vasculitis, and erythromelalgia.

6. **Gout,** secondary to rapid cell turnover or tumor lysis, is seen mainly in leukemias and lymphomas. Institution of allopurinol helps prevent this complication. The dosage of azathioprine and 6-mercaptopurine must be reduced if the patient receives concomitant allopurinol therapy.

D. **Paraproteinemias.** Amyloid arthropathy attributed to deposition of AL protein is associated with dysproteinemias, such as multiple myeloma. It occurs in up to 5% of myeloma patients and is more common in men and those with λ light chains. This arthropathy can mimic RA and is associated with carpal tunnel syndrome, shoulder pad sign, and nodules. Erosions are rarely noted. Additional clinical clues that warrant consideration of amyloidosis are hepatosplenomegaly, congestive heart failure, macroglossia, pinch purpura, raccoon eyes, and nephrosis. Biopsy sites to establish a tissue diagnosis include abdominal fat, rectum, synovium, and bone marrow. (see Chapter 51, section **I**.)

E. **POEMS syndrome** (plasma cell dyscrasia with **p**olyneuropathy, **o**rganomegaly, **e**ndocrinopathy, **m**onoclonal protein, and **s**kin changes) can mimic a systemic, multiorgan rheumatic disorder. The skin changes are similar to those of scleroderma.

   Raynaud's syndrome, digital ischemic necrosis, and vasculitis may occur in patients with dysproteinemias.

   Tendon xanthomas, typically seen in familial hypercholesterolemia, have been reported with near-normal lipid levels in patients with dysproteinemias such as multiple myeloma and monoclonal gammopathy of unknown significance (MGUS).

F. **Metastatic carcinomatous arthritis associated with solid neoplasms.** Metastatic deposits of solid neoplasms in bone, synovium, or periarticular tissue can masquerade as monarthritis or polyarthritis. This is a rare occurrence. The synovial membrane can either react nonspecifically to adjacent malignant deposits or, less commonly, contain tumor itself. In general, the incidence of appendicular bone metastases lessens with increasing distance from the axial skeleton. Phalangeal metastases are usually caused by bronchogenic or gastrointestinal carcinomas and can mimic gout, osteomyelitis, osteoarthritis, or even RA. Metastatic breast carcinoma is the most common cause of metastatic carcinomatous arthritis in women. Joint effusions can rarely be associated with solid tumors in the absence of radiographically apparent periarticular osseous metastasis. In such cases, synovial fluid cytology or synovial tissue biopsy specimens may be positive for tumor cells in two-thirds of patients. In patients with unresponsive or progressive unilateral sacroiliitis, additional imaging and biopsy should be considered to detect metastatic carcinoma.

   In children, neuroblastoma should be considered as a cause of metastatic carcinomatous arthritis. In most instances, the primary neoplasm is evident.

If the tumor is occult, tomography, bone scan, or biopsy becomes necessary for accurate diagnosis. In general, therapy is directed toward the underlying neoplasm.

G. Hypertrophic osteoarthropathy

1. The **clinical presentation** is one of periostitis and chronic periosteal reaction. Periostitis occurs predominantly at the distal ends of the long bones. The term periostosis may more accurately describe these radiologic changes without necessarily implying an inflammatory mechanism. If early periostitis is not evident on plain radiographs, bone scan is useful in demonstrating its presence. Patients present with symmetric painful tenderness and swelling near the wrist and ankle regions. The discomfort is typically exacerbated by dependency of the limb and relieved by elevation.

   Note: Periostitis without clubbing does not constitute hypertrophic osteoarthropathy. Periostitis alone can occur in hypervitaminosis A, thyroid acropathy, retinoic acid toxicity, hyperphosphatemia, sarcoidosis, and Caffey's disease.

2. **Clubbing of the fingers.** Although finger clubbing is invariably present, it may develop only after pain in the distal long bones occurs. The characteristic bulbous deformity or drumstick appearance of the fingertips is easy to recognize. However, before obvious clubbing develops, the only abnormality may be a nail that can be rocked or floated upon its nail bed to produce a spongy sensation. Next, the ungual-phalangeal angle (the angle between the nail plate and the proximal digit) increases beyond 160 degrees and becomes obliterated at 180 degrees. Alternatively stated, the normal nail plate forms an angle of 20 degrees or more dorsally with the axis of the digit. The circumference of the nail bed becomes greater than the circumference of the distal interphalangeal joint. The nail may eventually appear convex, like a watch crystal. A very rare, familial form of hypertrophic osteoarthropathy is pachydermoperiostitis. This is not associated with any underlying disorder and is typically associated with coarse facial features and painless periostitis.

   In synovial hypertrophy, with or without joint effusions, synovitis affects predominantly the knees and ankles but may also involve metacarpophalangeal and proximal interphalangeal joints. Effusions, if present, are typically not inflammatory.

   Underlying disorders should always be considered in patients with hypertrophic osteoarthropathy (Table 50-1). Associated conditions include pleural, pulmonary, cardiovascular, gastrointestinal, hepatic, and miscellaneous diseases. Although clubbing occurs in the majority of patients with cyanotic congenital heart disease and cystic fibrosis, it is seen in fewer than 5% of patients with the other disorders listed. Neoplasms and chronic suppurative diseases predominate. Overall, pulmonary problems dominate in most series of patients with hypertrophic osteoarthropathy. Bronchogenic carcinoma and suppurative lung disease are the two most common associated pulmonary conditions. The incidence of hypertrophic osteoarthropathy in these diseases is 2% and 5%, respectively.

3. **Treatment.** If a neoplasm can be successfully resected, the presenting musculoskeletal symptoms of hypertrophic osteoarthropathy often resolve within weeks. A patient with inoperable bronchogenic carcinoma may respond to chemotherapy or radiation therapy. In those patients with an untreatable underlying disorder, chemical or surgical vagotomy may be beneficial. NSAIDs can be helpful in the control of local joint symptoms.

H. Rheumatoid arthritis and carcinomatous polyarthritis

1. **Rheumatoid arthritis.** Classic RA has never been clearly documented as a sign of occult malignancy. Some reports in which RA was purported to be an initial manifestation of malignancy likely included patients with hypertrophic osteoarthropathy. The detection of a solid neoplasm shortly after the onset of RA most probably represents a chance occurrence. Rheumatoid factors occur in the serum of up to 20% of patients with solid neoplasms.

Table 50-1. Conditions associated with hypertrophic osteoarthropathy

I. Neoplasms
- **A.** Pulmonary and pleural
  - **1.** Primary lung tumors—squamous cell carcinoma, large- and small-cell carcinoma, lymphoma
  - **2.** Metastases from soft-tissue, muscle, and bone sarcomas; nasopharyngeal, gastrointestinal, and renal carcinomas
  - **3.** Mesothelioma of pleura
  - **4.** Fibromas
- **B.** Gastrointestinal
  - **1.** Stomach and colonic mucus-producing carcinomas
  - **2.** Esophageal carcinoma
  - **3.** Hepatoma
  - **4.** Small-intestinal carcinoma
  - **5.** Polyposis of colon, esophagus
- **C.** Miscellaneous
  - **1.** Secondary myelofibrosis
  - **2.** Thymoma
  - **3.** Neurilemmoma
  - **4.** Chronic myelogenous leukemia

II. Chronic suppurative diseases
- **A.** Pulmonary and pleural
  - **1.** Bronchiectasis
  - **2.** Cystic fibrosis
  - **3.** Empyema
  - **4.** Lung abscess
  - **5.** Other: tuberculosis, sarcoid, hydatid cyst
- **B.** Gastrointestinal
  - **1.** Inflammatory bowel disease (Crohn's disease and ulcerative colitis)
  - **2.** Other: bacillary and amebic dysentery, ascariasis, subphrenic abscess, tuberculosis

III. Cardiovascular
- **A.** Cyanotic congenital heart disease
- **B.** Subacute bacterial endocarditis
- **C.** Other: pulmonary hemangioma, infected aortic prosthesis, aortic aneurysm, Takayasu's arteritis

IV. Miscellaneous: primary biliary cirrhosis, nontropical sprue, blood dyscrasias, myxedema, amyloidosis, syringomyelia, thyroid acropathy

V. Familial and idiopathic

Seropositivity and RA-like nodules have on occasion been described in patients with leukemia, including hairy-cell leukemia.

2. Carcinomatous polyarthritis. The concept of a rheumatoid-like arthropathy that heralds a malignancy remains controversial (Table 50-2). Typically, the diagnosis of a seemingly related malignancy—usually prostate, breast, or lung cancer—is made about 3 to 10 months after the onset of arthropathy. This arthritis typically differs from RA in that it is sudden in onset and is typically an asymmetric polyarthritis of predominantly the lower extremities; the wrist and small joints are spared. Subcutaneous nodules and rheumatoid factor are absent. Distinctive radiographic and synovial fluid findings have not been reported. The arthropathy may respond to anticancer therapy. In general, an age-appropriate malignancy assessment is appropriate in patients presenting with new-onset arthritis.

3. Dermatomyositis and polymyositis

a. Clinical presentation. Overall, malignancy occurs in 5% to 20% of persons with myositis. Dermatomyositis has a stronger association with cancer than does polymyositis. The association is most apparent in men older

Table 50-2. Rheumatic syndromes and the cancers they may herald

Rheumatic syndrome	Cancer type
Established associations	
Hypertrophic osteoarthropathy	Intrathoracic neoplasms, colon and hepatic neoplasms
Dermatomyositis	All tumor types
Secondary gout	Lymphoproliferative disorders, leukemia
Amyloid arthropathy/carpal tunnel syndrome	Plasma cell dyscrasias
Metastatic carcinomatous arthritis	Lung, breast, large-intestinal tumors predominate
Migratory arthritis	Acute lymphocytic leukemia
Raynaud's phenomenon; digital ulcers	Plasma cell dyscrasias, lymphoma
Palpable purpura	Lymphoproliferative disorders, other
Subcutaneous fat necrosis/polyarthritis	Pancreatic tumors
Possible associations	
Palmar fasciitis/polyarthritis	Ovarian, other
Carcinomatous polyarthritis	Prostate, other
"Lupuslike antibody syndrome"	Hypernephroma, gastric and cervical; breast carcinoma; gastrointestinal lymphoma; testicular seminoma
Progressive systemic sclerosis	Breast, uterus, prostate, other
Polyarteritis nodosa	Hodgkin's disease, hairy-cell leukemia
Temporal arteritis	Malignant histiocytosis, myeloma

than 40 years. Myositis may precede the discovery of a malignancy by several months to a few years. Among the many types of malignancies that present with myositis, lung, breast, and ovarian carcinoma are the most common. In the absence of an easily detectable neoplasm defined as part of an age-appropriate malignancy assessment, an exhaustive search for an occult malignancy may not be cost-effective. Patients with interstitial lung disease and antibodies to Jo-1 appear less likely to have an associated malignancy.

b. **Treatment.** Corticosteroids, with or without cytotoxic agents, remain the mainstay of therapy. Severe, progressive myositis that responds poorly to steroid therapy may improve after successful treatment of the neoplasm.

4. **Subcutaneous fat necrosis, arthritis, and eosinophilia.** Panniculitis, with or without monarthritis or polyarthritis, may herald pancreatic carcinoma. Painful nodules or periarticular fat necrosis often precedes the onset of abdominal pain. Eosinophilia is variably present. In a male patient with subcutaneous fat necrosis and monarthritis or polyarthritis, pancreatic carcinoma should be strongly suspected, especially when eosinophilia is present.

   Endocrine tumors can mimic a variety of rheumatic disorders. Pituitary tumors causing acromegaly mimic polyarthritis; carcinoid can mimic scleroderma; pheochromocytoma can mimic vasculitis.

5. **Vasculitis**

   a. **Palpable purpura.** An unexplained necrotizing cutaneous vasculitis warrants consideration of, or surveillance for, an underlying lymphoreticular or myelodysplastic disorder. Vasculitis, including giant cell arteritis, is also rarely associated with solid neoplasms. The mechanism is likely immune-mediated and not attributable to direct vascular involvement by tumor, except in the rare case of **intravascular lymphoma** (see section **I.C.3**). Cutaneous vasculitis as a paraneoplastic syndrome is unusual. Only 8 of 192 patients (4.2%) with cutaneous vasculitis had an underlying malignancy. Six of the eight were hematologic malignancies.

b. **Raynaud's disease, digital ulcers, purpura, and gangrene.** Serum cryoproteins associated with plasma cell dyscrasias and lymphomas should be considered. Cryofibrinogen, evident in plasma, is associated with metastatic malignancy. Anti-cardiolipin antibodies may also be associated with malignancy (see below).

c. **Polyarteritis nodosa** may rarely develop in patients with hairy-cell leukemia or Hodgkin's disease.

d. **Temporal arteritis and polymyalgia rheumatica.** Temporal arteritis as the initial manifestation of malignant histiocytosis may occur. Biopsy-proven arteritis has also been associated with follicular small cleaved-cell lymphoma, hairy-cell leukemia, lymphoplasmacytoid lymphoma, multiple myeloma, amyloidosis, and Waldenström's macroglobulinemia.

e. **Polymyalgia rheumatica** should not prompt an extensive workup for occult malignancy above and beyond an age-appropriate malignancy assessment. Associated neoplasia is usually a chance occurrence and may involve any primary site. When polymyalgia rheumatica-like symptoms predate neoplasia, the latter is usually apparent within 3 months of onset of symptoms.

Mimics of vasculitis associated with protean, multiorgan symptoms and signs can occur in patients with pheochromocytoma, left atrial myxoma, intravascular lymphoma, tumor emboli, and anti-cardiolipin antibodies.

f. **Anti-cardiolipin antibodies** can be seen in patients with neoplasia. Anti-cardiolipin antibody syndromes are associated with thrombocytopenia and arterial or venous thrombotic events in the absence of disseminated intravascular coagulation. Such syndromes warrant consideration of underlying malignancy but probably do not justify an exhaustive search for underlying occult neoplasia.

6. **Systemic lupus erythematosus and scleroderma**

a. **Systemic lupus erythematosus.** There are no well-documented cases of occult malignancy presenting as SLE. Although antinuclear antibodies can be present in patients with solid neoplasms or leukemias who lack other evidence of a rheumatic syndrome, the significance of this is not understood. LE cells or antinuclear antibodies can be seen in patients with lymphoma or **angioimmunoblastic lymphadenopathy with dysproteinemia (AILD)**. Diagnostic confusion may arise, as lymphadenopathy and splenomegaly are features also common in SLE.

A "lupuslike antibody syndrome," manifested by typical SLE serologic and laboratory abnormalities but lacking clinical criteria for SLE, has been associated with certain tumors and myelodysplastic disorders. For example, hypernephroma has been found in a peripartum woman, but this may have been an incidental finding because a similar lupuslike antibody syndrome can occur during pregnancy. Other tumors include gastric, cervical, and breast carcinomas, gastrointestinal lymphoma, AILD, and testicular seminoma.

In general, a diagnosis of clinical SLE should not prompt a search for occult malignancy. However, lupuslike serology and unexplained Coombs'-positive anemia, thrombocytopenia, or circulating anticoagulants without clinical features of SLE warrant consideration of an occult neoplasm. In addition, in a patient with a known tumor who presents with pleural effusions, pericarditis, or nondeforming polyarthritis, an associated lupuslike illness should be considered.

b. **Scleroderma.** Rarely, hematologic malignancies, bladder cancer, and breast or stomach carcinoma become apparent shortly after the onset of scleroderma. The scleroderma may improve following treatment of these malignancies. Carcinoid tumors are associated with scleroderma-like changes of the lower extremities. POEMS may also be associated with scleroderma-like skin changes. Scleroderma may be erroneously diagnosed before these disorders are considered.

7. **Miscellaneous.** Rheumatic syndromes that may be a harbinger of neoplasia include eosinophilic fasciitis and the following disorders. Patients should be followed for development of hematologic disorders (e.g., aplastic anemia and lymphoid malignancies).

I. Reflex sympathetic dystrophy may occur secondary to brain tumor, ovarian carcinoma, or Pancoast lung tumor.

J. Erythromelalgia (burning, red, warm feet) may be associated with myeloproliferative disorders in 10% of cases.

K. Sweet's syndrome, or acute neutrophilic dermatosis, is associated with malignancy in at least 15% of cases, most commonly with acute myelogenous leukemia.

L. Palmar fasciitis and polyarthritis. Originally described in women with ovarian carcinoma, this differs from reflex sympathetic dystrophy. Palmar fasciitis and polyarthritis has also been associated with other malignancies. Plantar fasciitis may be associated with this syndrome. Polychondritis may rarely predate the discovery of a neoplasm.

M. Osteomalacia may develop in patients with a variety of benign or malignant mesenchymal tumors, giant cell tumor, hemangioma, angiosarcoma, hemangiopericytoma, neurilemmoma, and nonossifying fibroma. Epidermal nevus syndrome is also associated with this condition. Patients exhibit hypophosphatemia, normal or slightly decreased serum calcium, and usually normal serum parathyroid hormone concentrations. Abnormalities revert to normal following successful removal of tumor tissue.

Unclassified rheumatic disorders in hospitalized patients may be associated with an underlying occult neoplasia in up to 24% of cases during a 2-year period. The frequency may be higher in men and patients over 50 years old. The malignancy is usually discovered on routine physical examination.

N. Miscellaneous musculoskeletal problems in patients with neoplasia

1. **Bone and joint infections.** Patients with malignancy, especially those receiving cytotoxic therapy, are predisposed to septic complications such as pyarthrosis and osteomyelitis. Organisms include both common and opportunistic pathogens. Pyogenic arthritis caused by *Streptococcus bovis* or enteric organisms may signal an occult colonic neoplasm.
2. **Referred pain to the joints, neck, or back.** Knee pain exacerbated by recumbency has been attributed to diffuse histiocytic lymphoma of the spinal cord. Back pain and radiculitis may be secondary to leukemic meningeal involvement or be the initial manifestation of Hodgkin's disease. Shoulder pain with normal findings on shoulder examination may be referred pain caused by infradiaphragmatic, intraabdominal neoplasms. Alternatively, intrathoracic neoplasms (e.g., Pancoast tumor) may extend into the brachial plexus and cause pain in a shoulder with a normal range of motion but evidence of muscle atrophy and loss of deep tendon reflexes.

   Mimics of vasculitis such as subacute bacterial endocarditis, cholesterol emboli, and anti-cardiolipin syndrome may occur in any patient with concomitant neoplasia.

II. Malignancies associated with an established rheumatic syndrome. The risk for certain types of cancer appears to be increased in some of the rheumatic syndromes. The increased incidence of malignancy does not appear to be related to antirheumatic therapy in the following instances:

A. Polymyositis is associated with all types of neoplasm. Although the increased risk for cancer after the diagnosis of polymyositis is consistent with cancer detection bias, clinical vigilance for associated neoplasia is indicated. Routine urinalysis, complete blood count, examination of stools for occult blood, sigmoidoscopy, mammography, prostate and testicular examinations, chest radiography, and Papanicolaou's smear are recommended screens. A more extensive search for occult malignancy may be indicated in patients at greatest risk, such as older men or patients with severe, refractory dermatomyositis.

B. **RA,** even in the absence of treatment with potentially oncogenic drugs, appears to be associated with an increased risk for hematologic malignancies, including lymphoma and myeloma. There is also an increased risk for leukemia in some cohorts of RA patients. In certain patients with Felty's syndrome, there is a twofold increase in total cancer incidence and a 12-fold increased risk for non-Hodgkin's lymphoma. There is also an increased risk for CD16+ large granular lymphocytes and leukemia. RA patients with secondary Sjögren's syndrome are at a 33-fold increased risk for non-Hodgkin's lymphoma. Paraproteins are an additional marker of increased risk for hematopoietic neoplasms.

The overall risk for malignancy is reduced in some RA cohort studies. Prospective, longitudinal cohort studies of RA patients have demonstrated a lower incidence of stomach and colon carcinomas, the latter possibly related to use of nonsteroidal antiinflammatory drugs.

C. Patients with **Sjögren's syndrome** are at increased risk for the development of non-Hodgkin lymphoma. Waldenström's macroglobulinemia also appears to be more frequent in these patients. The risk is increased in both primary and secondary Sjögren's syndrome in National Institutes of Health (NIH) cohorts. In Italian studies, women with primary Sjögren's syndrome are at greatest risk. Risk factors such as disappearance of rheumatoid factor were predictive of the evolution in the NIH cohort but not in a Vanderbilt cohort.

D. **Systemic sclerosis** patients with pulmonary fibrosis and "honeycomb" lung are at increased risk for bronchoalveolar cell carcinoma.

Discoid lupus erythematosus lesions may develop into epidermoid carcinoma. Patients with eosinophilic fasciitis are at increased risk for associated aplastic anemia and lymphoproliferative disease.

E. **Immunodeficiency states.** Patients with X-linked hypogammaglobulinemia, common variable immunodeficiency, ataxia-telangiectasia, and Wiskott-Aldrich syndrome are at increased risk for the development of lymphoreticular malignancy. Leukemia, medulloblastoma, and adenocarcinomas may also occur with increased frequency. Asymptomatic patients with isolated immunoglobulin A deficiency do not appear to have an increased risk for neoplasia.

F. Patients with **systemic lupus erythematosus** do not appear to be at increased risk for malignancy, except for neoplasia complicating cytotoxic therapy (Table 50-3).

G. **Mixed cryoglobulinemia** associated with vasculitis and hepatitis C was associated with non-Hodgkin's lymphoma in 14 of 200 patients. Monitoring for hepatocellular carcinoma should also be considered.

H. **Paget's disease.** Osteogenic sarcoma may complicate Paget's disease in 1% of patients and present with persistent, severe pain. Bone biopsy may be necessary for accurate diagnosis.

I. **Multicentric reticulohistiocytosis** may herald a subsequent malignancy.

J. **Chronic osteomyelitis.** Squamous cell carcinoma may occur in adjacent cutaneous tissue in up to 2% of cases.

Table 50-3. Malignancies associated with established connective tissue disorders

Connective tissue disorder	Malignancy
Progressive systemic sclerosis	Bronchioalveolar cell
Discoid lupus erythematosus	Epidermoid
Sjögren's syndrome	Lymphoma
Polymyositis	All types
Eosinophilic fasciitis	Aplastic anemia, perhaps lymphoproliferative neoplasia
Mixed cryoglobulinemia associated with hepatitis C	Lymphoma, hepatoma

III. Malignancy as a complication of antirheumatic therapy. The influence of immunosuppressive drug therapy in altering the incidence of cancer in the rheumatic population is unclear, but an increased risk for neoplasia is apparent with some regimens.

A. Alkylating agents such as cyclophosphamide and chlorambucil can increase the risk for leukemia and myelodysplastic syndromes. Cytogenetic abnormalities of chromosome 5/7 are associated with therapy-related myelodysplastic syndromes seen in rheumatic disease. In addition, cyclophosphamide is associated with bladder and other genitourinary cancers. As the latter may occur 20 years after exposure, ongoing surveillance should be considered. Sodium-2-mercaptoethane sulfate can bind the toxic metabolite acrolein and may diminish the incidence of bladder carcinoma.

B. Immunosuppressive Agents

1. **Purine antimetabolites** such as azathioprine are associated with an increased risk for lymphomas and non-melanoma skin carcinomas in renal transplant recipients. The possibility of a similar increased incidence of malignancy in rheumatic disease patients treated with azathioprine remains to be firmly established. An increased incidence of non-Hodgkin's lymphoma and cervical carcinoma in SLE patients on azathioprine has been suggested. There is no apparent relationship between the amount and duration of cytotoxic therapy and the development of malignancy.
2. **Folic acid antagonists.** Methotrexate, a folic acid antagonist, may rarely be associated with the development of B-cell non-Hodgkin's lymphoma in RA patients. Many, but not all, of these tumors are positive for Epstein-Barr virus. Some regress on withdrawal of the drug. Interestingly, the tumors of up to 30% of methotrexate-naïve RA patients with lymphoma are positive for Epstein-Barr virus.
3. **Cyclosporine,** although not mutagenic, is associated with lymphoproliferative disorders in up to 3% of renal transplantation patients treated with concomitant azathioprine and prednisone. Whether patients with rheumatic diseases who are taking cyclosporine, with or without methotrexate, have an increased risk for lymphoma and brain or skin cancers remains to be determined. In one review of more than 1,000 RA patients treated with cyclosporine, tumors developed in 17 of them.
4. **Novel or biologic agents.** It remains unresolved whether agents to block tumor necrosis factor-alpha, such as Enbrel, which are available to treat refractory RA, are associated with a higher risk for non-Hodgkin's lymphoma. It also remains to be determined whether any of the other new agents with immunomodulating effects [e.g., leflunomide (Arava), mycophenolate mofetil, interleukin-10 (IL-10), or interleukin-1 receptor antagonist (IL-1ra)] will increase the relative risk for development of a malignancy in RA. Increased surveillance is certainly indicated in RA patients on combination therapies including methotrexate, anti-TNF agents and cyclosporine.
5. **Radiation therapy.** Ankylosing spondylitis patients treated with spinal irradiation have an increased frequency of leukemia. The risk for myeloproliferative disorders and osseous sarcoma is likely increased in RA patients treated with total nodal irradiation.

IV. Chemotherapeutic agents that may induce rheumatic-like disorders are the following:

A. Busulfan can cause a syndrome resembling sicca syndrome.

B. Cisplatin (Platinol) has been associated with Raynaud's phenomenon.

C. Bleomycin (Blenoxane) can produce scleroderma-like features involving the skin and lungs.

D. Fluorouracil is associated with a hand-foot syndrome characterized by palmar-plantar erythrodysesthesia.

E. Anthracyclines can cause transient polyarthritis. Liposome-encapsulated doxorubicin used to treat human immunodeficiency virus-related Kaposi's sarcoma is associated with a painful hand-foot syndrome. Painful, reddened, swollen hands and feet may ulcerate, fissure, and desquamate.

F. Cytosine arabinoside (ara-C). Most vascular reactions have been noted after combination chemotherapy, but treatment with ara-C as a single agent has also been associated with necrotizing cutaneous vasculitis.

G. Any immunosuppressive therapy may predispose a patient to bone and joint infections.

H. Hormonal manipulation. Tamoxifen is reported to be associated with cases of vasculitis and polyarthritis.

I. Luteinizing hormone-releasing hormone (LHRH) agonists, such as leuprolide, buserelin, and nafarelin, and nonsteroidal anti-androgens, such as flutamide, may be associated with myalgia and arthralgias.

J. Antibacterial and antiviral agents used in the treatment of opportunistic infections may cause a variety of rheumatic problems. For example, zidovudine (AZT) is associated with a syndrome resembling dermato-myositis-polymyositis.

K. Cephalosporins are associated with serum sickness-like reactions.

L. Ciprofloxacin has been associated with tendon ruptures and flares of SLE.

M. Radiation therapy may be associated with a delayed obliterative radiation arteritis and avascular necrosis.

N. Growth factors and biologic response modifiers

1. Granulocyte colony-stimulating factor (G-CSF) may be associated with Sweet's syndrome. Interleukins and interferons have been associated with the development of signs and symptoms of autoimmune disease or autoantibodies. Treatment with interferon-alfa is associated with Raynaud's syndrome and SLE-like illness. The manifestations vary depending on the underlying disease being treated. When used to treat myeloproliferative disorders, interferon-alfa can induce formation of antinuclear antibodies and rheumatoid factor, polyarthritis, or polyarthralgia. The incidence for these complications appears to be much lower in patients treated for carcinoid or viral hepatitis. Ongoing clinical trials of IL-4, IL-10, IL-1ra, and other biologic response modifiers should continue to monitor for any increase in autoantibodies or autoimmune complications.

O. Bone marrow transplantation may be associated with chronic graft-versus-host disease that includes scleroderma-like skin changes, alopecia, xerostomia, keratoconjunctivitis sicca, photosensitivity, myositis, and joint contractures.

P. Anti-thymocyte globulin is associated with a serum sickness reaction that consists of arthralgia/arthritis and a distinctive erythematous, serpiginous rash on the hands and feet at the margins of the palmar and plantar skin ("moccasin" distribution).

Q. Intravesical therapy with bacille Calmette-Guérin for bladder cancer can be associated with a reactive or RA-like arthritis.

V. General recommendations. It is important to remain alert to the development of malignancy in any patient with a rheumatic syndrome, either as a complication of immunosuppressive therapy or secondary to the disease process itself. However, patients who **require special attention or surveillance for malignancy** include those on/with:

A. Hypertrophic osteoarthropathy.

B. Dermatomyositis or polymyositis.

C. Cytotoxic or immunosuppressive therapy.

D. Immunodeficiency states (patients with lupuslike serology and unexplained Coombs'-positive anemia, thrombocytopenia, or circulating anticoagulants without clinical features of SLE).

E. Hepatitis C-associated mixed cryoglobulinemia/vasculitis.

Bibliography

Abu-Shahra M, Guillemin F, Lee P. Cancer in systemic sclerosis. *Arthritis Rheum* 1993;36:460.

Ahmed I, et al. Cytosine arabinoside-induced vasculitis. *Mayo Clin Proc* 1998;73:239.

Arellano F, Krupp P. Malignancies in rheumatoid arthritis: conclusions of an international review. *Br J Rheumatol* 1994;33[Suppl 1]:72.

Brooks PM. Rheumatic manifestations of neoplasia. *Curr Opin Rheumatol* 1992;4:90.

Burstein HJ, Janicek MJ, Skarin AT. Hypertrophic osteoarthropathy. *J Clin Oncol* 1997;15:2759.

Caldwell DS, McCollum RM. Rheumatologic manifestations of cancer. *Med Clin North Am* 1986;2:385.

Cash JM, Klippel JH. Is malignancy a major concern in rheumatoid arthritis patients? *J Clin Rheumatol* 1995;1:14.

Cibere J, Sibley J, Haga M. Rheumatoid arthritis and the risk of malignancy. *Arthritis Rheum* 1997;40:1580.

Falcini F, et al. Corona arthritis as a presenting feature of non-Hodgkin's lymphoma. *Arch Dis Child* 1998;78:367.

Farhey Y, Luggen M. Seropositive, symmetric polyarthritis in a patient with poorly differentiated lung carcinoma—carcinomatous polyarthritis, hypertrophic osteoarthropathy or rheumatoid arthritis. *Arthritis Care Res* 1998;11:146.

Garcia-Porrua C, Gonzalez-Gay MA. Cutaneous vasculitis as a paraneoplastic syndrome in adults. *Arthritis Rheum* 1998;41:1133.

Gaudin P, et al. Skeletal involvement as the initial disease manifestation in Hodgkin's disease: a review of 6 cases. *J Rheumatol* 1992;19:146.

Georgescu L, et al. Lymphoma in patients with rheumatoid arthritis: association with the disease state or rheumatoid arthritis. *Semin Arthritis Rheum* 1997;26:794.

Kaell AT. Is it arthritis or metastases? *Prim Care Cancer* 1989;9:15.

Keung YK, et al. Association of temporal arteritis, retinal vasculitis, and xanthomatosis with multiple myeloma: case report and review of the literature. *Mayo Clin Proc* 1998;73:657.

LaCivita L, et al. Mixed cryoglobulinemia as a possible paraneoplastic disorder. *Arthritis Rheum* 1995;38:1859.

Levy Y, et al. Subcutaneous T-cell lymphoma in a patient with rheumatoid arthritis not treated with cytotoxic agents. *Clin Rheumatol* 1997;16:606.

Maoz CR, et al. High incidence of malignancies in patients with dermatomyositis and polymyositis—an 11-year analysis. *Semin Arthritis Rheum* 1998;27:319.

Martinez-Lavin M. Hypertrophic osteoarthropathy. *Curr Opin Rheumatol* 1997;9:83.

McCarthy CJ, et al. Cytogenetic abnormalities and therapy-related myelodysplastic syndromes in rheumatic disease. *Arthritis Rheum* 1998;41:1493.

Mertz LE, Conn DL. Vasculitis associated with malignancy. *Curr Opin Rheumatol* 1992;4:39.

Mody G, Cassim B. Rheumatologic manifestations of malignancy. *Curr Opin Rheumatol* 1997;9:75.

Naschitz JE, et al. Cancer-associated rheumatic disorders: clues to occult neoplasia. *Semin Arthritis Rheum* 1995;24:231.

Needlemen M. Childhood leukemia mimicking arthritis. *J Am Board Fam Pract* 1996;9:56.

Nesher G, Ruchlemer R. Alpha-interferon-induced arthritis: clinical presentation, treatment, and prevention. *Semin Arthritis Rheum* 1998;27:360.

Sigurgeirsson B, et al. Risk of cancer in patients with dermatomyositis or polymyositis: a population-based study. *N Engl J Med* 1992;326:363.

Smalley W, DuBois R. Colorectal cancer and nonsteroidal antiinflammatory drugs. *Adv Pharmacol* 1997;39:1.

Von Kempis J, et al. Intravascular lymphoma presenting as symmetric polyarthritis. *Arthritis Rheum* 1998;41:1126.

Wallendal M, Stork L, Hollister J. The discriminating value of serum lactate dehydrogenase levels in children with malignant neoplasms presenting as joint pain. *Arch Pediatr Adolesc Med* 1996;150:70.

Yoe J, et al. Development of rheumatoid arthritis after treatment of large granular lymphocyte leukemia with deoxycoformycin. *Am J Hematol* 1998;57:253.

Zantos D, Zhang Y, Felson D. The overall and temporal association of cancer with polymyositis and dermatomyositis. *J Rheumatol* 1994;21:1855.

51. MISCELLANEOUS DISEASES AND COMPLICATIONS

Giovanna Cirigliano and Stefano Bombardieri

I. Amyloid arthropathy

Amyloidosis is a disorder characterized by the extracellular deposition of an insoluble fibrous protein in the connective tissues or in one or more organs. Based on its staining with iodine and sulfuric acid, and on the mistaken belief that it was similar to cellulose, Virchow in 1854 designated this protein as amyloid.

During the past 25 years, the belief that a single amyloid substance appears during the course of several diseases has been refuted by a body of evidence showing that there are actually many "types" of amyloidosis. Each type is associated with a specific protein, and the resulting organ failure can be linked to the location, quantity, and ratio of deposition. The protein (P) itself consists of a homogeneous hyaline, eosinophilic material identifiable pathologically by three features: Congo red binding with a unique green-yellow birefringence under polarized light; a characteristic ultrastructure distinguished by fine, nonbranching, rigid fibrils 70 to 100 Å in diameter; and the presence of the serum amyloid P component, which belongs, together with C-reactive protein, to a family of proteins termed pentraxins because of their characteristic structure (made up of paired pentagonal subunits). Several different molecules have been associated with all forms of amyloid deposition—the P component, apolipoprotein E, and heparan sulfate proteoglycan—but the role of these molecules is still unclear.

The amyloidoses may be classified clinically as follows:

1. **Primary amyloidosis and myeloma-associated amyloidosis,** which show no evidence of predisposing disease and are characterized by the deposition of **amyloid AL protein** (immunoglobulin:κ or λ light chains).
2. **Secondary or reactive amyloidosis,** which is associated with chronic infectious or chronic inflammatory diseases and is characterized by the deposition of **protein AA.**
3. **Heredofamilial amyloidosis.**
4. **Hemodialysis-associated amyloidosis.**
5. **Senile amyloidosis.**
6. **Localized amyloidosis.**

The amyloidoses are of interest to rheumatologists because of their demonstrated association with long-standing inflammatory joint disease accompanied by amyloid deposition in the kidneys, liver, and spleen. However, the clinical presentation of arthropathy is rare; it has been seen in association with the deposition of AL protein, the amyloid associated with the immunoglobulin light chain; β_2-microglobulin in patients with chronic renal failure. Arthropathy is occasionally associated with transthyretin (TTR) amyloid (transthyretin is the precursor of amyloid protein).

A. Primary and myeloma-associated amyloidosis. These two forms of amyloidosis are characterized by the deposition of fibrils of AL amyloid made up of the monoclonal chain of immunoglobulin, the production of which indicates an underlying monoclonal plasma cell dyscrasia. Recent data also suggest the presence of structurally abnormal light chains.

1. Clinical picture. Amyloid fibrils may localize in the synovial membrane and tendon sheaths, in the synovial fluid, and in the articular cartilage in a small percentage of patients with AL deposition. Clinical arthropathy in not common, although when seen it is chronic and may involve the small or large joints (shoulders, wrists, knees, or fingers) either symmetrically or asymmetrically. Stiffness (but not pain) is characteristic, together with swelling, limitation of motion, and subcutaneous nodules. Shoulder involvement may be particularly striking, with accumulation of amyloid at the joint producing the "shoulder pad" sign.

2. **Diagnosis.** Radiography may show soft-tissue swelling and generalized osteoporosis with or without lytic lesions; joint space narrowing is not seen, and erosions are rare. The diagnosis can be confirmed by an examination of the synovial fluid and, when necessary, by synovial biopsy. The synovial fluid is noninflammatory and yellow or xanthochromic, and it may contain fibrils that have the tinctorial and ultrastructural features of amyloid. Clinicians must keep in mind the importance of the differential diagnosis with rheumatoid arthritis; a biopsy of the involved tissue may be needed. Careful evaluation for the presence of primary plasma cell dyscrasia and systemic organ involvement must also be carried out.

B. **Hemodialysis-related amyloidosis.** The second form of amyloid deposition associated with significant articular involvement is the deposition of β_2-microglobulin in patients with chronic renal failure undergoing long-term dialysis treatment. Use of the cellulose-based cuprophane dialysis membrane appears to be associated with a higher incidence of amyloidosis; the incidence is lower in patients undergoing peritoneal dialysis. Rarely does β_2-microglobulin amyloidosis develop in patients with renal failure before they begin dialysis.

1. **Clinical picture and diagnosis.** β_2-Microglobulin amyloidosis involves the musculoskeletal system, with infiltration of the carpal ligaments, formation of bone cysts (frequently in apposition to the joints), scapulohumeral periarthritis, stiff and painful fingers, and destructive cervical spondyloarthropathy with cyst formation and occasional odontoid fracture. Cervical disease usually takes the form of vertebral end plate erosion without osteophyte formation. Rapid joint destruction then usually follows. Median nerve compression is very common with its attendant carpal tunnel syndrome.

   Ultrasonography of the wrist is useful to identify the characteristic thickening of the carpal ligaments. Sonograms of the shoulder can help to distinguish amyloidosis from other forms of shoulder disease.

   Radiographs will often show subchondral radiolucent bone cysts consisting of amyloid deposits and erosion. Systemic deposits are rare, and specimens obtained by abdominal fat pad aspiration (the simplest screening test) are usually negative for amyloid deposits. In patients with chronic renal failure, other conditions, such as secondary hyperparathyroidism, aluminum overload, and apatite crystal deposition, may occasionally play a contributory role in arthropathy, and such conditions should be identified.

2. **Therapy.** In patients with either the primary or myeloma-associated form of the disorder, amyloidosis is treated directly, the goal being to reduce the number of cells producing the amyloid precursor, with a resultant reduction in the protein product and fibril formation.

   In hemodialysis-associated amyloidosis, renal transplantation can halt the disease progression but will not relieve the symptoms caused by already existing lesions. Pain cannot be relieved with surgery, but functional improvement may be obtained in joints that are accessible by arthroscopy. Proper monitoring of both the dialysis procedure and the patient's phosphate-calcium metabolism can help decrease the risk for destructive arthropathy.

II. **Arthropathy in hemochromatosis.** Hemochromatosis is one of the most common genetic disorders characterized by excessive body stores of iron and by the deposition of hemosiderin, both of which can cause tissue damage and organ dysfunction. Approximately one in every 250–300 persons is homozygous for this mutation. Idiopathic hemochromatosis is an autosomal recessive disorder associated with two-point mutations on the HFE gene located on the short arm of chromosome 6. It rarely appears before the age of 40 unless there is a family history, and men are affected 10 times more frequently than women, who are protected by physiologic blood losses.

Increased intestinal iron absorption and visceral deposition can lead to the classic features of hepatic cirrhosis, cardiomyopathy, diabetes mellitus ("bronze" diabetes), pituitary dysfunction, sicca syndrome, and skin pigmentation. Liver abnormalities are probably the most constant manifestation. However, hemochromatosis is usually symptomless and is often detected only accidentally.

Other presenting manifestations include constitutional symptoms such as weakness, lethargy, and increased sleep requirements.

Arthropathy is present in 40% to 60% of patients. It sometimes constitutes the first manifestation but more often occurs later, even following treatment. The expression of hemochromatosis with arthritis is most common in homozygotes, although the pathogenesis of the arthritis is unknown. Prolonged excessive iron ingestion, as practiced by the South African Bantu tribesmen or as the result of repeated blood transfusions for chronic hypoproliferative anemia and thalassemia, may also result in iron deposition. When not associated with tissue damage, this disorder is known as hemosiderosis; when organ damage is present, it is called secondary hemochromatosis.

A. Clinical picture. Chronic progressive arthritis, predominantly affecting the second and third metacarpophalangeal and proximal interphalangeal joints and resembling rheumatoid arthritis, is the presenting feature in about one-half of all cases. Hemochromatosis can also affect the larger joints, such as the shoulders, hips, knees, and ankles. A progressive destructive osteoarthritis may be seen. The arthropathy causes stiffness and pain in the hands, often after excessive use, and symmetric, mildly tender joint enlargement without erythema or increased warmth. Sometimes, acute episodes of inflammatory arthritis may occur secondary to calcium pyrophosphate deposition. This form of chondrocalcinosis occurs in 15% to 30% of patients and involves the cartilage of the knees, wrists, intervertebral disks, and symphysis pubis.

Yersinia septic arthritis is an unusual complication that may arise because of the predilection of this microbe for an iron-rich environment.

B. Diagnosis. The erythrocyte sedimentation rate is normal and rheumatoid factor is absent. The synovial fluid shows good viscosity, with leukocyte counts below 1,000/mm^3. During acute episodes of pseudogout, synovial fluid leukocytosis and calcium pyrophosphate crystals may be found. Radiographs show cystic lesions with sclerotic walls, joint space narrowing, sclerosis, osteophytes, and osteoporosis. These radiologic changes may mimic those of osteoarthritis. Hemochromatosis should be suspected in the presence of raised serum iron and ferritin concentrations and increased saturation of transferrin, a plasma iron-binding protein. An effective screening algorithm includes a fasting morning transferrin saturation. If the percentage is > 50% and a serum ferritin is high, HFE testing is appropriate. Needle biopsy of the liver will confirm the diagnosis. Synovial biopsy in hemochromatosis will show iron deposition in the type B cell linings of the synovium.

C. Therapy. The arthritic symptoms may be brought under control by nonsteroidal antiinflammatory drugs (NSAIDs), although sometimes arthroplasty is required. Excess iron can be removed from the body by weekly phlebotomy. Phlebotomy usually does not relieve the arthropathy, however, and the damage to the synovial membrane and cartilage seems to be irreversible.

III. Rheumatic manifestations of hematologic disorders

A. Hemophilic arthropathy. Hemophilia is an inherited, X-linked recessive disorder of blood coagulation found almost exclusively in males. Female heterozygotes are asymptomatic carriers of the disease. Hemophilia A is caused by a factor VIII deficiency and hemophilia B (Christmas disease) is caused by a factor IX deficiency. Recurrent joint hemorrhages resulting in a synovial proliferative response and chronic inflammation are responsible for the arthropathy associated with hemophilia.

Hemarthrosis, the most common bleeding manifestation, occurs in up to two-thirds of all patients affected by hemophilia. It may occur spontaneously or as the result of minor trauma, and the onset includes stiffness, pain, warmth, and swelling. The joints usually affected are the knees, elbows, and ankles.

The pathogenesis of hemophilic arthropathy is not yet completely understood, but it may result from excessive iron deposition in the synovial tissue and articular cartilage. Because prothrombin and fibrinogen are absent, the blood in the joint remains liquid. The plasma is gradually resorbed and the remaining red cells undergo phagocytosis by the synovial lining cells and macrophages. Hemosiderin is found in synovial lining cells, where it may be toxic, causing chronic inflammation with proliferation of the synovium and pannus formation.

1. **Clinical features.** Three stages of hemophilic arthropathy can be distinguished:
   a. Stage 1. **Acute hemarthrosis** is often the initiating event in hemophilic arthropathy, occurring when a child begins to walk. It is manifested by pain, warmth, swelling, and limitation of motion. The episodes can vary in severity from mild subsynovial hemorrhage to tense hemarthrosis. The age at onset and the frequency of these acute episodes depend on the severity of the factor deficiency.
   b. Stage 2. **Subacute hemophilic arthropathy** often follows repeated episodes of intraarticular hemorrhage. It manifests in the form of persistent synovitis with synovial thickening, chronic joint effusion, and varying degrees of pain. Polyarticular involvement is rare. Muscle weakness and joint laxity contribute to bleeding from the friable synovium, which causes chronic damage.
   c. Stage 3. **Chronic hemophilic arthropathy** is characterized by joint deformity, fibrous ankylosis, and osteophytic overgrowth. Soft-tissue swelling and joint effusion are less common in this stage, and the pain is fluctuating and variable. Late manifestations include muscle hemorrhage, muscle cysts, and osseous pseudotumors.
2. **Diagnosis.** Hemophilia can be detected on the basis of laboratory tests measuring factor VIII and factor IX levels, which are directly correlated with the severity of the hemophilia and the ensuing hemarthrosis. The complete absence of either factor is associated with spontaneous bleeding in the muscles and joints; a level of 1% to 5% is associated with either spontaneous bleeding or bleeding after minor trauma; a level of 5% to 25% may be associated with excessive bleeding after minor surgery; and a level of 25% to 50% can result in excessive bleeding after major surgery or injuries. In patients with acute hemarthrosis, other diagnoses that must be considered include pigmented villonodular synovitis, the use of anticoagulant drugs, and joint trauma.

   Conventional radiology shows the typical findings of degenerative arthritis: joint space narrowing, subchondral sclerosis, and subchondral cysts. In children, radiographic findings include epiphyseal irregularities, squaring of the inferior patella, and enlargement of the proximal radius in the elbow. Ultrasound examination and magnetic resonance imaging (MRI) can provide detailed information regarding the degree and rate of progression of the articular disease.
3. **Treatment.** Replacement therapy is essential to improve the longevity and prognosis of hemophiliac patients. Prompt, appropriate treatment for the hemarthrosis is vital and may include cold applications, analgesics, and joint immobilization followed by a carefully designed physiotherapy program. Aspiration (after factor replacement) is less commonly performed unless the joint is very tense or sepsis is suspected. Corticosteroids, whether oral or intraarticular, do not seem to be effective. Chronic arthropathy may be treated with NSAIDs. Joint replacement arthroplasty can be performed in those patients with advanced joint destruction. It demands a team approach with optimal factor replacement.

B. Sickle cell disease and β-thalassemia. In the hemoglobinopathies, osteoarticular symptoms may arise as a result of bone and joint involvement secondary to juxtaarticular-periarticular bone infarcts or synovial ischemia and infarction. Sickle cell crises can produce a painful arthritis of the large joints with effusion; the synovial fluid is typically noninflammatory. Local bone ischemia resulting from *venous* occlusion by sickle cells may cause osteonecrosis of the femoral head in up to one-third of patients; this osteonecrosis, when advanced, can be successfully treated with total arthroplasty. In about one-third of infants with sickle cell disease, dactylitis secondary to vascular occlusion in the bones of the hands and feet may represent the first manifestation of the disease. Children with sickle cell disease are prone to infection, and *Salmonella* osteomyelitis is seen with increased frequency in all stages of the disease.

Thalassemia is associated with musculoskeletal complications. In β-thalassemia minor, recurrent asymmetric arthritis may be seen, whereas in β-thalassemia major, manifestations may include osteoporosis, pathologic fractures, and epiphyseal deformities. **Treatment of the arthritis associated with sickle cell disease** consists of supportive therapy, intravenous hydration, oxygen, folate supplementation, and analgesics.

C. **Arthritis and monoclonal gammopathies.** An association of the paraproteinemias and arthritis has been widely reported in the literature, in particular during the course of myeloma, Waldenström's macroglobulinemia, and primary amyloidosis. The presence of an erosive arthritis has also been described in patients affected by monoclonal gammopathies of uncertain significance. In these cases, arthritis may occur either as a rheumatoid-like symmetric polyarthritis or as an atypical oligoarthritis. The course is generally slow but progressive. The pathologic mechanism potentially responsible for the arthritic process is the deposition of paraprotein-derived material in the synovium with consequent activation of the inflammatory response. (See section **I.** above.)

D. **Cryoglobulinemia.** The cryoglobulins are immunoglobulins that reversibly precipitate at low temperatures. They are present in a variety of autoimmune, neoplastic, and infectious disorders and may be divided into two categories. The type 1 cryoglobulins are single monoclonal proteins, usually immunoglobulin G (IgG), sometimes IgM, and rarely IgA, that are generally associated with myeloma and macroglobulinemia.

The type 2 cryoglobulins consist of a macromolecular complex of more than one class of immunoglobulin; hence, they are termed mixed cryoglobulins. One component of the mixed cryoglobulins is usually an IgM rheumatoid factor, which is responsible for the formation of the complex and for its precipitation properties. The mixed cryoglobulins have been further subdivided into those in which one component is monoclonal and those in which all the components are polyclonal.

Mixed cryoglobulinemia is a systemic vasculitis characterized by the presence of cryoglobulins with rheumatoid factor activity. Although mixed cryoglobulinemia is a disease of multifactorial origin, the hepatitis C virus has been shown to play a central role in its pathogenesis. The disease is an immune complex-mediated disorder with a number of immunologic phenomena that are often triggered by hepatitis C.

1. **Clinical picture.** The most common clinical manifestations of mixed cryoglobulinemia are arthralgias and purpura. Arthralgias are present in the majority of cases, usually recurring intermittently during the course of the disease. They most frequently involve the small and medium-sized joints such as the hands, knees, ankles, and elbows. Mild, transient, nonerosive arthritis is far less common. Other organs that may be involved in mixed cryoglobulinemia are the liver and kidneys.

   Liver involvement is present in more than two-thirds of patients with mixed cryoglobulinemia but is generally asymptomatic. It may precede the onset of mixed cryoglobulinemia and can evolve—more or less insidiously—into liver cirrhosis. Renal involvement affects about one-third of patients with mixed cryoglobulinemia. It takes the form of a membranoproliferative glomerulonephritis characterized clinically by proteinuria, which may evolve to an overt nephritis syndrome and, if not appropriately treated, end in renal failure.

   Other manifestation of mixed cryoglobulinemia are sensorimotor peripheral neuropathy, Raynaud's phenomenon, sicca syndrome, hyperviscosity syndrome, and lung involvement.

2. **Diagnosis.** The diagnosis of cryoglobulinemia is based on the typical triad of symptoms: purpura, arthralgias, and weakness, and on the presence of type 2 cryoglobulins. Complement levels (C1, C2, C4) are low. Rheumatoid

factor is present. Hepatitis B and C viruses frequently have been associated with mixed cryoglobulinemia.

3. **Treatment.** Mixed cryoglobulinemia is characterized by a broad spectrum of clinical manifestations ranging from mild (arthralgia and weakness) to severe (renal involvement), and the course of disease is characterized by spontaneous remissions and exacerbations. As a consequence, no single treatment protocol can be established.

For the minor clinical manifestations (arthralgias, purpura, arthritis), therapies aimed at treating the symptoms are sufficient: NSAIDs and low-dose corticosteroids (<10 mg of methylprednisolone daily). The major manifestations of mixed cryoglobulinemia (central nervous system involvement, kidney involvement, hyperviscosity syndrome) require more aggressive treatment, such as high-dose corticosteroids (1 mg/kg or pulse therapy), cytotoxic drugs (2 to 3 mg of cyclophosphamide per kilogram pulse therapy), or plasma exchange with or without immunosuppressive drugs. The aggressive use of cytotoxic agents is no longer recommended in view of their immunomodulatory properties and the potential to promote viral replication. Interferons have been used in the management of mixed cryoglobulinemia; in our experience interferon-β can have a positive effect. Controlled short-term trials have clearly shown that the interferons can reduce many of the signs (hepatitis C virus and cryoglobulin levels) and symptoms (purpura, abnormal liver enzymes), but its long-term effect on the natural history of the disease has not yet been established.

E. **Leukemias.** Rheumatic manifestations occur in a small percentage of adults with either acute or chronic leukemia, but they are common in children with acute lymphoblastic leukemias. In some cases, bone pain, arthralgias, and periarthritis are caused by leukemic infiltration of the periosteum, synovium, or periarticular bone and may predate the diagnosis of leukemia. The arthritis is asymmetric, additive, and polyarticular and the joint pain can be prominent at night. The knees, ankles, and shoulders are most commonly affected. In children, the association of arthritis and fever can mimic Still's disease. In hairy-cell leukemia, both polyarthritis and polyarteritis nodosa have been described. Symptomatic skeletal involvement is uncommon in the lymphomas, although bone lesions may be found at autopsy.

IV. **Multicentric reticulohistiocytosis.** Multicentric reticulohistiocytosis is a systemic disorder of unknown etiology characterized by the infiltration of tissues by histiocytes and multinucleated cells. It primarily affects the skin, mucous membranes, and joints. The disease has a worldwide distribution with a female predominance. It usually begins during the fourth decade of life with polyarthritis, cutaneous lesions, or concurrent arthritis and skin manifestations. Up to 25% of cases have been associated with malignancies, but the condition is not considered to be paraneoplastic.

A. **Clinical picture.** The polyarthritis is symmetric, progressive, and destructive, attacking the small and large peripheral joints. The joints most frequently affected are the interphalangeal joints of the hands including the DIP joints, shoulder, knee, wrist, hip, elbow, and spine. The clinical picture can mimic that of rheumatoid arthritis. In one-half of all patients, severely deforming arthritis mutilans may develop.

The skin lesions are usually asymptomatic, discrete, firm, pinkish brown or purple, hemispheric, nonpruritic papulonodules that occasionally coalesce. They are most numerous over the dorsum of the hands, on the face, and behind the ears. Lesions of the buccal mucosa, nasal septum, or lips occur in about half of the patients with skin nodules. Involvement of bone, tendon sheath, muscle, liver, lung, and other organs has been reported but is not common.

The course of disease is not well defined; it may be either mild and slow in progression or aggressive, and spontaneous remissions may be seen.

B. **Diagnosis.** The diagnosis is based on histology of the cutaneous nodules; characteristic findings are infiltration by histiocytes and large, multinucleated giants cells with a ground-glass appearance, which stain positively for lipids and glycoproteins (periodic acid–Schiff).

The diagnosis of joint disease is usually indicated by radiographs showing extensive bone destruction rather than articular cartilage loss, and very mild osteopenia around the affected joints. The findings on joint fluid analysis may be quite variable; most often, the effusions are inflammatory. The erythrocyte sedimentation rate is normal or slightly raised, and rheumatoid factor is absent.

C. **Treatment.** Because of the flares and spontaneous remissions that characterize this disorder, the efficacy of different drug therapies is difficult to assess. Immunosuppressive drugs such as corticosteroids and cyclophosphamide have been claimed to be effective. Low-dose pulse methotrexate has also been shown to be useful as a maintenance therapy.

V. **Pigmented villonodular synovitis (PVNS)** is a rare disorder of unknown etiology characterized by a slowly progressive, yet potentially invasive, benign proliferation of the synovial tissue. It is more common in females than in males. The salient histologic features are the deposition of hemosiderin and the infiltration of histiocytes and giant cells in a fibrous stroma within the synovium of the tendon sheaths and large joints.

A. **Clinical features.** PVNS may present in three different clinical forms:

1. **Pigmented villonodular tenosynovitis** (also referred to as giant cell tumor of the tendon sheath), the most common expression of PVNS, typically presents in adults and is more prevalent in women. The lesion is isolated, discrete, and usually painless but is slowly progressive and may cause erosion of the adjacent bone. The hand, especially the fingers, is the most common site of involvement.
2. **Diffuse intraarticular pigmented villonodular synovitis** primarily affects young adults. It takes the form of a chronic monarticular arthropathy, with the knee being the most commonly involved joint, followed by the hip and ankle. Less frequently, the hand, shoulder, wrist, or vertebrae may be affected. Progression is slow, with initially intermittent and later persistent joint swelling and pain. Joint effusion is usually present. Histologically, the lesion resembles that of pigmented villonodular tenosynovitis. This form can mimic the chronic synovitis of rheumatoid arthritis.
3. **Localized pedunculated villonodular synovitis** is the least common presentation of PVNS. The knee is the most frequently involved joint, the lesion being localized in the medial or lateral compartment. The patient presents with mechanical symptoms of locking and clicking. Synovial effusions may be slightly bloody.

B. **Diagnosis.** In both diffuse and localized joint synovitis, radiographs may show soft-tissue swelling without calcifications, a useful clue for the differential diagnosis from synovial osteochondromatosis. Osteophytes and juxtaarticular osteoporosis, typical of degenerative joint disease and rheumatoid arthritis, respectively, are absent. Sonography and MRI may show synovial proliferation. The diagnosis can be confirmed by arthroscopy and synovial biopsy, which show fibroblasts, giant cells, hemosiderin deposits, and areas of hemorrhaging with a mild inflammatory component.

C. **Treatment.** PVNS may be treated surgically, but recurrences are frequent. Radiotherapy, alone or in association with synovectomy, can reduce the risk for recurrence. Surgical excision in cases of the localized form involving the knee is usually more successful. Total arthroplasty is required when extensive joint destruction is present.

VI. **Sarcoidosis.** Sarcoidosis is a systemic disease of unknown etiology characterized by the presence of noncaseating granulomas of the involved tissue. The disease is most common in subjects 20 to 40 years of age and generally involves the lung, although any organ may be affected and the condition can mimic rheumatic disease. The sarcoid granuloma may arise in the lung (86% of patients); lymph nodes (86%); liver (86%); spleen (63%); heart, kidney, or bone marrow (17% to 20%); or pancreas (6%). The etiopathogenesis is unknown, but it appears that the cellular immune response plays a central role.

A. **Clinical picture.** The most frequent clinical manifestations of sarcoidosis are pulmonary symptoms, asymptomatic hilar adenopathy, constitutional symptoms, and extrathoracic manifestations, which may include rheumatologic manifestations.

1. **Pulmonary involvement.** Pulmonary symptoms include dry cough, dyspnea, and chest pain; pleural effusions are rare. Four types of findings may be revealed on chest radiography: type 0, no abnormalities; type 1, enlargement of the hilar and mediastinal lymph nodes; type 2, adenopathy and pulmonary infiltrates; and type 3, infiltrates without adenopathy.
2. **Rheumatologic manifestations.** Acute polyarthritis is the most common and is often the first manifestation of the disease. Erythema nodosum is strikingly associated with early arthritis.

   The association of acute arthritis, erythema nodosum, and bilateral hilar adenopathy is called Lofgren's syndrome; it has an excellent prognosis with a 90% remission rate. The acute arthritis is usually symmetric and generally involves the larger joints, especially the ankles and knees, although the small joints of the hands and feet and the shoulders, hips, wrist, and elbow can also be affected. Periarticular swelling is more common than joint effusions. When effusions occur, the synovial fluid is not inflammatory. The symptoms of arthritis may resolve in a few weeks or may persist for several months. Few patients suffer more than one isolated attack, however.

   The second form of arthritis that may occur in sarcoidosis appears 6 months or more after the onset of disease; the knee is the most frequently involved joint, followed by the ankles and proximal interphalangeal joints. Monarthritis can also occur. The arthritis may be transient or chronic and is not associated with erythema nodosum. The synovial fluid shows little or no signs of inflammation; synovial biopsy occasionally reveals granulomas. The chronic form often manifests as dactylitis. The symptoms of sarcoid dactylitis are swelling of the soft tissue over the affected digits, tenderness, and painful stiffness: the overlying skin may be erythematous. Radiographic changes are uncommon but destructive, and bone cystic changes can occur.

   Myopathy in sarcoidosis is rare; the affected patient may have a chronic, progressive muscle disease that resembles polymyositis or muscular dystrophy. Acute myositis and palpable nodules can occur. Muscle biopsy may reveal a sarcoid granuloma, even in the presence of asymptomatic muscle involvement. Other rheumatologic manifestations that may be associated with sarcoidosis include parotid gland enlargement and keratoconjunctivitis, similar to Sjögren's syndrome, or upper airway disease (sinusitis, laryngeal inflammation, saddle nose deformity), similar to Wegener's granulomatosis. Eye involvement is seen in about 22% of patients, anterior uveitis being more common than posterior uveitis.

   Other extrathoracic manifestations include peripheral lymphadenopathy, skin involvement (erythema nodosum, papules, nodules, plaques, lupus pernio), and renal and central nervous system involvement. Most patients have hepatic granulomas, but only 20% show hepatomegaly or elevated liver enzymes. Constitutional symptoms such as malaise, fever, and fatigue are often present.

B. Diagnosis. The diagnosis of sarcoidosis is made on the basis of the clinical findings, histologic evidence of noncaseating granulomas, and the exclusion of other diseases. Biopsy of lesions, scalene muscles, or mediastinal lymph nodes is necessary to confirm the diagnosis. Liver biopsy may also be helpful. Skin anergy is typical but not diagnostic. Bronchoalveolar lavage is another useful indicator, with specimens showing an increased number of T lymphocytes during active disease.

Levels of ACE (angiotensin-converting enzyme) inhibitor, produced by the cells of sarcoid granulomas, are elevated in two-thirds of all patients.

A gallium citrate scan may show increased uptake in the pulmonary parenchyma; this is not specific for sarcoidosis but is helpful in following the disease activity and course, as well as the effects of therapy.

C. Treatment. The treatment may consist of short courses of corticosteroids at moderate doses (20 to 40 mg of methylprednisolone). Methotrexate and hydroxychloroquine can be used as a corticosteroid-sparing agent in patients with chronic disease. NSAIDs may be useful to treat acute episodes of arthritis.

The disease course is generally mild, and treatment usually results in long-term remission. Chronic or aggressive disease develops in only a small number of patients and may demand equally aggressive immunosuppressive therapy.

VII. Storage diseases

A. Gaucher's disease. Gaucher's disease is an autosomal recessive disease resulting from the accumulation of glucocerebroside in organs and tissues, mainly throughout the reticuloendothelial system in characteristic storage cells (Gaucher's cells). The condition is caused by a deficiency of the lysosomal enzyme glucocerebrosidase.

Clinically, patients with the disease may be divided into three subgroups. Rheumatologic manifestations may constitute the first symptoms in the neuropathic adult form (type 1) and in the juvenile form (type 3). Acute severe pain (bone crisis) may be accompanied by tenderness, swelling, erythema, and fever, thus resembling osteomyelitis (pseudo-osteomyelitis). Osteonecrosis of the hip and talus have been described. Pathologic fractures of the long bones and low back pain can also occur.

1. **Diagnosis.** The diagnosis is established by bone marrow biopsy and analysis of the peripheral blood leukocytes for residual β-glucocerebrosidase and β-glucosidase activity.
2. **Treatment.** The principal treatment is enzyme replacement therapy with macrophage-targeted glucocerebrosidase purified from human placental tissue. Other options include splenectomy for thrombocytopenia and total hip arthroplasty for osteonecrosis. The possible efficacy of bone marrow transplantation and organ transplantation for end-stage disease involving the failure of a single organ is presently being explored.

B. Fabry's disease. Fabry's disease is a lysosomal lipid storage disease in which glycosphingolipids accumulate in nerve cells, organs, skin, and osteoarticular tissue. It is a sex-linked disease caused by deficiency of the enzyme α-galactosidase. Rheumatologic features include painful crises of burning paresthesias of the extremities, and degenerative changes and flexion contractures of the distal interphalangeal joints of the fingers. Systemic features include renal disease with progressive renal failure and cardiovascular, cerebrovascular, and ocular disease.

C. Farber disease. Farber disease is a rare sphingolipidosis of early childhood caused by the accumulation of ceramide. The initial manifestations may include hoarseness of the voice secondary to thickened vocal cords and various rheumatologic manifestations (pain and swelling of the joints of the fingers, wrists, elbows, ankles, and knees; joint contractures; and nodular masses or tendon sheaths in the periarticular tissues). Death often occurs before the age of 2, usually from respiratory disease.

Bibliography

Buxbaum J. The amyloidoses. In: Klippel J, Dieppe PA, eds. *Rheumatology,* 2nd ed. St. Louis: Mosby–Year Book, 1998:1–10.

Della Rossa A, Trevisani G, Bombardieri S. Cryoglobulins and cryoglobulinemia. Diagnostic and therapeutic considerations. *Clin Rev Allergy Immunol* 1998;16(3):249.

Husby G. Amyloidosis and rheumatoid arthritis. *Clin Exp Rheumatol* 1985;3:173.

Liang G, Granston A. Complete remission of multicentric reticulohistiocytosis with combination therapy of steroid, cyclophosphamide and low dose pulse methotrexate. *Arthritis Rheum* 1996;39:171.

Olsson KS. Hemochromatosis. In: Klippel J, Dieppe PA, eds. *Rheumatology,* 2nd ed. St. Louis: Mosby–Year Book, 1998:1–4.

Steven MM, et al. Hemophilic arthritis. *J Med* 1986;58:181.

Vitali C, et al. Erosive arthritis in monoclonal gammopathy of uncertain significance: report of four cases. *Arthritis Rheum* 1991;34:1600.

Zuber M, et al. Ulnar deviation is not always rheumatoid. *Ann Rheum Dis* 1996; 55:786.

52. PSYCHOSOCIAL ASPECTS OF THE RHEUMATIC DISEASES

Tracey A. Revenson

I. Overview

This chapter addresses psychological and social issues that many patients face in the course of living with rheumatic diseases. Most patients are mentally healthy at the time their illness is diagnosed, but they may show signs of being under great psychological stress throughout the course of their illness.

Living with rheumatic disease involves facing a number of psychosocial stresses and challenges. In addition to coming to terms with the meaning of the illness for one's life and the more existential issues of disease progression and deformity, persons with rheumatic disease must cope with pain, stiffness, fatigue, and physical activity restrictions on a daily basis. Many of these adaptive challenges require help from others. Thus, patients with rheumatic disease need an available and satisfying network of interpersonal relations on which they can count for both emotional sustenance and more practical help during periods of pain and disability.

Although, from a medical point of view, the rheumatic diseases may differ in regard to presentation and treatment, they are all associated with several psychosocial coping tasks. These include (a) pain, (b) disability and loss of role functioning (real and anxiety over anticipated losses), (c) increased risk for depression, (d) ongoing and often frustrating interactions with the health care system, (e) the need to adhere to a prescribed and often changing treatment regimen, (f) changes in life-style and appearance, (g) changes in interpersonal relationships, (h) the need to tolerate uncertainty, and (i) in some, the possibility of death. Patients also must work to maintain their self-esteem, mastery, and interpersonal relationships. As symptoms, disease course, and prognosis are unpredictable and may change over time, the salience of these coping tasks changes as well. However, the need to tolerate uncertainty is an ever-present issue and one that can be both frustrating and frightening.

II. Psychosocial effects of rheumatic disease

A. Depression

1. Background. Most persons with arthritis do not experience clinical depression, although a significant minority of them do. People with arthritis are more likely to experience depression than people without any serious chronic illness. If depression does occur, it can augment the pain and disability associated with arthritis. Depressed patients may feel unsupported by others; this may reflect reality, as it is difficult to be with depressed people.

Although depression is often linked to pain, it is the loss of the ability to perform valued roles and activities (as a result of that pain, inflammation, and subsequent disability) that is a risk factor for the development of depressive symptoms. Patients' psychological interpretations of the *meaning of their limitations* and role changes may be more significant than their actual disease status.

Depression by itself can be a devastating condition. People with symptoms of depression, in the absence any other health problems, function at a lower level physically and emotionally than do people with any one of a number of diseases. When depressive symptoms occur in combination with or as a result of illness, declines in functioning can be exaggerated.

In addition to being at greater risk than men for some of the more common and serious rheumatic diseases, women also are at greater risk for depression. Within the U.S. population, depression is about twice as prevalent among women than among men. Health practitioners need to be especially alert for depression in women so that both the depression and the rheumatic disease are treated. If depression in women with rheumatic diseases is overlooked, declines in functioning caused by depression can be attributed mistakenly to the rheumatic disease and result in overtreatment or unwarranted changes in therapy. Alternatively, if symptoms of depression are perceived as symptoms of arthritis, female patients may suffer needlessly, given the availability of effective treatments for depression. It is important that health care professionals monitor their patients for depressive symptoms and treat them appropriately, rather than assume that depression is a "normal" and anticipated part of rheumatic disease. Also, the physician should be aware of the fact that steroids may both trigger or worsen depression.

2. **Definition.** A **major depressive episode** involves at least 2 weeks of depressed mood or loss of interest or pleasure in nearly all activities, accompanied by at least four of the following symptoms: (a) feelings of worthlessness; (b) excessive or inappropriate feelings of guilt; (c) fatigue or loss of energy; (d) difficulty thinking, concentrating, or making decisions; (e) recurrent thoughts of death or suicide; (f) changes in appetite or weight (not caused by dieting); (g) changes in patterns of sleep or fatigue; (h) decrease or increase in psychomotor activity (e.g., agitation). In addition, the following criteria must be met: the symptoms must appear to cause clinically significant distress or impairment in social, occupational, or other important areas of functioning; are not a consequence of direct physiological effects of medication or a general medical condition; and are not better accounted for by bereavement.
3. **Dysthymic disorder** involves at least 2 years of a depressed mood that occurs for most of the day on more days than not. At least two of the following symptoms must be present: poor appetite or overeating; insomnia or hypersomnia; low energy or fatigue; low self-esteem; poor concentration or difficulty making decisions; feelings of hopelessness. Additional criteria to be met: The person has never been without the symptoms for more than 2 months at a time, and the mood disturbance is not easily distinguished from the person's "usual" functioning. (In contrast, a major depressive episode represents a change from the person's previous functioning.)

B. **Life-style changes.** Living with a rheumatic disease not only magnifies the stresses of everyday life but also creates additional ones. Most life-style changes are a direct or indirect result of frequent episodes of pain and increasing physical disability. The majority of patients report decreases in social, recreational, and leisure activities at one time or another. Some of these changes may seem trivial to the health care provider but may have great psychological significance for the patient. These include problems with activities that previously might have been taken for granted, such as performing household chores or getting around one's community easily. These "smaller" problems should not be dismissed offhand, as they accumulate over time and may lead to maladjustment.

1. **Changes in paid and unpaid work.** Rheumatoid arthritis (RA) has a profound effect on employment status, with many people unable to maintain their jobs as the disability worsens. This may exacerbate financial concerns. "Forced" retirement, medical leave, or the need to change careers in mid-life because of physical limitations can increase psychological distress.

   Rheumatic disease affects the ability to perform regular activities of daily life, such as child care, cleaning, personal hygiene, and sports. For many women, loss of the valued roles of care giver and nurturer leads to a decline in self-worth. Patients should be reassured that decreases in activity levels are normal, as is feeling frustrated with one's level of ability. Patients must be encouraged to find new ways to perform tasks, to find new leisure activities, or to redefine roles at home and work.
2. **Changes in marital and intimate relationships.** The evidence is mixed on whether divorce is more prevalent among persons with rheumatic disease than in the general population. Patients with RA are no more likely to be divorced when compared with patients having other inflammatory rheumatic disorders, but they are more likely to be divorced than are patients with *noninflammatory* disorders, particularly osteoarthritis of the hip or

knee. There is little evidence to suggest that RA precipitates divorce, or that the lower rate of remarriage among patients with RA is associated with disease severity.

Communication, everyday life, and sexual satisfaction seem to be the areas of marriage that are disrupted most. The degree of disability is a major determinant of the extent to which the marital relationship is affected. Spouses may feel frustrated about a reduction in shared pleasurable activities, helpless in response to seeing their wife or husband in pain, and fearful regarding their future.

Positive effects on the marriage are as likely to be experienced as negative ones, although they are seldom reported to physicians. People with RA rate their close relationships (primarily family) at least as favorably as do people in comparison groups. When the onset of the illness is later in life, marital and family relationships may be less vulnerable to disruptions caused by the illness. This may be a result of the long-term nature of these marriages, or because illness onset in late life is a more predictable "on-time" life event, shared by one's peers. For widowed women, however, rheumatic disease may have even greater costs, in terms of reduced sources of support.

3. **Sexuality.** Persons with rheumatic diseases may be vulnerable to sexual problems because of the physical changes caused by the illness and their attendant emotional distress. However, studies comparing rheumatic disease patients with healthy persons in comparison groups have found no differences in sexual satisfaction, although arthritis patients do report declines in sexual satisfaction with time. Sexual dissatisfaction is greater for those with severe joint involvement or greater functional disability. In one study, some spouses reported not having sex for fear they would hurt their partners.

Some studies conclude that male patients are more dissatisfied and experience greater sexual dysfunction than do female patients, but in others, women reported greater sexual dissatisfaction. In a study of female patients with systemic lupus erythematosus, poor sexual adjustment was best predicted by severe disease, older age, poor premorbid sexual relationships, and poor quality of the current relationship.

Many biologic and psychological factors may lead to sexual problems. Insufficient vaginal lubrication may develop secondary to Sjögren's syndrome or menopause; artificial lubrication may help. If pain is interfering with sexual satisfaction, an extra (or earlier) dose of medication (within the hour) may be helpful. Some patients find it helpful to take a warm bath to relax and minimize stiffness. If pain is less at certain times of day, suggest having sex at those times. Some patients report postcoital pain relief, perhaps as a consequence of feeling loved and the release of endorphins.

Depression itself may lead to fatigue, malaise, and decreased libido. Medications, particularly those for depression and hypertension, may adversely affect libido and sexual arousal.

Sexual problems are not uncommon in the general population, although couples with rheumatic disease often blame such problems on their illness. Long-standing sexual dysfunction unrelated to the rheumatologic illness will be uncovered by a careful premorbid sexual history.

Avoidance of sex because of embarrassment about joint deformities or steroid-induced changes in appearance have been overemphasized in the clinical literature. Partners may be less interested in sex because of exhaustion or anger created by role changes or added household demands resulting from the illness. This can be addressed by fostering communication between the partners (see section **VI.A**).

Sexuality is seldom addressed within the context of the medical visit. Men and women may have very different concerns regarding sexuality; concerns may also vary with age and disease severity. Health care providers should be sensitive to patients' questions and concerns regarding sexuality, and not dismiss them or immediately initiate a psychological referral.

Physicians should discuss these issues openly and frequently with both patients and their partners as a routine part of care.

4. **Social life.** Relations with friends are at more risk than those with family. Reduced mobility and increased pain make social relations outside the home more difficult to maintain; more than half of RA patients report that they visit people less often because of their disease. In addition, patients are less satisfied with these relationships when they do continue. In some cases, social isolation may arise because a patient prefers to avoid the stigma and embarrassment associated with the condition.

   Changes in the quantity and quality of close relationships frequently occur. In the years following diagnosis and with initiation of a new treatment, family and friends are quite helpful. With the passage of time, however, friends and family may tire of providing help, and patients may interpret this as withdrawal from them or criticism of their coping strategies. This may occur at a time when patients are becoming less able to care for themselves and actually need more help.

5. **Effect of rheumatic disease on family members.** Spouses or live-in partners play a dual and sometimes conflicting role; they serve as the primary provider of support to the patient, but at the same time, they experience stress because of the illness. Spouses often encounter anxiety, marital communication difficulties, and problems at work, but they do not appear to manifest clinical levels of psychopathology. Spouses report the greatest intrusion of illness in the areas of social and leisure activities, family activities, and sex.

   Frequent episodes of pain, increasing disability, an unpredictable course of illness, and financial pressures brought on by the illness may affect the spouse's ability to be supportive for the long-haul. The societal pressures embodied in marriage vows ("In sickness and in health, 'till death do us part") may create feelings of resentment, anger, and guilt. If the patient is depressed, it is difficult to provide empathy and help, and when one does, the task is unrewarding. With advancing age, many spouses have health limitations themselves, which makes tending to their mates' physical and emotional needs more difficult.

   There is little research on families of children with juvenile rheumatoid arthritis (JRA) or on children of parents with rheumatic disease. Having a child with JRA creates many new stressors and coping tasks, similar to those experienced by adults but handled differently in terms of the child's cognitive abilities and life context (school, team sports, dating). Compliance problems with treatment can create family conflict, and healthy siblings may vie for attention. Many families, however, are pulled closer together in coping with the illness.

   The children of a parent with rheumatic disease do not show a greater level of depression than do the children of healthy parents; however, in adolescence, they may be embarrassed by a parent's illness.

III. Factors promoting psychological adaptation to rheumatic disease

A. Sense of personal control over the illness. The extent to which patients maintain a sense of control over their illness appears to have a significant impact on their adjustment. Perception of personal control over treatment is related to positive mood, and perceived control over pain is related to less daily pain with time. Patients who perceive having little control over their illness *and* who attribute the cause of an arthritis flare to personal rather than external factors are more likely to experience depression.

B. Coping mechanisms. Coping is defined as both cognitive and behavioral efforts to manage specific external and internal demands that are viewed as exceeding a person's psychological, social, and financial resources. Coping is not synonymous with adaptational outcomes. Coping efforts may have good or poor results and should not be judged *a priori* as adaptive or maladaptive.

Coping efforts can be directed toward dealing with the stressful situation itself, managing psychological distress aroused by the situation, or maintaining interpersonal relationships. Most stressful situations evoke all three modes of coping. On learning of their diagnosis, patients may need to minimize the seriousness of their situation or they will be flooded with emotions and not be able to act. Slowly, the patient can acknowledge emotions and deal with the situation in a more adaptive fashion, such as by seeking information to make a treatment decision. Many patients try to "normalize" or pass as healthy, performing activities that are not advisable.

People tend to have fairly stable coping styles. For example, some are optimists and others are pessimists; some perceive a good deal of control over their illness, whereas others believe it is better left to fate; some want to know everything about the illness (monitors), yet others prefer not to know (blunters). However, aspects of a patient's current life and medical situation, such as pain, disease progression, level of disability, any concomitant diseases, financial resources, and availability of social support all influence coping.

Whereas men use more active strategies, women's strategies are more focused on managing their emotions, such as seeking social support. Women tend to have more flexible coping repertoires and thus may be more willing to try new approaches.

C. Effectiveness of coping strategies. Strategies such as actively seeking information about the illness, seeking support from others, and trying to view one's situation in a more positive light have been associated with better psychological functioning. Coping strategies that involve wishful thinking, fantasizing, self-blame, avoidance, and denial are associated with poorer psychological functioning. However, reports of emotion-focused coping strategies such as self-blame may reflect levels of distress rather than actual coping efforts.

The effectiveness of particular ways of coping depends on the degree of personal control the patient has over the situation and whether the patient believes that the coping strategy will be effective. A particular coping strategy might result in good outcomes in some areas and poor outcomes in others. For example, strategies to reduce tension, such as drinking or sleeping, may make patients feel better temporarily but diminish their overall physical health status. Similarly, a coping strategy that has worked in a similar situation in the past (such as a pain flare) may not work the next time that the situation occurs. The effects of a patient's coping efforts may not appear immediately. Daily diary studies indicate that the effects of any particular coping strategy may not appear until one or more days after it is employed.

A person's coping efforts may not be effective if they conflict with the coping styles of family members. For example, expressing anger at a spouse may reduce a patient's tension but increase the spouse's tension, which may in turn lead to reduced support. Patients also may feel depressed if family members criticize their coping efforts. The families of children with JRA that cope in a unified fashion and keep channels of communication open fare better than do families in which the styles of individual members conflict with one another. However, dissimilar coping styles between husbands and wives do not result automatically in adjustment problems, greater psychological distress, or lower levels of marital adjustment.

D. Social support. Social support refers to interpersonal exchanges that provide information, emotional reassurance, material assistance, and a sense of continued self-esteem. The family is an important source of support, but this can also be provided by friends and health professionals.

Social support from friends and family can bolster the coping efforts of patients, particularly those with severe pain and disability. Patients who receive more support from friends and family exhibit greater self-esteem, psychological adjustment, and life satisfaction, cope more effectively, and are less depressed. Social support also has been shown to affect immune functioning. Family support can serve as an adjunct to professional treatment. Support from family members has been shown to enhance the effects of psychological treatment and help patients maintain initial treatment gains. Emotional support is most beneficial during periods of great illness-related stress.

Most simply, social support provides coping assistance. It provides feedback and new information; helps patients come to a better understanding of the problem faced; increases their motivation to take instrumental, problem-focused action; and reduces emotional stress, which may impede more adaptive coping efforts. Support reinforces the performance of positive health behaviors and compliance with treatment recommendations, which leads to greater overall health and control of disease.

Different types of support, from different sources, may be more helpful at various points in the illness. Early in the disease, there is a strong desire for information. As patients begin to adjust to the medical management of their illness, emotional support is most helpful. As the illness progresses and patients often have to cope with increasing physical limitations and changes in prescribed treatment, greater tangible assistance with the chores of everyday living in addition to continued emotional support is most helpful. It is likely to be important throughout the course of the illness because support makes patients feel loved, valued, and part of a family or community.

Requesting social support does have costs as well as benefits. Common types of unhelpful support are minimizing the severity of an illness or the patient's pain; making pessimistic comments about the patient's ability or health status; criticizing the patient's coping efforts; pitying the patient; and offering help when it is not wanted. Even well-intentioned support from close friends and family may backfire if patients do not want the help or comfort that is offered. For example, if a patient is not too disabled, she may resent offers of help because it interferes with her self-image as a healthy person and usurps social roles she values. In these circumstances, the patient may reject the emotional support or tangible help being provided.

For patients to benefit from social support, the type of support offered must fit in with what the patient needs at that time. Unwanted or unhelpful support leads to negative affective states, diminished self-esteem, loss of autonomy, and decreased psychological well-being. New tensions within a relationship may emerge. Patients who receive little positive support at the same time that they receive a lot of unhelpful support from their friends and family are at highest risk for depression. At all periods of an illness, it is important to stress that patients must communicate clearly their feelings and needs for help, and that family and friends must learn to listen and respond to patients' needs, not their own. Patients experiencing a good deal of pain and disability are most affected by others' critical comments. Low levels of spousal support may be an indication of marital discord and deeper psychological problems, which may warrant psychological referral.

Support for family members. Support from naturally occurring social ties enables family members to cope as well. Spouses who receive support outside the marital relationship are able to be more supportive to a sick partner. Outside support may alleviate some of the burden of providing care or provide a safe outlet for expressing negative feelings.

E. Compliance with treatment

1. **Generic issues.** Treatment efficacy depends on patients' carrying out therapeutic recommendations. Treatment often includes behavioral recommendations, such as daily exercise and wearing splints, keeping regularly scheduled appointments for medical checkups, and physical or occupational therapy. Sometimes, treatment involves major life-style changes, such as changing diet or work habits.

   Compliance with the appropriate use of prescribed medication ranges from 30% to 78% for rheumatic disease patients. Rates of noncompliance with exercise regimens are equivalent to or higher than those for oral medication, with values as high as 34% to 62%. Both patients and physicians overestimate compliance, possibly because direct and specific questions regarding compliance are rarely asked during a medical visit.

   Risk factors for noncompliance are numerous, some logged within the person, and others related to the treatment or the patient-physician relationship. Characteristics of the treatment regimen include duration, complexity, number of changes, and extent of somatic and emotional side effects. Patient characteristics include age, social class, beliefs about treatment efficacy, and cultural concepts about disease.

Characteristics derived from the patient's social context include support or criticism from friends and family, and encouragement and interest from persons in the health care setting. Because physicians have more kinds of power than allied health professionals, patients are more likely to listen to them. Patient-physician communication may be the single most important variable affecting compliance and satisfaction with medical care. Patients are not active in seeking information, and physicians are not active in giving it. Poor patient-physician communication is a result of the time constraints of most medical visits, impersonal health care environments, and inequity in power and status residing within the patient-physician encounter. Physicians tend to use medical terms when providing information, and patients are unfamiliar with the medical language. Patients and physicians may not speak the same language or may be of different ethnic backgrounds; in these cases, it is essential to ascertain that the information is being provided clearly and understood. Often, reading materials may be written at a level above the patient's comprehension.

Physicians often underestimate how much information patients want, and patients often fail to inform the physician when they do not understand the information presented. Physicians often do not understand the amount and type of information that patients want, and the methods they prefer for obtaining it.

Perceptions of a physician's caring, warmth, sensitivity, concern, friendliness, interest, and respect also affect adherence to treatment regimens. Satisfaction with care increases when the physician addresses the patient's concerns before the end of the visit. Physicians may not elicit or discuss psychosocial concerns because they believe they are irrelevant, time-consuming, or outside their field of expertise.

2. Increasing compliance

a. **Treatment partnership.** Make patients partners in their treatment. Talk about models of disease progression and treatment goals so that patients can share those goals with you. It is important for patients and physicians to share the same "cognitive models" of the disease and its treatment.

b. **Describe the treatment rationale.** Help the patient understand why treatment is necessary, and what the short- and long-term goals of treatment are (functional improvement, decreased pain, decreased inflammation). The expected time course for improvement should be made explicit.

c. **Set goals.** Set short-term goals that can be accomplished by the next visit.

d. **Explain and clarify.** Present information clearly. It is equally important for patients to feel comfortable asking the physician to clarify anything that they do not understand (see section **E.1**). Dispel any false beliefs about the treatment (e.g., that medication loses its efficacy over time, that medication should be used only when symptoms are present or when pain is unbearable).

e. **Describe possible adverse effects.** It is a good idea to warn patients of any anticipated side effects and provide methods to minimize them. Common perceived side effects include decreased libido, fatigue, and depression.

f. **Simplify treatment regimens** (e.g., by prescribing, if appropriate, daily medication in one dose instead of in multiple administrations, or by recommending exercises that can be fitted into the patient's daily schedule). This is likely to enhance self-efficacy beliefs and treatment adherence.

Identify potential and real difficulties with compliance. Before the end of the visit, make a plan incorporating the patient's input to overcome these difficulties by the next visit.

Provide written treatment information. As physicians' handwriting is often illegible, have handouts prepared in advanced to cover the most common situations. The Arthritis Foundation also can provide materials.

g. **Respect the patient.** Respect a patient's use of holistic remedies if they do not interfere with treatment. They may help and, at a minimum, may increase a patient's sense of well-being.

Never threaten a patient. Threats or warnings, such as "You're killing yourself by not taking your medications," are not effective, particularly when patients are given concrete strategies to change such behavior. Furthermore, threats may jeopardize the patient's satisfaction with medical care and trust in the physician.

h. **Medication reviews.** Patients should be asked periodically to review their medication dosage and schedule with the physician, even in the absence of changes. Such reviews will uncover unintentional noncompliance resulting from simple misunderstanding. This and other behavioral technologies, such as putting tracking caps on pill bottles, may increase compliance by reinforcing its importance. Make clear that the purpose of such monitoring is to help patients with difficulties in adhering to a medication schedule, and not to punish or humiliate them.

Forgetful persons should be taught to leave themselves notes in prominent places or elicit the aid of a family member. There are many new pill containers that separate the administrations by day and time, and programmable watches with beepers have been used successfully as reminders. If manual dexterity is severely limited, be sure that patients obtain medication bottles with easy-open caps.

i. **Family participation.** Having family members remind patients to take medication or do exercises does not work consistently. In some cases, it can be extremely helpful; in others, in creates feelings of social control, which often result in a psychological reaction of doing what one wants in the face of loss of personal freedoms. This often occurs during early adolescence for JRA patients, when parents are transferring responsibility for taking medication or doing exercises to their children.

j. **Appreciate costs.** Be attentive to patient concerns about out-of-pocket expenses. Explain the short- and long-term benefits. Suggest that the patient calculate the cost per day. Prescribe a generic drug, if possible, or contact the patient's managed care organization if necessary. Many pharmaceutical companies have special plans to make drugs available to those patients who need, but cannot afford, a medication. Contact your pharmaceutical representative to find out about such programs.

k. **Fit treatment into the patient's life.** For increasing compliance with exercise regimens, ask the physical therapist if the exercises can be made more congruent with the patient's daily schedule or with other physical activities.

3. **Open up lines of communication.** Aside from the importance of listening carefully to you patient during a visit, some patients also like to communicate with you via fax or e-mail. Employing these technologies can foster a relationship that fits into you and your patient's schedules.

IV. **Gender myths.** Gender differences have been discussed in several places within this chapter. However, we know little about psychological differences between the sexes in terms of their adjustment to rheumatic disease. This is, in part, because most research has studied only patients of one sex—most often women. Thus, it is important to acknowledge areas in which gender differences do not occur and note those for which we have evidence of important gender differences.

A. **Reporting symptoms.** When men and women are compared, women report more symptoms than men do. However, when differences between men and women regarding disease severity (e.g., joint appearance) and sociodemographic characteristics (e.g., age, income) are taken into account, women report fewer symptoms than men. Given comparable severity of disease, women do not exaggerate symptoms and may, in fact, report RA symptoms more conservatively than men.

B. Impact on work. Arthritis may have an even more severe effect on employment for women than for men. The economic impact of women's work disability is probably underestimated because their nurturing, teaching, and housekeeping work in the paid labor market is economically undervalued. Furthermore, the economic value of work that women do at home without pay is undervalued even more. Women with RA who have more significant homemaker responsibilities are less likely to be disabled than women with fewer responsibilities (even after disease severity and functional status are equalized statistically). In fact, having a greater number of homemaker responsibilities may enhance a woman's sense of self-worth and social functioning. An ergonomic prescription is as important as one for medication. The physician should attempt to improve the work environment or recommend work-share programs in order to optimize the patient's ability to maintain their desired position or occupation.

C. Effects of gender on treatment. Some recent research suggests that gender may affect the nature and quality of treatment across a variety of medical conditions. However, there is currently little information on whether specific procedures, drugs, or treatment strategies differ for female and male patients with rheumatic disorders.

Any disparities may result from a number of factors. Physicians may base treatment outcomes on differential expectations of treatment success for men and women or may have stereotyped expectations about male and female patients. For example, female patients with fibromyalgia syndrome are often told at first that their symptoms are imagined or psychological in origin. One study found that women undergo major orthopedic surgery at a more advance stage in their disease, and this gender difference could not be explained by other medical variables, such as disease severity. One explanation is that women wait longer for surgery because of family care-giving demands.

V. Psychological interventions. In addition to biomedical treatment, participation in psychological interventions can contribute to decreases in physical symptoms and improvements in quality of life. A wide variety of psychological and educational interventions for people with rheumatic disease have been developed. The overall aim of these interventions is to minimize the impact of arthritis on patients' physical, psychological, and social functioning. Most psychological interventions are multimodal and usually include one or more of the following components: provision of general information about arthritis, instruction in arthritis self-management and coping skills, sharing of concerns, biofeedback, cognitive-behavioral techniques, relaxation techniques, and hypnosis to aid relaxation. There is little evidence that providing information about arthritis, by itself, has a beneficial effect on therapeutic outcomes.

A. Cognitive-behavioral therapy is a type of psychological intervention in which patients are taught specific skills, including relaxation techniques, goal setting, and activity pacing, and receive training in coping skills to help them control problems such as pain. Cognitive-behavioral therapy can occur within either group or individual settings. Controlled studies of RA patients who participated in cognitive-behavioral therapy interventions have found positive effects at the end of treatment, which sometimes are sustained through subsequent follow-up assessments.

B. The **Arthritis Self-Management Program (ASMP),** offered through local chapters of the Arthritis Foundation, is a structured group intervention led by trained lay persons with arthritis. Reported benefits of the program include increased knowledge, improved self-care behaviors, such as exercise and relaxation, and decreased pain. The ASMP teaches basic arthritis self-management skills, such as the development of individualized exercise regimens and cognitive pain management strategies. Recent revisions of the ASMP emphasize the enhancement of patients' self-efficacy to manage their arthritis.

Mutual help or support group discussions provide avenues for discussing problems and coping solutions. They also reassure members that they are not alone. People who are coping well with their illness may serve as strong role models.

Multimodal treatments have beneficial effects in terms of decreasing disease activity, joint swelling, pain, and impairment, and anxiety. They also have been shown to increase self-efficacy and improve perceptions of pain control. Most of these benefits are short-lived, however, and dissipate in the months following treatment unless follow-up "booster" sessions are provided. Psychological interventions may be most helpful during flares or surgery to replace joints, or when treatment does not seem to be working. Families occasionally participate in multicomponent programs or in the ASMP, and this participation often augments the benefits of individual treatment.

VI. **Practice guidelines.** Guidelines for attending to the psychological well-being of your patients, improving your communication skills, and increasing compliance are presented:

A. **Increasing the psychological well-being of your patients**

1. **Be on the lookout** for symptoms of dysthymia or a major depressive episode, so that professional treatment can be obtained immediately.
2. **Serve as a source of information** concerning mental health problems before patients have to ask for it. Have information available on community resources, psychological counseling within the hospital, and support groups or patient education programs offered through the local chapter of the Arthritis Foundation. Patients may also be directed to websites with current information. This resource sharing is best presented early in the illness. A brief list of resources can be found at the end of this chapter. It may be advantageous to have a printed list to hand to patients.
3. **Offer emotional support.** Physicians can offer emotional support during medical visits with little effort. During medical visits, physicians can ask patients about the stresses in their lives and simply listen. This not only increases patient satisfaction but may provide early clues regarding the onset of depression.

   Help patients to evaluate the meaning of illness in their lives more positively, and not to see only the negative aspects.
4. **Actively involve family members in the patient's care.** On the most basic level, patients with stronger support systems are more compliant with treatment. Involve family members in treatment from the beginning, not merely during a crisis. Family members need to understand the nature and severity of the patient's illness and the details of treatment if they are to be helpful. Informing family members about such simple things as what to expect when flares occur and potential side effects of medication may serve to minimize problems. Encourage family members to join in discussions during medical visits. Encourage family members to reinforce patients' coping efforts and learn to offer help that does not undermine patients' self-esteem.

   Strengthen communication skills among family members. Many of the unintended consequences of helping result from faulty communication or misinterpretation of the patient's need for support. Focus on how the illness affects the marriage or how it affects the family's daily life. Discussions can be started with questions such as, "How do you feel when your daughter provides help to you? Or when she asks what you're thinking?" Or to the husband, "How do you feel when your wife is complaining about her pain?"

   Encourage patients and family members to build support networks outside the family. Stress to patients and family members the importance of having people available to provide emotional support in addition to those living in the household. Suggest that they start with people in existing networks, such as groups involved in neighborhood activities, local churches or synagogues, and the patient's workplace. Encourage families to use joint support groups or telephone help lines. This should begin early in the illness, as social networks must be built up and strengthened in the early stages of the illness so that they are available during crises. This advice may be even more important for men, for whom their spouse is often the primary or sole source of support. Men have fewer close ties and are less likely to seek support from them. Encourage male patients and male spouses to attend support groups and "open up," even though it might be difficult.

It is worthwhile to attend to family members' difficulties in supporting your patient. Only about one-third of patients and partners seek any kind of help from mental health professionals or participate in support groups. Although the practitioner may feel responsible for the patient's physical health, the psychological well-being of family members may directly or indirectly affect the patient's response to treatment.

B. **Improving communication with your patients and their families.** The manner in which physicians inform patients about their illness plays an important role in how they form their beliefs about the implications of their illness, their views of treatment, and their impression of the physician. It has been linked in numerous studies to patients' satisfaction with their physician and treatment, and compliance with prescribed treatment.

1. **Assess the disease knowledge of patients with newly diagnosed arthritis.** Dispel any false beliefs, such as that the patient "brought on" the disease or that their is no treatment for the disease.
2. **Ensure understanding of treatment.** Ensure that the patient understands the basic details of treatment by giving instructions that are explicit, clear, and unambiguous. This may not be as obvious as it sounds, as it has been demonstrated that many patients do not even know the names of their medications.
3. **Optimize communication of information.** Do not give too much or too little information. People can remember only 7 ± 2 bits of information at a time, and this number is probably reduced by the anxiety of being in a physician's office.
4. **Stress basic issues.** Go over basic issues slowly and clearly and provide any information necessary for making decisions about treatments. Do not be evasive, but do not overwhelm the patient with information either.
5. **Avoid jargon.** Work hard not to use medical jargon without defining terms.
6. **Assess feedback.** To see how well you have done, ask patients to paraphrase the instructions that they have been given before the end of the visit.
7. **Repeat and utilize information.** Repeat the most important information again at the close of the visit. Provide a written handout from your office and supplement it with pamphlets from the Arthritis Foundation.
8. **Encourage questions.** Encourage patients to write out questions for you before they arrive for their checkups; that way, they do not have to worry about remembering their concerns.
9. **Consider communicating by electronic mail or fax.** Some physicians have found that communicating with their patients by electronic mail or fax is useful for responding to questions forgotten during the medical visit and providing a sense of "being there" between visits.

C. **Communicating about sex**

1. **Initiate a discussion.** Do not leave it to patients to initiate discussions of sex. Physicians are responsible for broaching the topic in a sensitive manner, and this can be deferred until the patient and physician have developed a relationship.
2. **Be educational.** Start with questions that are relevant to the patient and have the potential to be educational. For a patient with severe hip arthritis, the physician may say, "Many people with hip arthritis find that pain and limitation of motion interfere with their sex life; has this happened to you (and your spouse)?" This can be followed by a more general probe about sexual satisfaction based on the patient's response.
3. **Review medications** with the patient to determine the possibility of eliminating any that potentially may interfere with sexual functioning.
4. **Sexual counseling.** Some physicians may be interested in and feel comfortable providing sexual counseling. Others may wish to refer patients to a marriage or sex therapist. A useful publication is *Living and Loving with Arthritis,* published by the American College of Rheumatology.

D. Increasing satisfaction with care

1. **Optimize the doctor-patient relationship.** Enough cannot be said about the importance of a good doctor-patient relationship. What makes for a good relationship varies from patient to patient. Clearly, empathy, trust, and communication are most important. The effects of friendly versus casual styles of interacting vary according to the gender match of the patient and the physician.
2. **Determine the patient's personality style.** Some patients find it important to be involved in a major way in any decision-making process; others want no part in it. It may take several visits to peg the patient's style. This may vary with age, socioeconomic background, and ethnic group and may change with time.
3. **Minimize waiting, and listen to the patient's responses to questions.** Minimize waiting time for medical visits. Perceived waiting time is inversely correlated with satisfaction and compliance. Some physicians have receptionists call patients several hours in advance if they are running extremely late, offering the opportunity to make a new appointment within the week.

   Always treat a patient as you would wish you and your family to be treated. Apologize for long delays and do not rush the visit to make up time. Both satisfaction with care and compliance increase if patients feel that they have been given adequate time with the physician. "Feel" is a key word. Perceived time spent with the physician frequently does not have to correlate with real time. Asking patients if there are any issues of importance to them that were not covered or whether they have questions yields considerable benefits. Address all the psychosocial concerns a patient voices, even those that may seem to be of little importance.

VII. Resources

A. For the physician

Arthritis Care and Research. This bimonthly, peer-reviewed journal of the Association of Rheumatology Health Professionals presents the best research on nonmedical aspects of arthritis and musculoskeletal disease. It is published by the American College of Rheumatology.

Daltroy LH. Doctor-patient communication in rheumatological disorders. *Baillieres Clin Rheumatol* 1993;7:221.

DeVellis BM, Revenson TA, Blalock SJ. Rheumatic disease and women's health. In: Gallant SJ, Keita GP, Royak-Schaler R, eds. *Health care for women: psychological, social, and behavioral influences.* Washington, DC: American Psychological Association, 1997:333.

Newman S, et al. (1996). *Understanding rheumatoid arthritis.* London: Routledge, 1996.

Newman S, Shipley M, eds. *Psychological aspects of rheumatic disease.* London: Bailliere Tindall, 1993.

B. For the patient

Arthritis Today. This monthly magazine, written for people with arthritis and those who take care of them, features articles on many of the issues discussed in this entry. It is published by the Arthritis Foundation.

The Arthritis Self-Management Program (ASMP) is offered through local chapters of the Arthritis Foundation.

Lorig K. *The arthritis helpbook: a tested self-management program for coping with arthritis and fibromyalgia,* 4th ed. Reading, MA: Addison-Wesley, 1995.

53. REFLEX SYMPATHETIC DYSTROPHY

James Halper and Michael Rubin

I. Introduction

A. Definition. Reflex sympathetic dystrophy (RSD) is a disorder in which an inciting noxious event—most often an injury to an extremity, a visceral disorder such as myocardial infarction, or a brain insult such as cerebrovascular accident—is followed by the development of a constellation of signs and symptoms in a regional distribution. These include the following:

1. Pain (both spontaneous and in response to ordinarily non-noxious sensory stimulation).
2. Swelling and stiffness.
3. Vasomotor and sudomotor changes.
4. Trophic skin changes.
5. Marked functional disability that initially results from pain, edema, and stiffness but later from less reversible changes (e.g., soft-tissue atrophy, osteopenia, and capsular-ligamentous joint changes).

An abbreviated definition of RSD is a syndrome associated with (a) pain, (b) autonomic changes, (c) trophic changes, and (d) functional impairment that are not attributable to a discrete nerve injury and are *out of proportion to the apparent precipitating noxious event.*

B. Localization and variants. Hands and feet are typically affected, although it becoming increasingly appreciated that RSD may occur in other areas, particularly the knee. There are also localized variants (i.e., "segmental forms") limited to individual rays of the hand or foot or parts of joints (e.g., patella, femoral condyle, or hip). The manifestations of RSD may spread to affect contiguous and even contralateral areas. Movement disorders and psychiatric disturbances frequently develop. Other disorders that have been proposed to be variants of RSD include transient regional osteoporosis, migratory regional osteoporosis, and palmer fasciitis, but the appropriateness of including these under the rubric of RSD remains controversial.

C. Diagnostic criteria. Advances in the understanding of and treatment of RSD have been hampered by a lack of consistent laboratory findings associated with the disorder and the absence of a standardized set of diagnostic criteria accepted by the many specialties that deal with this type of pain syndrome. A given patient may vary in presentation within a short time scale (minutes to hours), reflecting reactive increases and decreases of different autonomic functions, or during a longer term as the picture evolves through the stages discussed below. Heterogeneity also results from the fact that that a multiplicity of neuropathic mechanisms, involving both sympathetic and somatic nerves, can cause different components of RSD or simultaneously contribute to a single manifestation. This has led to the appreciation that RSD is associated with both "sympathetically" and "nonsympathetically" maintained pain, the relative importance of which fluctuates over time. Thus, although amelioration of signs and symptoms by sympathetic blockade has been held by some to be an important criterion for RSD, this is too restrictive a criterion because of the potential for technical factors to cause false-negative results and also because of the natural history of the illness.

The International Association for the Study of Pain has proposed that RSD, as defined by items 1 through 5 above, should be named type 1 complex regional pain syndrome. Causalgia, a disorder in which similar symptoms, especially pain, are found in a distribution that can be attributed to a neuroanatomically defined nerve injury, is classified as type 2 complex regional pain syndrome. Either type of complex regional pain syndrome may be associated with sympathetically mediated and nonsympathetically mediated pain. At present, RSD is probably both underdiagnosed and overdiagnosed.

II. Clinical presentations

A. Cardinal signs and symptoms

1. Pain and an exaggerated, painful response to sensory stimuli

a. Pain is variously described, but commonly used adjectives include "constant," "burning," "aching," "tearing," and "intense," and the pain is characteristically out of proportion to the initiating injury. Patients also report subjective stiffness and a feeling of coldness in the affected region.

b. Response to sensory stimulation

(1) Hyperalgesia—an exaggerated response to a painful stimulus.

(2) Allodynia—pain resulting from a stimulus that does not normally cause pain.

(3) Hyperpathia—persistent delayed pain, especially following repetitive stimuli.

(4) Marked sensitivity to thermal stimuli.

These pathologic sensory responses may contribute to the lancinating paroxysms of pain that may follow the slightest movement of or touch to the affected area. Joint movement may be particularly capable of inducing these paroxysms. Spontaneous paroxysms also occur.

In general, both pain and sensitivity are decreased by elevation of the extremity and increased by physical loads, movement, emotional excitement, and temperature changes.

2. Edema. This is initially pitting but later becomes brawny. It may be more marked in periarticular regions, interfere with blood flow, and lead to pain from nerve compression and decreased mobility. These problems may then exacerbate the RSD.

3. Vasomotor and sudomotor changes. These reflect sympathetic activation and may vary dramatically between patients and with time and in location in the same patient. This is because RSD is associated with sympathetic instability and hyperreactivity rather than simply a statically increased sympathetic tone. Mediators released by nociceptors (e.g., substance P) also affect blood flow.

a. Alterations in skin temperature. Skin temperature may be increased or decreased in comparison with the contralateral area, reflecting impaired thermoregulation. Initially, skin temperature is most commonly increased, but it often fluctuates over the affected area both spontaneously and in response to the triggering factors described above. As time passes, hypoperfusion with decreased skin temperature becomes more prominent. It should be noted that "increased" perfusion does not indicate an increase in nutrient blood flow, which is often decreased because of shunting and microcirculatory abnormalities.

b. Alterations in skin color. Skin color, which also reflects blood flow, is similarly variable, ranging from red (hyperemia) to pale or cyanotic (diminished perfusion). These hyperemic and cyanotic alterations are usually associated with warmth and coldness of the affected areas, respectively. Marked local flow variations that lead to a livedoid, reticulated appearance are often seen.

c. Hyperhidrosis, anhidrosis, and piloerection. Increased or decreased sweating and piloerection may occur, reflecting changes in autonomic tone.

d. Trophic changes. Nails may be brittle, ridged, and abnormally colored and may show increased curvature. Hair may be coarse and increased. Skin may be thin and atrophied or hyperkeratotic. Atrophy or edema can lead to loss of skin folds, and finger pulp may be lost. Bony resorption is prominent from the onset and increases with disease duration.

e. Functional impairment initially results from pain and swelling. This leads to disuse, which produces a synergistic effect with the pathophysiologic concomitant features of RSD, so that anatomic alterations and permanent functional impairment ensue. Such changes include severe atrophy of skin and other soft tissues, osteoporosis, nerve damage from compression, and joint capsular and ligamentous fibrosis.

B. Stages of reflex sympathetic dystrophy. The natural history of RSD is often divided into three stages (Steinbrocker classification). However, it should be noted that patients frequently may not demonstrate the full picture at each stage or an orderly progression from one stage to another.

1. **Stage 1 (acute, months 1 to 3)** is usually dominated by pain and tenderness, edema, and temperature changes, particularly increases. Patchy areas and periods of temperature decrease may, however, be seen. Sudomotor alterations, typically hyperhidrosis, tend to appear later in this phase. Signs and symptoms are initially limited to the region of injury or the surrounding areas but may spread to adjacent or even contralateral areas, reflecting changes at the spinal or even more central areas of the central nervous system.
2. **Stage 2 (dystrophic).** The pain usually extends beyond the area initially affected. Although still prominent, it may be either increased or decreased in comparison with pain in stage 1. Edema may take on a more brawny quality. Loss of hair and dystrophic nail changes become apparent, and muscle wasting and osteoporosis become more prominent. At this stage, a decreased range of motion (ROM) reflects capsular changes and contractures, in addition to pain and edema. The affected area is usually cool, pale, or cyanotic, reflecting a decrease in blood flow, although as usual marked fluctuations may occur.
3. **Stage 3 (atrophic or chronic).** Skin and soft-tissue atrophy, bony demineralization, and capsular thickening progress, as does functional impairment. The latter results from and leads to contractures, decreased passive movement, and apparent stiffness of joints. In extreme cases, a "claw hammer" hand or "frozen" shoulder may result.

   The importance of staging in treatment is controversial, at least in regard to stages 1 and 2. However, patients who have reached stage 3 are clearly distinct in that they have suffered irreversible damage and will respond poorly to any modality.

C. Movement disorders. Movement disorders become more prominent in the advanced stages (e.g., stages 2 and 3) and may even initially present after pain has subsided. Rarely, they may precede other changes. Abnormalities include tremor with resting, postural, and action components; spasms; myoclonus; focal dystonias; and an inability to initiate movements and complete complex movements that may develop into apraxia.

Hyperreflexia and decreased strength may cause or result from the guarding postures commonly assumed by the patient. However, the dysphasia and difficulty in swallowing that may be found in RSD affecting the upper extremities indicate cortical changes. The "neglect" reported to account for some cases of movement disorder in RSD is also consistent with cortical involvement. This is characterized by delayed, slowed, low-amplitude movements and a decrease in spontaneous movements. The patient feels disconnected from the involved region and may even refer to the affected extremity as "it."

Movement disorders may interfere with physical therapy or become independent causes of morbidity. Dystonias, for example, may lead to total loss of hand function and the development of pressure sores in the "clenched-fist" syndrome, or problems of ambulation resulting from inversion and an equine position of the foot.

Movement disorders result from sympathetic hyperactivity and from plastic changes at spinal and peripheral neurons and muscle spindles induced by sympathetic activity and products of nociceptors. Cortical changes are also involved.

D. Psychiatric disorders. Affective disorders (e.g., depression or anxiety) and behavioral disturbances (e.g., social withdrawal, physical inactivity, chronic invalidism) are extremely common both in patients with RSD and in those with causalgia. It has been suggested that psychological features may be involved in the initiation of the disorder, but this is controversial. However, it is widely agreed that psychological disturbances commonly occur secondary to the pain and disability associated with the disorder. Both "adjustment disorders" (subsyndromal presentation of depressive or anxiety symptoms felt to occur as a reaction to stress) and major depressive disorders (full syndrome felt to be precipitated by the stress of the illness) may occur. Suicidal thoughts may occur in either instance.

Demoralization and frustration with the medical system (because of the not uncommon delays in the diagnosis of RSD and minimization of the significance of this poorly understood illness) on top of chronic pain may make the patient argumentative and otherwise difficult to deal with. This leads to patterns of escalating negative interactions with health care professionals and family members. The family members may be similarly difficult.

Thus, the relationship between RSD and psychological symptoms is complex and variable. However, regardless of the etiology, the psychological concomitant features of RSD must be addressed early in the treatment because psychological factors, such as tolerance of pain, methods of coping with stress and pain, and beliefs and expectations, have a major effect on the patient's willingness and ability to (a) tolerate often painful treatments, (b) avoid the extremes of too much mobilization and too much immobilization, and (c) cope with transient or permanent functional impairments.

The clinical observation that emotional stress may cause disease exacerbations and data linking flares with elevation of catecholamines further underscore the importance of dealing with psychological issues.

Addiction is often overdiagnosed but sometimes does occur.

E. Complications. In a small but significant number of patients, infections, ulcers, and chronic edema may develop. Unrecognized or resistant infections may be diagnosed as refractory RSD or even malingering. Severe dystonias have been discussed above. It has been suggested that complications and motor disorders may be more common in younger female patients with multiple involved sites in the lower extremities and in patients who present initially with decreased blood flow ("cold presentation").

On the other hand, rarely, ulcerative lesions and infections have been the result of self-mutilation.

F. Possible atypical variants of reflex sympathetic dystrophy.

1. **Transient regional osteoporosis.**
2. **Transient migratory osteoporosis.** They are marked by a sudden onset of pain that is intensified by weight bearing. As the names imply, transient regional osteoporosis is limited to a single joint or part thereof. Hip pain in middle-aged men or in women in the third trimester of pregnancy is a common presentation of transient regional osteoporosis. Transient migratory osteoporosis most often affects the knee, ankle, and foot. As the name implies, it attacks a variety of joints, most often sequentially but occasionally with some temporal overlap. These conditions present with prominent focal areas of osteoporosis, unexplained severe pain (particularly on motion and weight bearing), positive findings on bone scans, and occasionally dependent rubor and muscle atrophy (from disuse). Thus, they may be diagnosed as RSD and have been considered by some authorities to be atypical forms of the disorder. However, a relation to an inciting insult can rarely be documented and physical changes are usually absent, as are the manifestations of neuropathic pain. Most importantly, neither transient regional nor transient migratory osteoporosis has a protracted course. Although there are scattered reports of responses to treatment with steroids, calcitonin, biphosphonates, estrogen, and even sympathetic blocks, there is no convincing body of evidence that these treatments actually alter the typically self-limited course of these entities. Hence, most authorities distinguish these disorders from RSD. It has been recently suggested that because of their association with characteristic changes on magnetic resonance imaging (increased intensity on T_1-weighted MRI and decreased intensity on T_2-weighted scans), bone marrow edema may be responsible for these syndromes. It is important to

exclude infections (particularly tuberculosis), osteonecrosis, stress fractures, and neoplasms of bone and joints as cause of the complaints. Treatment is focused on reassurance, rest and crutch use, medications noted above, and gentle ambulation—a very different approach from that taken with RSD.

III. Etiology. RSD results from conditions that cause (alone or together) regional tissue damage, pain and immobilization, and direct injury to the central nervous system. Local or central nervous system injury and immobilization lead to long-lasting changes at both the peripheral and central nervous system level in pain processing and control of sympathetic function. This neural plasticity explains the severity and persistence of the signs and symptoms that comprise the disorder.

Inciting events include local trauma, particularly fractures and or improper casting. Colles' fracture is a common cause of RSD of the hand, and this association is a good example of how RSD may affect an area adjacent to but not totally overlapping the site of injury. Other precipitants include apparently minor injuries ("sprains"); arthroscopic procedures and surgery (arthroplasty and carpal tunnel release); painful peripheral conditions (burns, herpes zoster); diseases of the spinal cord or brain (stroke); visceral disorders associated with pain and immobilization (myocardial infarction); local effects of metastatic cancer (which also may cause RSD as a paraneoplastic syndrome); pregnancy; and certain medications (phenobarbital, ergotamine, cyclosporine, and isoniazid) (Table 53-1). However, up to one-third of patients may not recall an inciting event.

Table 53-1. Precipitating factors and diseases associated with reflex sympathetic dystrophy

Peripheral triggers
- Soft-tissue injury
- Fractures, sprains, dislocations, operative procedures
- Immobilization with cast or splint
- Inflammatory and soft-tissue disorders (e.g., rheumatoid arthritis, polymylagia rheumatica, vasculitides, tendinitis, bursitis)
- Infection (e.g., necrotizing fasciitis)
- Vascular disorders: venous or arterial thrombosis

Visceral triggers
- Malignancy
- Myocardial infarction
- Aortic injury
- Pulmonary fibrosis
- Weber-Christian disease

Neurologic disorders or procedures
- Spinal cord disease or injury
- Myelography
- Spinal anesthesia
- Paravertebral alcohol injection
- Subacute combined degeneration
- Syringomyelia
- Poliomyelitis
- Amyotrophic lateral sclerosis
- Post-herpetic neuralgia
- Brachial plexopathy
- Scalenus anticus syndrome
- Radiculopathy
- Brain tumor
- Severe head injury
- Cerebral infarction
- Subarachnoid hemorrhage

As alluded to above, the lack of agreement on standard diagnostic criteria has hampered precise quantification of the overall incidence of RSD and its association with the different conditions thought to trigger it.

The potential for development of RSD after surgery is greater in patients who have had previous episodes of RSD, diabetic neuropathy, or depression, or in whom secondary gain may be important.

IV. Pathophysiology.

A. Nervous system insult. The initial insult, including local tissue injury, pain, and immobilization, is thought to cause functional and structural alterations at peripheral, spinal, and even cortical levels of the nervous system, resulting in spontaneous pain and exaggerated painful responses to mildly noxious or non-noxious stimuli. Changes at the spinal level include a decrease in descending inhibitory influences, hyperexcitability, increase in size of receptive fields of neurons, and reorganization of pain reflexes, including those involving sympathetic neurons. An alteration of a wide range of dynamic neurons has been proposed as an important occurrence, resulting in their signaling pain in response to ordinarily non-noxious stimuli. The decrease in normal sensory input resulting from the decreased activity of the affected region "opens the gate" to ongoing pain and leads to further neural reorganization.

In the peripheral nervous system, nociceptors begin to generate ectopic or exaggerated discharges. These may result from microscopic injury and alterations in the milieu, including edema, decreased nutrient flow, and release of products by activated sensory neurons themselves (e.g., substance P).

The sympathetic nervous system, which is normally linked to pain by spinal and more central reflexes, assumes a more prominent role in pain generation and becomes less able to regulate vascular tone, sweating, and other functions normally. One component of sympathetically mediated pain is the development in nociceptors of α-adrenergic receptors and synaptic connections with sympathetic neurons, so that they become inappropriately activated by sympathetic neuronal activity and circulating catecholamines.

B. Sympathetic dysfunction. Sympathetic function, including sudomotor and vasomotor activity, may be both increased and decreased abnormally (i.e., the key abnormality is instability and dysregulation). Periods of sympathetic hypofunction may lead to receptor hypersensitivity. This is why, in most patients, the affected region may at different times be warm and red (hypervasular), blue and cold (hypoperfused), or mottled. It should be noted that even in areas of hypervascularity nutrient flow will often be diminished (because of dysregulation of microvasculature and arteriovenous anastomoses), which contributes to pain and weakness. These changes explain both the effectiveness of treatments designed to decrease sympathetic nervous activity and the variability of the response.

C. Edema occurs when venous outflow is compromised either mechanically or in response to the products of sympathetic or sensory neurons (e.g., prostaglandins, substance P). Edema itself can cause pain through nerve compression, interference with blood flow and diffusion of nutrients, and interference with motion. All of these in turn can further increase edema and lead to dystrophic changes.

The synergistic effects of substance P and prostaglandins with abnormal blood flow patterns cause the rapid development of osteopenia. Atrophic changes result from the above abnormalities and disuse.

D. Movement disorders result from the effects of sympathetic hyperactivity and of neuropeptides released by nociceptors on motor neurons in the spinal cord and preganglionic sympathetic nerves. These, in turn, affect muscle spindles and muscle itself and nociceptor function in the affected region. Tremor is the movement abnormality most tightly linked to sympathetic activity. Changes at the cortical level may also play a role, particularly in neglect.

E. Mechanical derangements. The injury triggering RSD or the changes resulting from RSD can lead to "mechanical derangements" and secondary nerve injuries (e.g., compression and neuromas); these cause pain and further perpetuate the disorder.

A major and still unanswered question is why RSD develops in a particular person—in other words, what is the diathesis? Psychiatric components have been suggested but have never been convincingly demonstrated. It has been suggested that sympathetic reactivity as evidenced by a personal history of vasomotor instability, blushing or blanching, palmar perspiration in response to emotions, or a family history of Raynaud's syndrome may be a marker of susceptibility, but this remains to be firmly established.

V. Diagnosis. The **diagnosis is clinical** and based primarily on the development of the symptoms and signs described above in an appropriate temporal relation to an inciting event. The time required for symptoms to develop ranges from a day or two to 2 weeks or longer. In the early phase, the excessive pain may be attributed to the injury, whereas in the delayed presentation, the original injury may have been forgotten, especially if minor. Because the early signs and symptoms are vague and nonspecific, the clinician must have a high index of suspicion for RSD in the setting of conditions associated with it.

There are no diagnostic tests specific for RSD. Levels of acute-phase reactants are abnormal only if they are secondary to an associated illness. Hence, they may alert the clinician to consider alternative diagnoses. Radiographs and technetium bone scans are the modalities most commonly used in routine clinical practice. Increasing attention is being given to the incorporation of more sophisticated tests of blood flow and sympathetic function.

Most series emphasize the frequency with which diagnosis is delayed. The earlier the treatment is initiated, the better the response, because neural changes and osteopenia may take a while to reverse and RSD is perpetuated by the vicious cycle of pain and immobilization. There is some uniformity in the marked decrease in response to treatment after RSD has been present for a year or even 6 months.

A. Differential diagnosis includes the large number of conditions that in themselves cause pain, immobility, and swelling with or without inflammation. These include injuries (crush wounds, fractures, stress fractures, osteonecrosis); infections of both bone and soft tissue, which, like RSD, may result from injuries; thromboangiitis obliterans; Raynaud's syndrome; and inflammatory disorders, including crystal-induced and other arthritides. Pain and swelling may of course result from an injury *per se,* but their duration and severity and the associated vasomotor and sudomotor changes help in the differentiation. Thoracic outlet syndrome and cervical or thoracic spine disorders must be considered. It has been suggested that the former, particularly if associated with prominent subclavian stenosis, may be associated with true RSD. RSD may also be confused with scleroderma in cases that initially present with skin changes late in stages 2 or 3.

B. Radiography and laboratory tests

1. **Radiographs** reveal osteopenia with various patterns of bone loss, including patchy, bandlike periarticular loss, irregular cortical outlines, cortical tunneling and striation, scalloping of inner cortical surfaces, surface erosions of subchondral and subarticular surfaces, and other subchondral changes. These may occur late and are nonspecific. Joint spaces are preserved until late in the course.

   Quantitative bone density studies such as dual-energy x-ray absorptiometry indicate that substantial bone loss may occur early. Much of this is irreversible, at least in adults.

2. **Technetium bone scans.** The third (delayed, static) phase of the bone scan is considered the most useful study in the investigation of RSD. Diffuse bony uptake with periarticular accentuation is generally considered the most characteristic finding. Although this pattern has been quite specific (>90%) and sensitive (>90%) in some series, it is considered neither necessary nor sufficient for the diagnosis. However, if present, it may provide corroborative evidence, and if absent, it may prompt re-

examination of the diagnosis. The blood flow (immediate) component of the scan and the blood pool (early phase) are often asymmetric when the affected limb is compared with the normal one. As expected from blood flow and autonomic variability, the affected area may show either an increase or decrease in uptake.

3. **Measures of autonomic function.** Results will vary, as one might expect from the autonomic variability discussed above. Thermography and other techniques to measure temperature are most commonly employed and are often used to assess the efficacy of therapeutic manipulations (e.g., sympathetic blockade). Again, asymmetry is the most typical finding. Sudomotor function can be assayed by galvanic skin resistance (GSR), resting output, or quantitative sudomotor axon reflex test (QSART); these have been advocated both for diagnosis and for following response to treatment modalities.

   Certain specialized centers emphasize the importance of "stress tests" of autonomic function to uncover the degree of autonomic hyperreactivity or the specific stimuli most relevant to a particular patient.

   Inclusion of at least a semiquantitative assessment of sweating and some measurement of temperature is strongly recommended whenever sympathetic blocks are performed.

4. **Measures of pain** are required to follow a patient's response to treatment. At a minimum, these should include (a) a semiquantitative assessment of pain (e.g., Visual Analog Scale, with pain intensity graded on a scale of 1 to 10) for spontaneous pain and allodynia in response to gentle touch with a cotton swab; (b) a test of temperature sensitivity (e.g., to cold produced by evaporation of a drop of acetone placed on the skin); and (c) a rough "map" of the distribution of abnormalities. More quantitative measures, such as filaments and algometers, may be useful.

5. **Synovial biopsy** is no longer used except to rule out other diagnoses, as it reveals only nonspecific findings, including subsynovial fibrosis, synovial proliferation, and occasionally mild inflammatory changes.

6. **Response to sympathetic blockade as a criterion for diagnosis.** Although many earlier series made a response to "diagnostic" sympathetic blockade a *sine qua non* for the diagnosis of RSD, the role of this procedure has been reconceptualized. It is now employed to identify the contribution of sympathetically mediated pain in a given patient and to assess the utility of sympathetic blockade and related modalities for treatment. Thus, rather than being a diagnostic tool, sympathetic blocks are considered more of a therapeutic trial. As is the case for any test, misleading negative and positive results can occur. For example, failure to respond may result from the dominance of nonsympathetically mediated pain at the time the block was performed or the effect of high levels of circulating catecholamines (which may be increased in response to pain, depression, and anxiety). These will continue to induce sympathetically mediated pain even when local catecholamine release is blocked. False-negative results can also be caused by technical problems. In the case of stellate ganglion block for RSD of the upper extremity, it must be remembered that Horner's syndrome may occasionally result from blocks that fail to affect the sympathetic nerves controlling the upper limb. Thus, stellate ganglion blocks must be evaluated by a careful assessment of autonomic function of the relevant area, even when Horner's syndrome is noted. False-positive results can occur through the placebo response. It should also be remembered that some sympathetic blocks may affect somatic nerves (i,e., pain relief may reflect anesthesia of somatic afferents). This leads to a "false-positive" result from the perspective of assessment of the importance of sympathetically mediated pain and the decision regarding whether to continue treatment targeted at the sympathetic nervous system. Criteria for a "successful" blockade vary between centers (which vary in the sophistication of assessment of pain and autonomic function). At the minimum,

evaluation should include a semiquantitative assessment of pain (e.g., on the Visual Analog Scale of 1 to 10, both spontaneous and in response to gentle pressure with a cotton swab), measurement of skin temperature, and global estimation of sweat production function, which demonstrate substantial pain relief and reversal of autonomic features. This is indicated by elevation of fingertip temperature by more than 1° to 3°F, venous engorgement, dryness of the skin, and a subjective feeling of warmth. Doppler fluxometry may be particularly informative.

When the diagnosis of RSD is strongly suspected, the effects of several blocks on pain that meet the above criteria for technical adequacy should be assessed before any decision regarding treatment is made. This is because a large number of patients who fail to respond to one (technically successful) block may do so after three or occasionally more are performed. Implications of partial and brief responses are discussed below.

It has recently been suggested that high-dose IV phentolamine (an α-adrenergic receptor antagonist) infusions with demonstration of adequate α-adrenergic receptor blockade may be particularly useful for the demonstration of sympathetically mediated pain. Blockade of α-adrenergic receptors will antagonize the effects of circulating catecholamines not affected by sympathetic block as well as those released by the neurons innervating the area. Because this is a technically easier and less invasive procedure than sympathetic blockade, it is more suitable for placebo-controlled trials and for repeated trials followed by careful quantitative assessment of spontaneous and laboratory-induced pain and autonomic function in individual patients. Although well tolerated, blood pressure and electrocardiographic monitoring should be performed during and after the procedure, and the procedure should be performed in an area capable of handling cardiovascular emergencies. An absent or partial response indicates the presence of a nonsympathetically mediated pain component, a β-adrenergic component, or both. Some proponents stress the importance of high-dose (1 mg/kg) phentolamine and advocate inclusion of β-adrenergic blockers.

VI. General treatment concepts. It is hard to provide a treatment protocol for a disorder in which a consensus regarding either diagnostic criteria or etiology has not yet been reached and that is associated with so much variability between and within individual patients. Many outcome studies, particularly those using invasive procedures, have been poorly controlled. Interpreting the findings of other studies and applying their recommendations to an individual patient is complicated by the inclusion of subjects with different presentations. This refers not only to the Steinbrocker stages (which are relatively stable over time) but also to day-to-day fluctuations and region-to-region variations.

A. General concepts of therapy. Despite these caveats, agreement has been reached regarding certain general features of treatment. These include the following:

1. Early diagnosis.
2. Aggressive multimodal treatment by a multidisciplinary treatment team, including an anesthesiologist and physical therapist in addition to the orthopedist or rheumatologist.

B. Educational and psychological modalities. Gaining the confidence of patients is key because they will have to participate in a long and grueling program. This is best accomplished by devoting time to education, reassurance, and the assessment of maladaptive coping mechanisms, sleep disturbances, psychiatric disorders, and issues of compensation and litigation. On occasion, a psychiatrist or psychologist should be consulted. Treatment is focused on restoring functioning as rapidly as possible while avoiding an increase in pain, which will merely perpetuate the cycle of "pain, neuronal change, dysfunction, and more pain." The severe pain and exquisite sensitivity of the affected area to touch and movement together with the necessity for early mobilization and functional restoration puts the treatment team between Scylla and Charybdis. The patient and family are often frustrated and frustrating, but they must be enlisted as part of the team at the very onset of therapy.

Priority must be given to treating pain and edema. This in turn will allow ROM and strength to be addressed. In addition, it must always be kept in mind that RSD is a dynamic disorder with rapid fluctuations in autonomic tone and tolerance to manipulations. Modalities that were used yesterday to reduce blood flow in a hyperemic hand may have no place for today's cold, vasoconstricted hand. Procedures that a patient tolerated the day after a successful block can be excruciating as the block wears off. Thus, treatment requires sensitivity and flexibility, which in turn require careful ongoing assessment and utilization of a myriad of modalities, either sequentially or in combination. As so pithily put by Ficat and Hungerford, "It [RSD] is not a disease to be beaten into submission but to be gently seduced." The patient must be fully informed and convinced of the rationale behind the often painful modalities, and the patient should participate in the development of discrete and well-defined goals.

C. **Monitoring progress or lack thereof.** Progress should be carefully monitored. Whereas some centers attempt to quantify parameters as described above, others rely on more subjective descriptions. However, whatever method is used, the measurement of such milestones must be consistently and regularly applied.

D. **Pain control and physical therapy.** Occasionally, early cases will respond to simple analgesics, local measures such as transcutaneous electrical nerve stimulation (TENS), judicious use of heat and cold, elevation, and active ROM exercises.

E. **Use of sympathetic blocks as initial treatment.** This is indicated if (a) no improvement is seen in 1 to 4 weeks, (b) patients cannot tolerate even the most gentle application of these measures, or (c) a patient presents after 6 months of symptoms, a time at which the "window of opportunity" is rapidly closing. A recommended approach is shown in Fig. 53-1.

VII. Specific treatment modalities

A. Pain control

1. Nonsteroidal antiinflammatory drugs and analgesics are often insufficient for pain control (although the combination of ketorolac and amitriptyline may be efficacious). There has been an increase in the use of narcotics, including opioids, by either the oral or parenteral route. As is always the case, once a decision regarding these medications has been made, they should be given in adequate doses and at appropriate intervals. Transdermal fentanyl also has been found useful. Exercises should be coordinated wit h the pain medication. The early use of sympathetic blockade may be indicated if opioid/narcotic tolerance appears to be developing.
2. TENS is used in many centers for pain control, and according to some authorities, it may also be helpful with vasomotor phenomena. Stimulus parameters (frequency, pulse width, and amperage) and site of application must be chosen for tolerability and efficacy. Although stimulation to the site of discomfort is often most efficacious, patients frequently cannnot tolerate this location, and proximal or even contralateral sites may be initially employed. Acupuncture or trigger points have also been used.

B. **Physical therapy.** Physiotherapists/physiatrists experienced in this disorder are key because of the delicate balance required between appropriate mobilization of the affected region and pain relief. Allodynia may make certain manipulations (e.g., splinting) particularly difficult. Small, defined goals should be set and shared with the patient, and specific physical efforts should be prioritized. Initial focus is on pain and edema because their control allows increased focus on ROM (both active and passive). This then allows strengthening exercises and functional restoration.

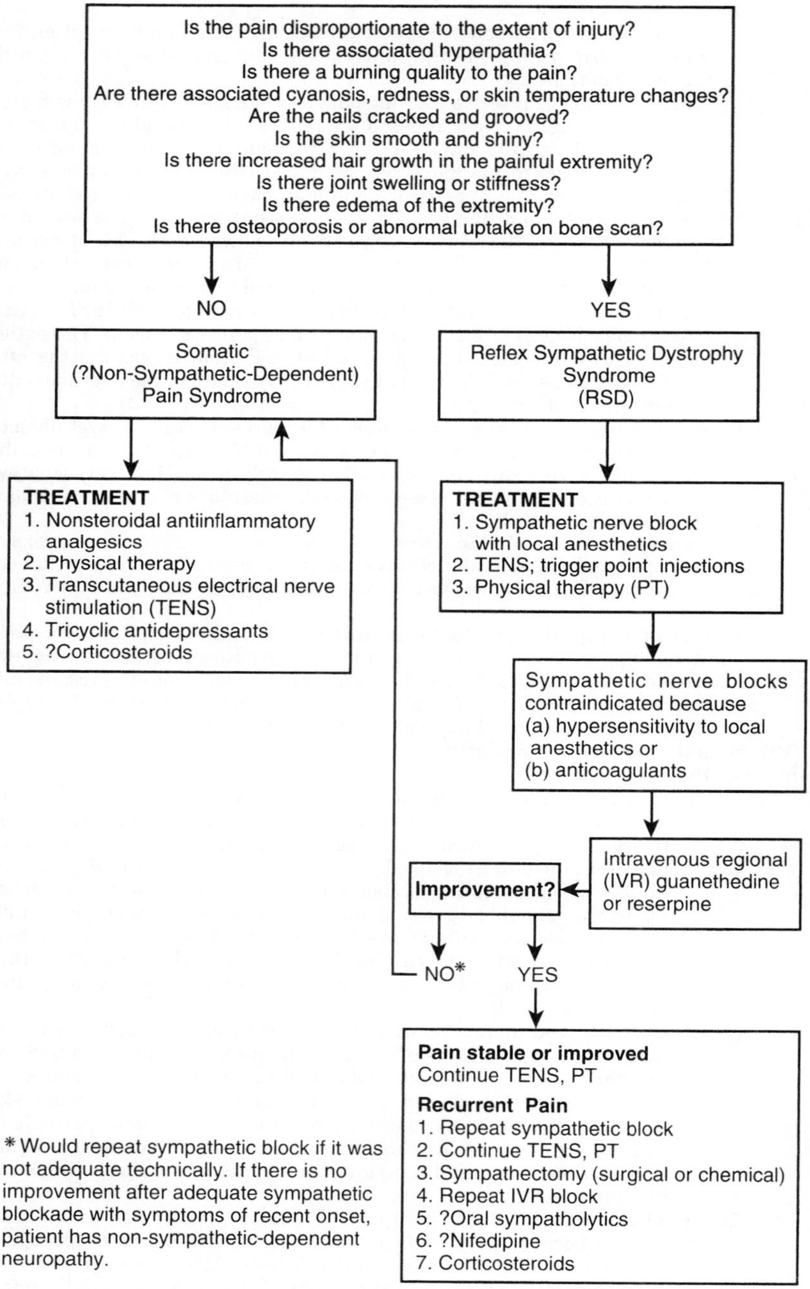

FIG. 53-1. Pain following injury (which may be trivial) to bone, soft tissue, or peripheral nerve; an approach to the diagnosis and treatment of the reflex sympathetic dystrophy syndrome. (From Payne R. Neuropathic pain syndromes with special reference to causalgia and reflex sympathetic dystrophy. *Clin J Pain* 1986;2:59.)

1. **Desensitization.** This must be carried out in a graded fashion and, when possible, in a functionally relevant way. Patients may be encouraged to rub their hand on the back of a couch while watching television. Vibration has also been advocated.
2. **Exercise** as tolerated may help by "gating out" pain, leading to release of opioids peripherally and stabilization of the autonomic nervous system. It may also increase the general sense of well-being of these often deconditioned patients.
3. **Thermal modalities**
   a. **Heat.** Heat may be useful during the times when the affected region is cold and vasoconstriction predominates. Many authorities discourage the use of a whirlpool because the dependent position of the affected area tends to increase edema. Paraffin and fluidotherapy are useful alternatives, and it is useful to combine them with stretching and ROM exercises. The often exquisitely increased sensitivity of these patients to heat must be kept in mind. Some patients may be able to tolerate application of heat only to remote areas. This may lead to vasodilation of the affected areas if thermoregulatory reflexes are even partially preserved.
   b. **Cold.** The application of cold packs may be useful for the warm, hyperemic limb, with caveats similar to those for the use of heat. Again, remote cooling may be useful.
   c. **Contrast baths.** When careful attention is given to determining tolerated temperature, these may be useful in the treatment of pain and edema and may be taken at home.
4. **Elevation, decongestive massage, and intermittent Jobst pneumatic compression.** These techniques are useful for edema, and the massage also provides desensitization. Again, many patients will have difficulty tolerating massage and compression because of allodynia and hyperpathia. For some patients in whom temporal summation of pain is prominent, pain can be minimized if care is taken to ensure continuous rather than intermittent contact during massage. It has been suggested that deep massage may lead to histamine release and increased inflammation.

   For patients who tolerate Jobst compression, this modality should be not be allowed to interfere with mobilization. Compressive garments and wraps if tolerated are advantageous with respect to motility.
5. **Range of motion.** Movement is necessary to prevent contractures, reduce edema, "gate out" pain, help restore normal neuronal architecture, and strengthen muscles. The necessity of the potentially painful exercises should be explained, and the therapist needs to monitor the patient's response constantly. The exercises should be coordinated with pain treatment and performed at appropriate intervals after pain medication. Failure to tolerate exercise even after that may be an indication for more aggressive treatment, including sympathetic blockade. A stress-loading approach involving compression and distraction while joint movement is minimized has been found to be particularly useful (e.g., scrub and carry for the upper extremity and standing with graduated weight bearing for the lower).

   Generally, active and assisted active ROM exercises are emphasized. On those occasions, when it is deemed that passive ROM exercises are indicated, it should be remembered that these are more likely to lead to pain and interference by allodynia. The ideal ROM exercises are those relevant to activities of daily living (e.g., walking with crutches for RSD of the lower extremity).
6. **Splinting.** Static and dynamic splinting may be useful, but only if employed judiciously. Too many or too complicated splints will overwhelm the patient. Static splints may be necessary to prevent contractures and may be useful at night to prevent joint motion from disturbing sleep. It

may also help position the affected areas to allow appropriate strengthening exercises. Of course, they will also contribute to the undesirable sequelae of immobilization if overused. Dynamic splinting, if carefully crafted, may decrease pain through stimulation of large afferents, reduce edema, and maintain ROM. Static progressive splinting is indicated when ROM is limited by contractures and stiffness and pain is relatively quiescent.

7. **Ultrasound** may be helpful by providing pain relief and inducing vasodilation.
8. **Biofeedback** may be useful for vasomotor instability and movement abnormalities, including hypertonicity, spasticity, and dystonias.

C. **Treatment of movement disorders.** Interventions that decrease sympathetic function may be useful in the treatment of tremor but have inconsistent effects on dystonias. Benzodiazepines may be helpful for spasms. Visual and verbal cues may be helpful in cases in which features of neglect are prominent.

D. **Psychiatric and psychological interventions.** Many patients with RSD present with a history of mistaken diagnoses, perceptions (which may or may not be accurate) that their pain has been dismissed (by professionals and family), irritability, demoralization, and sleep deprivation because of pain. These often lead to anger at the medical system and strained relations between the patient and family members. "Stress," anxiety, and depression, which are common in these patients, are well-known to exacerbate pain from any cause, and because of their effects on the autonomic nervous system (association with increase or dysregulation of circulating catecholamines), they also may play a more specific role in RSD.

Many psychological interventions can be performed by any member of the multidisciplinary team. These include developing a supportive relationship; carefully educating the patient about pain, including explicitly acknowledging its disabling effects and adverse effects on interpersonal relationships; and making the patient aware of the interaction of pain with mood. Certain antidepressant drugs that may be used for sleep and pain also have adrenergic-blocking effects.

Concerns about an associated depression or other psychiatric disorder that perhaps requires treatment with psychotropic agents, behavioral problems that severely compromise the treatment, or medical issues that complicate the use of an antidepressant may indicate the need for a more formal psychiatric consultation. This must be accomplished tactfully and after good rapport has been established (to the extent that this is not prevented by the psychological problems). Both patient and family may resist the suggestion of a psychiatric consult because, in addition to the usual stigma associated with such a consult, they may feel that this is another example of the dismissal of symptoms as being "all in the head." Indeed, this might be a good starting place for psychological education to begin: "Yes, pain is in your head, all of our feelings are in our head. Pain affects mood and mood affects pain. We all have heard stories of soldiers wounded in battle who do not feel the wound until the battle is over. On the other hand, we all know that minor pains (and I'm not talking about RSD) are 10 times more annoying when we're tired or upset." Another approach is to explain that the psychiatrist is a specialist in helping people deal optimally with stressful conditions and that many of the medications they use are effective in treating pain. The psychiatrist may also play a role as a neutral party in helping to monitor the use of narcotics, ensuring that the patient receives adequate dosage yet watching for inappropriate dosage escalation. Support groups may be useful for patient and family. Antidepressants are discussed below.

E. **Therapies directed at the nervous system.** The importance of factors other than sympathetic function in RSD has been discussed above. Nevertheless, interventions to decrease the activity of sympathetic neurons, such as ganglionic blocks and regional IV catecholamine depletion, still play an important role in assessment (see section **V.B.6**) and treatment. Again, it must be emphasized that only some of the adrenergic activity in a given region is caused by the local release of catecholamines, the target of these procedures. Circulating catecholamines (which may be increased in response to pain, depression, and anxiety), including norepinephrine released from sympathetic neurons in other regions and epinephrine from adrenal medullary activity, may stimulate the adrenergic receptors relevant to the manifestations of RSD.

α-Adrenergic blockade (e.g., phentolamine) will prevent the action of catecholamines, whether they are locally or systemically produced. Hence, a case could be made for the combined or sequential use of modalities. Somatic blockade may be required for patients in whom a major component of pain is nonsympathetic in origin.

Important note: Any pain relief provided by sympathetic or somatic blockade should be followed immediately by intensive mobilization and other physical therapy modalities.

1. **Sympathetic ganglion blockade.** Sympathetic blocks with local anesthetic agents are used for both diagnostic and therapeutic purposes. Stellate ganglion block is utilized for the upper extremities. However, as stated above, care must be taken to ensure that blockade of sympathetic nerves to the arm has actually been accomplished, even in the presence of Horner's syndrome. This is indicated by elevation of fingertip temperature by 1° to 3°F venous engorgement, dryness of the skin, and a subjective feeling of warmth. Although many use lidocaine for the initial treatment, bupivacaine block may last considerably longer than lidocaine block. Lumbar (L-2 through L-4) blocks are used for the lower extremities. It is generally agreed that the procedure should be repeated at least three times within 7 to 10 days before it should be considered to have failed. It is often performed even more frequently (every other day) and tapered when the response has plateaued, typically after six to 12 successful blocks.
2. **Epidural block.** The epidural route is also useful, particularly for the lower extremity, because of the technical difficulties and pain associated with lumbar ganglionic block. Further, the ease and safety of placement of epidural catheters make it an attractive procedure. Continuous epidural blocks may relieve pain even when repeated lumbar blocks have failed to do so. They can be performed quite selectively with respect to level and nature of neurons (sympathetic, somatic, or both). Some groups advocate initial infusion with local anesthetic followed by agents such as narcotics or ketamine; in this way, motor function is left intact so that active ROM exercises can continue. On the other hand, sparing of motor fibers is not as important when this procedure is used to "cover" passive ROM exercises or manipulations. Of course, epidural blocks also have their side effects, including hypotension, urinary retention, and rarely seizures or infection. Respiratory depression is rare unless morphine is used. Recently, epidural clonidine has been used alone and in combination with other agents because its α_2-adrenergic agonism will inhibit the release of norepinephrine.
3. **Intravenous regional "chemical sympathectomy."** In the past, IV regional chemical sympathectomy was recommended for patients in whom sympathetic or somatic ganglion block and epidural block were contraindicated (hypersensitive or on anticoagulants). Additionally, it represented an alternative to surgical sympathectomy in high-risk patients. In chemical sympathectomy, an IV infusion of agents depletes noradrenaline from sympathetic terminals. The agents are confined to the affected region by placement of a blood pressure cuff or other compressive device inflated above systolic pressure proximal to the site of injection. After a period of time, during which the agents are taken up by the sympathetic nerve terminals, the tourniquet is released. How-

ever, the place of this procedure in the modern armamentarium remains undefined. As is the case for so many modalities used in RSD, enthusiastic reports are counterbalanced by negative ones. This variability may result from patient heterogeneity and technical factors. Review of the studies indicates variation in the rigor with which sympathetic blockade was demonstrated. Guanethidine and to a lesser extent reserpine were used in virtually all the studies, and these agents are no longer routinely available in the United States. However, bretylium, another catecholamine-depleting agent, has been reported to be safe and efficacious. With respect to technical factors, the simplicity of the technique is more apparent than real. Because of the possibility of side effects (e.g., hypotension) resulting from systemic leakage before and after the cuff is released, this procedure should be carried out with continuous monitoring of vital signs. Electrocardiographic equipment in a suite equipped for resuscitation is mandatory, and a well-functioning IV line should be placed in an uninvolved area. In addition, application of the tourniquet may be quite painful and cause phlebitis.

These regional catecholamine depletion techniques do not relieve pain caused by circulating catecholamines. This problem has been addressed by the use of regional blockade of α-adrenergic receptors. The reversible antagonist phentolamine may be infused regionally in patients who cannot tolerate the marked autonomic side effects accompanying systemic infusion. The use of IV phenoxybenzamine, an irreversible antagonist that should in theory have a longer duration of action, was reported recently. Although the results were positive, the study must be considered preliminary.

4. **Intravenous α-adrenergic blockade** is the simplest technique to block the effects of circulating and locally produced catecholamines. Infusion of phentolamine and phenoxybenzamine has been used more often as a "diagnostic technique" than as an ongoing treatment because of the autonomic side effects of these drugs when administered systemically rather than regionally. Brief but reproducible and perhaps partial responses to abrogation of sympathetic activity may be indications to consider more permanent and invasive approaches to abrogating sympathetic function.
5. **Role of surgical sympathectomy or chemical sympatholysis.** Short-lived or partial responses to the above measures have in the past been considered indications for sympatholytic procedures, such as injection of phenol or alcohol into ganglia or surgical sympathectomy. Recently, radiofrequency ganglionic ablation has been reported. These techniques can be guided with imaging. However, their role is controversial because of technical considerations, because the results are irreversible (particularly in the case of surgical procedures), and because pain may paradoxically recur or even increase ("sympathalgia"). The latter may reflect aberrant regeneration or receptor hypersensitivity. Reliance on surgical sympathectomy and sympatholysis has decreased because of the availability of techniques for more continuous sympathetic blockade, the development of newer concepts regarding the importance of nonsympathetic pain in RSD, and the realization that the plasticity of the nervous system allows it to remodel in response to normalization of function and diminution of pain resulting from even temporary interruption of the pain cycle.
6. **Somatic blocks.** Patients in whom suboptimal pain relief is obtained with the above modalities may have an important nonsympathetic component to their pain and hence may benefit from somatic blocks. For them, continuous infusions may be considered, either directly into the relevant plexus or the epidural space. Again, this procedure is often used to facilitate physical therapy, so it is crucial to coordinate the modalities with respect to timing and technique. For example, lower concentrations of anesthetic (0.125% to 0.25% rather than 0.5% bupivacaine) to mini-

mize motor block are used if active exercises are to be undertaken following the block.

7. **Oral adrenergic receptor antagonist.** α-Adrenergic blockers (prazosin, phentolamine, phenoxybenzamine, terazosin) have been reported to be useful, although no controlled trials have been performed. Side effects include hypotension, reflex tachycardia, and impaired sexual function. β-Adrenergic blockers (with concern for their well-known side effects) may be used to treat the reflex tachycardia or occasionally alone (propranolol).
8. **Clonidine.** Clonidine decreases norepinehrine release through its agonist effect on inhibitory α_2-autoreceptors. Oral, transdermal, and epidural routes have been recommended. Aside from its potential to decrease peripheral catecholamines, it is also anxiolytic through a central effect. Hypotension and sedation are major side effects.
9. **Anticonvulsants.** Carbamazepine (Tegretol) has been used for RSD. Although carbamazepine has been extensively studied in neuropathic pain, it is difficult to use because of its narrow therapeutic margin, profile of side effects (most notably central nervous system, liver, and blood; rarely, syndrome of inappropriate secretion of antidiuretic hormone, or SIADH), and myriad drug interactions (it is a potent enzyme inducer). Its quinidine-like properties must be remembered in patients with heart disease who are taking anti-arrythmics and related compounds. Gabapentin (Neurontin) is a more recently introduced anticonvulsant that does not have these disadvantages but has not been as extensively used in the treatment of pain. Phenytoin and valproate have been used. As is typical for RSD, reports are anecdotal.
10. **Antidepressants.** It should be noted that tricyclic antidepressants, which may be used to treat depression and relieve pain while also leading to a transient increase in norepinephrine, may cause a decrease in norepinephrine turnover and hence be considered sympatholytic. Indications for their use in RSD include treatment of depression, insomnia, and pain *per se.* A fuller description of their use in depression may be found in Chapter 49. Tricyclics have been shown to be effective in neuropathic pain, with amitriptyline being the most frequently prescribed agent. The dosages for pain are usually but not always lower (25 to 75 mg) than those for depression (150 mg and higher); their effects are also evident more quickly (days rather than weeks). Even at these lower doses, side effects, including orthostatic hypotension, anticholinergic actions, and electrocardiographic (quinidine-like) abnormalities, make these drugs problematic. The sedative effects of amitriptyline and doxepin may be helpful with regard to sleep. The selective serotonin receptor inhibitors [Zoloft (sertraline hydrochloride), Prozac (fluoxetine hydrochloride), and Paxil (paroxetine hydrochloride)] are easier to use and hence are first-line drugs in the treatment of depression. However, their efficacy in the treatment of pain has not been as well demonstrated as that of the tricyclics. Trazodone (Desyrel), a heterocyclic antidepressant, is advocated by some because of its sedative effects and because it is a potent α-adrenergic blocker. However, it may cause severe gastrointestinal distress, hypotension, and rarely priapism.

F. Corticosteroids. The use of corticosteroids is controversial. Advocates claim that they are especially useful when joint involvement is prominent or bone scans show increased uptake. One protocol consists of 4 days of 60, 40, 30, 20, 15, 10 (in divided doses for the first six doses), and 5 mg. Relapsers may be re-treated with low-dose steroids or a second tapering course with the above doses but with 8 days at each dose. The risks of steroids, particularly the 8-day schedule, must be carefully considered in the light of the paucity of controlled trials regarding their benefit. There have been reports of benefit from regional IV corticosteroids.

G. Miscellaneous. Calcium channel blockers such as nifedipine (10 to 30 mg three times daily) were beneficial in one uncontrolled trial in 7 of 11 patients.

Presumably they act by reducing vascular myogenic hyperactivity. Calcitonin has been given, based on the marked degree of osteoporosis in some stages of RSD. Thus, it has been suggested that calcitonin would be particularly useful in the presence of marked bony changes or increased hydroxyproline excretion. Human recombinant calcitonin (0.5 to 1 g daily) is a first-line treatment in many European centers. Some advocates feel that intranasal calcitonin is markedly less effective.

Note: Although oral preparations of local anesthetic agents have been suggested, they are associated with potentially dangerous side effects and cannot be generally recommended.

H. Surgery. Surgery may be required in patients with RSD, but only for carefully defined indications, as there is no such thing as "minor" surgery. These patients have already demonstrated a diathesis for overreaction to injury, and in some cases, it was surgery that led to their RSD. However, under certain circumstances, surgery is indicated. As RSD resolves, it becomes evident that a previously obscured mechanical problem requires surgical correction, or that deformities (requiring capsulotomy, tenolysis) have arisen as a sequela of the RSD. Alternatively, mechanical pain triggers or triggers resulting from nerve injuries, including neuromas and nerve compression, may develop as a sequela of fibrosis and edema and serve to perpetuate the pain cycle. In the case of deformities and mechanical derangements, surgery should be delayed until the RSD is in remission. However, pain triggers will perpetuate RSD and must be addressed as soon as the treatment team is convinced that the RSD has plateaued and further improvement is unlikely to occur unless the pain triggers are addressed.

Surgery should be performed under sympathetic blockade, with particular attention to hemostasis and avoidance of mechanical stress on nerves. Postoperative pain control and elevation are critical, but a tourniquet effect from the overly zealous use of splints and casting should be avoided. Exercises (especially stress-loading exercises) should be started as soon as possible.

I. "Refractory" reflex sympathetic dystrophy. Potentially treatable, unrecognized causes of RSD, such as occult infection and triggers, must be identified and addressed. The potential contribution of secondary gain and associated noncompliance, in which the site is purposefully subjected to harmful stressors and even frank self-mutilation may be involved, also must be considered. Although amputation is fortunately rarely necessary and unpredictably useful in refractory cases, all too often it is associated with recurrence of RSD in the stump and poor tolerance of prosthesis or phantom limb pain. Neurosurgical interventions for pain, such as peripheral nerve stimulation and even cord or thalamic stimulation, may be successful.

VIII. Reflex sympathetic dystrophy of the knee is described in a separate section because until recently it was insufficiently appreciated and rarely considered. It may present as unexpectedly severe knee pain on walking and weight bearing and stiffness and temperature sensitivity following minor injuries (including falls, "sprains," or dashboard injuries). Vasomotor signs may be subtle. There may be relatively little limitation of motion, and gait disturbances are variable. The patellofemoral joint is invariably involved, and tenderness of the medial aspect of patellofemoral joint and medial capsule are characteristic. It has been suggested that severe knee pain and edema without effusions and mechanical allodynia along the margins of the patella and tibial joint lines either with or without a decreased ROM should alert the clinician to this diagnosis.

On the other hand, patients may present with locking and buckling knees because of mechanical derangements resulting from an injury. These may overshadow the RSD that has also resulted from the injury.

It has been suggested that not infrequently surgery or arthroscopy may be performed in cases of unrecognized RSD. This is liable to exacerbate the condition. On the other hand, RSD may be precipitated by knee surgical procedures ranging from arthroscopy to arthroplasty. It may be a common cause of "stiff knee" following arthroplasty. Prolonged pain (mistaken by the unwary for post-surgical pain but usually differentiated from that by the patient) and a poor response to rehabilitation after surgery are suggestive of RSD. Knee infections, meniscal tears, osteochondritiis dissecans, chondromalacia, and neuroma may be considered in the differential diagnosis of RSD or as precipitants of RSD.

This diagnosis must be considered whenever recovery from trauma or surgery is delayed for an unexpectedly long time. As with any type of RSD, the diagnosis is clinical. Increased uptake on the third phase of the bone scan provides corroborative evidence, but this may occur relatively late in the course. Interestingly, other joints in the lower extremities not infrequently show abnormalities. Osteoporosis develops after several weeks. It is diffuse, does not generally involve joint margins, and is often best seen on a skyline view of the patella. MRI is helpful in excluding other conditions. The role of sympathetic blockade in assessment is similar to its role in RSD affecting other locations. Treatment includes the modalities described above. Standing stress therapy and walking with crutches are frequently useful in patients who cannot tolerate other modalities (e.g., active or assisted active ROM exercises). Arthroscopy should be avoided unless it is required for correction of an underlying mechanical disturbance, and it should be delayed until patient is in remission. Arthroscopy, other surgery, or manipulations that may be required if capsular fibrosis occurs should be performed under the protection of sympathetic blockade.

Bibliography

Cooney, LA. Upper extremity pain dysfunction: somatic and sympathetic disorders. *Hand Clin* 1997.

Kozin F. Reflex sympathetic dystrophy syndrome [Editorial Review]. *Curr Opin Rheumatol* 1994;6:210.

O'Brien SJ, et al. Reflex sympathetic dystrophy of the knee: causes, diagnosis and treatment. *Am J Sports Med* 1995;23:655.

Payne R. Sympathetically maintained pain: diagnosis and treatment. Presented at the annual meeting of the American Academy of Neurology, Boston, April 21–27, 1991.

Pierce PA, Brose WG. Causalgia/reflex sympathetic dystrophy. In: Yaksh T, et al., eds. *Anesthesia: biologic foundations.* Philadelphia: Lippincott–Raven Publishers, 1998:889.

Portenoy RK. Issues in the management of neuropathic pain. In: Basbaum A, Besson JM, eds. *Towards a new pharmacotherapy of pain.* New York: John:Wiley and Sons, 1989.

Schwartzman RJ, McLellan TL. Reflex sympathetic dystrophy: a review. *Arch Neurol* 1987;44:555.

[illegible]

[illegible]

[illegible]

[illegible]

[illegible]

[illegible]

[illegible]

IV. ORTHOPEDIC SURGERY AND REHABILITATION: PRINCIPLES AND PRACTICE

54. PROSTHETIC JOINT REPLACEMENT

Harry E. Figgie, III

I. Definitions

A. Total joint arthroplasty consists of resecting a damaged joint and replacing the articulating surfaces with prosthetic components. The convex side is usually a titanium or chrome cobalt alloy that articulates with a concave surface made of high-density polyethylene. The polyethylene component is usually reinforced by a metal tray consisting of titanium or chrome cobalt alloy. Traditionally, polymethylmethacrylate bone cement has been used as a grout between the implant and the bone. This material provides fixation by filling the irregular interstices of the bone and closely contacting the prosthetic surfaces. Recent prosthetic designs and technology have allowed the prosthesis to be attached to the bone without cement. The efficacy and long-term durability of uncemented fixation in total joint replacement are not yet known.

B. Resection arthroplasty consists of excision of the damaged joint for pain relief or control of infection. Stability and motion are achieved by the scar tissue that grows between the bone ends.

C. Interposition arthroplasty consists of excision of the damaged joint and interposition of a biologic or foreign nonarticular material between two bones. Commonly interposed materials have included fascia, muscle, or silicone spacers. Relief of pain is the primary goal. Motion and stability are variable depending on the joint involved and the material used.

D. Arthrodesis or fusion is obtained by denuding the articular cartilage and shaping the subchondral bone to maximize bone-to-bone contact. The process of fusion is similar to the healing of a fracture. When solid bony fusion is achieved, no motion is possible.

II. Reconstructive alternatives. The optimal artificial joint must allow for a stable, pain-free, functional arc of motion. Additionally, its expected longevity should be adequate with regard to material properties and security of fixation. In general, the performance of the more common types of joint replacement is superior to that of resection arthroplasty, interposition arthroplasty, or arthrodesis.

A. Arthrodesis. In arthrodesis, the elimination of joint motion places abnormal stresses on the joint above and below the fusion and on the contralateral extremity. In addition, arthrodesis may be difficult to achieve when metaphyseal bone loss is present. Fusion is used predominantly as salvage for a failed arthroplasty of the knee and primarily in the ankle, wrist, and hip.

B. Resection arthroplasty or intraposition arthroplasty has provided unpredictable pain relief, motion, and stability. It has been virtually abandoned in the knee and hip, except in salvage procedures, and is used most commonly in the wrist, carpometacarpal joint of the thumb, metacarpophalangeal joints of the hands, and metatarsophalangeal joints of the feet.

C. Total joint replacement usually provides a stable, pain-free, functional arc of motion. Joint replacements of the hip and knee provide the most predictable results and have demonstrated adequate performance for more than 10 years. A small percentage of patients will require reoperation after 10 years, usually for loosening of prosthetic fixation.

III. Indications for total joint replacement are severe, unremitting pain with loss of joint function in the presence of radiographic evidence of articular damage. The degree of joint dysfunction is evaluated by using one of several quantitative scoring systems with numeric grades for preoperative pain, motion, stability, and activity levels. Postoperatively, the same system can be used to evaluate the degree and durability of improvement.

IV. Contraindications to total joint replacement

A. Absolute contraindications. Active local or remote sepsis.

B. Relative contraindications

1. Neurologic disorders, including hemiparesis, parkinsonism, and Charcot's joint.
2. Technical considerations
   - **a.** Severe loss of bone stock.
   - **b.** Poor soft-tissue coverage.
   - **c.** Multiple revision procedures.
3. Systemic illness precluding elective surgery.
4. Nutritional factors.

V. Expected benefits

A. Pain relief. Replacement arthroplasty has given excellent pain relief, and this is the primary indication for surgery in all joints.

B. Motion. Range of motion following arthroplasty is closely related to the preoperative arc of motion.

C. Stability is related to the joint being replaced, type of prosthesis used, amount of bone resected, and the degree to which periarticular ligaments are preserved and balanced.

VI. Complications

A. Systemic complications include the risks of general or regional anesthesia, myocardial infarction, pneumonia, and urinary tract infection.

B. Joint-specific complications

1. **Deep venous thrombosis.** With regard to the hip and knee, the incidence of deep venous thrombosis may be as high as 60%. Pulmonary embolism occurs in 1% to 4% of cases and is the leading cause of mortality following elective total joint arthroplasty. Some form of anticoagulation is indicated in most patients undergoing total hip or total knee arthroplasty, but the type, duration, and time of initiation of the anticoagulation regimen remain controversial.
2. **Infection**
   - **a. Acute infection** results from bacterial inoculation of the wound at the time of surgery. This is treated with either open debridement, irrigation, and closure over drains or removal of the prosthesis followed by antibiotic administration in preparation for reimplantation. Appropriate parenteral antibiotic therapy depends on obtaining accurate culture and sensitivity reports and adequate blood levels of the antibiotic selected.
   - **b. Late infection** that occurs 6 to 12 months postoperatively most likely arises from the hematogenous spread of bacteria from a site of active infection to the prosthesis. The most common sources of such a bacteremia are the genitourinary tract, colorectum, teeth, and skin. Late infection usually results in prosthetic removal and either immediate exchange with use of an antibiotic-impregnated cement or delayed exchange following parenteral antibiotic therapy.

VII. Joint replacement in the lower extremity. It is necessary to evaluate the status of all joints of a lower extremity when replacement of one of them is planned. Correcting one problem may create another (e.g., correcting a valgus knee may accentuate a fixed varus ankle deformity).

A. Total hip replacement is the procedure with the most predictable and reliable results. A metal femoral component is anchored into the femoral canal with acrylic cement, and a polyethylene acetabular component is similarly fixed into the acetabulum. Newer techniques utilizing an uncemented prosthesis rely on tissue ingrowth into irregularities in the prosthetic surfaces for fixation. The efficacy of tissue ingrowth in preventing late loosening, which is the most common problem encountered with cemented implants, is not yet known.

B. Total knee replacement utilizes polyethylene tibial and patellar components and metal femoral components that are either cemented or uncemented. Recent reports of long-term follow-up in cemented implants have shown knee replacement to be as predictable and reliable as total hip replacement, although technically more difficult. Close attention must be paid to alignment and ligamentous balancing during this procedure. Depending on the degree of deformity and ligamentous laxity or contracture, varying degrees of linkage between the tibial and femoral components may be selected in different prosthetic systems. In general, a completely constrained hinged implant will create high torsional stresses at the interface between prosthesis and bone and, therefore, will have unacceptably high rates of loosening or failure of prosthetic material. In most cases, less constrained systems are used that depend on either ligaments or augmented prosthetic surfaces for stability.

C. **Total ankle replacement** has a limited application. It is useful in a patient with severe arthritis of both ankles and subtalar joints, when an ankle fusion would be severely disabling. Ankle replacement usually provides an arc of motion at the ankle that allows a more physiologic gait cycle than would a fusion.

Because of the high loads that cross the relatively thin components and cement, loosening may be a problem. This technically difficult procedure is reserved primarily for less active patients with polyarticular arthritis.

VIII. **Joint replacement in the upper extremity.** Planning any joint replacement in an upper extremity must be directed at relieving pain and providing a functional hand. When several joints in the upper extremity are involved, the wrist and hand should receive primary attention, unless severe pain demands the replacement of a more proximal joint first.

A. **Total wrist replacement** usually provides a functional range of motion in addition to pain relief. It is therefore superior to arthrodesis from a functional standpoint, but its long-term efficacy has not been proved. The high loads that cross the small prosthesis are capable of causing loosening in the cemented replacements or excessive wear debris and secondary synovitis in silicone interposition arthroplasty. If a patient is active and expects to perform significant manual labor, an arthrodesis is the treatment of choice.

B. **Finger implant arthroplasty.** Silicone interposition arthroplasty has been used successfully at the metacarpophalangeal joints in arthritic patients.

Pain relief, functional motion, and good stability may be obtained routinely provided the preoperative deformity is not too great and that **functioning muscle-tendon units are still operative.** Recent advances in cemented arthroplasty of small joints have made possible the replacement of proximal interphalangeal joints, but the surgical results have not been evaluated during a long-enough period to demonstrate a clear and long-lasting advantage over arthrodesis.

C. **Total elbow replacement.** The elbow is an especially complex joint because of its crucial role in moving the hand in space throughout a wide range and the requirements for stability that are placed on it. Loads of up to six times one's body weight cross the elbow during the activities of daily living. An arthritic elbow can be severely painful and stiff and, in some cases, unstable. This presents significant disability to a patient with polyarticular rheumatoid arthritis who uses a cane or crutches. Replacement of the elbow joint is a technically demanding procedure that may produce significant, long-lasting relief of pain in a relatively inactive patient. The linked prostheses have built-in stability against varus-valgus stress and can be used in severe joint deformity. Minimally constrained surface replacements require the integrity of ligamentous structures around the elbow for success.

D. **Total shoulder replacement.** The replacement of the humeral head with a stemmed metallic prosthesis and the glenoid with a polyethylene component provides the arthritic patient with relief of pain and, in many cases, restores a functional range of glenohumeral motion. Postoperative range of motion is largely determined by the preoperative condition of the rotator cuff. Therefore, rheumatoid patients with atrophic cuffs are less likely to gain significant motion than are patients with posttraumatic arthritis or avascular necrosis of the humeral head.

55. PERIOPERATIVE CARE IN THE RHEUMATIC DISEASE PATIENT

C. Ronald MacKenzie and Nigel Sharrock

Patients with chronic rheumatologic diseases such as rheumatoid arthritis frequently require orthopedic surgery in the course of their illness. Therefore, the internist or rheumatologist will often be called on to evaluate patients in this setting. This chapter reviews the basic concepts that underlie perioperative medical management, emphasizing problems that are relatively specific to the rheumatic disease patient.

The goals of preoperative medical evaluation and perioperative care are to (a) identify comorbid conditions that might affect surgical and anesthetic decision making or influence preoperative and postoperative care, (b) stratify patients according to surgical risk, and (c) identify potential postoperative problems that can be addressed before surgery to reduce the likelihood of their occurrence.

I. **Preoperative evaluation** should take place, whenever possible, in the office setting several weeks *before* the surgical procedure. This allows sufficient time for discussion with other physicians involved in the patient's care, further investigation or consultation, and the institution of therapy directed at optimizing the patient's status before the anticipated surgery. It should serve as a focal point for communication between all the members of the medical team who will be caring for the patient.

   There is no consensus regarding what constitutes an optimal preoperative medical evaluation, and the specific needs of a given patient will depend on a variety of factors, including the patient's age, comorbidities, and the type of anesthesia and surgery being planned. Practical guidelines have been suggested and provide a useful framework from which to approach such evaluations.

   A. **History and physical examination.** Except for young patients and those undergoing minor surgical procedures, patients with rheumatic disease should provide the physician with a complete medical history and undergo a physical examination before surgery.

   B. **Laboratory studies.** Although it has never been demonstrated that preoperative laboratory testing improves surgical outcome, a number of investigations seem appropriate for patients undergoing major surgery. These include a complete blood cell count, urinalysis, measurement of electrolytes, biochemical profile, a basic evaluation of clotting (in selected patients), and a urine culture in patients undergoing joint arthroplasty. A 12-lead electrocardiogram and chest radiograph are also helpful, particularly in the elderly and those undergoing major surgery.

II. **Assessment of risk.** The primary purpose of the preoperative medical evaluation is the identification of patients at high risk for postoperative complications. Although the standard clinical examination remains the best screening method for the detection of diseases likely to affect surgical outcome, rating systems do exist that have proved useful in predicting which patients are most likely to have a complicated postoperative course.

   A. The best known of these is the **American Society of Anesthesiologists (ASA) Physical Status Scale,** which is based on the presence of a systemic disturbance designated as absent (I), mild (II), moderate (III), severe (IV), or virtually certain to cause death (V); the subdesignation *E* denotes emergency surgery. This system, which has been in widespread use for more than 30 years, has demonstrated a high correlation with a patient's postoperative course.

   B. A second system, which focuses primarily on the risk for cardiac complications after surgery, is the **Goldman Cardiac Risk Index.** Table 55-1 presents the specific risk factors, their relative contribution to the overall index, and the corresponding rates of serious postoperative morbidity and mortality according to the total index score.

Table 55-1. Goldman cardiac risk index

Risk factor	Points
S_3 gallop, jugular venous distension	11
Previous myocardial infarction(<6 mo)	10
Premature ventricular contractions (>5/min)	7
Atrial dysrhythmias, rhythm other than sinus	7
Age >70 y	5
Emergency surgery	4
Severe aortic stenosis	3
Poor general condition	3
Intraperitoneal or intrathoracic surgery	3

No. points	Life-threatening complications (%)	Cardiac deaths (%)
0–5	0.7	0.2
6–12	5	2
13–25	11	2
>26	22	56

III. Anesthesia in patients with rheumatic disease. A variety of issues, including airway considerations, the site and anticipated duration of surgery, existing comorbidity, and the patient's emotional state, are important determinants of the type of anesthesia to be used, whether invasive monitoring will be necessary, and the length of time the patient will spend in a recovery room after surgery.

A. Type of anesthesia. Both general and regional anesthesia is commonly used in the surgical treatment of patients with rheumatic disease. General anesthesia with endotracheal intubation may present a particular danger in patients with rheumatoid arthritis or ankylosing spondylitis (see section **V**). In patients with cervical spinal instability or a rigid airway, fiberoptic intubation may be required. Regional anesthesia may take the form of limited local anesthesia for minor procedures, peripheral nerve block for surgery of the upper and lower extremity, and epidural/spinal anesthesia for arthroplasty in the lower extremity.

B. Monitoring techniques. Patients undergoing major surgical procedures should have continuous electrocardiographic and pulse oximeter monitoring intraoperatively. At the discretion of the anesthesiologist, arterial and Swan-Ganz catheter monitoring may be helpful in selected patients. Such monitoring is often employed in patients undergoing bilateral joint replacement surgery and in those with a history of prior cardiac disease.

C. Postoperative analgesia. A number of options exist for the control of postoperative pain, including the traditional IV or IM routes (systemic) versus the administration of epidural analgesia. Patient-controlled analgesia via an epidural route of administration is a very effective method of pain control postoperatively and often facilitates postoperative physical therapy, which is important in the restoration of range of motion in patients undergoing orthopedic surgery. This technique also reduces the systemic absorption of analgesics, thereby minimizing the problems of narcotic-induced respiratory depression. New, parenterally administered nonsteroidal antiinflammatory agents such as ketorolac are a useful alternative to traditional analgesia after surgery and can be used to reduce narcotic requirements after major surgery. These drugs should not be given to patients with the common contraindications to nonsteroidal antiinflammatory drugs (i.e., peptic ulcer disease, concomitant use of anticoagulants, renal disease).

IV. Considerations pertaining to specific chronic conditions

A. Hypertension. The preoperative evaluation should determine whether end-organ damage (cardiac, neurologic, renal) is present, as this would increase the risk of surgery. Blood pressure should be measured with the patient lying down and in a sitting position to determine the maximal orthostatic fall in blood pressure and the degree of control. Patients are then classified as untreated, hypertensive controlled on medication, or hypertensive despite therapy.

1. **Risk of surgery.** Controversy exists about whether mild to moderate hypertension increases the risk of surgery. However, patients whose blood pressure is above this range likely are at greater risk and should be stabilized with antihypertensive therapy before surgery.
2. **Drug therapy.** Patients on antihypertensive therapy should continue their medication through the morning of surgery, and it should be restarted postoperatively as soon as they resume oral intake. After surgery, owing to bed rest and fluid losses, some patients may temporarily require less antihypertensive medication.

   Generally, patients taking long-term antihypertensive therapy should be maintained on their medications up to the time of surgery. A cautionary note regarding two medications is required. In the rare patient taking guanethidine or a monoamine oxidase inhibitor, these medications must be discontinued and replaced with other antihypertensive agents several weeks before surgery, as they may cause a marked lability in the blood pressure during or following anesthesia.

B. Ischemic heart disease

1. **Risk of surgery.** Patients with ischemic heart disease undergoing surgery are at greater risk for perioperative myocardial infarction. This risk is significantly greater in patients with a recent infarction. Stable angina pectoris is not thought to increase the risk of surgery, but unstable angina does. A prior myocardial infarction also increases risk, particularly if the infarction has occurred 3 to 6 months before the surgery. Patients who have undergone coronary revascularization have a substantially lower risk for postoperative myocardial infarction. A number of factors contribute to the risk for postoperative death, including decompensated congestive heart failure, arrhythmias, and obstructive lung disease.
2. **Preoperative testing.** The precise role of stress testing, nuclear scanning, and ambulatory electrocardiography in the preoperative setting is not clear. Such testing may be helpful in selected patients, and a decision regarding their utility can be reached in conjunction with cardiology consultation. Nonetheless, patients with unstable angina or a recent myocardial infarction should not undergo elective surgery until their risk can be modified with appropriate medical and surgical management.
3. **Drug therapy.** For patients taking long-acting nitrates, the drug should be given on the morning of surgery; cutaneous nitrate preparations can be continued postoperatively until the patient resumes oral intake. Likewise, beta blockers and calcium channel blockers should be restarted as soon as possible postoperatively. Decisions to give cardioactive and vasoactive medication on the day of surgery should be fully discussed and sanctioned by the anesthesiologist.
4. **Postoperative testing.** Postoperative surveillance for the development of cardiac ischemia or myocardial infarction is required for patients at high risk for these complications. Although creatine kinase levels are usually elevated in these patients because of the muscle trauma associated with surgery, serial electrocardiograms and determination of creatine kinase isoenzymes are useful in the detection of interval ischemia.

C. Congestive heart failure. Patients with decompensated congestive heart failure and, to a lesser extent, those with a history of cardiac failure are at greatest risk in the postoperative setting. Therefore, it is important to assess the patient's intravascular volume status, and elective surgery should be postponed until any existing cardiac failure is controlled. Patients should be maintained on their usual program of medications, including diuretics and ACE inhibitors, throughout the perioperative period. Digitalization before surgery is reasonable in patients with a known congestive cardiomyopathy, and in patients with a history of atrial fibrillation.

D. Valvular heart disease. The risks of surgery in patients with valvular heart disease depend on the valve affected and on the nature and severity of the valvular lesion. Hemodynamically significant aortic stenosis is the most serious lesion, followed by hypertrophic cardiomyopathy (the latter being considered a relative contraindication to epidural or spinal anesthesia). Mild to moderate mitral lesions or aortic insufficiency is usually well tolerated, although hemodynamically significant valvular disease (New York Heart Association class 3 or 4) of any type creates major risks. When it is present, cardiology consultation and monitoring from 13 to 48 hours is prudent.

E. Pulmonary disease. Chronic obstructive lung disease and asthma are the two forms of pulmonary disease seen most frequently in the preoperative setting.

1. **Risk of surgery.** The risk of pulmonary complications can be attributed to various factors, both pulmonary and nonpulmonary. Minor pulmonary complications (atelectasis, bronchitis) are increased in patients who smoke or who have chronic cough or abnormal spirometry values. However, the risk for severe postoperative pulmonary complications (pneumonia, respiratory failure) is increased mainly in those patients with marked impairment in lung function (FEV_1 <1.5 L). Among the nonpulmonary factors that contribute to the risk for postoperative complications are age, obesity, longer duration of anesthesia, excessive sedation, poor patient effort, and the type of surgery. Respiratory dysfunction is less severe after orthopedic than after intraabdominal or thoracic surgery.
2. **Bronchodilator therapy.** Patients who are taking bronchodilators on a long-term basis before surgery should be given their standard dose the night before surgery, and bronchodilator therapy should be administered postoperatively either systemically or by nebulizer.
3. **Incentive spirometry and mobilization** are helpful in preventing postoperative atelectasis or pneumonia.

G. Endocrine disease

1. **Diabetes.** The most important endocrine disorder encountered in surgical patients is diabetes mellitus. Diabetics appear to be at slightly greater risk for postoperative death, likely because of the greater prevalence of ischemic heart disease in these patients. Several reports also suggest that diabetics with autonomic insufficiency (manifested by postural hypotension, impotence, nocturnal diarrhea) may be at risk for sudden cardiopulmonary arrest postoperatively. Numerous regimens for the management of diabetics in the perioperative setting have been reported. A common method is to give one-half of the patient's usual morning dose of NPH (neutral protamine Hagedorn) on the morning of surgery together with 5% dextrose.

   Supplemental short-acting insulin is then given as dictated by daily fingerstick determination of blood sugars. This approach can be continued until the patient resumes oral intake. For patients on oral hypoglycemic agents, these medications can be taken the day before surgery and resumed when the patient is eating. Chlorpropamide (Diabinese), because of its long half-life, should be discontinued 2 to 3 days before surgery.
2. **Patients on corticosteroids.** A relatively common problem in rheumatic disease patients on long-term corticosteroid therapy who are undergoing surgery is prophylaxis against adrenal insufficiency. Patients believed to be at increased risk in this regard include those currently taking a pharmacologic dose of corticosteroid (>20 to 30 mg of hydrocortisone daily, >5 mg of prednisone), those who have taken such doses for longer than 2 weeks in the preceding year, and those who are receiving replacement corticosteroid therapy for known adrenal insufficiency. Such patients undergoing major surgical procedures should receive their usual steroid dose by mouth the day before surgery. **On the day of surgery,** 100 mg of hydrocortisone should be given IV in the early morning, with a second 100-mg dose administered intraoperatively. Postoperatively, 100 mg is given IV q8h for 24 hours, followed the next day by 50 mg q8h, and on the third day by a single IV dose of 100 mg. At this point, the patient's usual daily dose can be reinstituted. In

patients undergoing relatively minor procedures (i.e., surgery of the distal extremities or those requiring only regional or local anesthesia), either the usual dose in a sip of water or a single preoperative dose of 100 mg of hydrocortisone IV is sufficient coverage.

G. Gastrointestinal disease. Gastrointestinal problems, both acute and chronic, may result in significant morbidity in the postoperative period.

1. **Peptic ulcer disease,** a common condition in rheumatic disease patients, may be exacerbated during the perioperative period and is particularly problematic in the arthroplasty patient who is to be placed on prophylactic anticoagulant therapy after surgery. Therefore, patients with a history of peptic ulcer disease, gastrointestinal bleeding, or active symptoms of dyspepsia should receive prophylactic histamine$_2$ blocker therapy throughout the postoperative period. If clinical suspicion is strong that an active peptic process is ongoing, the surgery should be canceled, a workup performed, and treatment instituted before the surgery is undertaken. In patients at risk for the development of gastrointestinal bleeding after surgery, serial stool guaiac tests are a good approach to surveillance.
2. **Inflammatory bowel disease,** an occasional accompaniment to rheumatic disease, poses nutritional problems and also increases the risk for postoperative ileus. Preoperative dietary consultation should be obtained if such patients continue appropriate medications. Postoperatively, the resumption of the patient's oral intake should be careful and slow.
3. **History of diverticulitis.**
4. **Patients with chronic constipation.** Narcotics taken for pain relief after surgery will greatly aggravate bowel motility in this setting.

H. Genitourinary conditions. Because of the effects of bed rest, the use of narcotics and epidural anesthesia, or the presence of prostatic disease, urinary catheters are frequently placed in patients after major joint and back surgery. Such catheters frequently remain *in situ* for up to 48 hours after surgery, increasing the risk for urinary tract infection. Urinary catheters should be removed at the earliest possible time after surgery and a surveillance urine culture performed to rule out the development of a urinary tract infection. Prostatic disease leading to urinary outflow obstruction is a common problem in men after orthopedic surgery. In patients with significant symptomatology, a urologic consultation should be obtained before surgery and therapy (including transurethral resection of the prostate) instituted if deemed necessary. In patients with nephrolithiasis, dehydration should be rigorously avoided to avoid the development of acute renal colic.

I. Infection. The risk for infection in a prosthetic joint is of great concern in patients undergoing total joint arthroplasty. Therefore, assiduous efforts directed at the detection and prevention of any infectious process are of the utmost importance in these patients. The skin and urinary tract are sites of specific concern, and infection can be ruled out by a careful physical examination and routine preoperative urine culture. In addition, a formal dental consultation may be appropriate in patients with poor oral hygiene and dentition. Appropriate local and antibiotic therapy should be completed before surgery is performed.

J. Neurologic problems

1. **Confusional states.** As a result of a variety of factors arising in the perioperative setting (e.g., sedatives, analgesics, anesthesia, fever, metabolic derangements, the disorienting effects of an unfamiliar environment), elderly patients and those with a history of central nervous dysfunction (e.g., parkinsonism) are particularly prone to the development of confusional states after surgery. Although these are usually a transient phenomenon and multifactorial in etiology, the investigative approach to this problem should focus on the detection and treatment of correctable causes such as metabolic disturbances (hyponatremia, hypoxemia) and infection, the discontinuation of possible offending medications, and the treatment of acute conditions (e.g., respiratory failure, myocardial infarction, cardiac

arrhythmias, congestive heart failure, pulmonary and fat embolism syndrome). Occasionally, a formal neurologic consultation and workup are necessary, although the results are generally unrevealing.

2. **Neuropraxias** arise particularly after surgery of the upper and lower extremities. These are generally a compression-related phenomenon resulting from prolonged positioning of the extremity during surgery or casting. All persons involved in the postoperative care of orthopedic patients must keep this problem in mind, as early detection is critical to the ultimate recovery of nerve function. Patients with antecedent subclinical neuropathy are prone to the development of these lesions following surgery. Peroneal nerve palsy may occur following complex knee surgery (valgus deformity) and sciatic nerve palsy after revision or complex total hip replacement.

V. Specific clinical problems

A. The rheumatoid neck. Some rheumatoid patients with sufficiently severe joint destruction to necessitate hip or knee replacement surgery may also have significant involvement of the cervical spine. Atlanto-axial or subaxial subluxation should be ruled out on flexion-extension films in patients with neck pain or crepitus on range of motion, radicular symptoms, or arm or leg weakness. These patients are at increased risk for cord compression during intubation or during uncontrolled neck movement while being positioned for surgery. All such lesions should be well-defined preoperatively and discussed with the anesthesiologist and surgeon. These patients should wear a soft cervical collar in the operating room for immobilization and to warn all involved in their care not to manipulate the neck excessively. If possible, epidural or spinal anesthesia should be used.

B. The spondylitic patient. Patients with ankylosing spondylitis may have spinal or peripheral joint involvement and may require surgical intervention in the course of their illness. A variety of problems may arise, primarily as a result of severe spinal involvement. Patients with a rigid or ankylosed cervical spine may present the most challenging cases of endotracheal intubation to anesthesiologists. Fiberoptic techniques can be helpful, even mandatory, in these patients. If the patients are rigid and osteoporotic, there is a risk for spinal fracture and paraplegia with uncontrolled movement. In addition, restrictive lung disease often arises as a consequence of thoracic spinal involvement and increases the potential for postoperative pulmonary complications. Aggressive pulmonary toilet is mandatory in patients with anklyosing spondylitis, irrespective of the type of surgery that they are undergoing. A small percentage of these patients may also have underlying aortic valve disease or conduction abnormalities, which can complicate perioperative management.

C. Fat embolism syndrome. Although generally thought to arise more commonly in young trauma patients, fat embolism syndrome is not uncommon after total joint arthroplasty, particularly in patients undergoing simultaneous bilateral procedures. The time of onset may vary, with hemodynamic instability developing almost immediately (presaged by a rise in pulmonary artery pressure as the prosthesis is cemented) or more insidiously during the first 2 to 3 postoperative days. Postoperatively, patients are moderately to severely hypoxemic, may be hypotensive, and, in the case of the elderly, often become confused.

Hematologic abnormalities such as transient thrombocytopenia are commonly seen. Frank adult respiratory distress syndrome may develop and become life-threatening. Treatment includes the administration of increased concentrations of inspired oxygen (possibly intubation), prevention of pulmonary hypertension by fluid restriction, use of diuretics and venodilators, and prevention of pain. The use of corticosteroid therapy is not recommended. In high-risk circumstances (i.e., patients undergoing bilateral total joint arthroplasty, those with preexisting cardiopulmonary dysfunction), pulmonary artery catheterization for 24 to 48 hours can be helpful to guide therapy. If the pulmonary artery diastolic pressure is maintained at below 20 mm Hg, respiratory insufficiency is usually prevented.

D. Prophylaxis for thromboembolic disease. The prevention of thromboembolic problems after orthopedic surgery has been extensively investigated clinically, and numerous protocols have documented efficacy. Epidural anesthesia has been demonstrated to reduce markedly the rate of proximal deep venous thrombosis (10% vs. 25%) after total hip replacement; the beneficial effect following total knee replacement in comparison with general anesthesia is less certain. Likewise, pneumatic compression stockings, low-dose warfarin (prothrombin time in the range of 14 to 16 seconds), an international normalized ratio 1.5 to 2 times normal, and adjusted-dose heparin have all been reported to prevent venous thrombosis in patients undergoing total joint arthroplasty. Aspirin *alone* is of questionable efficacy but is useful when combined with other modalities such as pneumatic compression devices or pneumatic compression plus epidural anesthesia in total hip replacement. An alternative approach is to perform venography on the fifth to seventh postoperative day and treat only those patients with evidence of deep venous thrombosis.

E. Integument

1. **Rheumatic disease.** Either as a result of therapy or as a manifestation of the underlying rheumatic disease, skin integrity may be compromised in these patients. In addition to the delayed wound healing and a propensity to infection that may result from chronic corticosteroid and immunosuppressive therapy, an even greater problem in the postoperative period is the potential for the development of decubitus ulceration (particularly heels and buttocks).

   The early institution of measures to combat the development of decubitus ulcers is vital to an uncomplicated postoperative course. Above all, we should strive to prevent bedsores so that we do not have to expend effort in treating them.

2. **Scleroderma.** Patients with scleroderma present major challenges both in terms of patient selection for surgery and in wound healing. Whether the use of local or systemic vasodilators plays a short-term role in the maintenance of blood flow to the skin is uncertain.

F. Immunosuppressive therapy. Although few data exist to guide recommendations for immunosuppressive therapy in the perioperative setting, the issue frequently arises in patients taking methotrexate and other immunosuppressive agents. Whether such agents increase the potential for infection or delay wound healing is uncertain, but it seems prudent to discontinue such therapy 1 to 2 weeks before surgery and restart approximately 1 to 2 weeks postoperatively. Acute disease flares resulting from the abrupt discontinuation of antiinflammatory therapy can usually be managed with a short course of corticosteroids.

G. Eye

1. **Medication.** In general, patients taking long-term ophthalmic medication should have their eye drops instilled before surgery, especially if prolonged surgery is anticipated. The one exception to this recommendation involves the use of phosphodiesterase inhibitors in the treatment of glaucoma. These agents may prolong the action of the neuromuscular blocker succinylcholine. This is particularly pertinent in patients with Sjögren's syndrome, who require artificial tears to prevent perioperative conjunctival injury.
2. **Risk for injury.** Patients in the prone position are at risk for sustaining ocular injury secondary to external pressure. Patients with underlying vasculitis of the optic vessels are at particular risk for ischemic injury to the eye.

56. PHYSICAL THERAPY

Sandy B. Ganz and Louis L. Harris

Management of the physical therapy of patients with musculoskeletal and rheumatic diseases is a challenging task, even for the most astute clinician.

I. The **goals of physical therapy** in the treatment of patients with rheumatic diseases are fourfold:
   - **A.** Preventing disability.
   - **B.** Restoring function.
   - **C.** Relieving pain.
   - **D.** Educating the patient.

II. **Evaluation.** Before these goals can be achieved, a thorough physical therapy evaluation is performed, which includes the following:
   - **A. Functional assessment**
     - **1. Bed mobility.** Observe the patient
       - **a.** Turn over from a supine position to the side and then to a prone position.
       - **b.** Move up and down in bed.
       - **c.** Move from a supine to a sitting position.
     - **2. Transfer status.** Observe the patient transfer to and from various surfaces (i.e., bed, chair, and toilet).
     - **3. Gait analysis**
       - **a. Observational.** Watch the patient ambulate with or without assistive devices on level surfaces and stairs.
       - **b. Instrumented,** with a foot switch stride analyzer or computerized video analysis.
   - **B. Range of motion (ROM) assessment of all joints**
   - **C. Strength assessment**
     - **1.** Manual muscle test of trunk, neck, and proximal and distal muscles to determine weak musculature.
     - **2.** Instrumental biomechanical muscle test.
     - **3.** Isometric/isokinetic objective strength measurement recorded to selected muscle groups performed with an isokinetic dynamometer (i.e., Cybex,[1] Lido[2]).
   - **D. Posture assessment.** Observe the patient both standing and ambulating during functional activities.
   - **E. Respiratory status.** Chest evaluation consists of the following:
     - **1.** Auscultation.
     - **2.** Chest expansion.
     - **3.** Description of cough.
     - **4.** Inspirometry.

III. **Components of treatment.** Once the physical therapy evaluation has been performed, the clinician has baseline data for future comparison and a basis for determining treatment goals. These specific goals are achieved through therapeutic exercise, modalities, functional activities, and perhaps the most important aspect of treatment, patient education (Table 56-1).

IV. **Therapeutic exercise**
   - **A. Goals of exercise**
     - **1.** Maintain or improve ROM.
     - **2.** Strengthen weak muscles.
     - **3.** Increase endurance.
     - **4.** Enhance respiratory efficiency through breathing exercises.

[1] Cybex, Ronkonkoma, NY.
[2] Loredan, Davis, CA.

Table 56-1. Components of treatment in musculoskeletal and rheumatic disorders

Therapeutic exercise	Modalities
Range of motion	Heat
Strengthening	Cold
Endurance	Relaxation
Breathing	Electrotherapy
Massage and mobilization	Hydrotherapy, traction
Functional activities	Patient education
Gait training	Joint protection
Transfer and bed mobility	Home program
Activities of daily living	Body mechanics

5. Improve balance and coordination.
6. Enable joints to function better biomechanically (Table 56-2).

B. **Therapeutic exercises** used in the treatment of musculoskeletal and arthritic conditions are as follows:
1. **Range of motion.** Excursion of a joint through available range.
2. **Passive range of motion (PROM).** Without active muscle contraction about the joint. The joint is moved through available ROM by another person, object, or other extremity.
3. **Active assisted ROM (AAROM).** The patient performs ROM exercises with the assistance of another person, object, or extremity.
4. **Active ROM (AROM).** The patient performs ROM exercises without assistance.
5. **Active resisted ROM (ARROM).** The patient performs ROM exercises with some form of resistance (manual or mechanical resistance, elastic bands, or weights).
6. **Strengthening exercises**
   a. **Static.** Isometric exercises in which the patient contracts or tightens the muscle around the joint without producing any joint motion.
   b. **Dynamic.** Some form of resistance is used, either manually or with an externally applied load (i.e., weight).
      (1) **Isotonic.** Concentric or eccentric contractions of variable speed with use of a set weight or resistance throughout the full ROM.
      (2) **Isokinetic.** A concentric or eccentric contraction at a set speed with use of a set weight or resistance throughout the full ROM.

Table 56-2. Treatment goals

Stages of disease	Treatment goals	Exercise
Acute	Control inflammation	Passive range of motion (PROM)
	Maintain range of motion (ROM)	Active assisted range of motion (AAROM)
	Minimize loss of function	
Subacute	Increase ROM	Active range of motion (AROM)
	Maintain strength	Isometric
Chronic	Increase ROM	AROM
	Increase strength	AAROM
	Increase endurance	Isokinetic
		Aerobic

C. General instructions to patients

1. Use pain as your guide. Pain or discomfort should not last longer than 1 hour after exercise.
2. Make the exercise part of your daily routine.
3. Try to do a complete set of exercises at least twice a day at a time convenient to you.
4. Prescribed medication and applications of heat or cold may precede exercises to enhance relaxation and decrease pain.
5. Perform only those exercises given to you by your physician or therapist.
6. Perform exercises on a firm surface.
7. Exercise slowly with a smooth motion. Do not rush.
8. Avoid holding your breath while exercising.
9. Modify the exercise regimen during an acute attack, and contact your physician or physical therapist if you have any complaints or problems with the exercises.

V. Physical agents (modalities). Various modalities/treatments are employed by the physical therapist, including the application of heat, cold, electrical stimulation, mechanical traction, and mobilization/massage. These are generally provided as an adjunct to a total rehabilitative program.

A. Superficial heating

1. **Hot packs** contain a silica gel that absorbs water. These packs are kept in thermostatically controlled water at 175°F. The literature demonstrates that hot-pack effectiveness reached at a depth of 1 cm increases skin temperature by 10°C.
   a. **Indications.** Relief of pain, muscle spasm, decreased ROM.
   b. **Contraindications.** Sensory involvement, open lesions, malignancy.
2. **Paraffin bath.** Paraffin wax is mixed with mineral oil and maintained at 118° to 126°F. It is most useful in the treatment of hands. The wax mold conforms to the hand and provides heat to all joint surfaces. The heating benefits are similar to those obtained with hot packs.
   a. **Indications.** Relief of pain, muscle spasm, decreased ROM.
   b. **Contraindications.** Sensory involvement, open lesions.
3. **Hydrotherapy** (whirlpool, therapeutic pool). Water is maintained at 94° to 96°F. Coupled with its ability to eliminate the effect of gravity (buoyancy), heated water can provide excellent moist heat and exercise simultaneously. Whirlpools for individual limbs are also beneficial to promote wound cleaning and healing. Hydrotherapy is a related form of heat treatment.
   a. **Indications**
      (1) Muscle spasms, relief of pain, decreased ROM.
      (2) **Whirlpool.** Open lesions.
   b. Contraindications
      (1) Patients with decreased heat tolerance.
      (2) **Therapeutic pool.** Open lesions, urinary tract infection, diarrhea; extreme care should be taken in patients with cardiopulmonary involvement.
4. **Fluidotherapy** is a dry application of heat. A bed of finely ground solids (e.g., glass beads with an average diameter of 0.0165 in.) are blown with thermostatically controlled warm air. This creates a warm, semifluid mixture for treatment of the hand or foot. The temperatures are within the same ranges as the paraffin wax.
   a. **Indications.** Relief of pain, muscle spasm, decreased ROM.
   b. **Contraindications.** Sensory involvement, open lesions.

B. Deep heating: ultrasound. The application of high-frequency sound waves to the musculoskeletal system causes a deep heating response. This response is deeper than that induced by other physical agents, and it has been demonstrated that the intraarticular temperature of the hip joint rises by 1.43°C after a properly applied therapeutic dose. Typical patient exposure is 1 to 2 W/cm^2 for 5 to 10 minutes. Ultrasound can also be combined with electrical stimulation.

1. **Indications.** Pain relief, muscle spasm, and decreased ROM.
2. **Contraindications.** Local malignancy, unstable vertebrae (after laminectomy), pregnancy, spinal cord disease; ultrasound should not be applied directly over the eyes, brain, or spinal cord.

C. **Cold.** Cryotherapy is very effective in promoting vasoconstriction, thus decreasing restricted joint ROM resulting from an inflammatory process and aiding with pain relief. Cold modalities include ice packs, frozen gel packs (cold packs), and ice massage.
1. **Indications.** Swelling and inflammatory reactions, spasms, contusions, traumatic arthritis.
2. **Contraindications.** Decreased sensation, sensitivity to cold, Raynaud's phenomenon.

D. **Mobilization** generally means moving joints, including spinal joints, through an ROM designed to stretch the joint capsule and, in some instances, move the joint beyond the norm of its associated muscles. The technique is primarily used in patients with musculoskeletal pain.
1. **Indications.** Joint hypomobility, decreased proprioception, restriction of accessory joint motion, ligamentous tightness, adhesions, joint dysfunction.
2. **Contraindications.** Ligamentous laxity, unstable joints.

E. **Massage** is a widely practiced modality. It is intended to relieve pain, soft-tissue tightness, and muscle spasm. It is often used in conjunction with heat or cold applications. Other forms of massage include acupressure, connective tissue massage, postural integration (rolling), and deep friction massage.
1. **Indications.** Muscle spasm, decreased extensibility of soft tissues.
2. **Contraindications.** Cellulitis, malignancy, phlebitis.

F. **Electrical stimulation** is one of the oldest and most effective physical agents. Its purpose is to contract or reeducate muscle, relax muscle spasms, stimulate nerves to promote motion and pain relief, and generally improve circulation. A wide range of current types (AC and DC) and a wide variety of electrical generators [low-volt, high-volt, biofeedback, transcutaneous electrical nerve stimulation (TENS)] are available. No individual system or model is ideal for all clinical situations, and the therapist's choice depends on the desired therapeutic response.
1. **Indications.** Muscle reeducation, denervated muscles, pain relief, decreased general circulation, decreased muscle strength during immobilization, decreased ROM.
2. **Contraindications.** Phlebitis, demand pacemakers, hemorrhage, recent fractures.

G. **Mechanical traction.** Intermittent traction is utilized for spinal disorders, generally in conjunction with other modalities. The amount of traction prescribed depends on the area being treated and on the patient's tolerance. Its effectiveness in promoting relaxation through muscle stretching, relieving nerve compression, and relieving pain has been demonstrated. Patients receive intermittent traction two to three times per week on average for 20 minutes.
1. **Indications.** Muscle spasm, mild nerve compression, vertebral osteoarthritis.
2. **Contraindications.** Unstable vertebrae, local malignancy, spinal cord disease, osteoporosis, osteomyelitis, pregnancy.

VI. **General guidelines for rehabilitation of specific rheumatologic disorders and areas of the body**

A. The **systemic rheumatic diseases,** including rheumatoid arthritis, juvenile rheumatoid arthritis, progressive systemic sclerosis, and systemic lupus erythematosus, are characterized by multisystem involvement. All are chronic, remitting, and relapsing with variable clinical courses that result in myriad clinical manifestations. Comprehensive rehabilitative management is necessary in the treatment of such systemic inflammatory diseases. Rest is essential in the management of active inflammatory joint or soft-tissue disease, and the amount of rest versus activity is the subject of extensive debate. Peripheral joint involvement in psoriatic arthritis, Reiter's syndrome, and colitic arthropathies should be treated in a similar manner to that in rheumatoid arthritis and juvenile rheumatoid arthritis, as noted below. The proper balance between rest and exercise is the key for successful treatment.

1. **Aims of treatment**
   - **a.** Preserve or increase functional level.
   - **b.** Decrease pain.
   - **c.** Improve joint mechanics.
   - **d.** Decrease joint inflammation.
   - **e.** Improve ROM, strength, and endurance.
2. **Therapy**
   - **a. Active inflammatory disease**
     - **(1)** Rest
       - **(a)** Systemic (body) rest.
       - **(b)** Articular (joint) rest.
       - **(c)** Emotional rest.
     - **(2)** Joint protection
       - **(a)** Splinting.
       - **(b)** Assistive devices.
       - **(c)** Ambulatory aids.
     - **(3)** Techniques for relaxation and stress reduction.
     - **(4)** Patient education.
   - **b. Pain**
     - **(1)** Superficial heat.
     - **(2)** Cryotherapy.
     - **(3)** TENS.
   - **c. Decreased range of motion**
     - **(1)** PROM.
     - **(2)** AAROM.
     - **(3)** Stretching.
   - **d. Weakness.** Muscle strengthening with the following:
     - **(1)** Isometric.
     - **(2)** Isotonic.
     - **(3)** Isokinetic.
   - **e. Ambulation**
     - **(1)** Ambulatory aid.
     - **(2)** Orthotic.
   - **f. Decreased endurance techniques**
     - **(1)** Energy conservation.
     - **(2)** Aerobic exercise program.
   - **g. Difficulty with activities of daily living (ADL)**
     - **(1)** Adaptive equipment.
     - **(2)** Assistive devices.

B. Spinal and sacroiliac disease in ankylosing spondylitis and other seronegative spondyloarthropathies. Maintenance of an erect posture is critical for all ADL, including sitting, standing, walking, and sleeping. Patients should sleep in a prone or supine position on a firm mattress with one small pillow or no pillow. (Pillows under the knees should be avoided at all times to prevent flexion deformities.) Breathing and chest expansion exercises are extremely important. In addition, stretching exercises that facilitate extension of the neck, spine, and peripheral joints should be taught and diligently followed.

1. **Aims of treatment**
   - **a.** Facilitate skeletal mobility.
   - **b.** Prevent contractures.
2. **Exercises.** Figures 56-1 through 56-7 are examples of appropriate exercises used in the treatment of patients with back involvement in ankylosing spondylitis and other seronegative spondyloarthropathies.

C. Osteoporosis. Weight-bearing activities such as brisk walking, biking, jogging, and working with a selected group of exercise machines can be an effec-

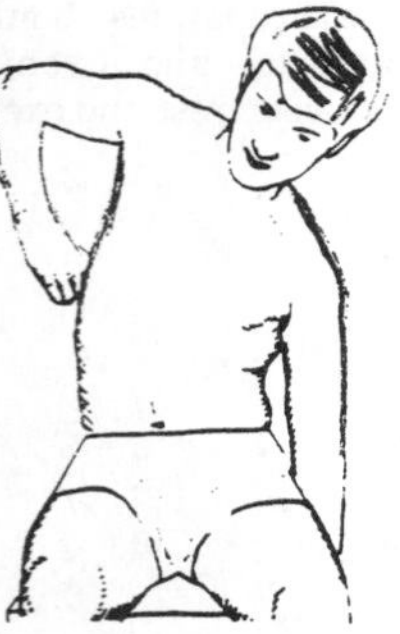

FIG. 56-1. Chest mobilization (inspiration). Bend away from right side during inspiration.

tive way to maintain and strengthen muscles while stimulating bone formation. These types of exercises and activities are referred to as impact-loading or weight-bearing exercises. An exercise program should consist of postural retraining, education in proper body mechanics, deep breathing, stretching, strengthening, and impact-loading activities. Extreme caution should be taken during forward flexion exercises of the spine because of the longer lever arm produced with increased flexion. An osteoporotic vertebral body may not be able to tolerate this load, and compression fracture with wedging may occur.

1. **Aims of treatment**
   - **a.** Strengthen abdominal muscles and extensor musculature of the spine.
   - **b.** Pectoral stretching.
   - **c.** Increase weight-bearing activities of lower extremities.
2. **Exercises.** See Figs. 56-18 through 56-20 for appropriate exercises used in the treatment of patients with osteoporosis.

D. Polymyositis and dermatomyositis. The degree of muscle weakness can be quite variable because muscle destruction during the acute inflammatory phase is variable, as is muscle regeneration during the recovery phase. Patients exhibit difficulty climbing stairs, rising from low surfaces, and performing various aspects of ADL. The emphasis of rehabilitation is on progressive proximal muscle-strengthening exercises. Vigorous and injudicious exercise of any type may be associated with a rise in serum enzyme levels,

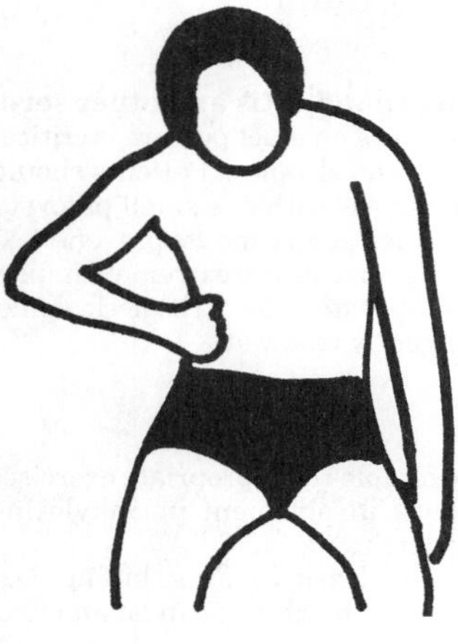

FIG. 56-2. Chest mobilization (expiration). Bend toward right side during expiration. Push fisted hand into the lateral aspect of chest as you bend toward the right side.

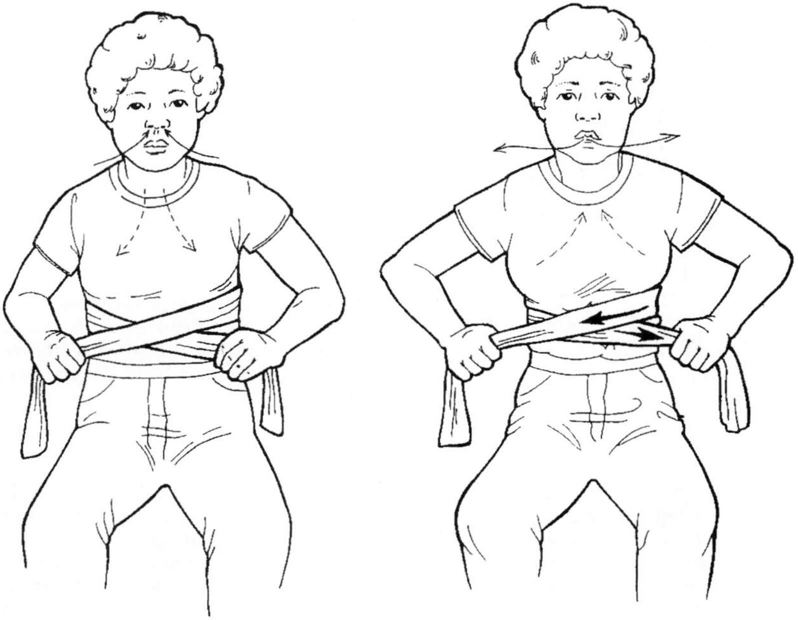

FIG. 56-3. Belt exercises for lateral costal expansion. Reinforce lateral costal expansion during inspiration. Assist with pressure along the rib cage during expiration. (Reprinted from the Saunders Group, Inc. © 1996.)

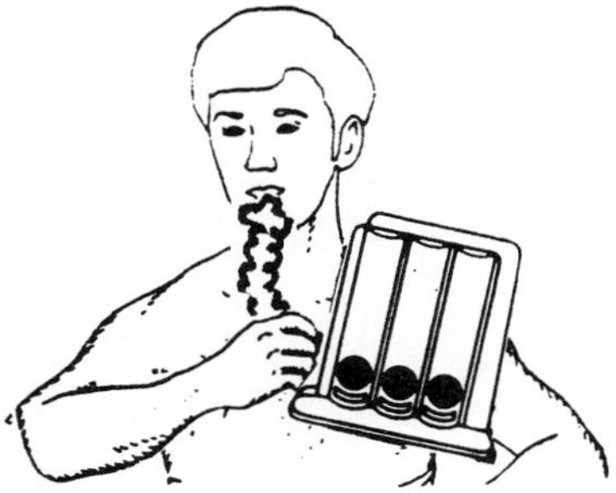

FIG. 56-4. Deep breathing with an incentive inspirometer. For inspiration, use right side up and breathe in. For expiration, use upside down and breathe out.

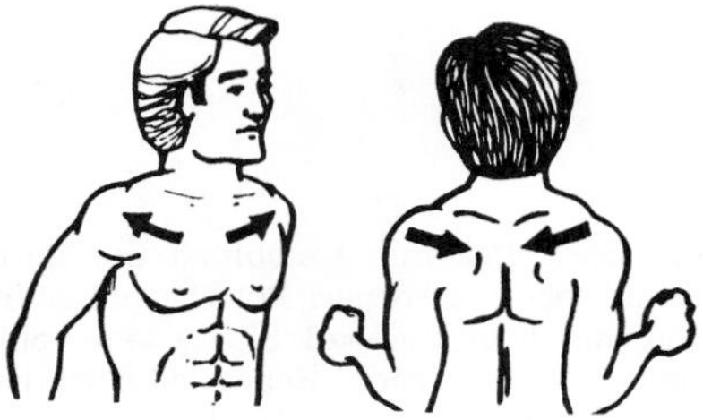

FIG. 56-5. Pectoral stretching (shoulder blade pinch). Stand or sit straight and tall. Pull your shoulders back, squeezing your shoulder blades together.

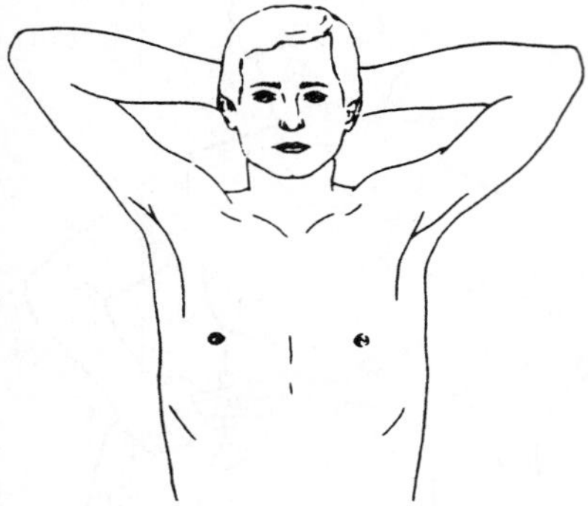

FIG. 56-6. Pectoral stretching (hands behind head). Stand or sit. Place your hands behind your head with elbows in front. Move your elbows back as far as possible.

increased fatigue, and a decrease in function and strength. Therefore, a balance between rest and exercise must be achieved. Overall, disease assessment involves a myositis functional assessment (Appendix 56-1), a biomechanical muscle test with isokinetics (Cybex or Lido), and monitoring of creatinine kinase. Physical therapy management and type of exercise are determined from the results of the above tests. It remains controversial whether exercise should be avoided during an increase in creatine kinase levels or overall disease activity.

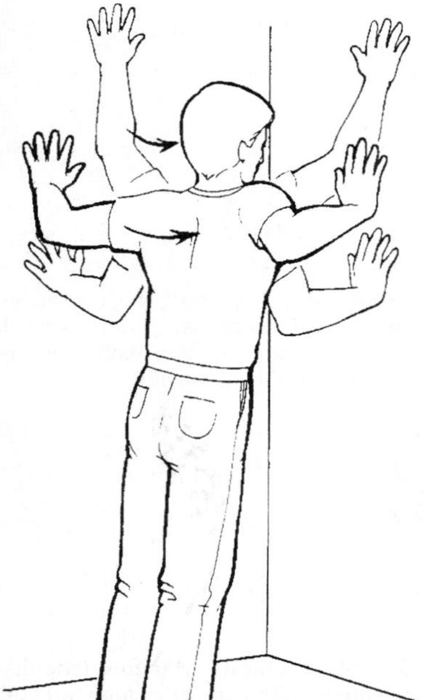

FIG. 56-7. Pectoral stretching (standing). Stand facing a corner. Put the palms of your hands on the wall. Slowly lean your chest into the corner. (Reprinted from the Saunders Group, Inc. © 1996.)

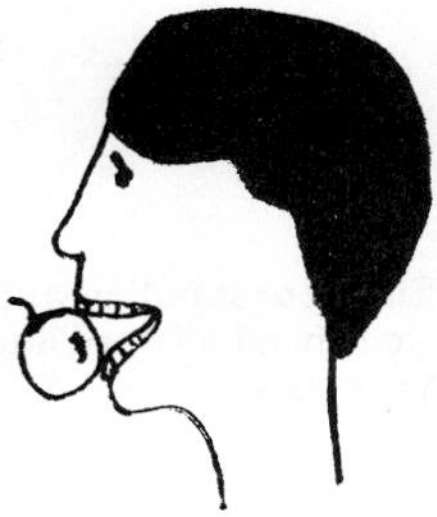

FIG. 56-8. Jaw excursion. Hold an apple in front of your mouth. Gradually open your mouth, sliding your top and bottom teeth on the apple and increasing the jaw's range of motion.

1. **Aims of treatment**
   a. Increase proximal muscle strength.
   b. Improve function.
   c. Decrease pain.
2. **Exercises.** See Figs. 56-10 through 56-17 and 56-23 through 56-32 for appropriate exercises used in the treatment of patients with polymyositis and dermatomyositis.

E. **Scleroderma (progressive systemic sclerosis).** Prevention of joint contractures is the primary goal in the physical therapy management of patients with progressive systemic sclerosis. An ROM program designed to stretch soft-tissue contractures should be instituted immediately. Passive stretching of all joints, soft-tissue mobilization, and massage are highly recommended. In addition, paraffin is used on the hands in an effort to decrease pain and increase finger ROM. Skin tightness around the jaw is extremely common. A series of temporomandibular joint exercises are routinely performed to increase jaw excursion. Deep breathing, use of incentive inspirometer, and mobilization of the chest wall to increase chest expansion should be incorporated into the physical therapy program. To assist with feeding and chewing activities, speech therapy is often instituted.

1. **Aims of treatment**
   a. Increase ROM.
   b. Prevent contractures.
   c. Improve chest expansion.
2. **Exercises.** Figures 56-1 through 56-4, 56-8, and 56-9 are appropriate exercises used in the treatment of progressive systemic sclerosis, in addition to PROM for all joints.

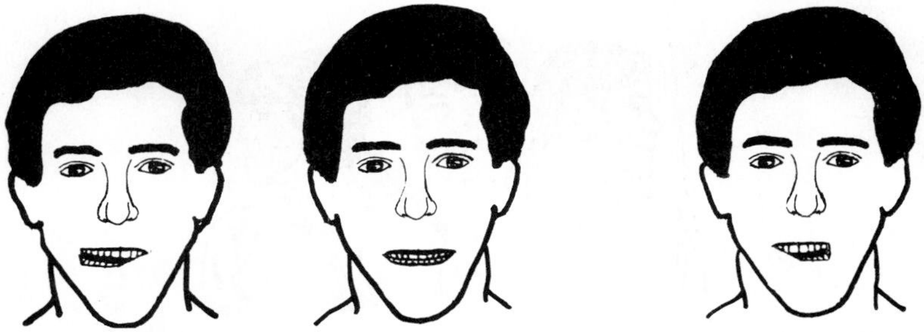

FIG. 56-9. Lateral jaw excursion. Smile so that your top and bottom teeth are touching. Move your mouth from right to left.

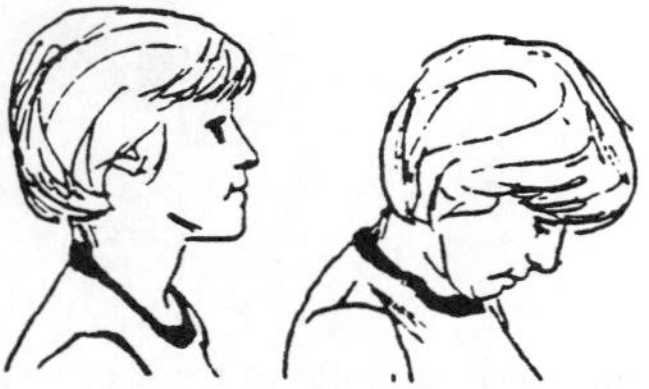

FIG. 56-10. Neck flexion. Sitting or standing with your back straight, bend your head forward and tuck your chin in toward your chest.

F. Neck pain

1. Aims of treatment

a. Promote a decrease in pain.

b. Increase muscle relaxation.

c. Improve head and neck posture.

2. Therapy

a. The **modalities** available to the physical therapist include heat and electrical stimulation.

b. Specific manual mobilization techniques include manual and motorized intermittent cervical traction, which provide muscle and soft-tissue stretching to promote relaxation of the neck and upper back and pain relief.

c. An **exercise program** consisting of gentle active exercises progressing to isometric exercises in the supine position, or with the head supported, are generally beneficial in increasing circulation, decreasing muscular tension, and improving posture. Figures 56-10 through 56-12 are examples of exercises used in the treatment of neck pain.

d. An educational component should also be provided to ensure the following:

(1) Proper postural awareness.

(2) Body mechanics.

(3) Preventive measures, which include an explanation of home or work activities to be avoided or that may contribute to the patient's complaints (e.g., driving, computer terminal/typewriter operation, sleeping postures).

G. Shoulder

1. Aims of treatment

a. Improve joint ROM.

b. Increase muscle strength.

c. Promote a decrease in pain.

2. Therapy

a. Exercise program. An ROM program initially consisting of manual joint mobilization and passive ROM should be instituted. As ROM increases, the patient is instructed in active exercise progressing to a

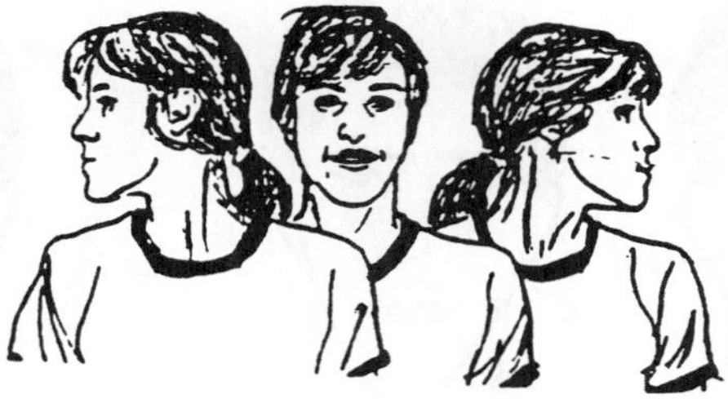

FIG. 56-11. Neck rotation. Sitting or standing with your back straight, tuck your chin in toward your chest. Look over your right shoulder, then over your left shoulder.

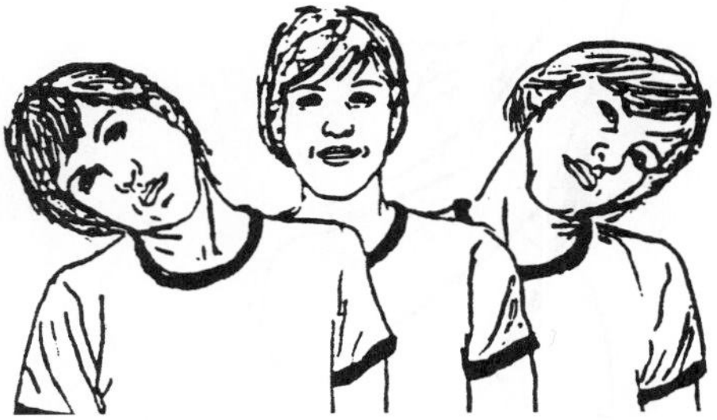

FIG. 56-12. Neck lateral flexion. Sitting or standing with your back straight, tuck your chin in. Bend your head so that your ear is moving toward your shoulder.

strengthening program as tolerated. As the patient progresses, an individual program can be guided by the needs of the patient. Figures 56-13 through 56-17 are examples of exercises used in the treatment of shoulder pain.

b. Physical agents that can be an adjunct to the exercise program are various heat modalities and electrical stimulation to promote a decrease in pain. Cryotherapy may also be utilized following an exercise session to decrease any physiologic response to treatment.

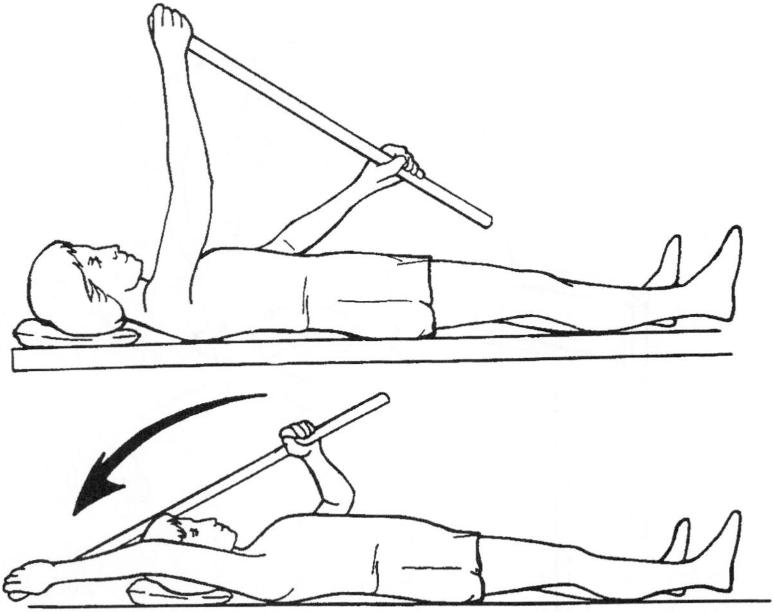

FIG. 56-13. Shoulder flexion. Lie on your back while holding a rod, with one hand at the top and the other near the bottom. Pull the rod back toward your head until your arm holding onto the top is straight. Return to starting position. Switch hands and repeat. (Reprinted from the Saunders Group, Inc. © 1996.)

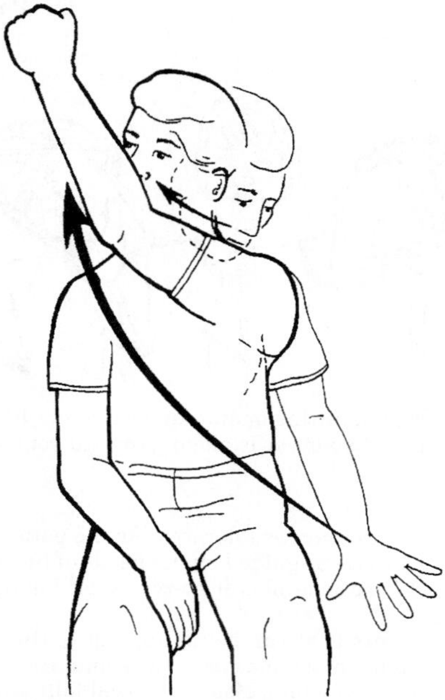

FIG. 56-14. Diagonal shoulder flexion. Keeping your elbow straight, bring your left arm down across your body with your thumb pointing toward your right hip. (Reprinted from the Saunders Group, Inc. © 1996.)

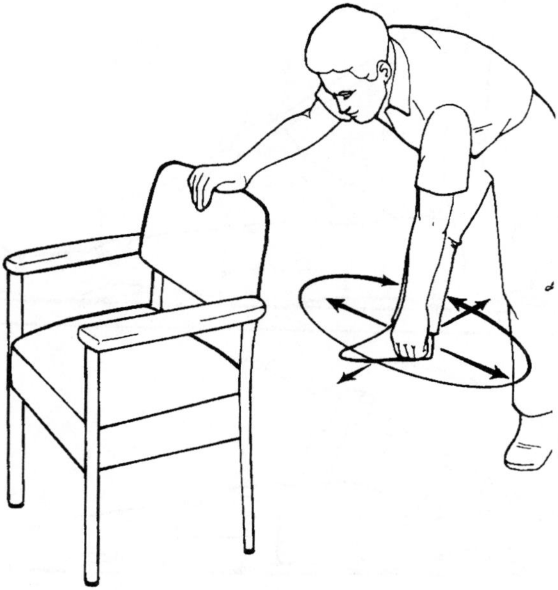

FIG. 56-15. Pendulum exercises. Stand holding onto a sturdy chair with your uninvolved arm. Bend forward at the waist and bend your knees to help protect your back. Let your involved arm hang limp. Keep your shoulder relaxed, and use your body motion to swing your arm in a circle. (Reprinted from the Saunders Group, Inc. © 1996.)

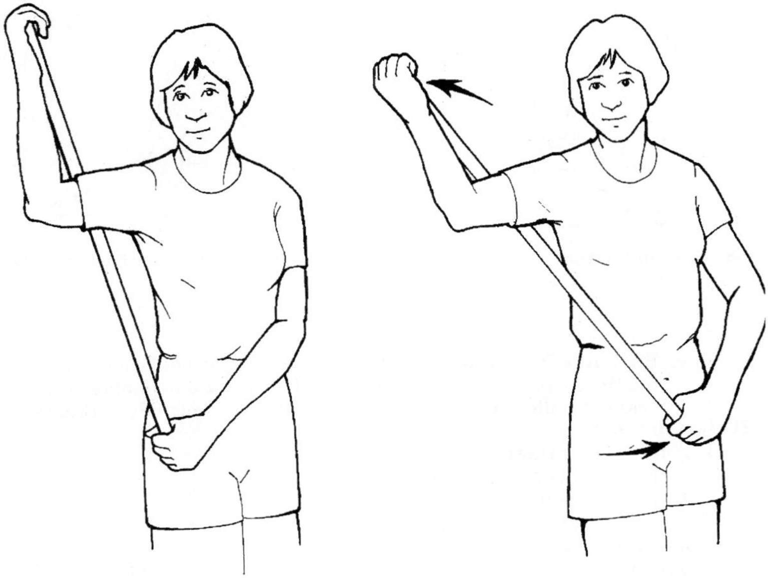

FIG. 56-16. Shoulder rotation exercise. While standing, hold a stick or towel as illustrated, with the uninvolved arm over your shoulder and holding the top and the involved arm holding the bottom. Slowly pull the top of the stick or towel with your uninvolved arm as shown. (Reprinted from the Saunders Group, Inc. © 1996.)

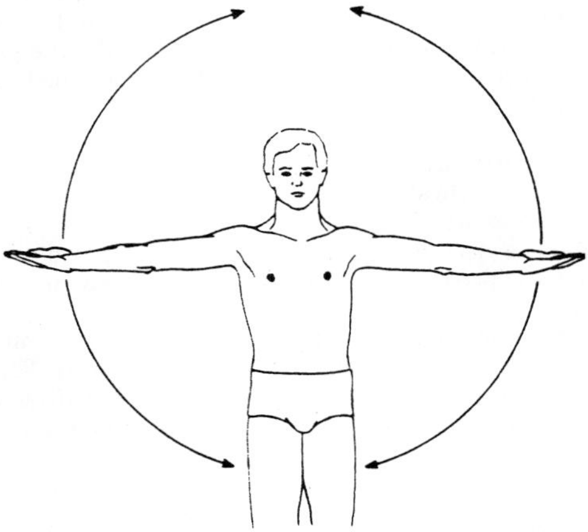

FIG. 56-17. Stand with your arm at your side and palm facing forward. (This can also be done while lying on your back with palm up.) Raise your weak arm out to the side and up toward your ear. Keep your elbow straight and palm facing forward.

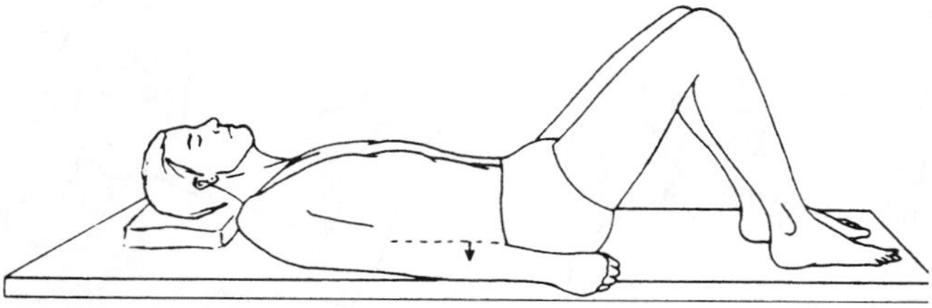

FIG. 56-18. Lying on your back with knees bent, press the small of your back into the bed. Tighten your abdominal and buttock muscles.

c. **Patient education.** It is essential that the patient be educated regarding the goals of physical therapy and be given a daily home exercise program. A pulley system is an excellent device to include in this program.

H. Low back pain

1. Aims of treatment

a. Promote a decrease in pain.
b. Increase muscle relaxation.
c. Strengthen abdominal muscles.
d. Normalize low back joint motion and posture.

2. Therapy

a. Physical agents (modalities) are available that can be incorporated to promote a decrease in pain. These include hot packs, ultrasound, and electrical stimulation. When indicated, passive joint and soft-tissue mobilization are also effective manual techniques to promote further decrease in pain, increase circulation, and aid in restoring normal joint motion.

b. An **exercise program** consists of exercises designed to stretch the pelvis, low back, and hamstrings and to strengthen the abdominal muscles. As the patient progresses, an individualized program can be guided by the patient's tolerance and need. Figures 56-18 through 56-28 are examples of exercises used in the treatment of low back pain.

c. Patient education. To restore function fully, the patient must be educated in preventive measures, including proper body mechanics, posture, and ADL.

I. Hip

1. Aims of treatment

a. Increase muscle strength.
b. Maintain ROM.
c. Promote a decrease in pain. A painful hip usually results in limited motions, which can further produce joint contractures and gait deviations.

2. Therapy

a. Exercise program. The primary emphasis with muscle strengthening is to optimize the extensor and abductor groups. These muscles help to stabilize the joint and normalize gait. ROM activities associated with this strengthening program should concentrate on stretching the hip flexors

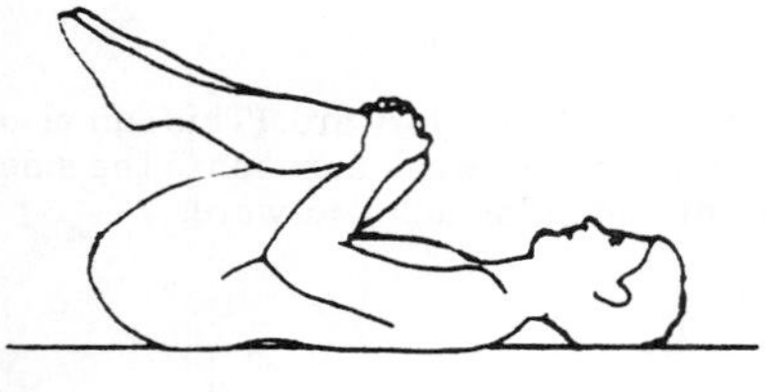

FIG. 56-19. Knees to chest. Lying on your back, slowly bring both knees up to your chest.

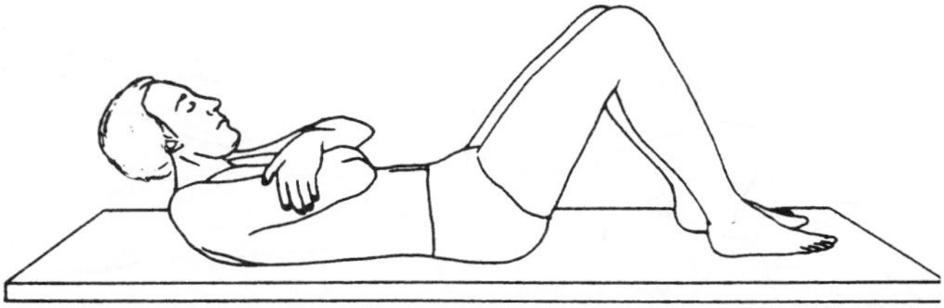

FIG. 56-20. Partial sit-ups. Lie on your back with knees bent and arms crossed. With chin tucked, slowly lift your head and shoulders toward your knees.

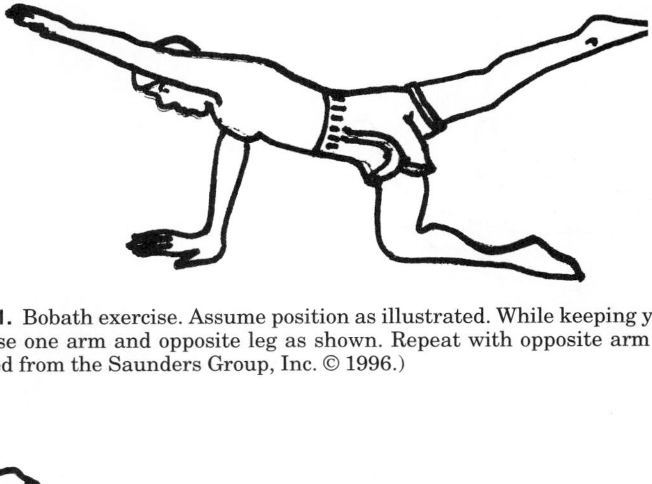

FIG. 56-21. Bobath exercise. Assume position as illustrated. While keeping your back level, raise one arm and opposite leg as shown. Repeat with opposite arm and leg. (Reprinted from the Saunders Group, Inc. © 1996.)

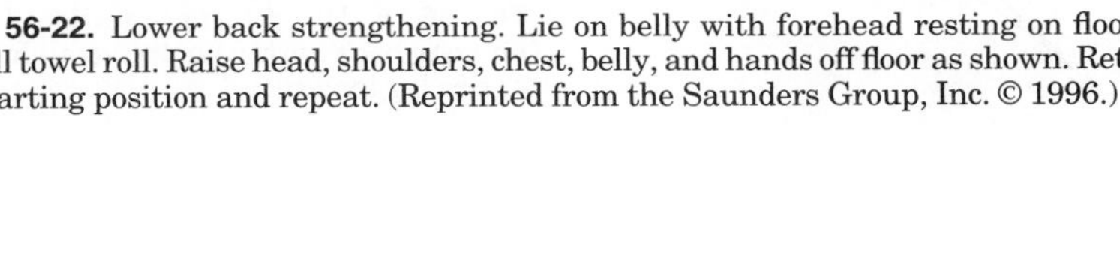

FIG. 56-22. Lower back strengthening. Lie on belly with forehead resting on floor or small towel roll. Raise head, shoulders, chest, belly, and hands off floor as shown. Return to starting position and repeat. (Reprinted from the Saunders Group, Inc. © 1996.)

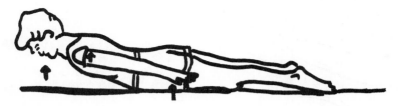

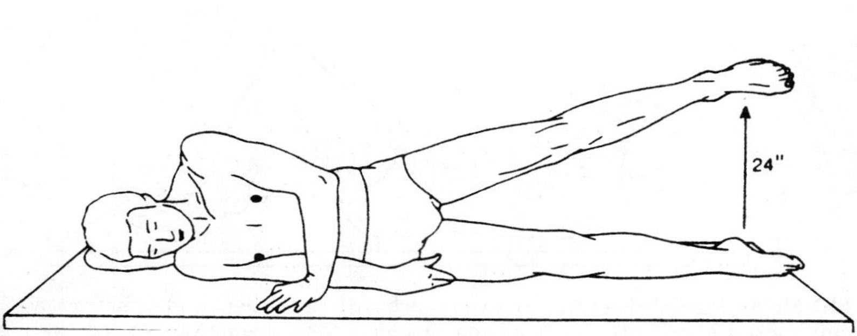

FIG. 56-23. Leg lifts while lying on side. Lie on your side, weak leg on top. The lower leg should be bent to help balance. Keep the top leg straight and in line with your body. Stay on your side and lift your leg up toward the ceiling. Do not bring your leg forward. Slowly lower it.

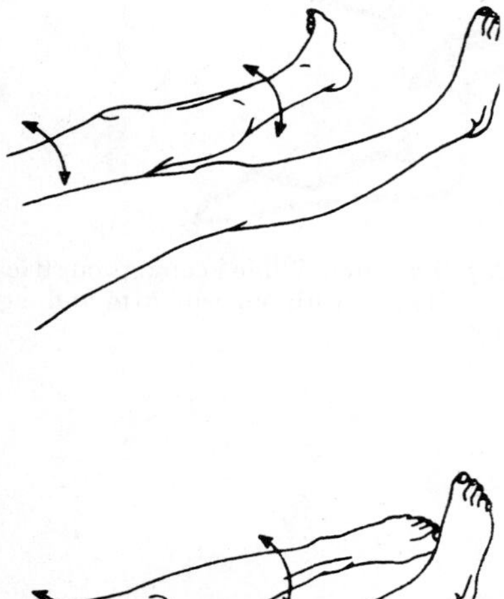

FIG. 56-24. Hip external rotation. Lying on your back with entire leg straight, roll entire leg outward.

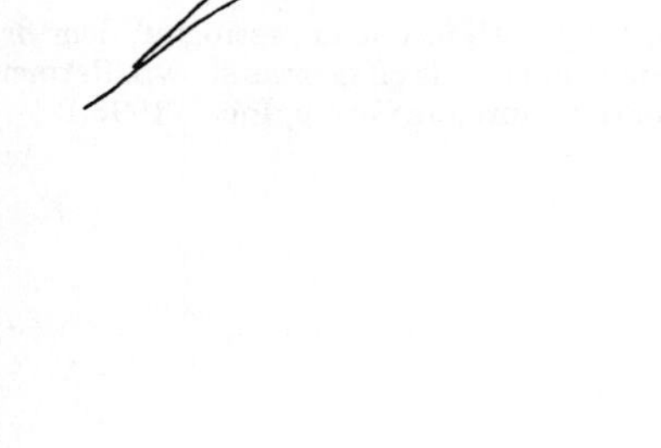

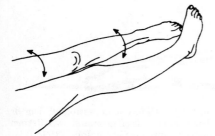

FIG. 56-25. Hip internal rotation. Lying on your back with your leg straight, roll entire leg inward.

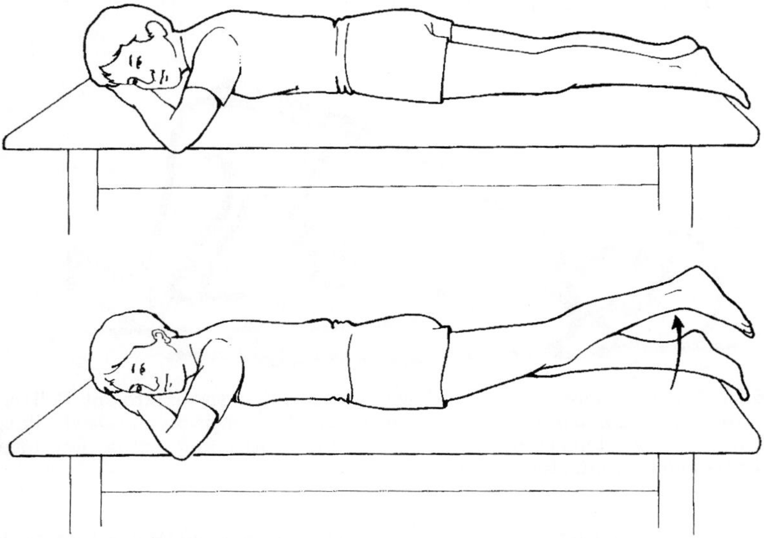

FIG. 56-26. Prone hip extension. Lie on your stomach with both legs straight. Lift one leg up toward the ceiling, keeping your knee straight. Slowly lower it. (Reprinted from the Saunders Group, Inc. © 1996.)

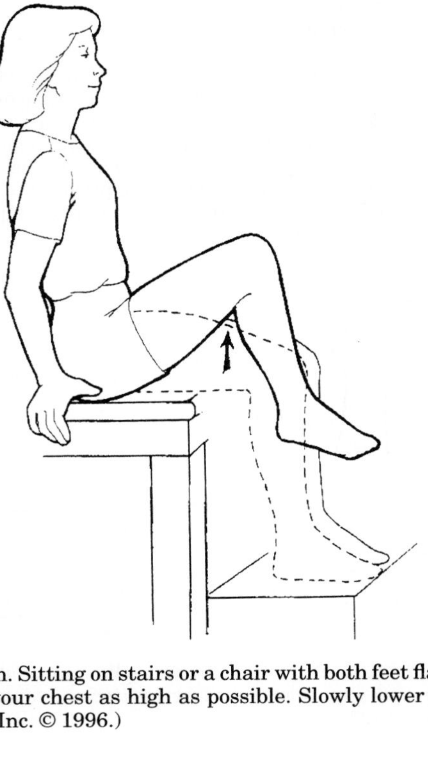

FIG. 56-27. Hip flexion. Sitting on stairs or a chair with both feet flat on the floor, raise one knee up toward your chest as high as possible. Slowly lower it. (Reprinted from the Saunders Group, Inc. © 1996.)

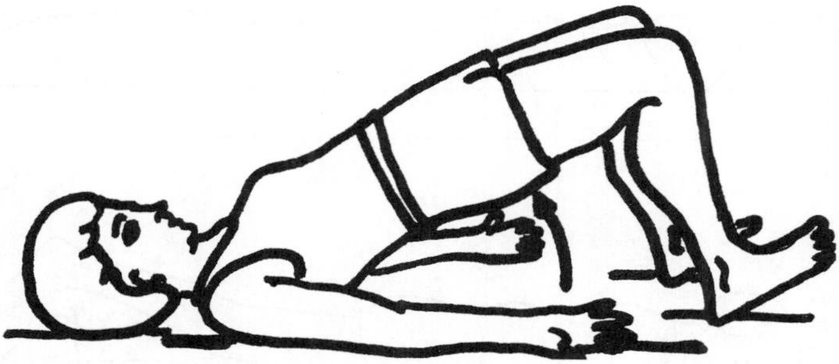

FIG. 56-28. Bridging exercise. Lie on back with knees bent and arms straight. Pull toes up toward the ceiling and push heels into the floor. Tighten buttocks and slowly lift up until hips are fully extended. Return to the starting position and repeat. (Reprinted from the Saunders Group, Inc. © 1996.)

and adductors and ensuring functional rotational ROM. See Figs. 56-23 through 56-28 for examples of exercises used in the treatment of hip pain.

b. **Heat modalities** such as hot packs and ultrasound can be employed to complement the exercise program and promote pain relief.

J. **Knee**

1. **Aims of treatment**
   a. Increase ROM.
   b. Improve muscle strength of the quadriceps and hamstrings.
   c. Normalize ambulation and function.
   d. Promote a decrease in pain.
2. **Therapy**
   a. A **therapeutic exercise program** should be established that concentrates on AROM and AAROM and progresses to muscle strengthening as tolerated. Many resistive exercise programs are available that utilize free weights and various types of exercise equipment. Isometric quadriceps sets and straight leg raising are excellent exercises to initiate quadriceps control, followed by an individualized program to meet the patient's specific needs. Figures 56-29 through 56-32 are examples of exercises used in the treatment of knee pain.

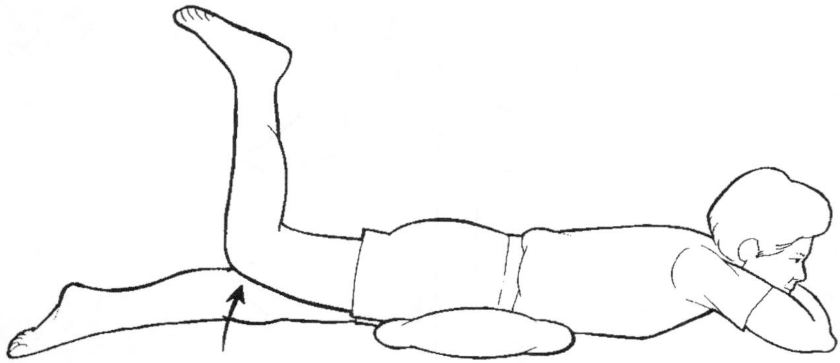

FIG. 56-29. Gluteal contraction. Lying prone, with pillow under abdomen, bend one knee and lift toward ceiling. Slowly lower to starting position and repeat. (Reprinted from the Saunders Group, Inc. © 1996.)

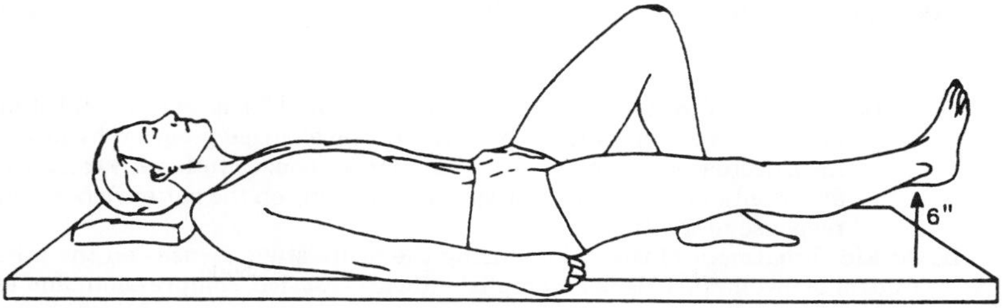

FIG. 56-30. Lie on your back with your weak leg as straight as possible. Bend the other leg as illustrated to protect your back. Tighten your thigh muscle. Raise your leg while keeping it straight. Keep your thigh muscles tight and leg straight as you slowly lower it.

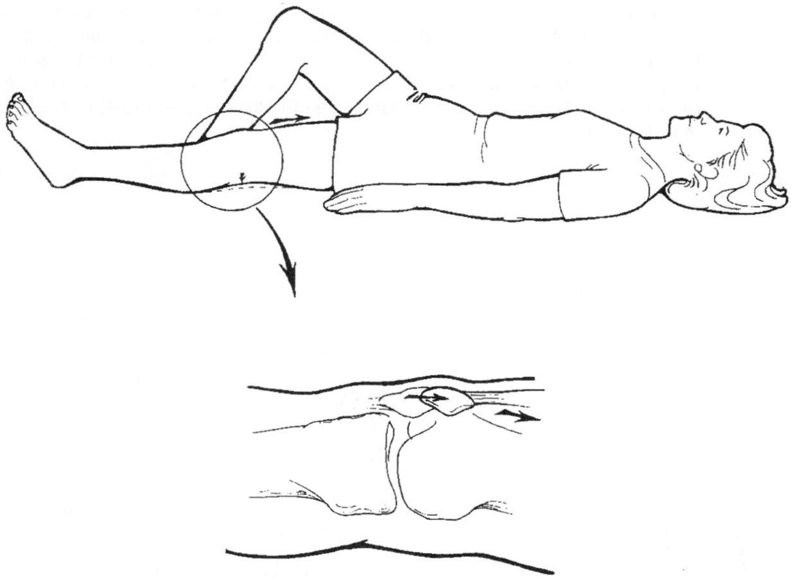

FIG. 56-31. Quad set. Half sitting with your involved leg straight, bend your other leg as illustrated. Tighten the muscles on the top of your thigh. This will make your knee cap move toward your hip. (Reprinted from the Saunders Group, Inc. © 1996.)

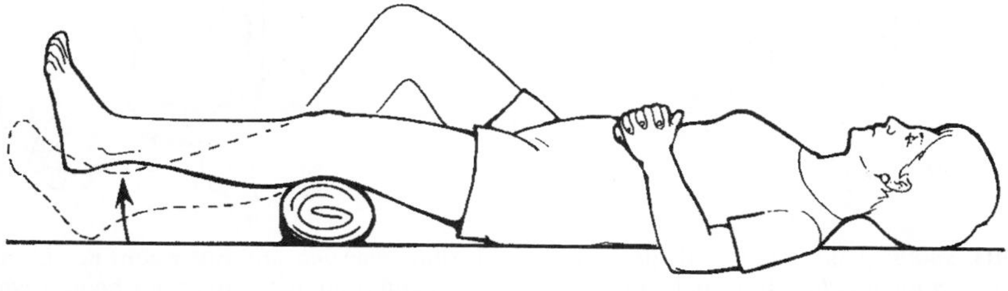

FIG. 56-32. Terminal knee extension. Lying on your back with a firm pillow under your involved knee, slowly lift your foot up. Your knee should remain on the pillow. Try to keep your leg as straight as possible. (Reprinted from the Saunders Group, Inc. © 1996.)

b. **Physical agents.** Various heat modalities and forms of electrical stimulation can be employed to complement the exercise program by promoting a decrease in pain before an exercise session. Cryotherapy can also be an essential part of a total program, depending on the patient's needs and response to treatment.

K. **Ankle.** Treatment of the ankle during the acute stage focuses on the initial control of swelling. This is accomplished with rest, ice, compression, and elevation. If no severe instability is present, the patient may be referred to physical therapy.

1. **Aims of treatment**
   - **a.** Increase muscle strength and function.
   - **b.** Increase and maintain ROM.
   - **c.** Promote a decrease in pain.
   - **d.** Normalize gait.
2. **Therapy.** An isometric program progressing to active resistive exercises encompassing functional and weight-bearing activities is important. These help to improve balance and coordination, and aid in preparing the patient for gait training and normalizing the ankle motion during ambulation. Figures 56-33 through 56-35 are examples of exercises used in the treatment of ankle pain.

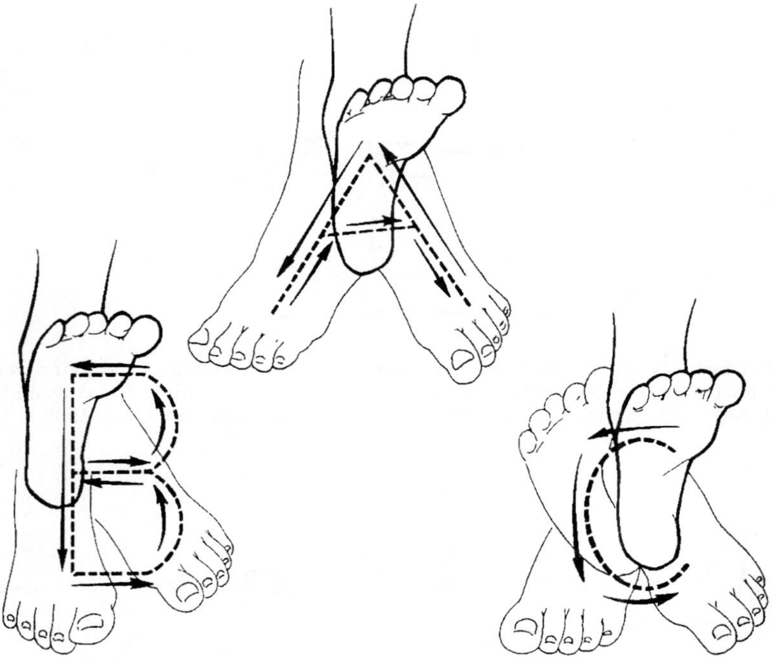

FIG. 56-33. Ankle plantar flexion and dorsiflexion, eversion and inversion. For plantar flexion and dorsiflexion, bring your toes down and then up toward your head. Also, try drawing an imaginary A. For eversion and inversion, push sole inward and then outward. Now, try drawing an imaginary B and C. (Reprinted from the Saunders Group, Inc. © 1996.)

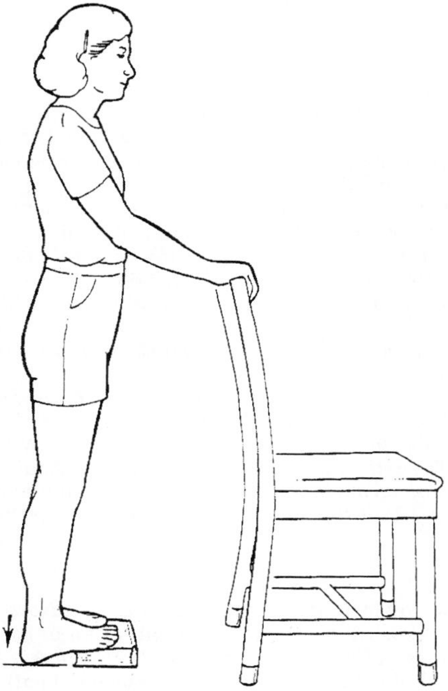

FIG. 56-34. Heel cord stretching. Stand with the ball of your foot on a book. Hold onto a firm chair or surface. Try to place your heel on the floor. Gently lean forward, keeping your knee straight. Hold, then stand on your toes, and return to starting position. (Reprinted from the Saunders Group, Inc. © 1996.)

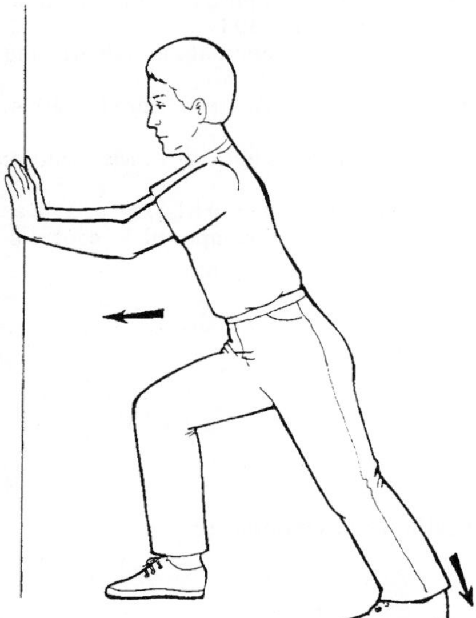

FIG. 56-35. Gastrocnemius (calf) stretch. Stand in front of a wall and bend one leg while keeping the other leg back. Lean forward and push against the wall and you will feel the stretch in your calf muscle, or gastrocnemius. (Reprinted from the Saunders Group, Inc. © 1996.)

Bibliography

Basmajian JV, ed. *Therapeutic exercise.* Baltimore: Williams & Wilkins, 1990.

DeLateur BJ. Therapeutic exercise to develop strength and endurance. In: Kotke FJ, Stillwell GK, Lehmann JF, eds. *Krusen's handbook of physical medicine and rehabilitation,* 3rd ed. Philadelphia: WB Saunders, 1982.

Ganz SB. Physical therapy. In: Spiera H, Oreskes I, eds. *Rheumatology for the health care professional.* St. Louis: Warren H. Green, 1991:210.

Hicks JE, Nicholas JJ, Sweezey RL, eds. *Handbook of rehabilitative rheumatology.* Atlanta: American Rheumatism Association, 1988.

Kahn J. Electrical stimulation. In: *Principles and practices of electrotherapy.* New York: Churchill Livingstone, 1987.

Kisner C, Colby LA. *Therapeutic exercise foundations and techniques.* Philadelphia: FA Davis Co, 1985.

Kotke FJ, Stillwell GK, Lehmann JF, eds. *Krusen's handbook of physical medicine and rehabilitation,* 3rd ed. Philadelphia: WB Saunders, 1982.

Lehmann JF, ed. *Therapeutic heat and cold,* 3rd ed. Baltimore: Williams & Wilkins, 1982.

Loring K, Fries JF. *The arthritis helpbook.* Reading, MA: Addison Wesley, 1986.

Michlovitz SL. *Thermal agents in rehabilitation.* Philadelphia: FA Davis Co, 1990.

Nelson RM, Currier DP. *Clinical electrotherapy.* East Norwalk, CT: Appleton-Century-Crofts, 1987.

Suggested Readings

Banwell BF. Exercise and mobility in arthritis. *Nurs Clin North Am* 1984;19:605.

Ganz SB, Harris LL. General overview of rehabilitation in the rheumatoid patient. Alexiades MM, Ranawat CS, eds. *Rheum Dis Clin North Am* 1998;24:181–201.

Gerber LH, Hicks JE. Rehabilitation in the management of patients with osteoarthritis. In: Moskowitz RW, et al., eds. *Osteoarthritis diagnosis and management.* Philadelphia: WB Saunders, 1984:287.

Hicks JE. Exercise for patients with inflammatory arthritis. *J Musculoskel Med* 1989;6:40.

Hicks JE. Syllabus update for joint and connective tissue disease: scientific basis for the use of exercise for rheumatoid disease. In: *Course supplements,* Annual Meeting of the American Academy of Physical Medicine and Rehabilitation, 1988:39 (vol 1).

Kreindler H, et al. Effects of three exercise protocols on strength of persons with osteoarthritis of the knee. *Top Geriatr Rehabilitation* 1989;4:32.

Minor MA, et al. Efficacy of physical conditioning exercise in patients with rheumatoid arthritis and osteoarthritis. *Arthritis Rheum* 1989;32:1396.

Semble EL, Loeser RF, Wise CM. Therapeutic exercise for rheumatoid arthritis and osteoarthritis. *Semin Arthritis Rheum* 1990;20:32.

Stenstrom CH. Therapeutic exercise in rheumatoid arthritis. *Arthritis Care Res* 1994; 7:190.

Wegener ST, Belza BL, Gall EP, eds. *Clinical care in the rheumatic diseases.* Atlanta: American College of Rheumatology, 1996.

Yelen E, et al. The impact of rheumatoid arthritis and osteoarthritis: the activities of patients with rheumatoid arthritis and osteoarthritis compared to controls. *J Rheumatol* 1987;14:710.

Resources: Arthritis Self-Help Products

1. Adaptability
   P.O. Box 515
   Colchester, CT
   1-800-243-9232
2. Aids for Arthritis, Inc.
   3 Little Knoll Court
   Medford, NJ 08055
3. American College of Rheumatology/Association of Rheumatology
   Health Professionals
   1998 Membership Directory
   Phone: 1-404-633-3777
   Fax: 1-404-633-1870

4. Guide to Independent Living for People with Arthritis
   Arthritis Foundation
   1314 Spring Street, N.W.
   Atlanta, GA 30309
5. Comfortably Yours
   61 West Hunter Avenue
   Maywood, NJ 07607
   1-201-368-0400
6. Enrichments for Better Living
   145 Tower Drive
   P.O. Box 579
   Hinsdale, IL 60521
   1-800-323-5547
7. Maddak, Inc.
   Pequannock, NJ 07440-19932
   1-201-628-7600
   1-800-443-4926
8. The Osteoporosis Book 1993
   (life-style tips for healthy bones)
   Gwen Ellert. Trelle Enterprises
   305-1775 W. 10th Avenue
   Vancouver, British Columbia V6J 2A4, Canada
9. Sammons-Preston
   P.O. Box 32
   Brookfield, IL 60513
   1-800-323-5547

Appendix 56-1

MYOSITIS FUNCTIONAL ASSESSMENT

NAME ___________________ DATE ___________________

THIS FORM IS DESIGNED TO EVALUATE LOWER EXTREMITY FUNCTION IN PATIENTS WITH MYOSITIS. ALL ACTIVITIES SHOULD BE RATED ON THE PATIENT'S ABILITY TO PERFORM A GIVEN TASK WITHOUT THE ASSISTANCE OF THE EXAMINER.

TRANSFER FROM SUPINE TO SITTING (5)

A. (5) Spontaneously, normal; on request, use of upper extremity is not required.
B. (4) Spontaneously, but use of upper extremity is required.
C. (3) Tentatively; use of upper extremity is required.
D. (2) Laboriously; props up on both elbows.
E. (1) Laboriously; rolls to side while lying and pushes to sitting with arms.
F. (0) Unable to assume sitting position.

TRANSFER FROM SITTING TO STANDING (4)

A. (4) Rises from low chair (knees 2 in. higher than hips) without use of arms or compensatory movements.
B. (3) Rises from standard chair (knees level with hips) spontaneously, without use of arms or compensatory movements.
C. (2) Rises from standard chair tentatively; must use arms.
D. (1) Rises from standard chair laboriously; use of upper extremity, compensatory movements, or both are required for transfers.
E. (0) Unable to assume standing posture from a standard chair.

RISING FROM A LOW BENCH (9 in.); to be evaluated only if scored A or B on transfers from sitting to standing (2)

A. (2) Able to sit and rise without difficulty; normal.
B. (1) Able to sit and rise, but with effort or difficulty.
C. (0) Unable to rise from a low bench.

STAIR CLIMBING—four 6-in. steps (14) UP/DOWN

A. (7) (7) Reciprocal (step over step), normal; on request, no use of arms.
B. (6) (6) Reciprocal; on request, no use of arms, but deviations present.
C. (5) (5) Nonreciprocal; on request, no use of arms.
D. (4) (4) Reciprocal; use of one arm is required.
E. (3) (3) Reciprocal; use of two arms is required.
F. (2) (2) Nonreciprocal; use of one arm is required.
G. (1) (1) Nonreciprocal; use of two arms is required.
H. (0) (0) Unable to negotiate stairs.

COMMENTS

____
____
____

57. OCCUPATIONAL THERAPY

Toni Golin

Occupational therapy provides assistance to persons whose functional level of performance has been affected by physical, psychological, or developmental disabilities. The role of occupational therapy in the treatment of rheumatoid arthritis is to improve or maintain the patient's maximum level of functioning. The overall goal of the treatment is to minimize the effects of pain, decreased mobility, and decreased endurance on a person's ability to perform activities of daily living (ADL). To achieve this goal, a variety of strategies are employed to:

1. Maintain or increase range of motion (ROM), strength, and endurance in the upper extremity.
2. Correct and prevent the development or progression of hand deformity.
3. Improve functional abilities in ADL.
4. Explore adaptation or alternatives in vocational or avocational interests.
5. Provide patient education, specifically in the area of joint protection and energy conservation.

I. Evaluation. The first step in treatment is the evaluation. Careful observation of the extremity for heat, redness, edema deformity, pain, and stage of disease process helps determine treatment plans and goals. Active and passive ROM of the upper extremity and muscle strength are evaluated by means of goniometry and individual and functional muscle testing. Objective means of measuring strength include the dynamometer, sphygmomanometer, pinch gauge, and computer-assisted equipment. Based on findings, an exercise program can be prescribed. A hand evaluation is performed to assess grasp and prehension patterns, strength, deformities, and pain. Joint and tendon crepitus, joint stability, tendon integrity, and muscle imbalance should be noted. This information is necessary also when a patient's splinting needs are being determined. An ADL evaluation is performed to determine the patient's past and present ADL skills and level of independence. ADL include feeding, writing, dressing, grooming, hygiene, homemaking, and work-related skills as appropriate. Noted in this evaluation is the ease with which a task is accomplished, any pain associated with performing the task, and potentially deforming stresses to the involved joints.

The goals of exercise are to strengthen muscles and increase ROM and endurance, all of which contribute to an improved overall level of functioning. Modalities such as heat, cryotherapy, paraffin, and fluidotherapy are often used to augment treatment. Active, active assisted, and passive ROM, along with resistive exercises, are employed depending on the amount of disease activity present.

A. In the **acute** stage, when the joints are swollen and inflamed, rest accompanied by splinting is generally indicated. Active and gentle passive ROM is employed to maintain joint mobility. Isometric exercises can be performed. No stretching or resistive exercises are attempted in this phase.

B. In the **subacute** stage, gentle passive stretch and active isotonic exercises with minimal joint stress can be added to the passive or active ROM exercise program. Their purpose is to regain lost active ROM and improve endurance.

C. In the **chronic** stage, stretch at the end of ROM, active ROM, and isometric exercises is employed. Patients are encouraged to maintain general conditioning by performing ADL to tolerance.

II. Splinting is frequently used as part of the treatment program.

A. Indications for splinting include the following:

1. Immobilizing painful, inflamed joints.

2. Preventing contractures by maintaining proper joint alignment.

3. Preventing repetitive stress in a joint during activities.
4. Improving function by increasing support and stability.
5. Maintaining surgical correction.

B. Choice of splints. Static splints contain no moving parts and maintain the affected part in the desired position. Dynamic splints assist movement in specific directions by the application of a nearly constant force. They may utilize hinges, springs, or outriggers with elastic tension. When determining the type of splint to be fabricated for a particular patient, it is important to keep in mind that splints can be awkward to wear. Despite some gains, they somewhat limit function. A functional splint that the patient can easily manage is a wiser choice than a more complicated splint that attempts to accomplish many goals at once but is cumbersome and unmanageable for the patient. Also, immobilization of one joint alters the biomechanical forces in adjacent joints, causing increased stress and possible inflammation.

Common problems that may require splinting, the types of splints used, and the rationale are listed in Table 57-1.

Table 57-1. Common problems requiring splinting

Problem	Type of splint	Splinting effects
Acute wrist synovitis	Volar wrist cock-up (Fig. 57-1)	Provides wrist support while allowing digital movement.
Wrist and hand synovitis	Resting hand splint (Fig. 57-2)	Provides support for wrist, MCP and IP joints, and thumb by resting hand in a functional position. For nighttime use or an acute flare.
Carpal tunnel syndrome	Volar or dorsal wrist cock-up (Fig. 57-1)	Holds wrist in neutral position. Relieves pressure on median nerve. Usually worn at night.
MCP ulna drift	Volar splint with finger separators; splint can incorporate wrist or be hand-based (Fig. 57-3)	Allows hand use while preventing ulnar deviation at the MCP joints.
de Quervain's tenosynovitis	Thumb spica splint (Fig. 57-4)	Restricts wrist deviation and thumb CMC flexion but allows IP flexion and some wrist flexion and extension.
Thumb CMC-MCP synovitis	CMP-MCP stabilizing splint ("shorty" thumb spica) (Fig. 57-5)	Restricts motion at CMC and MCP joints but allows motion at wrist and thumb IP.
Swan neck deformity/ boutonnière	Figure-of-8 or silver ring splint (Fig. 57-6)	Applies three-point pressure to restrict PIP hyperextension and permit or prevent PIP flexion.

MCP, metacarpophalangeal; IP, interphalangeal; CMC, carpometacarpal; PIP, proximal interphalangeal.

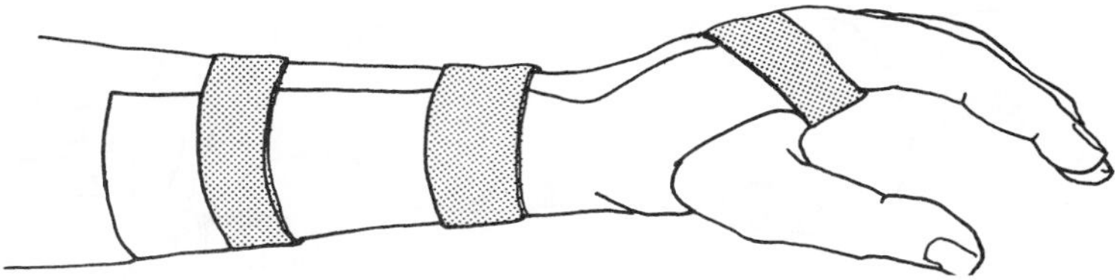

FIG. 57-1. Volar wrist cock-up.

III. Activities of daily living. At any stage of disease, the patient can experience functional limitations resulting from pain, decreased ROM, decreased muscle strength, deformity, or fatigue. ADL treatment includes instruction in alternate methods to perform a task and in the use of assistive devices to maintain independence and preserve joints.

Limited ROM in an upper extremity may make it difficult to bring food to the mouth. Weakness and deformity may make it difficult to manipulate utensils and cut food. Adapted utensils with enlarged or extended handles can compensate for decreased ROM and poor grip. Swivel or curved forks and spoons can compensate for lack of supination and wrist radial deviation. An insulated mug allows a patient to use two hands to bring cup to mouth when weakness or poor pinch is a problem. A long straw can eliminate the need to lift a glass from the table. A universal cuff can be used to hold utensils when hand use is severely limited. Rocker knives and Swedish-design knives make cutting foods easier.

IV. Dressing. Limited ROM in both upper and lower extremities may make it difficult to pull clothing over the head or feet. Poor grip and pinch strength and loss of fine prehension skills create difficulty in zippering, buttoning, and pulling up clothing. A dressing stick can help with putting on and taking off a shirt in cases of shoulder involvement and decreased ROM. A sock aid and a long-handled shoehorn can assist with dressing the lower extremity. A zipper pull and Velcro fasteners to replace buttons or the top button at the neck of a shirt are useful.

V. Bathing. Limitations in ambulation and transfer skills can make getting in and out of the bath or shower hazardous. Loss of strength and range in the upper extremity can make it difficult to reach body parts, manage faucets, and shampoo hair. Grab bars and tub or shower seats can aid in safe transfers. Lever-type faucet handles can replace traditional faucets, or tap-turning devices can be placed on existing faucets when hand strength and ROM are limited. A handheld shower head can be placed on the side of the tub for easy access and can aid in reaching body parts and washing hair.

VI. Homemaking. Reaching into cabinets, holding and opening containers, handling pots and pans, and chopping food are difficult for the person with arthritis. Many labor-saving appliances, such as a food processor, are useful when

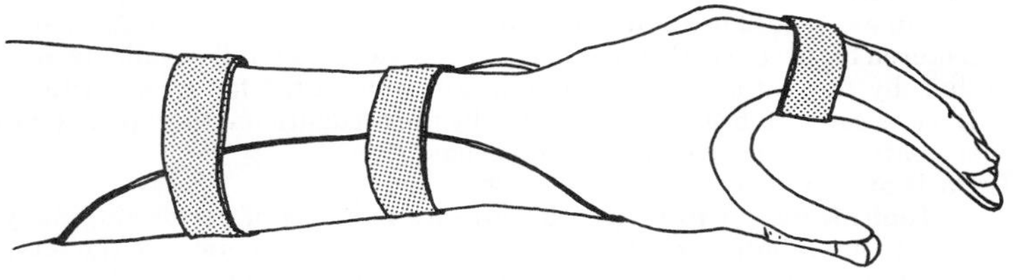

FIG. 57-2. Resting hand splint.

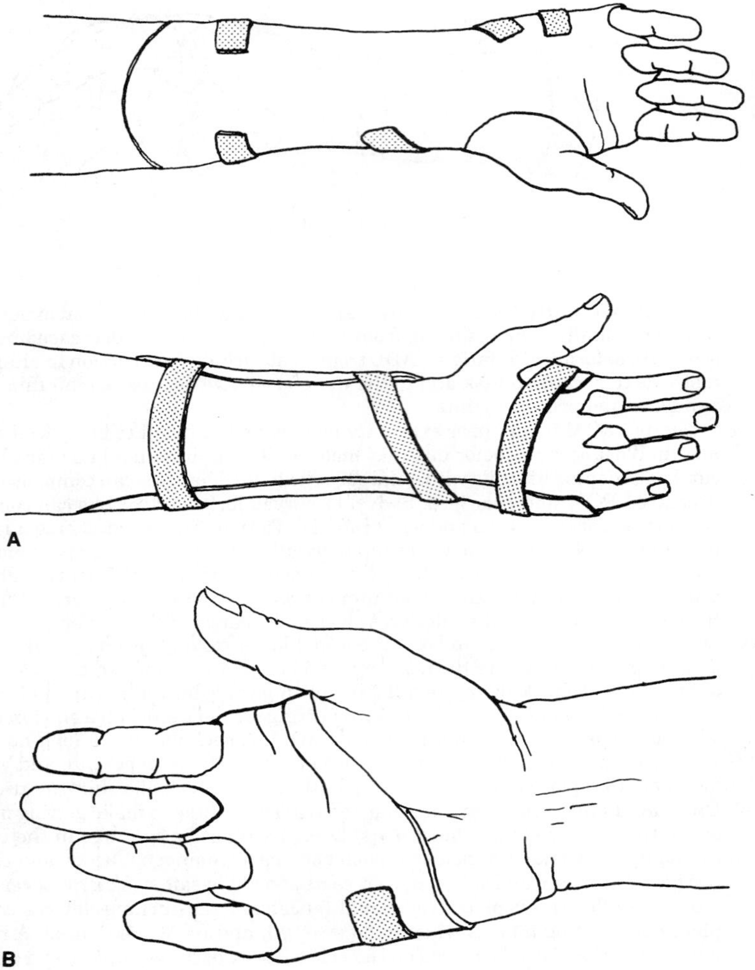

FIG. 57-3. A: Forearm-based ulna drift splint. **B:** Hand-based ulna drift splint.

lightweight and easy to operate. Roller knives or pizza cutters enable food to be cut with less stress placed on joints. A Zim jar opener easily opens tight lids. Items often used should be kept on low shelves, and small, easily managed food containers should be used. Many devices available to improve ADL are manufactured for people with disability. Many are commercially available appliances that, by the nature of their design, are well suited for an arthritic patient. Devices can be fabricated or adapted by the occupational therapist according to the patient's specific problems and needs.

VII. Patient education

A. Techniques of joint protection are methods of performing daily tasks with a minimum amount of stress on the joints. To preserve the integrity of the joint structures and reduce pain and inflammation, patients must be educated in how particular joints work biomechanically and how forces used dur-

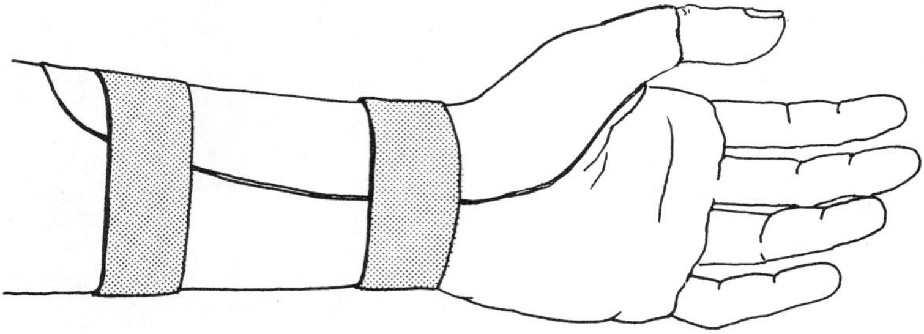

FIG. 57-4. Thumb spica splint.

ing activities can alter their function. Specific principles of joint protection are as follows:

1. Avoid deforming positions.
2. Avoid ulnar deviating pressures in the fingers.
3. Avoid activities involving a tight grasp.
4. Avoid holding joints in one position for an extended length of time.
5. Use the strongest joint available for any activity.
6. Respect pain.
7. Follow an ROM home program designed to prevent the development or progression of a fixed deformity.

B. Energy conservation techniques encourage the accomplishment of tasks with the expenditure of a minimal amount of energy. An appropriate balance of work and rest must be determined. Patients tend to try to get everything done on "good" days, when short rest breaks of 5 to 10 minutes during daily activities can be helpful in increasing overall endurance. Suggestions for conserving energy include the following:

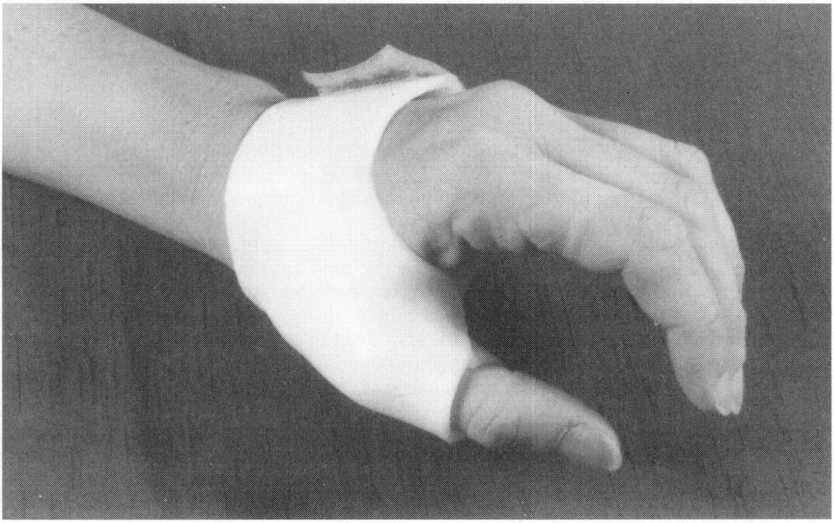

FIG. 57-5. "Shorty" thumb spica.

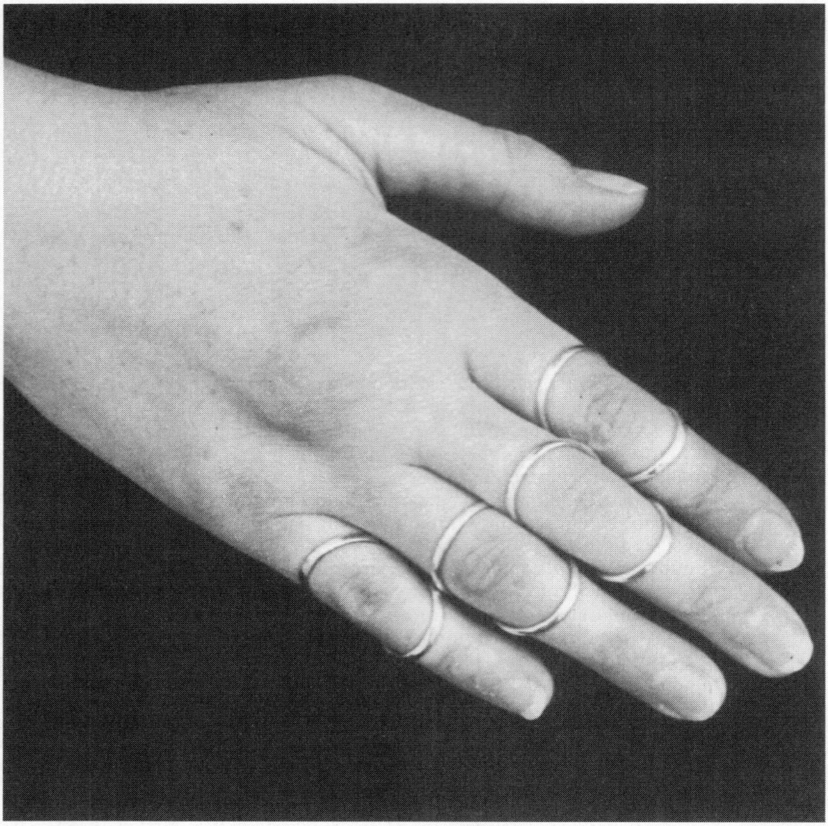

FIG. 57-6. Silver ring splints.

1. Plan work areas so that the most frequently used equipment is easily reached.

2. Use aluminum foil and other disposable utensils to cut down on dish washing.

3. Use lightweight equipment and small containers for cleaning and cooking.

4. Use a wheeled table or cart to move food, laundry, and so on. A cobbler's apron can be useful to carry objects from one room to the next.

5. Use prepared foods when possible.

VIII. Hand. Specific hand exercises are employed to counteract deforming or potentially deforming forces. Resistive hand exercises, such as squeezing a ball, are contraindicated, as they can add stress to already weak joints and tendons. An adequate grip strength necessary to perform ADL is approximately 20 pounds, as measured by a Jamar goniometer. Below this level, patients may have difficulty lifting a coffee cup or brushing their hair. A pinch strength of 5 to 7 pounds has been found to be adequate in performing most tasks. This is particularly applicable for self-care tasks, such as buttoning, writing, and holding a feeding utensil.

Bibliography

Hicks JE, et al. *Handbook of rehabilitative rheumatology.* Atlanta: American Rheumatism Association, 1988.

Hunter JM, et al. *Rehabilitation of the hand: surgery and therapy,* 3rd ed. St. Louis: Mosby, 1990.

Melvin JL. *Rheumatic disease in the adult and child.* Philadelphia: FA Davis Co, 1989.

Pedretti LW. *Occupational therapy practice skills for physical dysfunction.* St. Louis: Mosby, 1990.

58. THE FEMALE ATHLETE

Lisa R. Callahan and Jo A. Hannafin

Regular exercise has been shown to decrease the risk for multiple diseases, including coronary heart disease, hypertension, osteoporosis, obesity, depression, and some reproductive cancers. The U.S. Preventive Services Task Force and the Office of Disease Prevention and Health Promotion have emphasized that as the population ages (with women comprising the majority of the elderly), physical activity and fitness must be viewed as a health goal priority. Additionally, studies have demonstrated that girls who play high school sports are less likely to have an unwanted pregnancy or use drugs, are more likely to graduate from high school, and have lower levels of depression. Clearly, encouraging an active life-style among women is critical to their long-term health. Although many aspects of physical activity are similar in both male and female populations, some issues require special consideration in the female athlete.

I. Physiologic considerations

A. Body structure

1. Skeletal growth reaches its peak at an earlier age in girls (10.5 to 13 years of age) than in boys (12.5 to 15 years of age). Skeletal maturity occurs by age 17 to 19 in girls, and by age 21 to 22 in boys.
2. The female pelvis is wider than the male pelvis, causing an increased quadriceps (Q) angle, which commonly contributes to anterior knee pain (also called patellofemoral syndrome).
3. Women have thinner, lighter bones than their male counterparts, which may predispose them to osteoporosis and stress fractures.

B. Body composition

1. In general, women have approximately 10% more body fat than men do, and 60% to 85% of the total muscle cross-sectional area of men. Because muscle is more metabolically active than fat, women have on average a resting metabolic rate 5% to 10% lower than that of men.
2. The response to weight training, as measured by muscle hypertrophy and gains in strength, is similar in women and men.
3. The percentage of body fat can be estimated by a variety of methods; ideal body fat composition varies with age and sex.

C. Cardiorespiratory system

1. Women have a smaller thoracic cage and heart size, resulting in a lower lung capacity and maximal cardiac output.
2. Maximum oxygen consumption (VO_2max) is lower in women, largely because of differences in body composition and oxygen-carrying capacity. VO_2max is similar in boys and girls before puberty.

D. Circulatory system

1. Women have a smaller blood volume, smaller iron stores, and lower concentrations of hemoglobin. These factors are associated with a lower oxygen-carrying capacity and also increase the risk for anemia.
2. Both male and female élite athletes tend to have lower levels of hemoglobin than their sedentary counterparts. This may be secondary to both a low dietary intake and exercise-related blood loss, such as occurs from the gastrointestinal tract.

E. Endocrine system

1. There is no evidence that the phase of the menstrual cycle influences athletic performance.
2. Female athletes may experience a wide array of alterations in the menstrual cycle, ranging from suppression of the luteal phase to amenorrhea. The latter is especially prevalent in athletes at risk for the "female athlete triad" (see section **II**).

3. Pregnancy results in many physiologic changes, including increases in cardiac output, blood volume, and oxygen demand. There is a great deal of controversy surrounding exercise in the gravid athlete; the American College of Obstetrics and Gynecology has released guidelines that some researchers criticize as being more conservative than necessary. Much more research is needed to delineate safe volumes, types, and intensities of exercise in the pregnant athlete.

II. Female athlete triad

A. General considerations

1. The female athlete triad refers to the interrelatedness of three conditions: disordered eating, amenorrhea, and osteoporosis.
2. Traditionally, female athletes at risk were thought to be those whose activity emphasized leanness for aesthetic reasons (ballet, gymnastics), who associated a low body weight with improved performance (distance running), or those who were classified by weight (rowing, judo). However, girls at risk have been found in many other sports, including swimming, soccer, volleyball, and cycling.

B. Disordered eating

1. It is important that the clinician differentiates disordered eating from the eating disorders of anorexia nervosa and bulimia nervosa, which are psychiatric diagnoses with specific diagnostic criteria. Disordered eating is a much more common phenomenon, and restricting awareness to the extremes of anorexia and bulimia will result in failure to recognize girls at risk for the triad.
2. Disordered eating behaviors include the following:
   - **a.** Food restriction.
   - **b.** Fasting.
   - **c.** Bingeing (which may or may not be followed by purging).
   - **d.** Use of diet pills, diuretics, and laxatives.
3. Girls suffering from disordered eating are often
   - **a.** Preoccupied by thoughts of food.
   - **b.** Plagued by a distorted body image.
   - **c.** Afraid that any weight gain is the equivalent of "getting fat."

C. Amenorrhea

1. Primary amenorrhea is defined as the absence of menarche by the age of 16.
2. Secondary amenorrhea is the absence of three to six consecutive menstrual cycles in women who have experienced menarche.
3. It is believed that exercise in the setting of inadequate calorie consumption may contribute to an "energy-deficient" state, which may lead to amenorrhea.
4. In this setting, amenorrhea represents a hypo-estrogenic state, which can predispose to osteoporosis.
5. Exercise-related amenorrhea is a diagnosis of exclusion. Other causes of amenorrhea, such as pregnancy, must be considered before it is assumed that cessation of menses in an athlete is exercise-driven.

D. Osteoporosis

1. Osteoporosis refers to bone loss in addition to inadequate bone formation, which results in lower bone mass, increased skeletal fragility, and increased risk for fracture.
2. Premature osteoporosis occurring in the female athlete may be irreversible, even when treated with calcium supplementation, hormonal replacement therapy, and correction of amenorrhea.
3. Stress fractures may occur with more frequency and severity in female athletes at risk for the triad; although there are no current guidelines regarding screening, one should consider evaluation of bone density to screen for premature osteoporosis in an athlete identified as being at risk for the female athlete triad.

III. Orthopedic issues. Current knowledge suggests that most injuries sustained by athletes are sport-specific rather than gender-specific (see Chapter 22). However, several orthopedic issues of special concern in the female athlete deserve specific mention.

A. Anterior cruciate ligament (ACL) injuries

1. Epidemiologic data suggests that the incidence of severe knee injuries, especially ACL injuries, is higher in women than in men, particularly in the sports of soccer and basketball (threefold to fivefold increase).
2. The causes of increased ACL injuries are unclear. Factors thought to contribute to the higher rate of ACL injury are both intrinsic and extrinsic.
   - **a.** Intrinsic factors
     - **(1)** Ligament size.
     - **(2)** Intercondylar notch dimensions.
     - **(3)** Muscular strength and coordination.
     - **(4)** Limb alignment.
     - **(5)** Hormonal influences.
   - **b.** Extrinsic factors
     - **(1)** Shoe-floor interface.
     - **(2)** Level of skill and experience.
     - **(3)** Inadequate training and coaching.

B. Patellofemoral pain

1. **Injuries to the patellofemoral joint** are more common in women. Patellofemoral pain is often thought to be secondary to a variation in limb alignment ("miserable malalignment" syndrome) consisting of a combination of increased anteversion of the femoral head, internal rotation of the femur, external rotation of the tibia, and foot pronation. Other anatomic features often blamed for patellofemoral pain include an increased quadriceps angle and hypermobility of the patella.
2. **Patellofemoral pain** should be differentiated according to whether the patella is hypermobile or "tight" (lateral patella compression syndrome). This distinction is important because treatment varies depending on whether the patella needs to be restrained (in the case of hypermobility) or "loosened" (in the case of tight lateral structures causing lateral compressive pain). In the case of the hypermobile patella, strengthening of the medial quadriceps (vastus medialis obliquus) aids in restraining the patella. In the patient with tight lateral structures causing lateral pull of the patella, stretching lateral structures, including the lateral retinaculum and iliotibial band, is recommended. A patellar tracking brace may be helpful in the patient with hypermobility of the patella but may actually exacerbate pain in the patient with lateral patella compression syndrome.

C. Shoulder pain

1. **Adhesive capsulitis** is an idiopathic inflammatory synovitis in the glenohumeral joint. It occurs three to seven times more frequently in women than in men. The cause is not well understood, but the clinical entity is frequently associated with other conditions, such as diabetes and menopause. Four distinct stages have been recognized, which reflect the degree of synovitis. The cornerstones of treatment include intraarticular steroid injection and a rehabilitation program to maintain strength and range of motion. Manipulation under anesthesia and arthroscopy may be required.
2. **Impingement syndrome,** an overuse injury to the rotator cuff, occurs frequently in both male and female patients. However, in women, causative factors are often related to underlying glenohumeral laxity. Increased capsular laxity requires an increase in rotator cuff activity, leading to overuse and impingement. Another factor, especially in the novice female athlete, is deconditioning and weakness of the upper extremity, which leads to rapid fatigue of the rotator cuff, particularly with overhead activity.

D. Stress fractures

1. Although stress fractures occur in both male and female athletes, they are clinically considered more common in female athletes, especially in certain sports such as running and gymnastics.
2. The tibia is the most common site of stress fracture for all athletes; the pelvis and metatarsals are frequent sites of fracture only in female athletes.

3. Variables related to the increased rate of stress fractures in women include the following:
   a. Menstrual irregularity/amenorrhea.
   b. Low bone mineral density.
   c. Training errors.
   d. Biomechanical alignment of the lower extremity.
   e. Decreased muscle strength in the lower extremity.
   f. Diet.
4. Evaluation of the female athlete with a stress fracture *must* include a careful menstrual history; loss of menses or any change in frequency or duration of the menstrual cycle requires further evaluation.

IV. Medical considerations. Achieving fitness through moderate exercise has been linked to lower risks for heart disease, hypertension, cancer, depression, and osteoporosis—diseases that affect both women and men. General guidelines suggest that both women and men should be evaluated by a physician before embarking on an exercise program, especially after age 40. Although most medical considerations in the athlete are not gender-specific, a few issues are of special concern to those caring for the female athlete.

A. Osteoporosis. Moderate exercise may help to decrease the risk for osteoporosis, but exercise in the face of disordered eating and amenorrhea may contribute to premature osteoporosis. Low estrogen states are associated with an increase in urinary loss of calcium and a decrease in calcium absorption from the gastrointestinal tract, which lead to less calcium deposition in bone. In the female athlete, a stress fracture may be a warning sign of osteoporosis and warrants thorough evaluation. Additionally, illnesses such as hyperthyroidism (whether overt, subclinical, or iatrogenically induced by excessive replacement of thyroid hormone) are more common in the female population and may contribute to osteoporosis.

B. Rheumatologic disease. Most rheumatologic diseases, such as lupus, rheumatoid arthritis, and fibromyalgia, are reported to occur two to 10 times more frequently in women than in men. Often, the first manifestation of such an illness is mistaken for an athletic injury. The physician should be alert to this fact and should include rheumatologic disease in the differential diagnosis of musculoskeletal pain, especially in women.

C. Cardiovascular issues

1. Factors affecting the risk for sudden death include the following:
   a. Age and, to a small degree, cholesterol level (both sexes).
   b. Hematocrit, vital capacity, and glucose level (women only).
   c. Women who die suddenly are 50% less likely than men to have coronary artery disease.
2. In women, the incidence of false-positive findings on electrocardiographic exercise testing is much higher than in men; therefore, the use of additional imaging modalities is especially important in the female athlete suspected of having cardiovascular disease.

D. Exercise-related anemias. Anemia is more common in the female than in the male athlete, and in fact is more common in the female athlete than in the general population.

1. Dilutional pseudo-anemia is a natural dilution of hemoglobin that occurs as a result of the increase in plasma volume that is associated with regular exercise; it is often called sports anemia and is benign.
2. Exercise-induced hemolytic anemia may be secondary to macrocytosis (repetitive foot strike destroying red blood cells) or to intravascular hemolysis. Although the iron loss is usually insignificant, this may become a clinically important entity in the élite female athlete.
3. Iron-deficiency anemia may be caused by gastrointestinal, sweat, urinary, or menstrual losses; impaired absorption; and inadequate intake. This type of anemia has an adverse effect on performance and requires treatment.

E. Infections. Physicians treating female athletes should be aware that certain types of infection, such as urinary tract and vaginal/genital infections, are related to gender and anatomy and therefore are more common in the female population.

V. Nutritional concerns. Good nutrition is essential to athletic performance, and the basics of good nutrition are not gender-dependent. However, female athletes need to pay particular attention to a few special considerations.

A. Calcium

1. As mentioned previously, calcium is essential for bone health.
2. Recommendations for daily intake: 1,000 to 1,200 mg in premenopausal women, and 1,500 mg in postmenopausal women and adolescents.

B. Iron

1. See section **IV.D.**
2. Iron deficiency is often secondary to inadequate diet in addition to frequent losses, such as through menstruation.
3. A thorough evaluation is warranted before iron supplementation is prescribed.

C. Other dietary insufficiencies. Female athletes may have an inadequate intake of total calories, protein, and fat in efforts to avoid weight gain. Such dietary inadequacies are known to contribute to poor bone health and are thought to contribute to increased rates of certain injuries and possibly to decreased rates of healing. Extreme restriction of intake may not only affect performance but also have negative effects on health, similar to those seen in the patient with anorexia nervosa.

VI. Equipment and shoes

A. Equipment. Only recently has the athletic equipment industry begun to design exercise equipment intended for use by female athletes. In developing and choosing equipment, the physiologic differences between women and men mentioned briefly at the beginning of this chapter should be kept in mind. These factors should influence the future design of equipment such as bicycles, skis, racquets, and weight machines.

B. Shoes. A woman's foot is different from that of her male counterpart in both shape and size. It is only recently that shoe manufacturers have begun to take such factors into consideration, which has resulted in greatly improved technology that is specific to the female athlete's anatomy and biomechanics as well as specific to the sport.

Bibliography

Agostini R. *Medical and orthopedic issues of active and athletic women.* Philadelphia: Hanley & Belfus, 1994.

Agostini R, et al. The athletic woman. *Clin Sports Med* 1994;13:2.

Warren M, Shangold M. *Sports gynecology: problems and care of the athletic female.* Cambridge, MA: Blackwell Science, 1997.

A. AMERICAN COLLEGE OF RHEUMATOLOGY CRITERIA FOR DIAGNOSIS AND CLASSIFICATION OF RHEUMATIC DISEASES

Stephen A. Paget and Allan Gibofsky

I. Diagnostic criteria for rheumatoid arthritis (RA)[1,2]

A. Classic rheumatoid arthritis. This diagnosis requires seven of the following criteria. In criteria 1 through 5, the joint signs or symptoms must be continuous for at least 6 weeks. (Any one of the features listed under section **E** will exclude a patient from this and all other categories.)

1. **Morning stiffness.**
2. **Pain on motion** or tenderness in at least one joint (observed by a physician).
3. **Swelling** (soft-tissue thickening or fluid, not bony overgrowth alone) **of at least one joint** (observed by a physician).
4. **Swelling** (observed by a physician) **of at least one other joint** (any interval of time between the two joint involvements when the patient is free of joint symptoms may not be longer than 3 months).
5. **Symmetric joint swelling** (observed by a physician) with simultaneous involvement of the same joint on both sides of the body (bilateral involvement of proximal interphalangeal, metacarpophalangeal, or metatarsophalangeal joints is acceptable without absolute symmetry). Terminal phalangeal joint involvement will not satisfy this criterion.
6. **Subcutaneous nodules** (observed by a physician) over bony prominences, on extensor surfaces, or in juxtaarticular regions.
7. **Roentgenographic changes** typical of RA (which must include at least bony decalcification localized to or most marked adjacent to the involved joints and not just degenerative changes). Degenerative changes do not exclude patients from any group classified as having RA.
8. **Positive agglutination test result.** Demonstration of rheumatoid factor (RF) by any method that in two laboratories has not yielded a positive result in more than 5% of normal controls, or positive streptococcal agglutination test result (the latter is now obsolete).
9. **Poor mucin precipitate** from synovial fluid (with shreds and cloudy solution).
10. **Characteristic histologic changes in synovium** with three or more of the following: marked villous hypertrophy; proliferation of superficial synovial cells, often with palisading; marked infiltration of chronic inflammatory cells (lymphocytes or plasma cells predominating) with tendency to form lymphoid nodules; deposition of compact fibrin, either on surface or interstitially; foci of necrosis.
11. **Characteristic histologic changes in nodules.** Granulomatous foci with central zones of cell necrosis surrounded by a palisade of proliferated macrophages, and peripheral fibrosis and chronic inflammatory cell infiltration, predominantly perivascular.

B. Definite rheumatoid arthritis. This diagnosis requires five of the above criteria. In criteria 1 through 5, the joint signs or symptoms must be continuous for at least 6 weeks.

[1] It should be noted that these criteria were developed before the new classification of rheumatic diseases was adopted by the American Rheumatism Association in 1963, in which ankylosing spondylitis, psoriatic arthritis, and arthritis associated with ulcerative colitis and regional enteritis are listed as distinct from rheumatoid arthritis (Blumberg B, et al. ARA nomenclature and classification of arthritis and rheumatism. *Arthritis Rheum* 1964;7:93).

[2] Data from Ropes MW, et al. Revision of diagnostic criteria for rheumatoid arthritis. *Bull Rheum Dis* 1958;9:175.

C. Probable rheumatoid arthritis. This diagnosis requires three of the above criteria. In at least one of criteria 1 through 5, the joint signs or symptoms must be continuous for at least 6 weeks.

D. Possible rheumatoid arthritis. This diagnosis requires two of the following criteria, and the total duration of joint symptoms must be at least 3 weeks:

1. **Morning stiffness.**
2. **Tenderness or pain on motion** (observed by a physician) with a history of recurrence or persistence for 3 weeks.
3. History or observation of **joint swelling.**
4. **Subcutaneous nodules** (observed by a physician).
5. **Elevated erythrocyte sedimentation rate (ESR) or C-reactive protein (CRP).**
6. **Iritis** [of dubious value as a criterion except in the case of juvenile rheumatoid arthritis (JRA)].

E. Exclusions

1. **Typical rash of systemic lupus erythematosus (SLE)** (with butterfly distribution, follicle plugging, and areas of atrophy).
2. **High concentration of LE cells** (four or more in two smears prepared from heparinized blood incubated not more than 2 hours) or other clear evidence of SLE.
3. **Histologic evidence of periarteritis nodosa.** Segmental necrosis of arteries associated with nodular leukocytic infiltration extending perivascularly and tending to include many eosinophils.
4. **Weakness** of neck, trunk, and pharyngeal muscles or persistent muscle swelling or dermatomyositis.
5. **Definite scleroderma** (not limited to the fingers). (The latter is an arguable point.)
6. A clinical picture characteristic of **rheumatic fever** with migratory joint involvement and evidence of endocarditis, especially if accompanied by subcutaneous nodules or erythema marginatum or chorea. (An elevated anti-streptolysin titer will not rule out the diagnosis of RA.)
7. A clinical picture characteristic of **gouty arthritis.** Acute attacks of swelling, redness, and pain in one or more joints, especially if relieved by colchicine.
8. **Tophi.**
9. A clinical picture characteristic of acute **infectious arthritis** of bacterial or viral origin. Acute focus of infection, or in close association with a disease of known infectious origin; chills; fever; acute joint involvement, usually migratory initially (especially organisms are present in the joint fluid or there is a response to antibiotic therapy).
10. **Tubercle bacilli** in the joints or histologic evidence of joint tuberculosis.
11. A clinical picture characteristic of **Reiter's syndrome.** Urethritis and conjunctivitis associated with acute joint involvement, usually migratory initially.
12. A clinical picture characteristic of the **shoulder-hand syndrome.** Unilateral involvement of shoulder and hand, with diffuse swelling of the hand followed by atrophy and contractures.
13. A clinical picture characteristic of **hypertrophic osteoarthropathy.** Clubbing of fingers or hypertrophic periostitis along shafts of long bones, or both, especially if an intrapulmonary lesion (or other appropriate underlying disorder) is present.
14. A clinical picture characteristic of **neuroarthropathy.** Condensation and destruction of bones of involved joints with associated neurologic findings.
15. **Homogentisic acid** in the urine, detectable grossly with alkalinization.
16. Histologic evidence of **sarcoid** or positive Kveim test result.
17. **Multiple myeloma,** evidenced by a marked increase in plasma cells in the bone marrow, or Bence-Jones protein in the urine.
18. Characteristic skin lesions of **erythema nodosum.**

19. **Leukemia or lymphoma.** Characteristic cells in peripheral blood, bone marrow, or tissues.
20. **Agammaglobulinemia.**

II. Proposed 1987 revised American Rheumatism Association criteria for rheumatoid arthritis.[3] Four or more criteria must be present to diagnose RA:

A. Morning stiffness for at least 1 hour and present for at least 6 weeks.
B. Swelling of three or more joints for at least 6 weeks.
C. Swelling of wrist, metacarpophalangeal, or proximal interphalangeal joints for 6 or more weeks.
D. Symmetric joint swelling.
E. Hand roentgenographic changes typical of RA that must include erosions or unequivocal bony decalcification.
F. Rheumatoid nodules.
G. Serum RF by a method yielding positive results in fewer than 5% of normal controls.

III. Proposed criteria for clinical remission in rheumatoid arthritis

A. Four or more of the following requirements must be fulfilled for at least 2 months consecutively:

1. Morning stiffness not exceeding 15 minutes in duration.
2. No fatigue.
3. No joint pain (by history).
4. No joint tenderness or pain on motion.
5. No soft-tissue swelling in joints or tendon sheaths.
6. ESR (Westergren method) below 30 mm/h for a female patient or 20 mm/h for a male patient.

B. These criteria are intended to describe either spontaneous remission or a state of drug-induced disease suppression, which stimulates spontaneous remission. To be considered for this designation, a patient must have met the American Rheumatism Association criteria for definite or classic RA at some time in the past.

C. No alternative explanation may be invoked to account for the failure to meet a particular requirement. For instance, in the presence of knee pain, which might be related to degenerative arthritis, a point may not be awarded for "no joint pain."

D. Exclusions. Clinical manifestations of active vasculitis, pericarditis, pleuritis, or myositis, and unexplained recent weight loss or fever attributable to RA prohibit a designation of complete clinical remission.

IV. Jones criteria (revised) for guidance in the diagnosis of rheumatic fever[4]

A. Major manifestations[5]

1. **Rheumatic carditis** is almost always associated with a significant murmur. Consequently, the other manifestations listed below, when not associated with a significant murmur, should be labeled rheumatic carditis with caution.

   a. **Murmurs**

   (1) In a patient without previous rheumatic fever or rheumatic heart disease, a significant apical systolic murmur, apical mid-diastolic murmur, or basal diastolic murmur.

   (2) In a patient with previous rheumatic fever or rheumatic heart disease, a definite change in the character of any of these murmurs or the appearance of a new, significant murmur.

[3] Arnett FC, et al. The 1987 revised ARA criteria for rheumatoid arthritis. *Arthritis Rheum* 1987;30:S17.

[4] Data from Stollerman GH, et al. Jones criteria (revised) for guidance in the diagnosis of rheumatic fever. *JAMA* 1992;268:2069.

[5] The presence of two major criteria, or of one major and two minor criteria, indicates a high probability of the presence of rheumatic fever. Evidence of a preceding streptococcal infection greatly strengthens the possibility of acute rheumatic fever. Its absence should make the diagnosis doubtful (except in Sydenham's chorea or long-standing carditis).

b. **Cardiomegaly.** Unequivocal cardiac enlargement in a patient without a history of previous rheumatic fever, or an obvious increase in cardiac size in a patient with a past history of rheumatic heart disease.
c. **Pericarditis** is manifested by a friction rub, pericardial effusion, or definite electrocardiographic evidence.
d. **Congestive heart failure** in a child or young adult in the absence of other discernible causes.

2. **Polyarthritis** is almost always migratory and is manifested by swelling, heat, redness, and tenderness, or by pain and limitation of motion in two or more joints. (Arthralgia alone, without other evidence of joint involvement, may occur in rheumatic fever but is not considered a major manifestation.)
3. **Chorea.** Purposeless, involuntary, rapid movements often associated with muscle weakness are characteristic of chorea. These must be differentiated from tics, athetosis, and restlessness. Chorea is a delayed manifestation of rheumatic fever, and other rheumatic manifestations may or may not be present. In the latter case, one should make the diagnosis of "rheumatic fever, chorea only."
4. **Erythema marginatum.** This evanescent, pink rash is characteristic of rheumatic fever. The erythematous areas often have pale centers and round or serpiginous margins. They vary greatly in size and occur mainly on the trunk and proximal part of the extremities, never on the face. The erythema is transient, migrates from place to place, and may be brought out by the application of heat. It is not pruritic and not indurated, and it blanches on pressure.
5. **Subcutaneous nodules.** These firm nodules are seen or felt over the extensor surface of certain joints, particularly elbows, knees, and wrists, in the occipital region, or over the spinous processes of the thoracic and lumbar vertebrae. The skin overlying them moves freely and is not inflamed.

B. Minor manifestations

1. **Clinical.** Other clinical features occur frequently in rheumatic fever. Because they also appear in many other diseases, their diagnostic value is minor. They are useful in supporting the diagnosis of rheumatic fever when this diagnosis rests mainly on a single major manifestation.
   a. A **history of previous rheumatic fever** or evidence of preexisting rheumatic heart disease increases the index of suspicion in the evaluation of any rheumatic complaint. The history must be well documented or the evidence of preexisting rheumatic heart disease clear.
   b. **Arthralgia** constitutes pain in one or more joints (not in the muscles and other periarticular tissues) without evidence of inflammation, tenderness to touch, or limitation of motion. The presence of arthralgia, in addition to polyarthritis, does not make the latter any more indicative of rheumatic fever and should not be used for diagnosis when polyarthritis is a major manifestation. In the case of monarthritis, however, arthralgia in other joints strengthens the diagnosis of rheumatic fever and can be considered a minor manifestation.
   c. **Fever** (rectal temperature >38°C) is usually present early in the course of untreated rheumatic fever.
2. **Laboratory findings**
   a. **Acute-phase reactions** offer objective but nonspecific confirmation of the presence of an inflammatory process. The ESR and CRP tests are most commonly employed. Unless the patient has received corticosteroids or salicylates, the results of these tests are almost always abnormal in patients who present with polyarthritis or acute carditis, whereas they are often normal in patients presenting with chorea. The ESR may be markedly increased by anemia and may be decreased in congestive heart failure. The CRP test is a sensitive indicator of inflammation, and the result is negative in uncomplicated anemia. Heart

failure of any cause is often accompanied by a positive CRP test result. Sera from normal persons do not contain this protein, but relatively minor inflammatory stimuli may result in a positive reaction. Leukocytosis, anemia, or other nonspecific responses to inflammation may also occur in acute rheumatic fever.

b. **Electrocardiographic changes,** mainly prolongation of the PR interval, are frequent but may occur in other inflammatory processes. Furthermore, electrocardiographic changes, whether or not associated with clinical evidence of carditis, have no bearing on the ultimate development of rheumatic heart disease. Such changes by themselves, therefore, do not constitute adequate criteria for a diagnosis of carditis. The diagnosis of acute rheumatic fever should never be made solely on the basis of laboratory findings plus minor clinical manifestations. On the other hand, because laboratory indications of recent streptococcal infection and current inflammation occur so regularly with this disease, their unexplained absence should make the physician question the diagnosis of rheumatic fever.

C. **Supporting evidence of streptococcal infection**

1. **Laboratory evidence** of preceding streptococcal infection by specific antibody tests or by identification of the offending organism (positive throat culture) greatly strengthens the possibility of acute rheumatic fever. Clinical evidence of preceding streptococcal infection by a history of a recent attack of scarlet fever is the best clinical indication of antecedent streptococcal infection.
2. **Recent scarlet fever.**

V. **Current proposed revision of criteria for juvenile rheumatoid arthritis**[6]

A. **General.** The JRA Criteria Committee has reviewed the initial criteria approved by the American Rheumatism Association in December 1971 and published in 1973. The Committee has determined that the criteria be revised at this time, that the term juvenile rheumatoid arthritis be retained, and that the disease should be classified into three subtypes based on onset (systemic, polyarticular, and pauciarticular). Confusion would result from attempts at this time to change the name to *juvenile chronic polyarthritis* and to create subclassifications. The term *Still's disease,* which pays legitimate homage to Dr. George Frederick Still, has nonetheless become confusing in that it denotes different clinical patterns in different parts of the world, and it should not be used. The purpose of a working classification is to allow clinicians everywhere to report experiences that can be readily categorized. A classification with appropriate subtypes allows uniform multicenter evaluation of patients with different manifestations. Clusters can then be identified with regard to prognosis or therapy. The following classification enumerates requirements for a diagnosis of JRA and three subtypes based on clinical onset.

B. **General criteria for juvenile rheumatoid arthritis.** Persistent arthritis of one or more joints for at least 6 weeks is sufficient for diagnosis if the conditions listed under exclusions have been eliminated. Arthritis is defined as swelling of a joint or limitation of motion with heat, pain, or tenderness. Pain or tenderness alone is not sufficient for the diagnosis of arthritis. Joints are counted individually with certain exceptions. The cervical spine is considered one joint. The carpal joints of each hand are counted as one joint, as are the tarsal joints on each foot. The metacarpophalangeal, metatarsophalangeal, and proximal and distal interphalangeal joints are counted individually.

C. **Subtypes of juvenile rheumatoid arthritis according to onset.** The onset subtype is determined by manifestations during the first 6 months of disease. Although manifestations more closely resembling those of another onset subtype may appear later, the subtype present during the initial 6 months remains the onset subtype.

[6] Data from Brewer EJ Jr, et al. Current proposed revision of JRA criteria. *Arthritis Rheum* 1977;20:195.

1. **Systemic-onset juvenile rheumatoid arthritis.** This subtype is defined as JRA with persistent intermittent fever (daily intermittent temperature elevations to 103°F or more) with or without rheumatoid rash or other organ involvement. Typical fever and rash are considered *probable* systemic-onset JRA if not associated with arthritis. Before a definite diagnosis can be made, arthritis as defined must be present.
2. **Pauciarticular-onset juvenile rheumatoid arthritis.** This subtype is defined as JRA with arthritis in four or fewer joints. Patients with systemic-onset JRA are excluded from this onset subtype.
3. **Polyarticular-onset juvenile rheumatoid arthritis.** This subtype is defined as JRA with arthritis in five or more joints. Patients with systemic-onset JRA are excluded from this subtype.
4. **Other factors to be considered for purposes of continuing study.** The following factors may be important for better understanding and future classification:
   - **a.** Rheumatoid factors.
   - **b.** Antinuclear antibodies (ANAs).
   - **c.** Histocompatibility antigens.
   - **d.** Sex.
   - **e.** Age at onset.
   - **f.** Iridocyclitis (chronic or acute).
   - **g.** Sacroiliitis.
   - **h.** Number of affected joints.
   - **i.** Distribution of affected joints.
   - **j.** Family history of arthritis and related rheumatic manifestations.
   - **k.** Responses to drug therapy.
   - **l.** Immunologic abnormalities.

D. Definitions of certain manifestations

1. **Fever.** Any type of fever may be seen in JRA; however, a persistent intermittent fever with diurnal variation from normal to 103°F or more is suggestive of systemic-onset JRA if other diseases, such as infection, malignancy, inflammatory bowel disease, and SLE, are excluded.
2. **Rheumatoid rash** is an evanescent, pale, erythematous, usually circumscribed macular rash, with individual lesions varying in size from 2 to 10 mm. The larger lesions may have a pale center with peripheral pallor. The rash may become confluent and is found predominantly on the chest, axillae, thighs, and upper arms and less commonly on the face and distal extremities. It occurs most frequently in patients with systemic-onset disease, may occasionally precede arthritis, and is occasionally pruritic.
3. **Iridocyclitis.** An anterior nongranulomatous iridocyclitis is most common in patients with pauciarticular-onset JRA. One or both eyes may be involved. The onset of iridocyclitis is characteristically insidious, and initial physical findings may be difficult to detect. The earliest findings on slit-lamp examination are cells or increased protein in the anterior chamber. Sequelae include posterior synechiae, band keratopathy, cataracts, secondary glaucoma, and phthisis bulbi. Iridocyclitis should be considered a serious complication that may lead to blindness. Frequent ophthalmologic examinations should be performed to detect lesions in the earliest stages.
4. **Cardiac involvement.** Pericarditis is not common and can be asymptomatic. It is most frequently associated with systemic-onset JRA. Symptoms may include chest pain, dyspnea, and tachypnea. Signs include friction rub, tachycardia, and enlarged heart. Electrocardiography, echocardiography, and chest radiography may be helpful in diagnosis. Occasional patients may have myocarditis or valvular insufficiency.
5. **Rheumatoid nodules** occur in a small percentage of patients with JRA. They are usually subcutaneous, vary in size up to several centimeters, and can generally be found in or about tendons of the hands, below the elbow, and around the Achilles tendon. A lesion sometimes known as a pseudo-

rheumatoid nodule has been reported in children to have a pathologic appearance indistinguishable from that of the adult type of rheumatoid nodules. In children, these benign nodules usually appear on the anterior tibial surface or occiput.

6. **Stiffness** exists in the joints and muscles when they lack flexibility and ease of movement and is frequently observed after inactivity. Stiffness is noted as a physical sign in young children but later also constitutes a symptom or complaint.
7. **Tenosynovitis** may involve the sheaths of the finger extensors or flexors of the wrist in addition to the posterior tibialis and peroneal tendons of the ankle. Arthritis of the adjacent joint is a frequent association.
8. **Arthritis of the cervical spine.** Pain and limitation of motion of the cervical spine are frequent in systemic- and polyarticular-onset JRA and less common in the pauciarticular-onset JRA subtype. Clinical findings and the radiographic appearance frequently do not correlate well. Motion is usually limited in extension and lateral flexion and rotation rather than in forward flexion. Radiographic changes consist primarily of narrowing of the apophyseal joints with subsequent fusion. The C2-3 apophyseal joint is most often involved, with the other cervical vertebrae less frequently affected. Abnormalities of the vertebral bodies are much less frequent. When seen, they consist of decreased growth of the bodies and their intervertebral disks. An uncommon but potentially severe complication is subluxation of C-1 on C-2.
9. **Rheumatoid factors.** Agglutination tests for RF are persistently positive in 5% to 20% of all patients with JRA. Positive test results are more frequently found in older children with polyarticular-onset disease. The presence of RF appears to correlate with a more chronic destructive arthritis.
10. **Antinuclear antibodies.** Results of fluorescent antibody tests for ANAs are positive in 10% to 40% of children with polyarticular- and pauciarticular-onset JRA; the frequency depends somewhat on the sensitivity of tests in individual laboratories. In the majority of children with the chronic iridocyclitis of JRA, results of tests for ANAs are positive. ANAs are less commonly found in children with systemic-onset JRA or with juvenile ankylosing spondylitis.
11. **Growth disturbances** in JRA patients are a consequence of the disease itself. Total growth can be severely reduced. Localized growth disturbances may also occur, such as epiphyseal overgrowth at the knee or ankle, or undergrowth of the mandible. Growth can resume with remission. Prolonged corticosteroid therapy can also suppress growth.
12. **Anemia and leukocytosis** occur frequently in systemic-onset JRA. Peripheral leukocyte counts may be greatly elevated, with a predominance of early forms (left shift); anemia may sometimes be profound. Less pronounced leukocytosis and anemia may also be seen during periods of active disease in children with polyarticular JRA.
13. **Hepatosplenomegaly and lymphadenopathy.** Marked hepatosplenomegaly and generalized lymphadenopathy may occur in children with active systemic-onset JRA. Mild abnormalities of liver enzymes may be associated with the disease or with therapy. Less pronounced degrees of organomegaly and lymphadenopathy also occur at times with other onset subtypes of JRA.
14. **Amyloidosis** as a complication of JRA is rarely reported in the United States. In some countries in Europe, the incidence is said to be 4% to 6%. Amyloidosis may be a contributing factor in up to 50% of deaths in JRA patients reported in European countries.

E. Exclusions

1. **Other rheumatic diseases**
   - **a.** Rheumatic fever.
   - **b.** SLE.

- **c.** Ankylosing spondylitis.
- **d.** Polymyositis and dermatomyositis.
- **e.** Vasculitis
  - **(1)** Anaphylactoid purpura (Henoch-Schönlein).
  - **(2)** Polyarteritis.
  - **(3)** Serum sickness and other allergic reactions.
  - **(4)** Mucocutaneous lymph node syndrome; infantile polyarteritis.
  - **(5)** Other.
- **f.** Scleroderma.
- **g.** Psoriatic arthritis.
- **h.** Reiter's syndrome.
- **i.** Sjögren's syndrome.
- **j.** Mixed connective tissue disease.
- **k.** Behçet's syndrome.

2. Infectious arthritis

- **a.** Bacterial arthritis (including tuberculosis).
- **b.** Viral, fungal, and mycoplasmal arthritides.
- **c.** Nonbacterial arthritis associated with bacterial infections.
- **d.** Other.

3. Inflammatory bowel disease.

4. Neoplastic diseases, including leukemia.

5. Nonrheumatic conditions of bones and joints

- **a.** Osteochondritis.
- **b.** Toxic synovitis of the hip.
- **c.** Slipped capital femoral epiphysis.
- **d.** Trauma
  - **(1)** Battered child syndrome.
  - **(2)** Fractures.
  - **(3)** Joint, ligamentous, and muscular injuries.
  - **(4)** Congenital indifference to pain.
  - **(5)** Acute chondrolysis.
- **e.** Chondromalacia of the patella.
- **f.** Congenital anomalies and genetically determined abnormalities of the musculoskeletal system (including inborn errors of metabolism).
- **g.** Idiopathic tenosynovitis.

6. Hematologic diseases

- **a.** Sickle cell anemia.
- **b.** Hemophilia.

7. Psychogenic arthralgia.

8. Miscellaneous

- **a.** Immunologic abnormalities.
- **b.** Sarcoidosis.
- **c.** Hypertrophic osteoarthropathy.
- **d.** Villonodular synovitis.
- **e.** Chronic active hepatitis.
- **f.** Familial Mediterranean fever.

VI. Revised (1982) criteria for the classification of systemic lupus erythematosus.[7] The proposed classification is based on 11 criteria. For the purpose of identifying patients in clinical studies, a person is said to have SLE if any four or more of the 11 criteria are present, serially or simultaneously, during any interval of observation.

A. Malar rash. Fixed erythema, flat or raised, over the malar eminences, tending to spare the nasolabial folds.

B. Discoid rash. Erythematous raised patches with adherent keratotic scaling and follicular plugging; atrophic scarring may occur in older lesions.

C. Photosensitivity. Skin rash as a result of unusual reaction to sunlight, by patient history or physician observation.

[7] Data from Tan EM, et al. The 1982 revised criteria for the classification of systemic lupus erythematosus. *Arthritis Rheum* 1982;25:1271.

D. **Oral ulcers.** Oral or nasopharyngeal ulceration, usually painless, observed by a physician.
E. **Arthritis.** Nonerosive arthritis involving two or more peripheral joints, characterized by tenderness, swelling, or effusion.
F. **Serositis**
   1. **Pleuritis.** Convincing history of pleuritic pain or rub heard by a physician or evidence of pleural effusion.
   2. **Pericarditis.** Documented by electrocardiogram or rub or evidence of pericardial effusion.
G. **Renal disorder**
   1. **Persistent proteinuria** above 0.5 g/d or above 3+ if quantification not performed.
   2. **Cellular casts.** May be red cell, hemoglobin, granular, tubular, or mixed.
H. **Neurologic disorder**
   1. **Seizures** in the absence of offending drugs or known metabolic derangements (e.g., uremia, ketoacidosis, or electrolyte imbalance).
   2. **Psychosis** in the absence of offending drugs or known metabolic derangements (e.g., uremia ketoacidosis or electrolyte imbalance).
I. **Hematologic disorder**
   1. **Hemolytic anemia** with reticulocytosis.
   2. **Leukopenia.** Total below 4,000/mL on two or more occasions.
   3. **Lymphopenia.** Below 1,500/mL on two or more occasions.
   4. **Thrombocytopenia.** Below 100,000/mL in the absence of offending drugs.
J. **Immunologic disorder**
   1. **Positive LE cell preparation.**
   2. **Anti-DNA.** Antibody to native DNA in abnormal titer.
   3. **Anti-Sm.** Presence of antibody to Smith nuclear antigen.
   4. **False-positive serologic test for syphilis** known to be positive for at least 6 months and confirmed by *Treponema pallidum* immobilization or fluorescent treponemal antibody absorption test.
K. **Antinuclear antibody.** An abnormal titer of ANA by immunofluorescence or an equivalent assay at any point in time and in the absence of drugs known to be associated with drug-induced lupus syndrome.

VII. **Preliminary criteria for the classification of systemic sclerosis (scleroderma).**[8] Systemic sclerosis (progressive systemic sclerosis, systemic scleroderma) is a disorder of the connective tissues characterized by induration and thickening of the skin (scleroderma), by abnormalities involving both the microvasculature and larger vessels (e.g., Raynaud's phenomenon), and by fibrotic degenerative changes in muscles, joints, and viscera, most notably the esophagus, intestinal tract, heart, lungs, and kidneys. The disease must be differentiated from a variety of other conditions associated with similar cutaneous changes (Table A-1). Advanced systemic sclerosis with diffuse scleroderma and characteristic involvement of internal organs is unmistakable. However, the disease also exists in a form in which only limited skin change is present, often confined to the fingers and face. This variant is now generally known as the CREST syndrome (**c**alcinosis, **R**aynaud's phenomenon, **e**sophageal dysfunction, **s**clerodactyly, and **t**elangiectasia). Also included within the spectrum of systemic sclerosis are patients in whom scleroderma and other changes typical of progressive systemic sclerosis coexist with manifestations of one or more of the other connective tissue diseases—the so-called overlap syndromes, such as mixed connective tissue disease.

A. **Design of the American Rheumatism Association Scleroderma Criteria Cooperative Study.** A multicenter study was designed to gather detailed data from patients with an early diagnosis of systemic sclerosis and comparison patients with certain selected rheumatic disorders. Physicians

[8] Data from preliminary criteria for the classification of systemic sclerosis (scleroderma). *Bull Rheum Dis* 1981;31:1.

Table A-1. Classification of scleroderma

I. Systemic sclerosis	
A.	Classic disease with bilateral symmetric diffuse involvement of the skin (scleroderma) affecting face, trunk, and proximal as well as distal portions of the extremities; associated with tendency toward relatively early appearance of visceral involvement
B.	Relatively limited involvement of skin, often confined to fingers and face, and tendency to long-delayed appearance of visceral involvement (CREST syndrome)
C.	Overlap syndromes, including sclerodermatomyositis and mixed connective tissue disease
II. Localized (focal) forms of scleroderma	
A.	Morphea (plaquelike, guttate, or generalized; subcutaneous and keloid morphea)
B.	Linear scleroderma
C.	Scleroderma *en coup de sabre,* with or without facial hemiatrophy
III. Chemically induced scleroderma-like conditions	
A.	Vinyl chloride disease
B.	Pentazocine-induced fibrosis
C.	Bleomycin-induced fibrosis
IV. Eosinophilic fasciitis	
V. Pseudoscleroderma	
A.	Edematous (scleredema, scleromyxedema)
B.	Indurative (amyloid disease, porphyria cutanea tarda, carcinoid syndrome, phenylketonuria, acromegaly)
C.	Atropic (progeria, Werner syndrome, lichen sclerosis et atrophicus)

CREST: calcinosis, Raynaud's phenomenon, esophageal dysfunction, sclerodactyly, and telangiectasia.
Data from Preliminary criteria for the classification of systemic sclerosis (scleroderma). *Bull Rheum Dis* 1981;31:1.

submitting cases from each of the participating centers were requested to group these into one of three categories: (a) definite, (b) probable or early stage, or (c) overlap syndrome. Comparison patients were entered from these centers with diagnoses of (a) SLE, (b) polymyositis-dermatomyositis, and (c) Raynaud's phenomenon, either primary or secondary (not associated with progressive systemic sclerosis or any of the comparison disorders). Patients with various forms of localized (focal) scleroderma were *excluded* from the study.

B. Results

1. **Clinical features.** Seven clinical variables were found to be significantly more frequent in the patients with systemic sclerosis than in comparison patients (Table A-2). Interestingly, these variables all related to sclerodermatous skin changes, except for Raynaud's phenomenon. Cutaneous scleroderma in any location was the most sensitive variable, but as many as 9% of the patients considered to have primary Raynaud's phenomenon by center physicians also showed this change (sclerodactyly in all instances). The presence of proximal scleroderma, a term indicating bilateral and symmetric sclerodermatous changes in any area proximal to the metacarpophalangeal or metatarsophalangeal joints, was the most discriminating variable for systemic sclerosis, having been found in 239 (91%) of the definite systemic sclerosis cases but in only one (0.2%) of the comparison patients, a woman thought to have SLE.
2. **Other findings.** The frequency of digital tuft resorption and subcutaneous calcinosis, identified by clinical or roentgenographic examination (or both), was found to be several times higher among the systemic sclerosis patients than in the comparison patients. Lower esophageal hypo-

Table A-2. Frequency of promising clinical variables originally considered for criteria analysis

	Systemic sclerosis patients(%)			Comparison patients (%)		
Clinical variables	Definite ($n = 264$)	Probable ($n = 35$)	Overlap ($n = 85$)	SLE ($n = 172$)	PM-DM ($n = 120$)	Raynaud's phenomenon ($n = 121$)
Sclerodermatous skin changes						
Any location	98	74	75	1	3	9
Sclerodactyly[a]	96	74	71	1	3	9
Proximal scleroderma[a]	91	51	58	<1	0	0
Face or neck	79	21	41	0	0	0
Bilateral hand edema	70	76	70	24	24	28
Digital pitting scars (fingertip)[a]	49	43	38	9	7	15
Hand deformity or contractures	54	27	36	3	14	3
Abnormal skin pigmentation	56	29	35	21	13	8
Telangiectasia, fingers	47	26	32	8	10	8
Raynaud's phenomenon	82	71	86	29	19	100

SLE, systemic lupus erythematosus; PM-DM, polymyositis-dermatomyositis.
[a] Subsequently accepted criteria variable.
From: Preliminary criteria for the classification of systemic sclerosis (scleroderma). *Bull Rheum Dis* 1981; 31:1.

motility detected by radiographic or manometric study was also found chiefly in the systemic sclerosis group.

Colonic sacculations were confined to patients with systemic sclerosis but occurred with a relatively low frequency (17% of the definite cases). Bilateral basilar pulmonary fibrosis (determined by roentgenogram) was found in approximately one-fourth of the definite and overlap patients with systemic sclerosis and in a smaller proportion of patients with the comparison disorders. The shin biopsy findings of dermal collagen thickening, condensation, or homogenization were the most sensitive of the laboratory features studied. These occurred in the highest frequency among the systemic sclerosis cases, but some of these changes were also found in 18% to 25% of the comparison patients studied.

3. **Major criterion: proximal scleroderma.** Because of its high specificity in separating systemic sclerosis from the comparison disorders, proximal scleroderma was selected as the single major criterion for systemic sclerosis. It was found in 91% of definite and 51% of probable cases of this disease and in 58% of the cases of systemic sclerosis-overlap syndromes, but in only one (0.2%) of 413 patients with comparison disorders (see Table A-2). No other variable provided such powerful discrimination.
4. **Minor criteria.** Multivariate analytic techniques were applied to the remaining definite systemic sclerosis and comparison patients without proximal scleroderma to select that combination of fewest items (minor criteria) that allowed the greatest discrimination. For simplicity, the "probable" and "overlap" systemic sclerosis patients were eliminated from these and subsequent analyses to derive criteria for an early diagnosis of definite disease. Many of the remaining "clinically promising" variables were redundant because they correlated with one another or were rather nonspecific for systemic sclerosis. Three additional variables in combination provided the most information and were selected as minor criteria: sclerodactyly, digital pitting scars of the fingertips or loss of distal finger pad substance, and bilateral basilar pulmonary fibrosis demonstrated by chest roentgenogram. An additional 17 (6%) patients with definite and four (11%) patients with probable systemic sclerosis satisfied at least two of these criteria, but only nine (2%) of the combined comparison patients did so (Table A-3).
5. **Proposed classification criteria for definite systemic sclerosis.** One major criterion or two or more minor criteria were found in 97% of the definite cases (97% sensitivity) but in only 2% of the comparison patients (98% specificity). This combination of variables constitutes the proposed preliminary classification criteria for systemic sclerosis.
   - **a.** Proximal scleroderma is the single major criterion, with 91% sensitivity and greater than 99% specificity.
   - **b.** Sclerodactyly, digital pitting scars of fingertips or loss of substance of the finger pad, and bilateral basilar pulmonary fibrosis contribute further as minor criteria, in cases in which proximal scleroderma is absent.
   - **c.** One major or two or more minor criteria were found in 97% of patients with definite systemic sclerosis, but in only 2% of the comparison patients with SLE, polymyositis-dermatomyositis, or Raynaud's phenomenon. When the criteria were applied to patients grouped according to the original diagnoses of the participating centers (i.e., before any subcommittee recommended revisions), the results were essentially identical (96% sensitivity and 98% specificity). When these criteria were tested with data stored in ARAMIS from more than 1,300 systemic sclerosis and comparison patients, they yielded 92% sensitivity and 96% specificity.

C. Discussion: application of the classification criteria. The proposed classification criteria are not intended to apply to all forms of scleroderma, but only to systemic sclerosis.

Table A-3. Number of patients who satisfied major or minor criteria for systemic sclerosis

Criteria	Systemic sclerosis patients: Definite ($n = 264$)	Systemic sclerosis patients: Probable ($n = 35$)	Comparison patients: SLE ($n = 172$)	Comparison patients: PM-DM ($n = 120$)	Comparison patients: Raynaud's phenomenon ($n = 121$)
Major criterion					
Proximal scleroderma	239	18	1	0	0
Minor criteria[a]	(25)	(17)	(171)	(120)	(121)
Sclerodactyly	19	8	1	4	11
Digital pitting scars	15	7	15	8	18
Bilateral basilar pulmonary fibrosis	8	1	11	22	3
Two or more minor criteria	17	4	0	3	6
Proposed criteria satisfied	256 (97%)	22 (63%)	1 (1%)	3 (3%)	6 (5%)

SLE, systemic lupus erythematosus; PM-DM, polymyositis-dermatomyositis.
[a] Applies to the number of patients who did not satisfy the major criterion, as shown in parentheses.
From Preliminary criteria for the classification of systemic sclerosis (scleroderm). *Bull Rheum Dis* 31:1,1981.

1. Changes characteristic of scleroderma were reported in skin biopsy specimens of a high proportion of the patients with systemic sclerosis. These included atrophy of dermal appendages, flattening of rete pegs, and thickening, condensation, and homogenization of dermal collagen. Some of these changes were also found, however, in approximately one-fourth of patients with the comparison disorders. More subtle histologic evaluation, including grading of the abnormalities noted above and assessment of such features as the site of collagen deposition (localization and skin layer), small-vessel alterations, and collections of lymphocytes might provide better discrimination of the sclerodermatous change. However, these measures are not yet standardized.
2. When proximal scleroderma is absent, as was true in 9% of the definite cases of systemic sclerosis in this series, classification depends on a number of less discriminating minor criteria. However, critical judgment must be exercised in applying the minor criteria in view of the fact that they are detected more variably and can have other causes (e.g., comparison disorders, frostbite, trauma, or unrelated chronic lung disease).
3. Raynaud's phenomenon is important in the diagnosis of systemic sclerosis in the individual patient in view of its nearly uniform occurrence. However, this cold-reactive state is also found in 20% to 30% of the other connective tissue diseases studied and so is nonspecific. Similarly, typical gastrointestinal disturbances are frequent in systemic sclerosis but may also be found in related disorders.
4. The presence of serum anti-ribonucleoprotein (RNP) antibodies in very high titers was uncommon in patients with definite or probable systemic sclerosis but was found in 69% of patients with systemic sclerosis in overlap. The latter were chiefly patients with clinical findings typical of mixed connective tissue disease. Recent research has revealed certain serum antibodies that appear to be highly specific for systemic sclerosis (e.g., anti-Scl 70, anti-centromere), and continuing investigation is likely to uncover the existence of still more antigen-antibody systems closely associated with this and other connective tissue disorders.

VIII. Criteria for the classification of acute gouty arthritis[9]

A. Presence of characteristic urate crystals in the joint fluid, or

B. Presence of a tophus proven to contain urate crystals by chemical means or polarized light microscopy, or

C. Presence of six of the following clinical, laboratory, and radiographic phenomena:

1. More than one attack of acute arthritis.
2. Development of maximal inflammation within 1 day.
3. Attack of monarticular arthritis.
4. Observation of joint redness.
5. Pain or swelling in first metatarsophalangeal joint.
6. Unilateral attack involving first metatarsophalangeal joint.
7. Unilateral attack involving tarsal joint.
8. Suspected tophus.
9. Hyperuricemia.
10. Asymmetric swelling within a joint (roentgenogram).
11. Subcortical cysts without erosions (roentgenogram).
12. Negative culture of joint fluid for microorganisms during attack of joint inflammation.

[9] Wallace SL, et al. Preliminary criteria for the classification of the acute arthritis of primary gout. *Arthritis Rheum* 1977;20:895.

B. NEUROLOGIC DERMATOMES

Stephen A. Paget and Allan Gibofsky

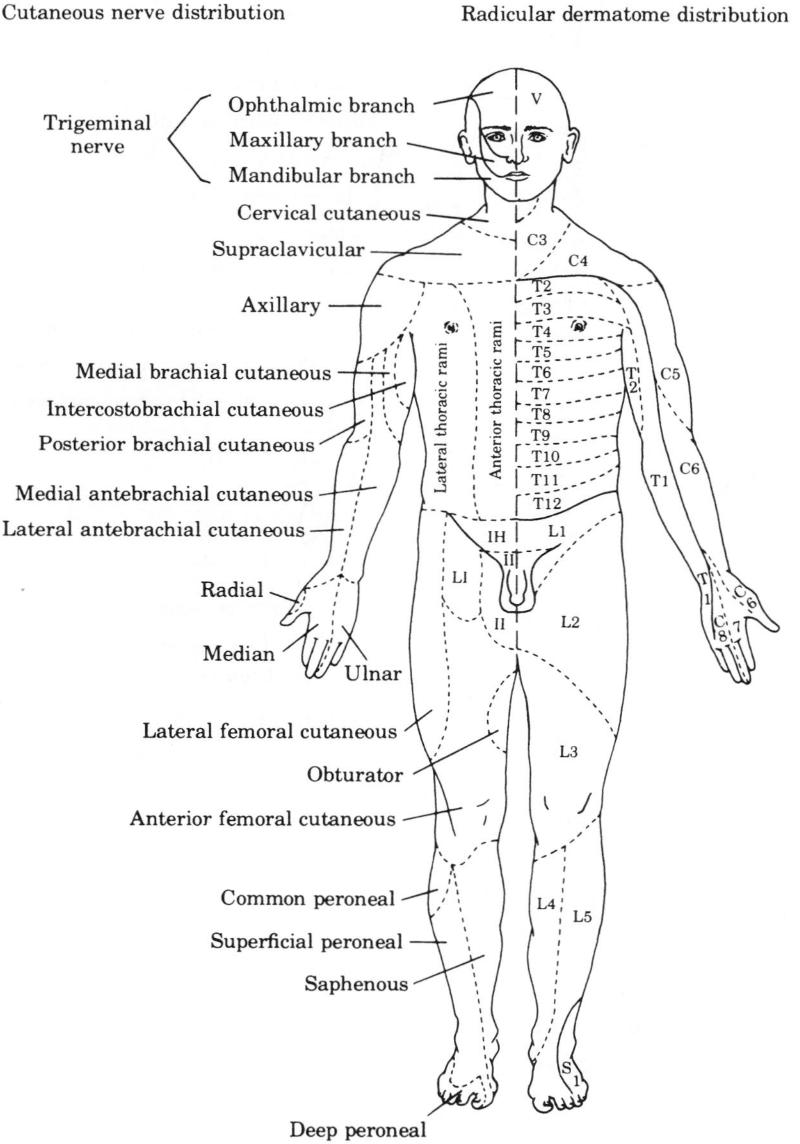

FIG. B-1. A: Radicular dermatomes and cutaneous nerve distribution, anterior view. **B:** Radicular dermatomes and cutaneous nerve distribution, posterior view. *IH,* iliohypogastric; *II,* ilioinguinal; *LI,* lumboinguinal.

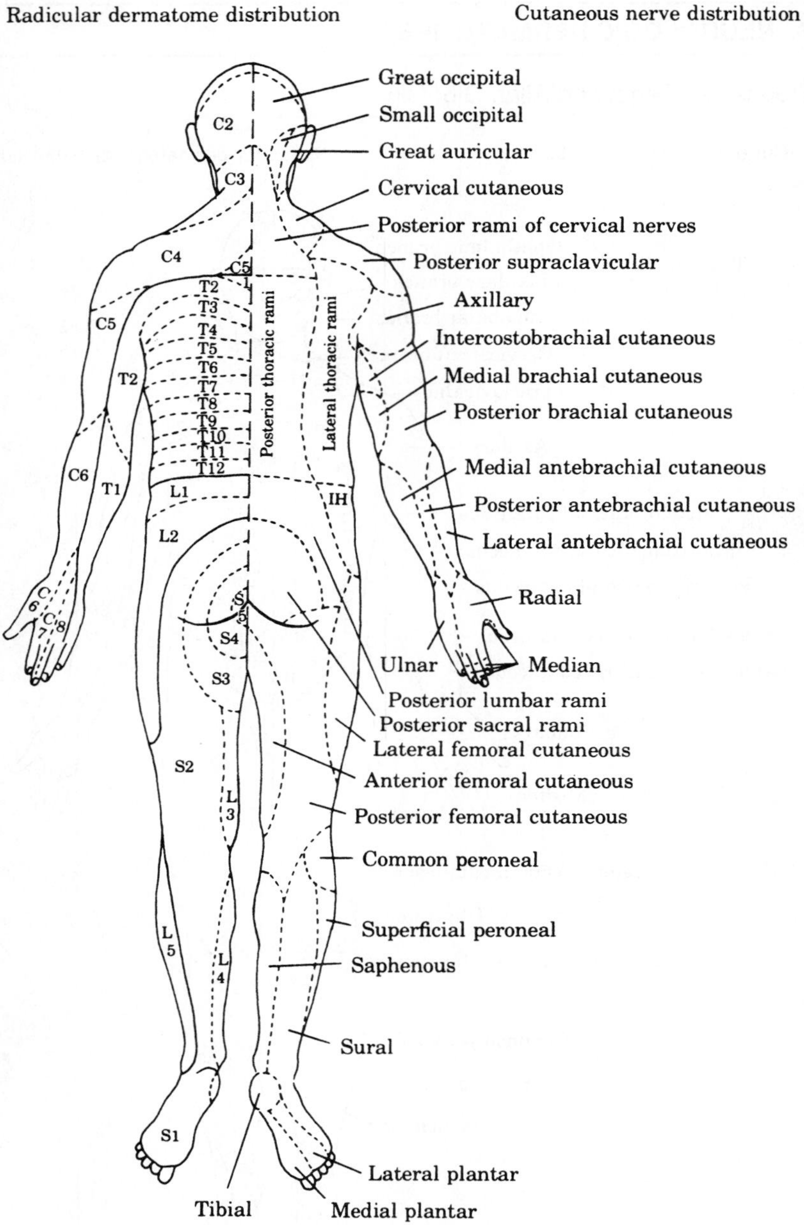
Radicular dermatome distribution
Cutaneous nerve distribution
C2
C3
C4
C5
C5
T1
T2
T3
T4
T5
T6
T7
T8
T9
T10
T11
T12
C5
T2
C6
T1
L1
L2
C6
C7
C8
S5
S4
S3
S2
L3
L5
L4
S1
Posterior thoracic rami
Lateral thoracic rami
IH
Great occipital
Small occipital
Great auricular
Cervical cutaneous
Posterior rami of cervical nerves
Posterior supraclavicular
Axillary
Intercostobrachial cutaneous
Medial brachial cutaneous
Posterior brachial cutaneous
Medial antebrachial cutaneous
Posterior antebrachial cutaneous
Lateral antebrachial cutaneous
Radial
Ulnar
Median
Posterior lumbar rami
Posterior sacral rami
Lateral femoral cutaneous
Anterior femoral cutaneous
Posterior femoral cutaneous
Common peroneal
Superficial peroneal
Saphenous
Sural
Lateral plantar
Tibial
Medial plantar

FIG. B-1. (*Continued*)

C. DESIRABLE WEIGHT OF ADULTS

Stephen A. Paget and Allan Gibofsky

Table C-1. 1983 Metropolitan height and weight tables[a]

Men					Women				
Height					Height				
Feet	Inches	Small frame	Medium frame	Large frame	Feet	Inches	Small frame	Medium frame	Large frame
5	2	128–134	131–141	138–150	4	10	102–111	109–121	118–131
5	3	130–136	133–143	140–153	4	11	103–113	111–123	120–134
5	4	132–138	135–145	142–156	5	0	104–115	113–126	122–137
5	5	134–140	137–148	144–160	5	1	106–118	115–129	125–140
5	6	136–142	139–151	146–164	5	2	108–121	118–132	128–143
5	7	138–145	142–154	149–168	5	3	111–124	121–135	131–147
5	8	140–148	145–157	152–172	5	4	114–127	124–138	134–151
5	9	142–151	148–160	155–176	5	5	117–130	127–141	137–155
5	10	144–154	151–163	158–180	5	6	120–133	130–144	140–159
5	11	146–157	154–166	161–184	5	7	123–136	133–147	143–163
6	0	149–160	157–170	164–188	5	8	126–139	136–150	146–167
6	1	152–164	160–174	168–192	5	9	129–142	139–153	149–170
6	2	155–168	164–178	172–197	5	10	132–145	142–156	152–173
6	3	158–172	167–182	176–202	5	11	135–148	145–159	155–176
6	4	162–176	171–187	181–207	6	0	138–151	148–162	158–179

[a] Weights at ages 25 to 29 based on lowest mortality. Weight in pounds according to frame (in indoor clothing weighing 5 lb for men and 3 lb for women; shoes with 1-in. heels).

From Metropolitan Life Insurance Company, 1983.

D. NORMAL LABORATORY VALUES

Stephen A. Paget and Allan Gibofsky

Table D-1. Normal laboratory values

Tests		Normal values
Immunologic		
Rheumatoid factor		
Latex fixation		<1.160 titer
Rate nephelometric		<30 IU/mL
Serum complement		
Total hemolytic complement (CH 50)		150–250 Us/mL
Complement components (immunoassays)		
C1q		11–22 mg/dL
C2		1.6–3.6 mg/dL
C3		64–210 mg/dL
C4		11.5–50.0 mg/dL
C5		7.1–20.4 mg/dL
C1 esterase inhibitor		14–30 mg/dL
Factor B		14.8–31.0 mg/dL
Antinuclear antibody (ANA)		Negative
Anti-DNA antibody (*Crithidia* immunofluorescence)		Negative
Anti-streptolysin O (ASO)		0–125 Todd units
Serum immunoglobulins (immunoassay)		
IgG		723–1685 mg/dL
IgA		69–382 mg/dL
IgM		63–277 mg/dL
Hematologic		
Blood counts	**Males**	**Females**
CBC (includes five-part differential)	3.5–10.7	3.5–10.7
RBC × 10^{12}/L	4.2–5.6	4.0–5.2
HGB (g/dL)	13–17	11.5–16.0
HCT (%)	38–52	34–46
MCV (fl)	82–98	82–98
PLT × 10^{9}/L	160 to 400	
Differential	%	**Absolute**
Neutrophils	40.0–74.0	1.90–8.00
Lymphocytes	19.0–48.0	0.90–5.20
Monocytes	3.4–9.0	0.16–1.00
Eosinophils	0.0–7.0	0.00–0.80
Basophils	0.0–1.5	0.00–0.20
Larger unstained cells	0.0–4.0	
Stained smears—bands		0–12 mm/h males <10%
Sedimentation rate (Westergren)		0–27 mm/h females

(continued)

Table D-1. (*Continued*)

Tests	Normal values
Activated partial thrombo-plastin time (aPTT)	Upper limit 38.0 sec
Prothrombin time (PT) (dependent on reagent lot No.)	Upper limit 13.0 sec
Fibrinogen	200–400 mg/dL
Biochemistry	
Acid phosphatase (spectro-photometry)	0–5.5 μ/L
Albumin (modified Doumas)	3.5–5.0 g/dL
Aldolase (ultraviolet, kinetic)	0–7.4 μ/L
Alkaline phosphatase (Bowers & McComb)	30–110 μ/L
Amylase (enzymatic/kinetic)	25–125 μ/L
Bicarbonate (enzymatic oxidation)	23–35 mEq/L
Bilirubin, total (azobilirubin)	0–1.0 mg/dL
Calcium (*o*-cresophthalein complex 1)	8.5–10.5 mg/dL
Chloride (ion-selective electrode)	97–107 mEq/L
Cholesterol (enzymatic)	150–240 mg/dL
Creatine kinase (enzymatic/kinetic)	40–175 females 40–225 μ/L males
Creatinine (modified Jaffe)	0.4–1.2 mg/dL
GGTP (modified Rosalki & Tarlow)	0–70 μ/L
Glucose (hexokinase)	70–105 mg/dL
Iron (ferrozine)	20–170 μg/dL females 20–200 μg/dL males
Iron-binding capacity (ferrozine)	250–450 μg/dL
LDH (modified Amador)	80–200 μ/L
5′-NT (enzyme kinetic)	4–11.5 μ/L
Phosphorus, inorganic (modified Fiske & Subbarow)	2.5–5.0 mg/dL
Potassium (ion-selective electrode)	3.5–5.0 mEq/L
Protein, total (Biuret)	6.0–8.0 g/dL
Salicylate (colorimetric You & Roe) therapeutic level	6–20 mg/dL
SGOT (AST) (modified Scandinavian)	10–45 μ/L
SGPT (ALT) (modified Scandinavian)	0–40 μ/L
Sodium (ion-selective electrode)	135–145 mEq/L
Triglyceride (enzymatic/colorimetric)	72–174 mg/dL
Urea nitrogen (modified Talke & Schubert)	5–25 mg/dL
Uric acid (uricase Trivedi)	2.0–9.0 mg/dL
Endocrine	
T_4 (immunoassay)	4.9–10.7 μg/dL
T_3 uptake (immunoassay)	28%–36%
T_3 RIA (immunoassay)	
0 to 14 y	125–250 ng/dL
14 to 23 y	100–220 ng/dL
>24 y	80–180 ng/dL
Intact PTH (immunochemiluminescent assay)	1.0–5.0 pmol/L
N-terminal PTH (immunochemiluminescent assay)	0–6.1 pmol/L
C-terminal PTH (radioimmunoassay)	0–50 mEq/mL
Quantitative urinary excretion	
Calcium	50–400 mg/24 h
Hydroxyproline, total	15–45 mg/24 h
Magnesium	75–150 mg/24 h
Sodium	43–217 mEq/24 h

Table D-1. (*Continued*)

Tests	Normal values
Potassium	26–123 mEq/24 h
Phosphorus (inorganic)	340–1,100 mg/24 h
Amylase (enzymatic/kinetic)	1–17 U/h
Protein	10–100 mg/24 h
Creatinine	800–1,900 mg/24 h
Creatinine clearance	70–180 mL/min
Uric acid (diet-dependent)	250–750 mg/24 h

E. FORMULARY

Arthur M. F. Yee and Jane E. Salmon

Recent progress in understanding the pathophysiology of rheumatic diseases and in the development of new therapeutic approaches has greatly expanded the pharmacologic armamentarium with which to treat these illnesses. Moreover, the spectrum of conditions that fall under the realm of rheumatology increasingly overlaps with that of other medical specialties, and so previously known medicines have frequently found new application. Thorough appreciation of the indications, contraindications, goals of therapy, and potential adverse effects of any medicine is essential for appropriate administration. Nonetheless, although the clinical situation may define the need for a given therapeutic category, the use of a specific agent is often determined by an empiric trial that considers patient response, tolerance, and compliance, as well as by drug expense. As with all medications, recognition of contraindications and careful monitoring of potentially adverse effects are of paramount importance, especially in children, the elderly, and pregnant women.

PREGNANCY AND MEDICATIONS

As many rheumatic diseases affect women of childbearing age, the clinician should be keenly aware of the many possible complications of medications and their effects on fertility and fetal development. A frank and thorough discussion with the patient is paramount *even before* pregnancy is attempted.

Although it is impossible to create absolute rules regarding the management of medications, the overriding principle will always be the weighing of the potential benefits of any drugs against the potential risks, to be considered on an individual case basis. Although minimizing drug intervention during pregnancy is always desired, there is very strong evidence for discontinuing the use of certain drugs, such as methotrexate (MTX) or cyclophosphamide (CTX), both before and during gestation. For other medications, such as azathioprine or hydroxychloroquine, the evidence is not as clear, although they are probably relatively safe. Warfarin should be discontinued because of its known teratogenic effects and should be substituted with heparin. Aspirin and nonsteroidal antiinflammatory agents should be discontinued in the latter part of pregnancy because of the potential for premature closure of the ductus arteriosus; nonetheless, in the anti-phospholipid syndrome, low-dose aspirin is an important treatment option in ensuring a successful pregnancy. Prednisone and methylprednisolone at low to moderate doses will not cross the placenta and are considered to be safe for fetal development. In contrast, the fluorinated corticosteroids (e.g., dexamethasone and betamethasone) will cross the placenta.

NONSTEROIDAL ANTIINFLAMMATORY DRUGS

Nonsteroidal antiinflammatory drugs (NSAIDs) exhibit antipyretic, antiinflammatory, and analgesic activity. They are used for degenerative musculoskeletal problems, systemic inflammatory illnesses, crystalline diseases, soft-tissue injuries, and hypercoagulable states, among others. All act by interrupting the arachidonic acid metabolic cascade, but therapeutic effects may involve actions other than, or in addition to, the inhibition of prostaglandin synthesis. NSAIDs are essentially equipotent, although individual responses may vary among patients. Most have similar side effects. Individual patient tolerance may vary between preparations. If an inadequate therapeutic response or intolerance occurs, a trial of an alternative agent, especially from a different chemical class, is often worthwhile. Compliance may be related to the schedule of administration (Table E-1). Concurrent use of aspirin and another NSAID or of multiple non-aspirin NSAIDs is not generally recommended. Side effects common to most NSAIDs include gastrointestinal intolerance, tinnitus, fluid retention, platelet abnormalities, and hepatic and renal dysfunction. In patients being treated on a long-term basis with NSAIDs, regular monitoring of hepatic and renal function is necessary.

Table E-1. Nonsteroidal antiinflammatory drugs

Drug	Tablet size (mg)	Dosing frequency (times per day)	Maximum dose (mg)
Aspirin	300, 325, 600, 650	3–4	6,000
Diclofenac	25, 50, 75	2–4	200
Diflunisal	250, 500	2–3	1,500
Fenoprofen	300, 600	3–4	3,200
Flurbiprofen	50, 100	3–4	300
Ibuprofen	200, 300, 400, 600	3–4	2,400
Indomethacin	25, 50, 75-SR	3	200
Ketoprofen	25, 50, 75	3–4	300
Meclofenamate	50, 100	3–4	400
Naproxen	250, 375, 500	2	1,000
Phenylbutazone	100	3–4	400
Piroxicam	20	1	20
Sulindac	150, 200	2	400
Tolmetin	200, 400	3	1,800

All NSAIDs should be used cautiously in patients with impaired renal or hepatic function and in the elderly. They are relatively contraindicated in patients with a history of peptic ulcer disease. If NSAIDs are needed in such patients or other high-risk groups, gastroprotective agents, such as misoprostol or proton pump inhibitors, should be used concurrently to reduce the risk for gastrointestinal complications. Asthma attacks, urticaria, and angioedema may be related to enzymatic inhibition of prostaglandin synthesis in susceptible persons or to immunoglobulin E (IgE)-mediated reactions, which usually occur with pyrazolone-type drugs. Patients who have these reactions to aspirin or other NSAIDs may be sensitive to all NSAIDs. Pregnancy is another relative contraindication to NSAID use, as NSAIDs may cause hemorrhagic complications or premature closure of the ductus arteriosus. The benefits of NSAID use in pregnant women must be weighed very carefully against the risks.

The platelet-inhibiting effects of aspirin are irreversible, whereas the effects of nonaspirin NSAIDs on platelet function are variable. However, in general, discontinuation of all NSAIDs for up to 1 week should be considered before any invasive procedure is undertaken.

Major recent advances have been made in the development of a new generation of NSAIDs that preferentially inhibit the activity of cyclooxygenase-2 (COX-2). Because of their relative sparing of constitutive COX-1 activity, which is necessary for mucosal protection, COX-2 inhibitors have been shown to have fewer adverse gastrointestinal effects than do traditional NSAIDs. Moreover, COX-2 inhibitors do not affect platelet function or increase bleeding time at therapeutic concentrations. Celecoxib and rofecoxib are the first COX-2 inhibitors to be approved for use in the United States, and it is anticipated that others will soon be available.

Aspirin

Action

Inhibits prostaglandin synthesis.

Metabolism

Aspirin (acetylsalicylic acid) is metabolized in the liver and excreted by the kidney. Its half-life increases with increasing doses. It is highly bound to albumin in plasma and widely distributed to all tissues, including synovium.

Adverse Reactions

Gastrointestinal discomfort with nausea and dyspepsia is common, especially in the elderly. Increased gastrointestinal blood loss occurs. Tinnitus, decreased hearing acuity, or both are related to mild toxicity and are reversible with a decrease in dosage. Central nervous system symptoms such as headache, vertigo, and irritability can occur in the elderly. Aspirin may induce mild, reversible hepatocellular injury in patients being treated for acute rheumatic fever, juvenile rheumatoid arthritis (JRA), and active systemic lupus erythematosus (SLE). Platelet adhesiveness and aggregation and adenosine diphosphate release are inhibited by irreversible acetylation of platelet membrane protein.

Caution
Idiosyncratic reactions such as asthma occur in 0.02% of patients. Patients with asthma and nasal polyps are at higher risk for this reaction. Cross-reactivity exists with other NSAIDs but has not been reported with sodium or magnesium salicylates. Aspirin is uricosuric at high doses (>45 g/24 h), but low doses (<2 g/24 h) may lead to urate retention. Aspirin may displace other drugs bound to albumin, thereby potentiating the effects of oral hypoglycemic agents, warfarin, and other medications. Because aspirin inhibits platelet aggregation and prolongs bleeding time, it should be avoided or used with great caution in patients receiving heparin or warfarin anticoagulants. In patients receiving large doses of salicylates, salicylate toxicity may occur during tapering of corticosteroids.

Supply
Tablets, 325, 500, and 650 mg. Buffered tablets, formulated with either absorbable (bicarbonate) or nonabsorbable antacids, are not associated with reduced gastrointestinal bleeding. Enteric-coated tablets are often better tolerated, with less dyspepsia and occult gastrointestinal blood loss, but also have more variable absorption rates than either buffered or nonbuffered tablets. Rectal suppositories are incompletely absorbed. Time-release tablets have delayed absorption with possibly more sustained plasma levels. The physician should be aware of the fact that a large number of over-the-counter drug combinations containing aspirin are widely available.

Dosage
The dosage is 600 to 1,200 mg every 4 to 5 hours, preferably with meals. For optimal antiinflammatory effects, blood levels between 20 and 30 mg/dL and a total daily dose of 3 to 6 g are usually required. Dosages necessary to achieve adequate therapeutic concentrations vary with the individual patient. The maximum tolerated dose must be reached slowly, so that waiting 1 week between dosage changes is appropriate. Salicylate levels are routinely available and may be useful to determine adequacy of dosage, patient compliance, and toxicity.

Celecoxib (Celebrex)
Action
Inhibits prostaglandin synthesis via preferential inhibition of COX-2.

Metabolism
Celecoxib is a diaryl-substituted pyrazole. Celecoxib may be generally administered without regard to timing of meals and will achieve peak plasma levels within 3 hours, although high-fat meals may delay peak plasma levels. About 97% of the drug is protein-bound, primarily to albumin. Metabolism is largely mediated via cytochrome P-450 2C9, and excretion is via both feces and urine. The effective half-life is about 11 hours.

Adverse Reactions
Dyspepsia and gastrointestinal intolerance are common, and vigilance for gastrointestinal hemorrhage is necessary. The renal effects are similar to those of other NSAIDs. Other forms of intolerance include hypertension, edema, and dermatologic reactions.

Caution
Lower initial doses are recommended in the elderly and in the setting of hepatic insufficiency. Potential drug interactions have been identified with lithium and fluconazole. Celecoxib may be taken with low-dose aspirin, warfarin, and MTX and appears to have no effect on platelet function at therapeutic levels. The drug is contraindicated in pa-

tients with known allergies to other NSAIDs or to sulfonamides and should also be avoided in pregnancy.

Supply
Capsules, 100 and 200 mg.

Dosage
The dosage is 200 mg in one or several divided doses daily. The maximum daily dose is 400 mg.

Diclofenac (Cataflam, Voltaren, Arthrotec)
Action
Inhibits prostaglandin synthesis.

Metabolism
Diclofenac is a phenylacetic acid derivative. Absorption is delayed by food. Peak plasma level after administration occurs in 2 to 3 hours. Ninety-nine percent is reversibly bound to plasma albumin. Half-life is approximately 2 hours. It is eliminated through metabolism and excretion in urine (65%) and bile (35%).

Adverse Reactions
Gastrointestinal ulceration, bleeding, and perforation occur in 1% of patients. Headaches and dizziness are common. Elevation in transaminases is present in 2% of patients and is generally reversible, although severe hepatotoxicity has been reported. Fluid retention, edema, and nephrotoxicity can occur. Cross-reactivity in patients with aspirin sensitivity occurs.

Caution
Because of potential hepatotoxicity, serum liver chemistries should be followed very closely. Signs and symptoms of gastrointestinal bleeding and renal dysfunction should be monitored. Diclofenac displaces albumin-bound drugs, which may lead to interaction with other drugs. Renal prostaglandin effects may increase toxicity of MTX, digoxin, and cyclosporine. In patients taking anticoagulants, extreme caution should be used, or the drug should be avoided altogether.

Supply
Tablets, 25, 50, and 75 mg. The 50-and 75-mg preparations are also available in combination with misoprostol.

Dosage
The dosage is 50 to 75 mg twice daily, which may be increased to a maximum daily dose of 200 mg.

Diflunisal (Dolobid)
Action
Inhibits prostaglandin synthesis.

Metabolism
Diflunisal is a difluorophenyl derivative of salicylic acid that is not metabolized to salicylic acid. Peak plasma level occurs 2 to 3 hours after ingestion. Ninety percent is excreted in the urine as glucuronides. Plasma half-life is 8 to 12 hours.

Adverse Reactions
See Aspirin. Diflunisal may cause less gastrointestinal irritation than aspirin does. The dose-related effect on platelet function is reversible.

Caution
See Aspirin. More than 99% of diflunisal is protein-bound and may displace other protein-bound drugs, with resultant drug interactions. Serious interaction with indomethacin has been reported.

Supply
Tablets, 250 and 500 mg.

Dosage
The dosage is 250 to 500 mg twice daily. An initial loading dose of 1,000 mg may accelerate attainment of steady-state serum levels. The maximum daily dose is 1,500 mg.

Etodolac (Lodine)
Action
Inhibits prostaglandin synthesis.

Metabolism
Etodolac is an indole acetic acid derivative. Food or antacids do not appear to compromise gastrointestinal absorption, although peak serum concentrations and time to peak concentration may be affected.

Adverse Reactions
Dyspepsia and gastrointestinal intolerance are common. Hepatic and renal toxicities should be concerns. Other forms of intolerance include hypertension, edema, malaise, depression, and dermatologic reactions.

Caution
Hepatic and renal function should be monitored closely with long-term use.

Supply
Capsules, 200 and 300 mg; tablets, 400 mg and 500 mg.

Dosage
The dosage is 200 to 300 mg two or three times daily. The maximum daily dose is 1,200 mg.

Fenoprofen Calcium (Nalfon)
Action
Inhibits prostaglandin synthesis.

Metabolism
Fenoprofen is a propionic acid derivative. It is rapidly absorbed, with peak plasma levels attained in 90 minutes and a half-life of 160 minutes; concomitant food ingestion decreases rate and extent of absorption. Enterohepatic circulation of the drug occurs. Ninety percent is excreted in the urine as glucuronides. Aspirin decreases the peak blood levels.

Adverse Reactions
Dyspepsia and gastrointestinal bleeding occur less commonly than with aspirin. Rash, headache, sodium retention, and, rarely, interstitial nephritis and nephrotic syndrome may occur.

Caution
Fenoprofen reduces platelet aggregation and may increase the risk for bleeding in patients on warfarin or heparin. Fenoprofen is 90% protein-bound and may displace other protein-bound drugs, with resultant drug interactions. The drug is not recommended in pregnancy. Cross-reactivity in patients with aspirin sensitivity occurs.

Supply
Tablets, 600 mg; capsules, 200 and 300 mg.

Dosage
The dosage is 300 to 600 mg four times daily. The maximum daily dose is 3.2 g.

Flurbiprofen (Ansaid)

Action

Inhibits prostaglandin synthesis.

Metabolism

Flurbiprofen is a phenylalkanoic acid derivative. It is well absorbed, with peak levels in 1.5 hours and an elimination half-life of 5.7 hours. It is extensively metabolized and excreted primarily in the urine. It is 99% protein-bound.

Adverse Reactions

Dyspepsia, nausea, diarrhea, and abdominal pain are common. Gastrointestinal ulceration and bleeding may occur. Headaches and fluid retention are also common. Renal and hepatic dysfunction may occur but usually are reversible on discontinuation of the drug.

Caution

Flurbiprofen may interfere with actions of diuretics and β-adrenergic blocking effects. Because it is protein-bound, it may modify levels of other protein-bound drugs. Flurbiprofen may affect bleeding parameters and should be used with caution in patients receiving anticoagulants.

Supply

Tablets, 50 and 100 mg.

Dosage

The dosage is 200 to 300 mg daily administered in three to four divided doses.

Ibuprofen (Advil, Motrin, Nuprin, Vicoprofen)

Action

Inhibits prostaglandin synthesis.

Metabolism

Ibuprofen is a propionic acid derivative. It is 38% protein-bound, and the half-life is 2 hours. It is primarily metabolized by the liver. Roughly equivalent amounts of the metabolized drug are excreted in urine and feces.

Adverse Reactions

Dyspepsia is common. Occult gastrointestinal bleeding may be less common than with aspirin. Occasionally, headaches, rashes, and salt retention occur. Aseptic meningitis and hypersensitivity reactions in patients with lupus erythematosus have been reported.

Caution

Ibuprofen decreases platelet aggregation and prolongs bleeding time. Caution must be used in patients taking anticoagulants. Cross-reactivity in patients with aspirin sensitivity occurs. It is not recommended during pregnancy. There is no clear evidence that exceeding 2,400 mg daily increases effectiveness.

Supply

Tablets, 300, 400, 600, and 800 mg (200 mg available over the counter). Also available in combination with hydrocodone bitartrate (7.5 mg).

Dosage

The dosage is 1,200 to 2,400 mg in three to four divided doses.

Indomethacin (Indocin)

Action

Inhibits prostaglandin synthesis.

Metabolism
Indomethacin is an indole acetic acid and is 90% bound to albumin. The kidneys excrete 65% of the metabolized drug. Probenecid may increase plasma levels of indomethacin by interfering with its excretion.

Adverse Reactions
Gastrointestinal side effects (dyspepsia, bleeding, nausea, and vomiting) occur in 10% to 40% of patients. Central nervous system effects, occurring in 10% to 25%, include headaches, vertigo, dizziness, and psychiatric disturbances. Less common effects include sodium retention, exacerbation of hypertension, hepatitis, and bone marrow suppression.

Caution
Indomethacin is not recommended for pregnant women or nursing mothers. It antagonizes the natriuretic and antihypertensive effects of furosemide. Indomethacin should be used cautiously in patients with coagulation defects or receiving anticoagulants because it inhibits platelet aggregation. Cross-reactivity in patients with aspirin sensitivity occurs.

Supply
Capsules, 25 and 50 mg; sustained-release capsules, 75 mg; oral suspension, 25 mg/mL; rectal suppositories, 50 mg.

Dosage
The dosage is 25 mg three or four times daily, taken with meals. The dosage can be gradually increased by 25-mg increments to 150 to 200 mg daily. The sustained-release preparation may be taken once or twice a day to a maximum daily dose of 150 mg.

Ketoprofen (Orudis, Oruvail, Actron)
Action
Inhibits prostaglandin synthesis.

Metabolism
Ketoprofen is a propionic acid derivative that is well absorbed after oral administration, but peak concentrations are delayed and reduced when the drug is administered with food. Peak plasma levels are reached at 0.5 to 2 hours, and the half-life is 2 to 4 hours. The drug is 99% bound to protein. The kidneys excrete 60% as glucuronide, and enterohepatic recirculation accounts for the other 40%.

Adverse Reactions
Dyspepsia, gastrointestinal ulceration, bleeding, and perforation may occur in up to 1% to 2% of patients. Central nervous system side effects such as headache, dizziness, and drowsiness are the second most common reaction. Impaired renal function (edema, increased blood urea nitrogen) and interstitial nephritis may occur. Reversible mild elevation of transaminase levels may be seen in up to 15% of patients, but marked elevations are seen in fewer than 1%. Cross-reactivity in patients with aspirin sensitivity occurs.

Caution
Ketoprofen displaces albumin-bound drugs, which may lead to interactions with MTX and other protein-bound drugs. It decreases platelet adhesion and aggregation and should be used with caution in patients on anticoagulation.

Supply
Capsules, 25, 50, and 75 mg; sustained-release capsules, 100, 150, and 200 mg (12.5 mg tablets are available without prescription).

Dosage
The starting dose is 75 mg three times daily or 50 mg four times daily. The daily dose is 150 to 300 mg in three or four divided doses.

Ketorolac (Toradol)

Action

Inhibits prostaglandin synthesis.

Metabolism

Ketorolac, a pyrrolizine carboxylic acid derivative, is available as a tromethamine salt that can be administered orally or parenterally for either IM or IV use. The bioavailability of the drug is very high regardless of the route of administration, although the rate of absorption is slowest following IM injection. When it is administered orally, the rate, but not the extent, of absorption may be diminished with food. The rate of absorption is also reduced in the geriatric patient or in the setting of hepatic or renal impairment. Peak plasma concentrations may be achieved within 3 minutes after IV administration. The drug is hydroxylated in the liver and mainly excreted in urine.

Adverse Reactions

Adverse nervous system reactions, including headache, somnolence, and dizziness, have been reported in up to 23% of patients. Gastrointestinal intolerance is reported in 13% of patients and may occur regardless of route of administration. Borderline elevations of serum liver enzymes may be detected in up to 15% of patients, although fewer than 1% have elevations more than three times greater than normal limits. Anaphylactoid reactions have been rarely reported.

Caution

Ketorolac is bound tightly to serum proteins. However, it does not displace digoxin and only slightly displaces warfarin. Gastrointestinal hemorrhage is a significant concern, and it is recommended that the use of ketorolac be limited to acute and severe pain and not exceed 5 days consecutively. Dosage adjustment is necessary with renal or hepatic impairment.

Supply

Tablets, 10 mg; injectable suspension, 15 and 30 mg/mL.

Dosage

The oral dose is 10 mg up to four times daily. The initial IV and IM doses are 15 to 30 mg and 30 to 60 mg, respectively. Up to 30 mg can then be used for maintenance parenteral administration every 6 hours.

Meclofenamate Sodium (Meclomen)

Action

Inhibits prostaglandin synthesis.

Metabolism

Meclofenamate sodium is an anthranilic acid derivative. Peak plasma levels occur in 30 to 60 minutes with a half-life of about 3 hours; concomitant antacid administration does not interfere with absorption. About two-thirds is excreted in the urine, mostly as the glucuronide conjugate, and about one-third appears in the feces.

Adverse Reactions

Gastrointestinal reactions occur more frequently than with aspirin. Diarrhea may occur in up to one-third of patients, and nausea in about 10%. Headache, dizziness, rash, and other reactions associated with NSAIDs may also occur.

Caution

Meclofenamate sodium enhances the effect of warfarin but has a smaller effect than aspirin on platelet aggregation. The drug is not recommended for use in pregnancy. Cross-reactivity in patients with aspirin sensitivity occurs.

Supply

Capsules, 50 and 100 mg.

Dosage
The dosage is 50 to 100 mg four times daily.

Mefenamic Acid (Ponstel)
Action
Inhibits prostaglandin synthesis.

Metabolism
Mefenamic acid is an anthranilic acid derivative that is rapidly absorbed after oral administration. After metabolism in the liver, about two-thirds of the drug is excreted in urine, and the remaining one-third is eliminated in the feces.

Adverse Reactions
Gastrointestinal adverse reactions are the most common and include diarrhea, nausea, dyspepsia, and peptic ulcer disease. Mild liver enzyme abnormalities are frequent (up to 15%) but rarely progress.

Caution
Mefenamic acid is highly protein-bound. It enhances the effects of warfarin and can elevate serum lithium concentrations.

Supply
Capsules, 250 mg.

Dosage
The loading dose is 500 mg, followed by 250 mg every 6 hours.

Nabumetone (Relafen)
Action
Inhibits prostaglandin synthesis.

Metabolism
Nabumetone, a naphthylkanone derivative, is a pro-drug that is activated by oxidation in the liver.

Adverse Reactions
Although it has been reported that gastrointestinal effects may be fewer than those seen with other NSAIDs, precautions should still be observed.

Caution
Because the drug is activated in the liver, it should be used cautiously in the setting of hepatic impairment.

Supply
Tablets, 500 and 750 mg.

Dosage
The dosage is 1,000 to 2,000 mg daily in single or divided doses.

Naproxen (Naprosyn, Naprelan, Aleve)
Action
An arylalkanoic derivative that inhibits prostaglandin synthesis.

Metabolism
Absorption is not significantly delayed by food. Ninety-eight percent is protein-bound. The half-life is 12 to 15 hours. The kidneys excrete 80% to 90% in conjugated form. Aspirin decreases peak plasma levels.

Adverse Reactions
Gastrointestinal bleeding, dyspepsia, headache, dizziness, and sodium retention occur less frequently than with aspirin. Interstitial nephritis rarely occurs.

Caution
Naproxen displaces albumin-bound drugs, which may lead to drug interactions. It inhibits platelet aggregation and should be used with caution in patients taking anticoagulants. Cross-reactivity in patients with aspirin sensitivity occurs.

Supply
Tablets, 250, 375, and 500 mg. Sustained-release formulations for once-daily dosing are available. Tablets are also available in nonprescription strength.

Dosage
The dosage is 250 mg twice daily, which may be increased to 500 mg twice daily. Up to 1,000 mg of the sustained-release form may be taken once daily.

Oxaprozin (Daypro)
Action
Inhibits prostaglandin synthesis.

Metabolism
Oxaprozin is a propionic acid derivative. The rate but not the extent of gastrointestinal absorption is reduced by food but not by antacids.

Adverse Reactions
Gastrointestinal precautions should be observed, as with other NSAIDs.

Caution
Geriatric patients may tolerate the drug less well because of the long half-life of the drug. Modification of the dosage is necessary in the setting of renal impairment and severe liver disease.

Supply
Tablets, 600 mg.

Dosage
The dosage is 600 to 1,800 mg daily in single doses.

Piroxicam (Feldene)
Action
Inhibits prostaglandin synthesis.

Metabolism
Piroxicam is an oxicam derivative that is well absorbed after oral administration with no effect of antacids on plasma levels. Peak levels are achieved 3 to 5 hours after administration with a long but variable half-life (range, 30 to 86 hours). The drug is excreted in urine and feces (in a ratio of about 2:1), with less than 5% unchanged by biotransformation. Piroxicam is highly protein-bound.

Adverse Reactions
Gastrointestinal bleeding, peptic ulceration, dyspepsia, tinnitus, dizziness, headache, edema, and other reactions associated with NSAIDs may occur.

Caution
Piroxicam can displace other protein-bound drugs, such as warfarin. Platelet aggregation may be affected. The drug is not recommended for use during pregnancy. Cross-reactivity in aspirin-sensitive patients may occur. As with other drugs having long half-lives, special care should be taken in the elderly.

Supply
Capsules, 10 and 20 mg.

Dosage
The dosage is 20 mg/d. Higher doses are not recommended and may be associated with increased gastrointestinal side effects.

Rofecoxib (Vioxx)
Action
Inhibits prostaglandin synthesis via preferential inhibition of COX-2.

Metabolism
Rofecoxib is a furanone derivative. Peak plasma levels are reached within 3 hours. Although high-fat foods may delay absorption after administration of the tablet form, rofecoxib may be generally administered without regard to timing of meals, and overall absorption is not affected. However, concomitant use of calcium- or magnesium-based antacids may impede absorption marginally. The effects of food and antacids on the absorption of the rofecoxib suspension have not been fully studied. About 87% of the drug is protein-bound. Elimination is largely mediated by hepatic metabolism and excretion in both urine and feces. The effective half-life is 14 hours. With continuous dosing, steady-state plasma concentrations are reached in 4 days.

Adverse Reactions
Dyspepsia and gastrointestinal intolerance are common, and vigilance for gastrointestinal hemorrhage is necessary. The renal effects are similar to those of other NSAIDs. Other forms of intolerance include elevations in liver enzymes, anemia, hypertension, edema, and fluid retention.

Caution
Lower initial doses are recommended in elderly patients and in the setting of hepatic or renal insufficiency. Rofecoxib may decrease the effectiveness of angiotensin-converting enzyme (ACE) inhibitors and may increase the risk for gastrointestinal complications when administered together with aspirin. Rofecoxib increases plasma concentrations of MTX and increases the prothrombin time in patients taking warfarin. The drug is contraindicated in patients with known allergies to other NSAIDs and in late pregnancy.

Supply
Tablets, 12.5 and 25 mg.
Suspension, 12.5 mg/5 mL and 25 mg/5 mL.

Dosage
The dosage is 12.5 to 25 mg daily. For acute pain and primary dysmenorrhea, 50 mg daily may be administered, although administration for more than 5 days has not been evaluated for safety and should be avoided.

Salicylate Salts (Trilisate)
Action
Inhibits prostaglandin synthesis.

Metabolism
See Aspirin.

Adverse Reactions
See Aspirin. Non-aspirin salicylates may cause fewer gastrointestinal disturbances and less gastrointestinal bleeding than aspirin does. They have less effect on platelet function.

Caution
Sodium salicylate may constitute a substantial sodium load for patients with heart failure or hypertension. Hypermagnesemic toxicity may develop with magnesium salicylate in patients who have renal insufficiency. See also Aspirin.

Supply
Sodium salicylate tablets, 325 and 650 mg; choline salicylate liquid, 870 mg/5 mL; magnesium salicylate tablets, 325, 500, 545, and 600 mg; choline magnesium trisalicylate tablets, 293 mg/363 mg, 440 mg/544 mg, 587 mg/725 mg; choline magnesium trisalicylate liquid, 293 mg/5 mL choline salicylate and 362 mg/5 mL magnesium salicylate; trolamine salicylate 10% cream or lotion.

Dosage
Sodium salicylate, 325 to 650 mg every 4 hours, maximum of 5,400 mg daily.

Choline salicylate, 435 to 870 mg every 4 hours, maximum of 7,200 mg daily.

Magnesium salicylate, 300 to 600 mg every 4 hours, maximum of 3,500 mg daily.

Choline magnesium trisalicylate, maximum of 4,500 mg total salicylate daily in divided doses.

Trolamine salicylate 10% cream or lotion for topical use, two to four times daily.

Salsalate (Disalcid, Argesic, Salflex, Salsitab)
Action
Inhibits prostaglandin synthesis.

Metabolism
Salsalate is the salicylate ester of salicylic acid and is activated after hydrolysis to salicylate. It is completely absorbed by the gastrointestinal tract, mostly in the small intestine. However, because up to 13% of the drug is conjugated with glucuronic acid in the liver and not hydrolyzed to active metabolites, the bioavailability of salsalate is less than that of a theoretically equivalent intake of salicylate. The drug is almost exclusively excreted in urine.

Adverse Reactions
See Salicylate Salts.

Caution
See Salicylate Salts.

Supply
Capsules, 500 mg; tablets, 500 and 750 mg.

Dosage
The dosage is 500 to 750 mg twice a day to a maximum daily dose of 4,000 mg.

Sulindac (Clinoril)
Action
Inhibits prostaglandin synthesis.

Metabolism
An indene acetic derivative of indomethacin, sulindac requires hepatic activation to the active sulfide metabolite. The half-life of sulindac is about 8 hours, whereas the half-life of the active sulfide metabolite is 16 to 18 hours. It is tightly protein-bound. The kidney excretes 45% to 50%, and 25% to 30% is found in feces.

Adverse Reactions
Dyspepsia, nausea, gastrointestinal bleeding, tinnitus, headaches, dizziness, hepatitis, rash, and edema may occur. There are reports of relative sparing of renal function in comparison with other NSAIDs, but these remain subject to debate and do not justify unmonitored use in patients at risk for renal impairment.

Caution
Sulindac may potentiate oral hypoglycemic agents, anticoagulants, and other protein-bound drugs. It prolongs bleeding time and should be used with caution in patients receiving anticoagulants. Cross-reactivity in patients with aspirin sensitivity may occur.

Supply
Tablets, 150 and 200 mg.

Dosage
The dosage is 150 mg twice daily, which may be increased to 200 mg twice daily.

Tolmetin Sodium (Tolectin)
Action
Inhibits prostaglandin synthesis.

Metabolism
The half-life of this pyrrole acetic acid derivative is 60 minutes. It is 99% excreted in urine and 99% protein-bound.

Adverse Reactions
Peptic ulcers occur in 2% to 3% of patients. Gastrointestinal bleeding occurs in 1%. Other reactions include diarrhea, abdominal pain, nausea, dyspepsia, rash, sodium retention, lightheadedness, headache, and dizziness.

Caution
False-positive test results for urinary protein are noted when sulfosalicylic acid, but not Albustix (tetrabromophenol blue), is used. It may decrease platelet adhesiveness and prolong bleeding time. Cross-reactivity in patients with aspirin sensitivity occurs.

Supply
Tablets, 200 and 600 mg; capsules, 400 mg.

Dosage
The dosage is 400 mg twice daily, preferably including doses on arising and at bedtime. Daily doses larger than 1,800 mg are not recommended. Tolmetin is approved for use in children.

CORTICOSTEROIDS AND CORTICOTROPIN

Corticosteroids are potent antiinflammatory agents capable of quickly suppressing many disease manifestations of systemic, autoimmune, and inflammatory disorders, and they are available in forms suitable for topical, locally injectable, and systemic use. Corticotropin, or adrenocorticotropic hormone (ACTH), has been used for the treatment of acute crystalline arthritides. Although their ability to modify the ultimate course of disease varies from disease to disease, their side effects with prolonged use are incontrovertible. Among the plethora of adverse effects associated with corticosteroid use are hypertension, weight gain, Cushing's syndrome, glucose intolerance, osteoporosis, osteonecrosis, emotional lability, premature atherosclerosis, immunosuppression, and others. Strong efforts should be made to employ disease-modifying agents to ensure that corticosteroids play as small role as possible in the management of inflammatory arthritis.

Corticosteroids differ with regard to relative antiinflammatory potency and to relative mineralocorticoid potency. A comparison of the properties of different selected corticosteroids is given in Table E-2.

Corticosteroids
Action
Glucocorticoids suppress inflammation in addition to humoral and cell-mediated immune responses.

Metabolism
Corticosteroids are well absorbed from the gastrointestinal tract. Prednisone is metabolized in the liver to prednisolone, the active compound. Further hepatic metabolism results in the inactivation of steroids. They are 90% protein-bound.

Table E-2. Glucocorticoid preparations

	Equivalent dose (mg)	Relative anti-inflammatory potency	Relative mineralocorticoid potency
Hydrocortisone	20	1.0	1.0
Cortisone	25	0.8	0.8
Prednisone	5	4.0	0.8
Prednisolone	5	4.0	0.8
Methylprednisolone	4	5.0	0
Dexamethasone	0.75	30.0	0

Dexamethasone vial, 4 mg/mL in 1-, 5-, and 25-mL containers; 24 mg/mL in 5- and 10-mL containers.
Intraarticular preparations:
Methylprednisolone acetate, 20- and 40-mg/mL suspension in 1-, 5-, and 10-mL containers.
Triamcinolone acetonide, 40-mg/mL suspension in 1-, 5-, and 10-mL vials; 10-mg/mL suspension in 5-mL vials.
Triamcinolone hexacetonide, 20-mg/mL suspension in 1- and 5-mL vials.
Prednisolone tertiary butylacetate, 20-mg/mL suspension in 1-, 5-, and 10-mL vials.
Topical preparations: See Table E-3.

Adverse Reactions

Cutaneous side effects include acne, hirsutism, striae, purpura, and impaired wound healing. Osteoporosis, myopathy, and aseptic necrosis of bone may occur. Gastrointestinal side effects include peptic ulceration with bleeding or perforation and pancreatitis. Hypertension and edema secondary to fluid retention occur. Steroid psychosis and benign intracranial hypertension are the central nervous system adverse reactions. Ocular effects include cataracts and glaucoma. Patients may suffer growth arrest, secondary amenorrhea, impotence, and suppression of the hypothalamic-pituitary-adrenal axis. Glucose intolerance, hyperosmolar nonketotic coma, and centripetal obesity occur. The risk for infection is increased. Intraarticular corticosteroids may cause a crystal-induced transient synovitis. Immobilization and ice compress will facilitate resolution;

Table E-3. Commonly used topical preparations

Very high strength
- Betamethasone dipropionate 0.05% (Alphatrex, Diprolene, Maxivate, Psorion)
- Clobetasol propionate 0.05% (Temovate)
- Diflorasone diacetate 0.05% (Psorcon)
- Halobetasol propionate 0.05% (Ultravate)

High strength
- Desoximetasone 0.25% (Topicort)
- Fluocinolone acetonide 0.2% (Synalar-HP)
- Fluocinonide 0.05% (Lidex)
- Halcinonide 0.1% (Halog)
- Triamcinolone acetonide 0.1% (Aristocort A)

Moderate strength
- Betamethasone valerate 0.1% (Valisone)
- Fluocinolone acetonide 0.025% (Synalar)
- Flurandrenolide 0.05% (Cordran)
- Hydrocortisone valerate 0.2% (Westcort)
- Triamcinolone acetonide 0.025% (Kenalog, Aristocort)

Low strength
- Hydrocortisone 0.25%, 0.5%, 1.0%
- Other preparations with cortisone, prednisolone, methylprednisolone acetate

persistence of the synovitis beyond 24 hours raises the possibility of an arthrocentesis-related infectious arthritis. Topical steroids, especially the more potent fluorinated compounds, may cause cutaneous telangiectasia, striae, epidermal and dermal atrophy, rosacea-like facial eruption, and senile-type purpura. When used with occlusive dressings, infection, folliculitis, and decreased heat exchange may occur.

Caution

Periodic determinations of blood sugar, complete blood cell counts, stool guaiac tests, and blood pressure measurements should be obtained. Diabetes mellitus, hypertension, pregnancy, and psychosis are relative contraindications. In patients receiving long-term steroids, the hypothalamic-pituitary-adrenal axis is suppressed, and they require glucocorticoid supplementation when undergoing surgical procedures or other physiologic stress. Repeated administration of intraarticular injections of corticosteroid may lead to disruption of cartilage and supporting soft-tissue structures. Soft-tissue injections may cause similar effects. Long-term steroid use demands appropriate immunizations and measures to ensure protection against osteoporosis.

Systemic absorption of topical steroid preparations may occur. Prolonged use, especially of the more potent compounds, may lead to suppression of the hypothalamic-pituitary-adrenal axis.

Dosage

The safest steroid regimen is the lowest effective dosage for the shortest time period. Numerous schedules for administering glucocorticoids have been developed to limit side effects and maximize therapeutic response. Single-dose, alternate-day regimens decrease the incidence of side effects but may not suppress disease activity adequately. In such cases, daily therapy (divided or single doses) may be administered. Dosage varies widely according to the specific disease. Intraarticular corticosteroids are useful in patients with involvement of only one or a few joints by inflammatory arthritis. Doses vary from several milligrams for small joints of the hand to 40 mg for large joints, such as the knee. The efficacy of topical steroids is related to both potency and percutaneous penetration. Adequate hydration of the skin, inflammation, and occlusion with plastic wraps enhance penetration. Better biologic activity is often obtained with ointment rather than cream or lotion preparations. As a general principle, therapy is started with stronger preparations and then reduced to less potent strengths once control of skin manifestations is achieved.

Supply

A. Selected oral preparations

Prednisone tablets, 1, 2.5, 5, 10, 20, and 50 mg. Prednisolone tablets, 1, 2.5, and 5 mg. Methylprednisolone tablets, 2, 4, 8, 16, 24, and 32 mg. Dexamethasone tablets, 0.25, 0.5, 0.75, 1.5, and 4 mg.

B. Selected parenteral preparations

Hydrocortisone vial, 100, 250, 500, and 1,000 mg. Methylprednisolone vial, 40, 125, 500, and 1,000 mg.

C. Selected intraarticular preparations

Methylprednisolone acetate, suspension of 20 and 40 mg/mL in 1-, 5-, and 10-mL containers. Triamcinolone acetonide, suspension of 40 mg/mL in 1-, 5-, and 10-mL vials; suspension of 10 mg/mL in 5-mL vials. Triamcinolone hexacetonide, suspension of 20 mg/mL in 1- and 5-mL vials. Prednisolone tertiary butylacetate, suspension of 20 mg/mL in 1-, 5-, and 10-mL vials.

D. Selected topical preparations

Very high strength

Betamethasone dipropionate 0.05% (Alphatrex, Diprolene, Maxivate, Psorion)
Clobetasol propionate 0.05% (Temovate)
Diflorasone diacetate 0.05% (Psorcon)
Halobetasol propionate 0.05% (Ultravate)

High strength

Desoximetasone 0.25% (Topicort)
Fluocinolone acetonide 0.2% (Synalar-HP)

Fluocinonide 0.05% (Lidex)
Halcinonide 0.1% (Halog)
Triamcinolone acetonide 0.1% (Aristocort A)

Moderate strength

Betamethasone valerate 0.1% (Valisone)
Fluocinolone acetonide 0.025% (Synalar)
Flurandrenolide 0.05% (Cordran)
Hydrocortisone valerate 0.2% (Westcort)
Triamcinolone acetonide 0.025% (Kenalog, Aristocort)

Low strength

Hydrocortisone 0.25%, 0.5%, 1.0%
Other preparations with cortisone, prednisolone, methylprednisolone acetate

Corticotropin

Action

Stimulates secretion of cortisol by adrenal glands.

Selected Indications

Acute crystal-induced arthritides.

Metabolism

Corticotropin is a polypeptide, usually extracted from the porcine pituitary gland, and is administered either IM or IV. Peak plasma cortisol levels are achieved usually within 1 hour of injection. The metabolism of corticotropin is not fully known, but it is rapidly removed from plasma by many tissues.

Adverse Reactions

Corticotropin may cause immediate hypersensitivity reactions, even without previous exposure; these may range from minor skin reactions to anaphylaxis. With prolonged use, typical toxicities associated with corticosteroid use may occur. Moreover, suppression of endogenous corticotropin release by the pituitary may result in hypothalamic-pituitary insufficiency.

Caution

Corticotropin is contraindicated in patients with known previous hypersensitivity reactions to the medication or to porcine proteins.

Supply

The supply is 25 or 40 units for IM, IV, or SC injection.

Dosage

The dosage is 40 units every 8 hours.

DISEASE-MODIFYING ANTIRHEUMATIC DRUGS

Disease-modifying antirheumatic drugs (DMARDs) are much more readily and promptly utilized than previously for the treatment of systemic rheumatic illnesses. Also called slowly acting antirheumatic drugs (SAARDs) or remittive agents in the medical literature, these drugs are certainly slowly acting but probably do not induce indefinite remissions. In rheumatoid arthritis (RA), for example, the capacity for these agents to modify disease varies greatly from drug to drug and from patient to patient. As a group, their modes of action are poorly understood and probably varied. Some are clearly immunosuppressive or cytotoxic, whereas others may act by reducing systemic inflammation. Their potential for and spectrum of adverse effects are diverse, and so careful monitoring for toxicities is crucial. Although their clinical effect generally becomes apparent only after several weeks to months, they appear capable of ameliorating the course of disease in a significant percentage of patients and reducing cumulative corticosteroid use. Accordingly, DMARDs are commonly used and are also known as steroid-sparing agents. Moreover, there appear to be advantages in using combinations of DMARDs in lower doses to maximize benefit while minimizing toxicities.

Azathioprine (Imuran) and 6-Mercaptopurine (Purinethol)

Action

Inhibition of purine synthesis.

Selected Indications

RA, SLE, vasculitis.

Metabolism

Azathioprine (AZA) is a pro-drug that is converted to the active compound 6-mercaptopurine (6-MP). However, because of better gastrointestinal absorption, AZA is more widely used. Urinary excretion, partial hepatic metabolism, and tissue uptake account for clearance from the blood.

Adverse Reactions

Hematologic toxicity is usually mild leukopenia and thrombocytopenia; aplastic anemia is rare. Drug fever may occur. Hepatitis and pancreatitis may also occur. Nausea, especially during initiation of therapy, is common. Stomatitis may be seen. An increased incidence of late lymphoreticular and hematopoietic malignancy is possible. The immunosuppressive effects of these drugs increases susceptibility to infections.

Caution

Complete blood cell counts and platelet counts should be obtained initially weekly and then monthly. A rapid fall in leukocyte count requires a decrease in dosage or discontinuation of the drug. Liver function tests should be performed periodically. Allopurinol inhibits the metabolism of both AZA and 6-MP, which causes high levels to accumulate; thus, concomitant use of allopurinol should be avoided, or else a significant reduction in the AZA dose by 75% is appropriate. AZA has been used safely in pregnancy, but as with any medication, discontinuation of the drug, if possible, is preferable. Dosages must be adjusted in patients with hepatic or renal impairment.

Supply

AZA tablets, 50 mg.
6-MP tablets, 50 mg.

Dosage

AZA, 2 to 3 mg/kg daily.
6-MP, 1 to 2 mg/kg daily.

Chlorambucil (Leukeran)

Action

Alkylating agent. Interferes with cell function and mitotic activity by inhibition of intracellular macromolecules.

Selected Indications

Severe RA, SLE, vasculitis.

Metabolism

Adequate and reliable oral absorption. Incomplete information concerning metabolism and excretion.

Adverse Reactions

Myelosuppression is usually moderate, gradual, and rapidly reversible. Gastrointestinal discomfort, dermatitis, and hepatotoxicity occasionally occur.

Caution

Frequent complete blood cell counts should be obtained. Delayed occurrence of acute leukemia is reported. Infertility in both sexes may occur.

Supply

Tablets, 2 mg.

Dosage
The dosage is 0.05 to 0.2 mg/kg daily. The total daily dose (usually 4 to 10 mg) is given as a single dose.

Chloroquine (Aralen)
Action
Mode of action is unknown. Potential actions include binding of nucleic acids, stabilization of lysosomal membranes, and trapping of free radicals.

Selected Indications
RA, SLE, cutaneous LE.

Metabolism
Chloroquine is well absorbed from the gastrointestinal tract. The drug is concentrated and retained in body tissues. Peak plasma concentrations are attained within 2 hours, which may be facilitated by administering the drug with food. Chloroquine and its metabolites are slowly excreted by the kidneys. Unabsorbed drug is eliminated in the feces.

Adverse Reactions
The most common side effects are allergic eruptions and gastrointestinal disturbances (anorexia, nausea, cramps, diarrhea). The most serious complication is ocular toxicity, which appears to be dose-dependent but more common than with hydroxychloroquine. Reversible corneal deposits of the drug are detectable by slit-lamp examination, but retinopathy affecting macular pigmentation may be irreversible. Less common side effects include hyperpigmented rash, hypopigmentation of hair, neuropathy, ototoxicity, and cardiomyopathy. Hematologic toxicity is rare.

Caution
Ophthalmologic examination (color testing, visual fields, funduscopy, slit-lamp examination) should be performed every 4 to 6 months. Complete blood cell count should be performed periodically. At the first sign of visual disturbance, the drug should be discontinued. Hydroxychloroquine may cause hemolytic anemia in patients with glucose-6-phosphate dehydrogenase deficiency. The drug is contraindicated in patients with significant visual, hepatic, or renal impairment, or porphyria, and during pregnancy.

Supply
Tablets, 300 mg.

Dosage
The dosage is 150 mg daily.

Co-trimoxazole (Bactrim, Septra)
Action
Co-trimoxazole is a fixed combination of sulfamethoxazole (SMX) and trimethoprim (TMP), both of which are synthetic folate antagonists. Although most widely used as an antiinfective agent, it has found use in some cases of limited Wegener's granulomatosis.

Selected Indications
Mild Wegener's granulomatosis, prophylaxis against *Pneumocystis carinii* infection.

Metabolism
Co-trimoxazole is rapidly absorbed after oral administration, and peak plasma levels of both components are reached within 4 hours. The liver converts TMP to oxide and hydroxylated metabolites, and acetylates and conjugates SMX to its metabolites. Almost all these metabolites are excreted in the urine. Elimination of co-trimoxazole is highly dependent on renal function.

Adverse Reactions
Gastrointestinal intolerance and hypersensitivity skin reactions of all degrees account for the majority of adverse effects. Hypersensitivity reactions may occur more commonly in patients with SLE. Cytopenias may occur, especially in patients with underlying hematologic abnormalities. In patients with renal impairment, potentially life-threatening electrolyte abnormalities may develop, particularly hyperkalemia.

Caution
Co-trimoxazole should be used with caution in the setting of liver or kidney impairment, underlying hematologic problems, and possibly folate or deficiency of glucose-6-phosphate dehydrogenase. Patients with sulfa allergies should not receive co-trimoxazole.

Supply
Tablets, TMP 80 mg/SMX 400 mg and TMP 160 mg/SMX 800 mg.

Dosage
For limited Wegener's granulomatosis, TMP 160 mg/SMX 800 mg twice daily.
For prophylaxis against *P. carinii,* TMP 160 mg/SMX 800 three times a week.

Cyclophosphamide (Cytoxan)
Action
Alkylating agent. Interferes with nucleic acids and proteins by cross-linking intracellular macromolecules. Cyclophosphamide (CTX) can inhibit secondary immune responses.

Selected Indications
Severe RA, SLE, vasculitis, interstitial lung disease.

Metabolism
Well absorbed from gastrointestinal tract. It requires activation by liver to produce active metabolites. Unchanged drug and metabolites are excreted in the urine.

Adverse Reactions
Bone marrow depression, primarily of white cell series, and predisposition to infection, both of which may be life-threatening but reversible with discontinuation of drug. Alopecia, drug-induced infertility with amenorrhea or defective spermatogenesis, hemorrhagic cystitis (in up to 25% of patients), fibrosing cystitis, carcinoma of the bladder, hematopoietic malignancies, anorexia, nausea, vomiting, and pulmonary fibrosis. Antidiuretic hormone-like activity may occur with large doses and result in hyponatremia.

Caution
Contraindicated in pregnant women and patients with hepatic impairment. Dosage requires adjustment in renal insufficiency. Frequent complete blood cell counts, platelet counts, and urinalyses must be obtained. Maintenance of high urine output and the use of 2-mercaptoethane sulfonate may reduce bladder complications.

Supply
Tablets, 25 and 50 mg; vials, 100, 200, and 500 mg for IV injection.

Dosage
Oral route: 0.5 to 3.5 mg/kg daily given as single morning dose. IV route: For treatment of diffuse proliferative glomerulonephritis associated with SLE or systemic vasculitides, begin with monthly IV treatments at an initial dose of 0.5 mg/m^2. Doses are then increased by 25% if the 7- to 10-day post-CTX white blood cell count is above 5,000/mL or decreased by 25% if that white blood cell count is below 3,000/mL. The highest dose is 1 mg/m^2. After six monthly treatments, the treatment interval is reduced to every 2 to 3 months for the second 6 months. Further treatments are defined by the clinical course. Appropriate hydration and anti-emetics are indicated.

Cyclosporin A (Sandimmune, Neoral)

Action

Cyclosporin A is a nonpolar, cyclic oligopeptide. It is a potent inhibitor of early steps in T-cell activation via suppression of early gene transcription.

Selected Indications

RA, psoriatic arthritis, autoimmune diseases.

Metabolism

The unmetabolized drug is active. The absorption of cyclosporin A is variable after oral administration, averaging about 30% of the ingested dose but varying from 2% to 89%, and it is reduced by simultaneous administration of food. Serum levels may followed if indicated. Two oral formulations of cyclosporin A are available, which differ in bioavailability and therefore do not exhibit equivalent dosing. The nonaqueous liquid formulation (Neoral) immediately forms an emulsion in aqueous fluids and has a bioavailability 1.2 to 1.5 times that of the conventional liquid preparation (Sandimmune). Peak levels appear between 3 and 4 hours, and the drug is metabolized on first pass though the liver. More than 90% of cyclosporin A is protein-bound, mostly to lipoproteins. It passes the placenta and into breast milk. About 95% is eliminated via feces.

Adverse Reactions

Nephrotoxicity is the most frequent and clinically significant adverse effect. At prior high doses for the treatment of RA, more than half of treated patients exhibit a significant elevation in serum creatinine, although fewer than 10% require discontinuation of the drug. New or exacerbation of preexisting hypertension is also frequently observed. Other common side effects include gastrointestinal intolerance, infections, gout, hypertrichosis, hyperesthesias, paresthesias, gingival hyperplasia, abnormal serum liver chemistries, and potential oncogenicity.

Caution

The dosage should not exceed 5 mg/kg of body weight; the usual starting dose in RA is 2.5 mg/kg of body weight daily. Renal function and arterial blood pressure should be monitored carefully. The serum creatinine should not be allowed to increase by more than 50% of baseline. Hypertension may be controlled with nifedipine or isradipine, but not with verapamil or diltiazem, both of which interfere with hepatic metabolism. Special caution should be taken with concomitant use of MTX, which can decrease the elimination of cyclosporin A. Additional medications to be avoided because of drug interactions include antifungal azole derivatives (ketoconazole, fluconazole, itraconazole), macrolide antibiotics (erythromycin, clarithromycin), and allopurinol, among many others. Grapefruit juice increases the bioavailability of the drug. Cyclosporin A is contraindicated in premenopausal women who do not practice effective contraception, during pregnancy, and in nursing mothers.

Supply

Capsules (Sandimmune), liquid-filled, 25, 50, and 100 mg.
Capsules (Neoral), liquid-filled, for emulsion, 25 and 100 mg.
Solution (Sandimmune), 100 mg/mL.
Solution (Neoral), for emulsion, 20 mg.

Dosage

The dosage is 2 to 5 mg/kg of body weight daily in twice-daily dosing.

Dapsone

Action

Possible antiinflammatory effects through inhibition of prostaglandin synthesis, complement activation, and myeloperoxidase-mediated pathways.

Selected Indications

Cutaneous LE, SLE.

Metabolism
Dapsone is well absorbed within the gastrointestinal tract. Peak levels are attained within 2 to 8 hours. The half-life of the drug is about 1 day. Dapsone is partially acetylated by the liver. It and its metabolites are mostly excreted in urine; about 20% is unchanged drug.

Adverse Reactions
Dose-dependent hemolytic anemia and methemoglobinemia are the most frequent adverse effects. Hemolysis may occur in patients with or without glucose-6-phosphate dehydrogenase deficiency but is more severe in those with glucose-6-phosphate dehydrogenase deficiency. Supplementation with ascorbic acid, folic acid, and iron may prevent some of the hematologic effects. Cutaneous hypersensitivity and gastrointestinal intolerance may occur. Elevated serum liver enzymes are common, but toxic hepatitis and cholestatic jaundice have been rarely reported.

Caution
Patients with significant anemia should not receive dapsone, and screening for glucose-6-phosphate dehydrogenase deficiency may be indicated in persons suspected to be at high risk for hemolysis (e.g., taking concurrent medications with adverse hematologic effects) or myelosuppression. Complete blood cell counts and serum liver chemistries should be followed weekly for the first month and then regularly thereafter with long-term administration.

Supply
Tablets, 25 and 100 mg.

Dosage
Initial dose of 50 mg daily; increases titrated according to response to a maximum of 400 mg daily.

Gamma Globulin, for Intravenous Use
Action
IV preparations of gamma globulin contain modified polyvalent antibodies with intact opsonic activity but with little or no aggregates. Action in thrombocytopenia may involve blockade of macrophage Fc receptors. Other proposed mechanisms of action include the activity of anti-idiotypic antibodies, effects on cytokine production and cytokine receptors, and induction of increased catabolism of pathogenic immunoglobulin.

Selected Indications
Inflammatory myositis, immune thrombocytopenia purpura, vasculitis.

Metabolism
Gamma globulin is distributed 50% intravascularly and 50% extravascularly after 6 days. Its half-life is 3 weeks. Disaccharides used for stabilization are excreted in the urine.

Adverse Reactions
In fewer than 1% of patients who are not immunodeficient, reactions develop 30 to 60 minutes after the start of infusions, including flushing, fever, dizziness, nausea, and hypotension. Patients should be observed and vital signs monitored throughout infusions.

Caution
Patients with selective IgA deficiency who possess antibodies to IgA should not receive intravenous gamma globulin.

Supply
Gamma globulin is supplied in 1-, 3-, and 6-g vials with sodium chloride for reconstitution.

Dosage
For treatment of inflammatory myositis or idiopathic thrombocytopenia purpura, 2 g/kg body weight (cumulative) in divided doses during 3 to 5 days.

Gold Compounds (Ridaura, Solganal, Aurolate)
Action
Mode of action in RA is unknown. Alters macrophage and complement functions.

Selected Indications
RA, psoriatic arthritis.

Metabolism
Approximately half of the administered IM dose is excreted within 1 week, 30% in the urine and the remainder in the stool. Gold in the circulation rapidly equilibrates with synovial fluid. It is stored by the reticuloendothelial system. It is 90% protein-bound. Approximately 25% of oral gold (auranofin) is absorbed and metabolized, with 15% excreted in urine and the remainder in feces. In blood, it is 60% protein-bound and 40% associated with red blood cells.

Adverse Reactions
Forty percent of patients experience some toxicity. Eosinophilia, although common, does not necessarily predict toxicity. The most common reaction is dermatitis, which may be heralded by pruritus or eosinophilia, or both. Both dermatitis and stomatitis are reversible with discontinuation of drug, and except for the rare instances of exfoliative dermatitis, gold therapy can be reinstituted with low doses. Hematologic abnormalities occur in 1% to 2% of patients. Thrombocytopenia is most common, followed by leukopenia, agranulocytosis, and pancytopenia. Gold should not be restarted. Proteinuria may be seen in 4% of patients, but nephrotic syndrome with membranous glomerulonephritis is much less common. Proteinuria of more than 0.5 g/d requires cessation of therapy. Mild proteinuria or celluria is a signal to interrupt therapy until urinalysis result is normal. Nitritoid reactions characterized by self-limited episodes of sweating, flushing, dizziness, nausea, and shortness of breath after administration of gold may occur with the thiomalate preparation. Treatment of nitritoid reactions involves switching to aurothioglucose and administering gold with the patient supine. Unusual problems include enterocolitis, intrahepatic cholestasis, skin hyperpigmentation, peripheral neuropathy, pulmonary infiltrates, and deposits of gold in the cornea.

Adverse reactions to oral gold (auranofin) are similar to but less common than those with IM gold and include the additional side effects of diarrhea in 50% of patients and abdominal pain in 14%.

Caution
Gold is contraindicated in patients with previous gold allergy or severe toxic skin, kidney, or bone marrow reaction to gold. Relative contraindications include functional impairment of kidneys or liver. Immunosuppressive agents and penicillamine, agents with a potential to suppress the bone marrow, should not be given with gold. Patients should have frequent complete blood cell counts (including platelets) and a urinalysis before each injection during the first few weeks of therapy and periodically thereafter.

Dosage
Initial dose is 10 mg IM to test for idiosyncratic reactions. Thereafter, 25 mg the second week and 50 mg at subsequent weekly intervals are given. In the absence of side effects, a total dose of 1 g may be given. If improvement has occurred, the drug is continued in 50-mg doses with an increasing time interval between injections: every 2 weeks for several months, then every 3 weeks, and finally 50 mg monthly for maintenance therapy. Improvement is gradual but usually begins when the cumulative dose is 300 to 700 mg. Dosage for children and adolescents is 1 m/kg up to 25 mg per injection. Oral gold (auranofin) is initially administered at 3 mg daily and increased to a maximum of 9 mg daily for maintenance therapy.

Supply
Gold thioglucose (Solganal), vials of 50 mg/mL in 10 mL.
Gold sodium thiomalate (Aurolate), 10, 25, 50, and 100 mg/mL in 1-mL ampules; 50 mg/mL in 10-mL ampules.
Auranofin (Ridaura), tablets, 3 mg.

Hydroxychloroquine (Plaquenil)
Action
Mode of action is unknown. Potential actions include binding of nucleic acids, stabilization of lysosomal membranes, and trapping of free radicals.

Selected Indications
RA, SLE, cutaneous LE.

Metabolism
Well absorbed from the gastrointestinal tract. The drug is concentrated and retained in body tissues. Excretion by the kidney is detectable months after therapy is discontinued.

Adverse Reactions
The most common side effects are allergic eruptions and gastrointestinal disturbances (anorexia, nausea, cramps, diarrhea). The most serious complication is ocular toxicity. Reversible corneal deposits of the drug are detectable by slit-lamp examination. Although retinopathy affecting macular pigmentation may be irreversible, it is extremely rare in patients with normal renal function receiving no more than recommended dosages. Less common side effects include hyperpigmented rash, hypopigmentation of hair, neuropathy, ototoxicity, and cardiomyopathy. Hematologic toxicity is rare.

Caution
When administered in daily doses of less than 6.5 mg/kg of body weight in patients with normal renal function, serious adverse effects are uncommon. Ophthalmologic examination (color testing, visual fields, funduscopy, slit-lamp examination) should be performed every 4 to 6 months. Complete blood cell count should be performed periodically. At the first sign of visual disturbance, the drug should be discontinued. Hydroxychloroquine may cause hemolytic anemia in patients with glucose-6-phosphate dehydrogenase deficiency. The drug is contraindicated in patients with significant visual, hepatic, or renal impairment, or porphyria. The question of safety of hydroxychloroquine during pregnancy remains unanswered. There are anecdotal reports of exacerbations of psoriasis with hydroxychloroquine.

Supply
Tablets, 200 mg.

Dosage
Initially, 400 mg in single or divided doses; after a good response (4 to 12 weeks), maintain at 200 mg/d.

Leflunomide (Arava)
Action
Inhibition of pyrimidine synthesis.

Selected Indications
RA.

Metabolism
Following oral administration, leflunomide is converted into its active metabolite, M1, which reaches peak levels after 8 to 12 hours. Administration of cholestyramine or charcoal reduces plasma titers of M1. The metabolite is extensively bound to albumin, and its half-life is about 2 weeks. M1 is excreted in both feces and urine.

Adverse Reactions
Gastrointestinal effects, including diarrhea, occur in more than one-fourth of patients, and elevated serum liver chemistries in 10%. Rash and alopecia are not uncommon. Adverse effects may be more common in patients taking concurrent hepatotoxic substances, such as MTX.

Caution
Leflunomide can cause fetal harm and is contraindicated in pregnancy and in nursing mothers. Women of childbearing potential should use reliable modes of contraception. Significant hepatic insufficiency is also a relative contraindication, and parameters of liver function should be followed regularly, especially during the initial part of therapy. Although concurrent administration with MTX does not demonstrate pharmacokinetic interactions, there may be additive hepatotoxic effects. In patients with renal insufficiency, the levels of M1 may be doubled. Cholestyramine or activated charcoal may be administered to accelerate the elimination of M1.

Supply
Tablets, 10, 20, and 100 mg.

Dosage
A loading dose of 100 mg is given daily for 3 days, followed by 10 to 20 mg as a daily maintenance dose.

Methotrexate (Rheumatrex)
Action
Folate antagonist that inhibits dihydrofolate reductase, resulting in pleiotropic effects that include immunosuppressive and antiinflammatory properties.

Selected Indications
RA, psoriatic arthritis, vasculitis, inflammatory myositis, systemic sclerosis.

Metabolism
MTX is readily absorbed from the gastrointestinal tract in dosages of less than 0.1 mg/kg of body weight. Approximately 50% is protein-bound and is susceptible to displacement by sulfonamides, salicylates, NSAIDs, and other drugs. The kidneys rapidly excrete 50% to 90%; this process is enhanced by urine alkalinization. Impaired renal function significantly affects elimination of MTX.

Adverse Reactions
Patients should be observed for marrow suppression (leukopenia, thrombocytopenia, or complete aplasia) and gastrointestinal injury (ulcerative stomatitis, diarrhea, hemorrhagic enteritis, and hepatic dysfunction, including cirrhosis). Pulmonary infiltrates and pneumonitis, osteoporosis, rashes, and alopecia may occur. Some of the mucocutaneous toxicities may be prevented by daily intake of 1 mg of folic acid.

Caution
Use in nonmalignant disease requires emphasis on long-term side effects. The risk for hepatic cirrhosis supports weekly administration of the drug and careful monitoring of hepatic function, which may include liver biopsy. Renal function, pulmonary function, and complete blood cell counts should also be monitored. Although serial liver biopsies before and during treatment are no longer universally recommended in patients with RA, their utility remains a subject of debate in other diseases, such as psoriatic arthritis. A baseline chest roentgenogram is suggested.

Supply
Tablets, 2.5 mg; vials, 5 and 50 mg for parenteral use.

Dosage
For RA and for psoriatic arthritis, 7.5 to 10 mg weekly may be used initially, administered orally or parenterally, and increased as clinically indicated. The optimal dose

for RA may fall in the range of 15 to 25 mg weekly. For inflammatory polymyositis and vasculitides, 10 to 15 mg IV weekly, with a gradual increase in 5-mg increments to 30 to 50 mg weekly. The dosage interval is subsequently increased to 2 weeks, then 1 month. The dosage should be increased for lack of responsiveness but cautiously because of increasing toxicity at higher levels.

Minocycline (Dynacin, Minocin)
Action
Semisynthetic tetracycline derivative that probably inhibits proteolytic enzyme activity in RA.

Selected Indications
RA.

Metabolism
Gastrointestinal absorption is excellent in the fasting state but is reduced with food and antacids. Peak serum levels are reached within 4 hours. The serum half-life is 11 to 26 hours and does not appear to be affected by mild hepatic or renal dysfunction, although dose adjustment may be necessary in severe renal impairment. Elimination is through both urinary and fecal excretion.

Adverse Reactions
As with other tetracyclines, a photosensitive skin rash may occur. Lightheadedness and dizziness may occur, especially early in therapy. Gastrointestinal intolerance is very common. Because minocycline is also an antibiotic, long-term use may result in overgrowth of nonsusceptible organisms, such as fungus or *Clostridium difficile.* A lupuslike syndrome has been reported in association with long-term use of minocycline.

Caution
Minocycline causes discoloration of dentin and should be avoided in children, pregnant women, and lactating mothers.

Supply
Tablets and capsules, 50 and 100 mg. Suspension, 50 mg/5 mL.

Dosage
The dosage is 100 mg twice daily.

Mycophenolate Mofetil (CellCept)
Action
Immunosuppression via inhibition of guanosine synthesis.

Selected Indications
RA.

Metabolism
Mycophenolate mofetil is rapidly absorbed and then hydrolyzed to its active metabolite, mycophenolic acid. Food does not affect absorption. Mycophenolic acid is later inactivated by hepatic glucuronidation. The inactive metabolites are mostly excreted in urine (93%), with the remainder excreted in feces.

Adverse Reactions
Gastrointestinal effects, including nausea, diarrhea, mucosal hemorrhage, and ulceration, can occur. Leukopenia and infections, especially by opportunistic organisms, are also potential problems. In the renal transplant population, there may be an increased risk for lymphoproliferative and non-melanoma skin carcinomas.

Caution
Complete blood cell counts should be obtained initially weekly and then monthly. A rapid fall in leukocyte count requires a decrease in dosage or discontinuation of the

drug. Serum liver chemistries should be checked periodically. Vigilance for infection and malignancy should be maintained. Mycophenolate should be avoided in pregnant and nursing women. Dose adjustment is necessary in severe renal insufficiency.

Supply
Tablets, 250 and 500 mg.

Dosage
Initially 500 mg twice daily; can be increased as indicated to 1,000 mg twice daily.

D-Penicillamine (Cuprimine, Depen)
Action
Mode of action in RA is unknown. D-Penicillamine decreases circulating immune complexes and rheumatoid factor titer and inhibits lymphocyte responsiveness to mitogens. A latent period of 2 to 3 months is often observed between initiation of therapy and clinical response.

Selected Indications
RA, systemic sclerosis.

Metabolism
Well absorbed from gastrointestinal tract and rapidly excreted in urine. It should be administered on an empty stomach (1 to 2 hours after a meal) to avoid interference of absorption by dietary metals.

Adverse Reactions
Pruritus and skin rash represent the most common side effects and can occur at any time. They can be treated by either lowering the dosage or administering antihistamines. If necessary, the therapy may be interrupted until the rash resolves. Stomatitis also occurs. Alteration of taste is frequent, independent of dosage, and self-limited, with resolution in 2 to 3 months despite continued drug administration. Bone marrow depression may occur precipitously at any time. If the platelet count falls below 80,000 to 100,000, therapy must be discontinued. The most common late toxic effect is immune complex nephropathy. Proteinuria may be seen in 20% of patients. If proteinuria exceeds 1 g/d, the dosage should be reduced. Nephrotic syndrome, hypoalbuminemia, or hematuria requires discontinuation of the drug. Less common side effects include autoimmune syndromes (lupus syndromes, Goodpasture's syndrome, myasthenia gravis, pemphigus, stenosing alveolitis, polymyositis), which necessitate prompt discontinuation of the drug.

Caution
Penicillamine administration is contraindicated in patients who are receiving gold compounds, immunosuppressive drugs, or phenylbutazone. Renal insufficiency and pregnancy are further contraindications. A history of penicillin allergy does not preclude use of penicillamine. All patients should have a complete blood cell count, including platelets, and a urinalysis at 2-week intervals for the first 6 months of therapy and monthly thereafter. An unreliable patient is a relative contraindication.

Supply
Capsules, 125 and 250 mg.

Dosage
Initially, a single daily dose of 250 mg, which is increased in 2 to 3 months to 375 or 500 mg daily if clinical response is insufficient. Further increases to the maximum dose of 750 mg daily may be made after 2 to 3 months.

Protein A Immunoadsorption Column (Prosorba)
Action
This is a device consisting of protein A from *Staphylococcus* bound to a silica matrix. By means of apheresis technology, potentially pathogenic IgG and IgG-containing immune complexes are removed.

Selected Indications
Refractory RA, immune thrombocytopenia purpura.

Metabolism
Extracorporeal passage of plasma through the immunoadsorption column is performed by means of an apheresis machine. The treated plasma is then returned to the patient.

Adverse Reactions
The most common adverse effects are joint pain and swelling, fatigue paresthesias, headache, hypotension, anemia, nausea, sore throat, edema, abdominal pain, hypertension, rash, dizziness, diarrhea, hematoma, flushing, chills, dyspnea, chest pain, and fever. Other complications associated with any procedure involving apheresis may occur, including blood loss, damage to blood cells, and problems arising from mismanagement of fluid balance (e.g., hypertension, hypotension, arrhythmias). In patients with RA, the rate of infection, local thrombosis, or both at the site of central venous catheters is greater than 40%.

Caution
A full discussion with the patient covering reasonable expectations and potential adverse effects of treatment is mandatory before therapy is initiated. This device should be used only at facilities with extensive experience in apheresis. Strict sterile technique is essential, and careful monitoring of vital signs and fluid status is crucial. Concurrent use of ACE inhibitors is contraindicated, and at least 3 days of drug withdrawal is recommended by the manufacturer before the procedure. Patients with previous intolerance to apheresis procedures, hypercoagulable states, or conditions that may become exacerbated by apheresis should not undergo treatment. Treatment may not be advisable in patients with poor peripheral access, impaired renal function, relative hypotension, significant vascular disease, intracranial disease, severe anemia, systemic infections, or significant risk for congestive heart failure and fluid overload. RA patients may be at particular risk for the development of severe anemia.

Supply
Prepackaged sterile polycarbonate columns containing 200 mg of protein A covalently bound to 300 mL of silica matrix.

Dosage
Individualized according to patient status. In general, weekly apheresis may be performed.

Quinacrine Hydrochloride (Atabrine)
Action
Mode of action is unknown. Potential actions include binding of nucleic acids, stabilization of lysosomal membranes, and trapping of free radicals.

Selected Indications
RA, SLE, cutaneous LE.

Metabolism
Well absorbed from the gastrointestinal tract and widely distributed into body tissues, where it is concentrated and retained. Excretion by urine can be detected months after therapy is discontinued.

Adverse Reactions
Common side effects include nausea, vomiting, anorexia, abdominal cramps, rash, and reversible yellow coloration of skin. Less common reactions include central nervous system stimulation, emotional changes, altered pigmentation of skin and nails (black and blue), and cardiomyopathy. Reversible corneal edema and deposits have been reported, but retinopathy is rare. Rare toxicity includes psychosis and aplastic anemia.

Caution
Ophthalmologic examination should be performed periodically. At any sign of visual disturbance, the drug should be discontinued. Quinacrine may cause hemolytic anemia in patients with glucose-6-phosphate dehydrogenase deficiency. It is contraindicated in pregnancy.

Supply
Tablets, 100 mg.

Dosage
The dosage is 100 mg/d.

Sulfasalazine (Azulfidine)
Action
Exact mechanism is unknown, but there is evidence for antiinflammatory, immunomodulatory, antibacterial (in the colon), and folate metabolism actions.

Selected Indications
RA, seronegative spondyloarthropathies.

Metabolism
Sulfasalazine is partially absorbed (one-third) from the small intestines and extensively metabolized. It is split into 5-aminosalicylic acid and sulfapyridine; the latter is metabolized in the liver. The metabolic products are excreted in the urine.

Adverse Reactions
The most common side effects, occurring in up to one-third of patients, include anorexia, headache, nausea, vomiting, gastric distress, and apparently reversible oligospermia. Rash, pruritus, urticaria, fever, and hemolytic anemia are less frequent. Rare reactions such as blood dyscrasia (especially leukopenia), hypersensitivity reaction, and central nervous system reaction have been reported.

Caution
Azulfidine is contraindicated in patients with porphyria and should be administered with caution in patients with hepatic or renal disease, blood dyscrasia, severe asthma, or allergies. Complete blood cell counts and liver function tests should be performed frequently. Urinalysis results should also be followed. Adequate fluid intake must be maintained to prevent crystalluria and renal stones. Patients with glucose-6-phosphate dehydrogenase deficiency should be followed closely for signs of hemolysis. Azulfidine should be avoided in patients with sulfa allergies and should not be given simultaneously with sulfa drugs.

Supply
Tablets, 500 mg.

Dosage
The dosage is 2 to 3 g/d in divided doses with meals.

BIOLOGIC AGENTS

Although biologic agents may be broadly defined and will certainly be subject to redefinition as their use evolves, they generally describe specific antibodies or recombinant forms of natural inhibitors against modulatory molecules of immunity or inflammation. These agents have been most widely studied in the setting of RA, but they represent a new approach to the treatment of all systemic inflammatory rheumatic diseases. Only etanercept has been approved by the Food and Drug Administration thus far, but many more agents specific for various target molecules are in development.

Etanercept (Enbrel)
Action
Inhibition of tumor necrosis factor-alpha (TNF-α).

Selected Indications
RA, psoriatic arthritis.

Metabolism
Etanercept is a dimeric recombinant protein consisting of two ligand-binding domains of the human 75-kd (p75) TNF-α receptor fused to the Fc domain of human IgG1. After SC injection, the median half-life is about 115 hours. Maximum serum concentration is reached in 72 hours. Pharmacokinetic differences have not been noted between male and female patients, or between adult and pediatric patients. The effects of hepatic and renal impairment are not known.

Adverse Reactions
Reactions at the local injection site occur in more than a third of patients but may respond to topical corticosteroids and generally do not result in discontinuation of the drug. Some controlled data suggest that minor upper respiratory tract infections may be increased, and there are few anecdotal cases of sepsis and death in patients taking etanercept. As with other immunomodulatory agents, vigilance for infections should be maintained, and discontinuation of the drug is recommended when severe infections are identified. The effects of etanercept in patients with a history of malignancies or on the risk for new malignancies are not known. The development of antibodies against etanercept are common, but only non-neutralizing antibodies have been detected and are not associated with clinical response or adverse effects.

Caution
Caution should be used during pregnancy, and the drug should be discontinued in nursing mothers. Etanercept is contraindicated in the setting of sepsis or in patients with known hypersensitivity to any component of the preparation or to latex. No drug interactions are known, but concurrent live vaccinations should not be given. The risk for the eventual development of neutralizing antibodies is not known.

Supply
Sterile lyophilized powder, 25 mg for reconstitution with 1.0 mL of sterile water.

Dosage
The dosage is 25 mg SC twice weekly.

MEDICATIONS FOR CRYSTALLINE ARTHRITIDES

NSAIDs and corticosteroids are the mainstays in the treatment of acute gout and crystalline arthritides. Colchicine may also be used in the acute setting, but it is more widely used for prophylaxis. Hypo-uricemic agents reduce serum uric acid levels by either inhibiting production or increasing excretion of uric acid and are used primarily in patients with chronic, recurrent gouty arthritis, tophaceous gout, nephrolithiasis, and urate nephropathy.

Allopurinol (Xyloprim, Lopurin)

Action
Allopurinol, an analog of the purine hypoxanthine, inhibits the enzyme xanthine oxidase, which converts hypoxanthine to xanthine and xanthine to uric acid. Plasma and urine concentrations of uric acid are lowered. Hypoxanthine, a more soluble product, and other purine metabolites are excreted in the urine rather than uric acid. Allopurinol also acts by a feedback mechanism to inhibit *de novo* purine synthesis. The efficacy of allopurinol decreases when the creatinine clearance falls below 20 mL/min.

Selected Indications
Refractory/recurrent gouty arthritis, tophaceous gout, nephrolithiasis, urate nephropathy.

Metabolism
Twenty percent is excreted in the urine unchanged, with the remainder excreted in the urine as alloxanthine. The half-life of the major metabolite, oxypurinol, which also inhibits xanthine oxidase, is 30 hours.

Adverse Reactions
Maculopapular rash is the most common side effect and occurs in 3% of patients. Immune complex dermatitis and hepatitis, occasionally with vasculitis and nephritis, can occur; pruritus is an important warning symptom. Side effects of allopurinol are increased in the presence of marked renal failure (creatinine clearance <20 mL/min).

Caution
Allopurinol inhibits the oxidation of 6-MP. Because 6-MP is the active metabolite of AZA, the concomitant use of either AZA or 6-MP should be avoided with allopurinol, or appropriate dosage reductions of 75% should be made. Allopurinol inhibits hepatic microsomal enzymes for drug metabolism; warfarin derivatives and other drugs metabolized by these enzymes should be given in lower dosages. Concurrent administration of ampicillin and allopurinol leads to a threefold higher incidence of drug rash. The toxicity of cytotoxic agents, such as CTX, appears to be enhanced by the concomitant administration of allopurinol. The dosage of allopurinol should be reduced in renal insufficiency and failure.

Supply
Tablets, 100 and 300 mg.

Dosage
For mild disease, 200 to 300 mg daily is usually adequate, but the dosage should be individualized to achieve the desired serum urate level. It is advisable to start with 100 mg/d and gradually build toward full dosage to lessen the probability of acute gout attacks that may be precipitated by sudden lowering of the serum uric acid. *Allopurinol is counterproductive and is to be avoided in acute attacks of gout.* For severe tophaceous gout, 400 to 600 mg daily can be used. The maximum single dose should be 300 mg. Total daily doses in excess of 600 mg are associated with increased toxicity. It is advisable to prescribe colchicine (0.6 mg PO daily or twice daily) during the first 3 months of therapy as prophylaxis against acute gout.

To prevent uric acid nephropathy during the treatment of neoplastic disease, a daily dose of 600 to 800 mg may be required, with the maintenance of large volumes of an alkaline urine.

Colchicine (ColBENEMID, Proben-C, Col-Probenecid)
Action
Colchicine inhibits microtubule assembly, which interferes with granulocyte mobility and the inflammatory response to precipitated crystals.

Selected Indications
Acute crystal-induced arthritis, prophylaxis for crystal-induced arthritis.

Metabolism
Although complete metabolism is unknown, colchicine is deacetylated in the liver to inactive metabolites; 10% is excreted unchanged by the kidney. The drug half-life is 90 minutes and is prolonged in patients with renal insufficiency.

Adverse Reactions
Gastrointestinal irritation producing nausea, vomiting, and abdominal pain occurs in up to 80% of patients receiving oral colchicine for acute gout. Bone marrow depression, renal dysfunction, and hemorrhagic colitis may occur, especially with overdose or in the setting of liver or renal disease.

Caution
IV colchicine should be diluted in 10 to 15 mL of normal saline solution and administered slowly during 5 minutes through a free-flowing IV route to decrease the chance of infiltration and soft-tissue necrosis. Fatalities have been reported with IV administration. Reduction in dosage is necessary in liver or renal impairment.

Supply
Tablets, 0.6 mg.
IV ampules, 2 mL containing 1 mg of colchicine.
Also available in combination with probenecid (ColBENEMID), tablets, colchicine 0.5 mg/probenecid 500 mg.

Dosage
For maintenance prophylaxis, 0.6 mg daily or twice daily. For acute attacks, oral colchicine, 0.6 to 1.2 mg initially followed by 0.6 mg hourly until symptoms abate or toxicity occurs. The total cumulative dose should not exceed 8 mg. IV colchicine, 1 to 2 mg initially followed by 0.5 mg every 3 to 6 hours up to a total of 4 mg. The dosage should be reduced significantly in the presence of renal or hepatic disease.

Probenecid (Benemid, ColBENEMID, Proben-C, Col-Probenecid)
Action
A uricosuric agent that inhibits renal tubular resorption of organic acids, including uric acid. Probenecid is not effective with a creatinine clearance of less than 40 mL/min.

Selected Indications
Hyperuricemia associated with refractory or recurrent gouty arthritis.

Metabolism
Excreted in urine in the glucuronide form and as oxidized metabolites. The half-life is dose-dependent and ranges from 6 to 12 hours.

Adverse Reactions
Gastrointestinal irritation occurs in 10% of patients; systemic hypersensitivity characterized by fever and rash is seen in about 3%.

Caution
A large alkaline urine output should be maintained, especially during the first week of therapy, to prevent urate renal stones. A history of renal calculi is a relative contraindication. Probenecid may alter the metabolism of other drugs by decreasing their excretion (indomethacin, ampicillin), reducing their volume of distribution (ampicillin), or delaying metabolism (heparin). Probenecid is antagonized by low-dose salicylates (<3 g/d).

Supply
Tablets, 500 mg.
Also available in combination with colchicine (ColBENEMID, Proben-C, Col-Probenecid), tablets, colchicine 0.5 mg/probenecid 500 mg.

Dosage
The dosage is 250 mg twice daily for 1 week, then 500 mg twice daily. Maintenance colchicine should be given during the first 3 months of probenecid therapy and then can be stopped if the patient is asymptomatic. Probenecid is not useful in acute attacks of gout.

Sulfinpyrazone (Anturane)
Action
A uricosuric agent that inhibits renal tubular reabsorption of organic acids.

Selected Indications
Hyperuricemia associated with refractory or recurrent gouty arthritis.

Metabolism
Rapidly and completely absorbed, with peak plasma levels in about 1 hour. Sulfinpyrazone is 98% protein-bound. The kidney excretes about 40% unchanged.

Adverse Reactions
Gastrointestinal irritation is common. Because sulfinpyrazone is similar in structure to phenylbutazone, it should be avoided in patients with known sensitivity to phenylbutazone.

Caution
A large alkaline urine output should be maintained, especially during the first week of therapy, to decrease the risk for urate calculi formation. Sulfinpyrazone inhibits platelet aggregation and potentiates the action of protein-bound drugs such as oral hypoglycemics and oral anticoagulants. The action of sulfinpyrazone is antagonized by low-dose salicylates, and the drug is ineffective in the presence of renal failure.

Supply
Tablets, 100 mg; capsules, 200 mg.

Dosage
Start with 50 to 100 mg twice daily with meals, and increase gradually during several weeks to a maintenance dosage usually of 300 to 400 mg/d in three to four divided doses. Maximum recommended daily dose is 800 mg. Maintenance colchicine should be given for the first 3 months of therapy to prevent precipitation of an acute attack of gouty arthritis.

ANALGESICS

Acetaminophen

Action
Centrally acting analgesic.

Metabolism
Acetaminophen is rapidly absorbed in the gastrointestinal tract and reaches peak levels within 1 hour. The drug is metabolized by the liver, largely to the glucuronide conjugate, and then excreted in urine.

Adverse Reactions
Although rare, hepatic toxicity, including hepatic failure, is the most dangerous potential adverse effect.

Caution
Alcohol use or abuse, fasting, concurrent use of medications that induce cytochrome P-450 activity, and preexisting liver disease increase the risk for liver toxicity. Reduced doses are necessary in children.

Supply
Tablets, caplets, gelcaps, 160, 325, and 500 mg; liquid, 500 mg/15 mL.
Multiple combinations with other medications are available.

Dosage
The dosage is 325 to 1,000 mg every 6 hours as necessary. Maximum adult daily dose is 4 g.

Amitriptyline (Elavil)

Action
Tricyclic antidepressant thought to block reuptake of a variety of neurotransmitters. Amitriptyline and other tricyclic antidepressants have been used for the adjuvant treatment of neuropathic pain.

Metabolism
Amitryptiline is rapidly absorbed by the gastrointestinal tract. The plasma half-life can range from 10 to 50 hours. Amitriptyline and its metabolites are primarily excreted in urine.

Adverse Reactions
The most common adverse effects are related to anticholinergic activity, such as xerostomia, mydriasis, constipation, and urinary retention, especially in geriatric patients. Central nervous system and neuromuscular symptoms are also common, including cognitive changes, somnolence, and exacerbations of underlying psychiatric disorders. Extrapyramidal symptoms ranging from minor involuntary movements and tardive dyskinesia to parkinsonism may occur. Cardiovascular effects include conduction disturbances and arrhythmias and postural hypotension.

Caution
Acute toxicities relate to extensions of adverse reactions. An acute withdrawal syndrome may result after sudden discontinuation of long-standing therapy. A baseline electrocardiogram is generally recommended. Amitriptyline should be used in elderly patients with extreme caution. Concomitant use of monoamine oxidase inhibitors, hypotensive agents, central nervous system depressants, sympathomimetics, and anticholinergic medications should be avoided.

Supply
Tablets, 10, 25, 50, 75, 100, and 150 mg.

Dosage
For neuropathic pain, initially 10 mg at bedtime, with escalating doses to a maximum of 300 mg daily.

Capsaicin (Zostrix, Dolorac)
Action
Inhibition of substance P.

Metabolism
No information is available.

Adverse Reactions
Capsaicin may cause local skin irritation, burning, and erythema.

Caution
Capsaicin is for external use only and should not be applied to open wounds. Contact with eyes should be avoided, and hands should be washed immediately after application. Dried material may cause irritation to nasal and respiratory mucosa and should not be inhaled.

Supply
Cream, 0.025%, 0.075%, and 0.25%.

Dosage
At lower doses, apply topically to skin up to four times daily; 0.25%, apply topically to skin up to twice daily.

Gabapentin (Neurontin)
Action
Gabapentin is a structural analog of τ-aminobulytic acid (GABA), which has been used for neuropathic pain syndromes. Although designed to mimic GABA activity at inhibitory neuronal synapses, gabapentin does not bind to GABA receptors, and its precise mechanism of action is not known.

Metabolism
At therapeutic doses, the bioavailability of gabapentin is about 60%. It is not significantly metabolized in humans and is excreted almost exclusively by the kidneys.

Adverse Reactions
Gabapentin is well tolerated. Nervous system effects are the most common forms of intolerance and include somnolence, dizziness, ataxia, and fatigue.

Caution
Concurrent use with other central nervous system depressants should be avoided. Dose adjustment is necessary in the setting of severe renal insufficiency.

Supply
Capsules, 100, 300, and 400 mg.

Dosage
Initially, 300 mg daily in divided doses, to be titrated up to 2,400 mg daily in divided doses.

Tramadol Hydrochloride (Ultram)
Action
Tramadol is a synthetic, centrally acting analgesic. Although it is not an opiate derivative, it is a selective opiate-receptor agonist. It may also have additional analgesic properties through inhibition of synaptic monoamine reuptake.

Metabolism
The absorption of tramadol is good and is not affected by food. Tramadol is partially metabolized by the liver, and about 90% of the drug and its metabolites are excreted in the urine.

Adverse Reactions
Tramadol shares similar adverse reactions with true opiates, including central nervous system effects (lightheadedness, somnolence), nausea, constipation, xerostomia, and pruritus. It may also potentially cause respiratory depression when administered at high doses and may lower seizure threshold. Tolerance, addiction, and manifestations of withdrawal may also occur, but risks are thought to be relatively small in comparison with those of other opiate agonists.

Caution
Tramadol should be used with extreme caution in conjunction with other medications that may depress the central nervous system, such as other opiates, alcohol, sedatives, and hypnotics, or medications that may reduce seizure threshold, such as monoamine oxidase inhibitors and antipsychotic agents. Patients receiving monoamine oxidase inhibitors should not receive tramadol also because of the drug's inhibitory effects on monoamine reuptake. Dosing should be less frequent in patients with renal or hepatic impairment.

Supply
Tablets, 50 mg.

Dosage
The dosage is 50 to 100 mg every 4 to 6 hours as needed.

DRUGS FOR OSTEOPOROSIS AND METABOLIC BONE DISEASES

Alendronate (Fosamax)
Action
Bisphosphonate that inhibits osteoclast activity and bone resorption but does not interfere significantly with bone mineralization.

Selected Indications
Osteoporosis prevention and treatment, Paget's disease of bone.

Metabolism
Alendronate is poorly absorbed by the gastrointestinal tract, especially when taken with food. Calcium-, aluminum-, and magnesium-containing supplements and antacids interfere with absorption. Absorbed drug is tropic for bone and will persist within the bony skeleton for years. The terminal half-life is about 11 years. Excretion is in the urine.

Adverse Reactions
Gastrointestinal intolerances are the most common adverse effects and include diarrhea, nausea, abdominal pain, and, most importantly, esophagitis and esophageal ulcerations. Adequate calcium repletion before the initiation of therapy may reduce the risk for arthralgias and other musculoskeletal complaints.

Caution
Alendronate must be taken on an empty stomach, while upright, at least a half-hour before eating. Patients with preexisting esophageal reflux or inflammation may not be good candidates for alendronate therapy. It is contraindicated in women of childbearing potential.

Supply
Tablets, 5, 10, and 40 mg.

Dosage
For osteoporosis prevention, 5 mg daily. For osteoporosis treatment, 10 mg daily. For Paget's disease, 40 mg daily with reassessment after 6 months.

Calcitonin (Calcimar, Miacalcin)
Action
Inhibits osteoclast activity and bone resorption.

Selected Indications
Osteoporosis prevention and treatment, Paget's disease of bone, analgesia for acute vertebral fractures, hypercalcemia.

Metabolism
Calcitonin is a protein that is rapidly metabolized to smaller, inactive fragments in the kidneys.

Adverse Reactions
Nausea and vomiting occur in 10% of patients with either the intranasal or SC route. Flushing of face and hands, peripheral paresthesias, urticaria, altered taste, and local skin reactions may be more common with SC calcitonin. Low-dose skin testing is recommended by some before full-dose SC treatment is administered. Irritation of the nasal mucosa, epistaxis, and rarely perforation can be seen with nasal inhalation, so that periodic nasal examinations are indicated.

Caution
Neutralizing antibodies may develop with partial loss of effectiveness.

Supply
Nasal spray, 200 U per spray (14-dose cannisters).
Sterile injectable solution, 1-mL vials.

Dosage
For postmenopausal osteoporosis, 100 U daily by SC or IM injection or 200 U daily intranasally. Each intranasal dose should be taken via the alternate nostril.

For Paget's disease, 100 U daily by SC or IM injection.

Calcium Preparations

Action
Increased calcium pool available for gastrointestinal absorption.

Selected Indications
Osteoporosis prevention and treatment.

Metabolism
Renal excretion of absorbed fraction.

Adverse Reactions
Nausea, constipation, and gastrointestinal irritation may occur.

Caution
Hypercalcemia may occur, especially in patients receiving concomitant vitamin D. Calcium carbonate is ineffective in patients with achlorhydria.

Supply
Calcium carbonate tablets, 500, 650, and 1,250 mg; calcium citrate tablets, 950 mg; calcium gluconate tablets, 450, 500, 600, 900, and 1,000 mg; calcium lactate tablets, 300 and 600 mg. Many preparations are now available with vitamin D.

Dosage
Supplement dietary calcium intake to achieve a total elemental calcium dosage of 1,000 mg/d in divided doses for male and premenopausal female patients; 1,500 mg/d in divided doses for postmenopausal women.

Estrogens

Action
Estrogens are bound by nuclear receptors in various tissues and ultimately affect the transcription of genes that bear the estrogen response element. In bone, inhibition of osteoclast activity is the eventual effect, resulting in reduced bone resorption.

Selected Indications
Prevention and treatment of postmenopausal osteoporosis.

Metabolism
Unconjugated estrogens are rapidly inactivated by the liver after oral administration and so are usually given parenterally. By contrast, conjugated estrogens may be administered orally. Estrogens accumulate in body fat and so may be cleared more slowly in obese patients. Steroidal estrogens are metabolized primarily by the liver via conjugation and then excreted in the urine. A substantial amount is recirculated through the liver from bile for further metabolism.

Adverse Reactions
Malignancies are the most feared potential complication of estrogen therapy (see Caution). It is clear that unopposed prolonged estrogen use increases the risk for endometrial carcinoma in postmenopausal women. However, an association with breast cancers remains a topic of great debate. Other potential adverse effects are manifold and include hypertension, hypercoagulability and thromboembolic disorders, fluid retention, nausea, vomiting, pancreatitis, skin rashes, glucose intolerance, hypercalcemia, hypertriglyceridemia, abnormal serum liver chemistries, cholestasis, gallbladder disease, breakthrough vaginal bleeding, menstrual-type cramping, fibroid enlargement, changes in affect, migraine headaches, mastodynia, and breast secretions.

Caution
Estrogens increase the risk for endometrial carcinoma in postmenopausal women; concomitant administration of progestin in women with intact uteri is recommended to reduce this risk. Estrogens are associated with developmental defects in fetal

reproductive organs and are contraindicated in pregnancy. Most physicians regard a past or current history of breast cancer as another contraindication. Other contraindications to estrogen therapy include estrogen-dependent neoplasias, undiagnosed abnormal vaginal bleeding, active or past thrombophlebitis, and severe liver disease. Use in women without a personal history but with a close family history of breast cancer requires careful discussion of the risks and benefits of initiating or withholding therapy. Caution should also be taken in patients with preexisting uncontrolled hypertension, cardiovascular disease, asthma, migraine headaches, seizure disorders, renal dysfunction, depression, gallbladder disease, hypercoagulable states, and fibroids.

Supply
Estradiol: tablets, 0.5, 1, and 2 mg; transdermal patch, 0.025, 0.05, 0.075, and 0.1 mg/24 h.

Estradiol/norethindrone acetate combinations: transdermal patch, estradiol 0.05 mg and norethindrone acetate 0.14 mg or 0.25 mg/24 h.

Conjugated estrogens: tablets, 0.3, 0.625, 0.9, and 0.125 mg.

Conjugated estrogens/medroxyprogesterone combinations:

Monophasic regimen, conjugated estrogens 0.625 mg and medroxyprogesterone 2.5 mg.

Monophasic regimen, conjugated estrogens 0.625 mg and medroxyprogesterone 5 mg.

Biphasic regimen, conjugated estrogens 0.625 mg in 28 tablets with medroxyprogesterone 5 mg in 14 tablets.

Estropipate: tablets, 0.75, 1.5, and 3.0 mg.

Esterified estrogens: tablets, 0.3, 0.625, 1.25, and 2.5 mg.

Dosage
The recommended initial dosages for prevention and treatment of postmenopausal osteoporosis are given. Women with intact uteri should receive concomitant cyclical or continuous progestin therapy; for example, oral medroxyprogesterone may be administered either in a cyclical fashion (5 mg daily during the last 2 weeks of a 4-week cycle) or continuously (2.5 mg daily). Women who have undergone hysterectomies may be given estrogen therapy without progestin.

Estradiol:

Oral regimen is 0.5 mg daily.

Transdermal regimen is 0.05 mg/24 h patch applied twice weekly. (Note: Combination patches containing norethindrone acetate 0.14 mg or 0.25 mg/24 h are available.)

Conjugated estrogens: 0.625 mg orally each day. (Note: combination regimens for concomitant continuous or cyclical medroxyprogesterone are available.)

Estropipate: 0.75 mg orally each day.

Esterified estrogens: 0.3 mg orally each day.

Etidronate Disodium (Didronel)
Action
Bisphosphonate compound that inhibits either osteoclast or osteoblast activity and diminishes bone resorption and new bone formation.

Selected Indications
Osteoporosis prevention and treatment, Paget's disease of bone.

Metabolism
Adsorbed to developing apatite crystals during bone formation. Excreted unchanged by the kidneys.

Adverse Reactions
Defective mineralization of bone with accumulation of unmineralized osteoid, and possible onset of new bone pain and pathologic fractures. Mild abdominal cramps, nausea, and diarrhea are common.

Caution
Patients with renal insufficiency should be treated cautiously. Like other bisphosphonates, etidronate is contraindicated in women of childbearing potential.

Supply
Tablets, 200 mg.

Dosage
For Paget's disease, 400 mg daily given as a single dose 2 hours before meals. Reassessment is indicated after 6 months of therapy. Dosages above 10 mg/kg daily should be used cautiously and reserved for suppression of rapid bone turnover or for prompt reduction in elevated cardiac output. For treatment of postmenopausal osteoporosis, the dosage is 400 mg of etidronate daily (2 hours before or after a meal) for 14 days every 3 months.

Fluoride, Sodium

Action
Incorporated into bone, rendering it less soluble. Stimulates new bone formation.

Selected Indications
Osteoporosis prevention and treatment.

Metabolism
Absorbed from gastrointestinal tract and incorporated into bone.

Adverse Reactions
Occasional gastrointestinal upset. Fluorosis, caused by chronic overexposure to fluoride, results in mottling of teeth and formation of thickened bones with poor mechanical quality (osteomalacia and osteosclerosis). Excessive doses, therefore, may result in an increased risk for fractures despite apparent improvement in bone density.

Caution
To prevent precipitation of calcium fluoride, calcium supplements and sodium fluoride are given at separate times of the day. Fluoride supplements should not be given to patients with renal insufficiency.

Supply
Tablets, 1 mg. Larger capsules and oral solution are also available in some pharmacies.

Dosage
The dosage is 10 mg of elemental fluoride twice daily.

Pamidronate (Aredia)

Action
Bisphosphonate that inhibits osteoclast activity.

Selected Indications
Hypercalcemia associated with malignancies, Paget's disease of bone.

Metabolism
After IV administration, pamidronate is immediately retained in bone, preferentially in areas of high turnover. The drug is then slowly cleared by the kidney, with a terminal half-life of about 300 days.

Adverse Reactions
Most adverse effects appear to be dose-related. These include fatigue, somnolence, reactions at the infusion site, anorexia, nausea, gastrointestinal hemorrhage, and electrolyte abnormalities (hypocalcemia, hypokalemia, hypomagnesemia, hypophosphatemia). Cardiopulmonary effects such as hypertension, atrial fibrillation, tachycardia, syncope,

and rales may occur with the highest doses. Fever occurs in about one-fifth of patients. Cytopenias may occur rarely.

Caution
Serum electrolytes should be followed closely. In patients with preexisting hematologic conditions, complete blood cell counts should also be followed. Pamidronate should not be given to women of childbearing potential.

Supply
Vials of lyophilized powder, 30 mg, 60 mg, and 90 mg, for reconstitution with sterile water.

Dosage
For Paget's disease, 30 mg daily IV given over 4 hours for 3 days. Higher doses are recommended for hypercalcemia associated with malignancies.

Raloxifene (Evista)
Action
Raloxifene, a benzothiophene compound, is a selective estrogen receptor modulator. It has estrogen agonist activity on bone and antagonist activity on breast and uterine tissue. Its anti-osteoporotic effects are probably a consequence of inhibition of osteoclast activity.

Metabolism
Sixty percent of ingested drug is absorbed. It is glucuronidated on first pass in the liver and excreted almost entirely in the feces. Its half-life is about 27 hours.

Adverse Reactions
Hot flashes and leg cramps occur. As with other estrogens, there is an increased risk for venous thromboembolism.

Caution
Men and premenopausal women are not candidates for raloxifene therapy. The drug is contraindicated in patients with histories of thromboembolic disease and in patients with known hypersensitivity to the drug or components of the tablets. Cholestyramine causes a 60% reduction in absorption and should not be administered together with raloxifene. Risks for breast and gynecologic malignancies have not been adequately studied.

Supply
Tablets, 60 mg.

Dosage
The dosage is 60 mg daily.

Risedronate (Actonel)
Action
Bisphosphonate that inhibits osteoclast activity and bone resorption but does not interfere with bone mineralization.

Selected Indications
Paget's disease of bone.

Metabolism
Risedronate is poorly absorbed by the gastrointestinal tract, especially when taken with food. Fasting absorption is less than 1%. Calcium-, aluminum-, and magnesium-containing supplements and antacids interfere with absorption. Absorbed drug is tropic for bone and will persist within the bony skeleton for years. Excretion is in the urine.

Adverse Reactions
Gastrointestinal intolerances are the most common adverse effects and include diarrhea, nausea, abdominal pain, and esophagitis. About a third of patients may experience arthralgias. Adequate calcium repletion before the initiation of therapy may reduce the risk for musculoskeletal discomfort.

Caution
Risedronate must be taken on an empty stomach, while upright, at least one-half hour before eating. Risedronate is contraindicated in women of childbearing potential.

Supply
Tablets, 30 mg.

Dosage
The dosage is 30 mg daily. For Paget's disease, reassessment is indicated after 2 months of therapy.

Tiludronate (Skelid)
Action
Bisphosphonate that inhibits osteoclast activity and bone resorption but does not interfere with bone mineralization.

Selected Indications
Paget's disease of bone.

Metabolism
Tiludronate is poorly absorbed by the gastrointestinal tract, especially when taken with food. Calcium-, aluminum-, and magnesium-containing supplements and antacids interfere with absorption. Absorbed drug is tropic for bone and will persist within the bony skeleton for years. The drug is not metabolized and is excreted in the urine.

Adverse Reactions
Gastrointestinal intolerances are the most common adverse effects and include diarrhea, nausea, and abdominal pain, but esophagitis and esophageal ulcerations have not been reported.

Caution
Tiludronate must be taken on an empty stomach, while upright, at least 2 hours before eating. Tiludronate is contraindicated in women of childbearing potential.

Supply
Tablets, 200 mg.

Dosage
The dosage is 400 mg daily. For Paget's disease, reassessment is indicated after 3 months of therapy.

Vitamin D
Action
Family of sterol derivatives that increase intestinal absorption of calcium and may increase mobilization of mineral from bone.

Selected Indications
Prevention and treatment of postmenopausal osteoporosis, prevention of drug-induced osteoporosis, osteomalacia, rickets, hypoparathyroidism, hypocalcemia, and renal osteodystrophy.

Metabolism
The activation of vitamin D is effected via sequential hepatic and renal hydroxylation. The metabolites of vitamin D are mostly excreted in bile.

Adverse Reactions
Vitamin D toxicity may produce elevated serum calcium and phosphorus levels, causing drowsiness, gastrointestinal symptoms, metastatic calcifications, renal failure, and hypertension.

Caution
Administration of exogenous calcium may also be necessary for desired effects of vitamin D therapy. Monthly monitoring of serum and urinary calcium to avoid manifestations of vitamin D toxicity is recommended. If urinary calcium rises above 120 mg/d, the dosage of vitamin D should be reduced.

Supply
Many options are available, including the following:
Vitamin D_3, 200 to 400 IU (contained in many multivitamin preparations).
Ergocalciferol (vitamin D_2), 25,000 and 50,000 IU.
Calcitriol capsules, 0.25 and 0.5 μg.
Calcifediol capsules, 20 and 50 μg.
Dihydrotachysterol tablets, 0.125, 0.2, and 0.4 μg.

Dosage
Postmenopausal osteoporosis: at least 400 IU of vitamin D_3 daily.
Prevention of drug-induced osteoporosis: 400 IU of vitamin D_3 twice daily.
The appropriate agent and dosing for other conditions should be adjusted on a clinical basis.

ANTICOAGULANTS

Indications for the use of anticoagulation have grown. In rheumatology specifically, some situations in which anticoagulants are widely utilized include primary treatment in the anti-phospholipid syndrome and other hypercoagulable states, adjuvant therapy in Raynaud's phenomenon and other low-flow states, and prophylaxis against deep venous thrombosis. Warfarin and heparins/heparinoids remain the primary agents currently available.

The major recent advances have been in the development and use of preparations of low-molecular-weight heparin, which appears to be as effective as traditional, unfractionated heparin and also safer and easier to use. All heparins act by enhancing the activity of antithrombin III, which neutralizes thrombin and factor Xa. Three preparations of low-molecular-weight heparin (ardeparin, dalteparin, enoxeparin) are currently available in the United States. They are all depolymerized heparins, but they differ in the degradation process by which they are obtained. An additional agent, danaparoid, is considered to be a low-molecular-weight *heparinoid;* it too enhances antithrombin III. One major difficulty in the current use of these preparations is the lack of standardization of activity. The drugs are not interchangeable on a milligram-for-milligram basis, and even attempts to standardize according to biochemical activity (e.g., anti-factor Xa activity) have been unsatisfactory. *At present, the only approved indication for the low-molecular weight heparins and danaparoid is prophylaxis of deep venous thrombosis. However, many studies have already shown that when administered at higher doses, these compounds are also effective in the treatment of acute deep venous thrombosis.*

Although these low-molecular-weight heparins/heparinoids are effective in a twice-daily regimen via the SC route and do not require monitoring of prothrombin times (PT) or partial thromboplastin times (PTT), physicians must appreciate that when they are used at therapeutic doses, they do induce full anticoagulation. Thus, as with IV heparin, significant risks for hemorrhage do exist.

Ardeparin (Normiflo)

Action
Ardeparin is a partially depolymerized heparin prepared by peroxide degradation of porcine intestinal heparin. It potentiates antithrombin III activity.

Selected Indications
Prophylaxis of deep venous thrombosis, hypercoagulable states.

Metabolism
The metabolic fate of ardeparin is not fully known. Most is probably removed by the reticuloendothelial system and by vascular endothelium. A small amount may be excreted in urine.

Adverse Reactions
Hematoma at injection sites is the most common adverse effect. Hemorrhage, although much less frequent than with unfractionated heparin, is still a concern. Hematomas at the site of epidural or spinal anesthesias may result in potentially devastating neurologic compromise, including permanent paralysis. Allergic reactions and skin necrosis are rare. Thrombocytopenia is much less common than with unfractionated heparin.

Caution
Monitoring of PT or PTT is not necessary. Use in patients with underlying thrombocytopenia or another potential bleeding diathesis should be monitored especially closely. Use in the setting of epidural or spinal anesthesia must be carefully considered. Ardeparin is contraindicated in patients with active hemorrhaging or in those with allergies to porcine products. It should not be administered IM.

Supply
Prefilled Tubex syringes, 5,000 U/0.5 mL and 10,000 U/0.5 mL.

Dosage
For deep venous thrombosis prophylaxis, 50 U/kg of body weight injected SC twice daily.

Dalteparin (Fragmin)
Action
Dalteparin is a depolymerized heparin prepared by nitrous acid degradation of porcine intestinal heparin. It potentiates antithrombin III activity.

Selected Indications
Prophylaxis of deep venous thrombosis, hypercoagulable states.

Metabolism
The metabolic fate of dalteparin is not fully known. Most is probably removed by the reticuloendothelial system and by vascular endothelium. A small amount may be excreted in urine.

Adverse Reactions
Hematoma at injection sites is the most common adverse effect. Hemorrhage, although much less frequent than with unfractionated heparin, is still a concern. Hematomas at the site of epidural or spinal anesthesias may result in potentially devastating neurologic compromise, including permanent paralysis. Allergic reactions and skin necrosis are rare. Thrombocytopenia is much less common than with unfractionated heparin.

Caution
Monitoring of PT or PTT is not necessary. Use in patients with underlying thrombocytopenia or another potential bleeding diathesis should be monitored especially closely. Use in the setting of epidural or spinal anesthesia must be carefully considered. Dalteparin is contraindicated in patients with active hemorrhaging and in those with allergies to porcine products. It should not be administered IM.

Supply
Disposable prefilled syringes, 2,500 anti-factor Xa U/0.2 mL and 5,000 anti-factor Xa U/0.5 mL.

Dosage
For deep venous thrombosis prophylaxis, 2,500 to 5,000 U of anti-factor Xa injected SC twice daily.

Danaparoid (Orgoran)

Action

Danaparoid is a depolymerized glycosaminoglycan isolated from porcine intestinal mucosa through a process that specifically excludes heparin and heparin fragments. It potentiates antithrombin III activity.

Selected Indications

Prophylaxis of deep venous thrombosis, hypercoagulable states.

Metabolism

The metabolic fate of danaparoid is not fully known. Most is probably removed by the reticuloendothelial system and by vascular endothelium. A small amount may be excreted in urine.

Adverse Reactions

Hematoma at injection sites is the most common adverse effect. Hemorrhage, although much less frequent than with unfractionated heparin, is still a concern. Hematomas at the site of epidural or spinal anesthesias may result in potentially devastating neurologic compromise, including permanent paralysis. Allergic reactions and skin necrosis are rare.

Caution

Monitoring of PT or PTT is not necessary. Use in patients with underlying thrombocytopenia or other potential bleeding diathesis should be monitored especially closely. Use in the setting of epidural or spinal anesthesia must be carefully considered. Danaparoid is contraindicated in patients with active hemorrhaging and in those with allergies to porcine products. Patients with sulfite sensitivity may also not be good candidates for danaparoid use. It should not be administered IM.

Supply

Disposable prefilled syringes, 750 anti-factor Xa U/0.6 mL.

Dosage

For deep venous thrombosis prophylaxis, 750 U of anti-factor Xa injected SC twice daily.

Enoxeparin (Lovenox)

Action

Enoxeparin is a depolymerized heparin prepared by alkaline degradation of porcine intestinal heparin. It potentiates antithrombin III activity.

Selected Indications

Prophylaxis of deep venous thrombosis, hypercoagulable states.

Metabolism

The metabolic fate of enoxeparin is not fully known. Most is probably removed by the reticuloendothelial system and by vascular endothelium. A small amount may be excreted in urine.

Adverse Reactions

Hematoma at injection sites is the most common adverse effect. Hemorrhage, although much less frequent than with unfractionated heparin, is still a concern. Hematomas at the site of epidural or spinal anesthesias may result in potentially devastating neurologic compromise, including permanent paralysis. Allergic reactions and skin necrosis are rare. Thrombocycotpenia is much less common than with unfractionated heparin.

Caution

Monitoring of PT or PTT is not necessary. Use in patients with underlying thrombocytopenia or other potential bleeding diathesis should be monitored especially closely. Use in the setting of epidural or spinal anesthesia must be carefully considered. Enoxeparin is contraindicated in patients with active hemorrhaging and in those with allergies to porcine products. It should not be administered IM.

Supply
Disposable prefilled syringes, 30 mg/0.3 mL.

Dosage
For deep venous thrombosis prophylaxis, 30 mg injected SC twice daily.

Heparin, Unfractionated
Action
Heparin is a heterogeneous mixture of anionic sulfated glycosaminoglycans, usually extracted from porcine intestinal mucosa or bovine lung. It potentiates antithrombin III activity.

Selected Indications
Prophylaxis and treatment of deep venous thrombosis, hypercoagulable states.

Metabolism
The metabolic fate of heparin is not fully known. Most is probably removed by the reticuloendothelial system and by vascular endothelium. A small amount may be excreted in urine.

Adverse Reactions
Hemorrhage and hematomas are the most common adverse effect. Hematomas at the site of epidural or spinal anesthesias may result in potentially devastating neurologic compromise, including permanent paralysis. Thrombocytopenia may occur in 15% of patients treated with bovine heparin and in 5% of patients treated with porcine heparin. Two reversible mechanisms of thrombocytopenia are identified, both of which are idiosyncratic and not dose-dependent: (a) a direct, non-immunologic effect and (b) a heparin-dependent IgG platelet-aggregating phenomenon. Rarely, a paradoxical thrombogenic "white clot" syndrome may occur with local or systemic manifestations. Prolonged heparin use may cause osteoporosis.

Caution
Although the PTT is most sensitive to heparin and is used for dose adjustment, the prothrombin time/international normalization ratio (PT/INR) may also be affected, especially at high dosages. Baseline values of PTT and PT/INR should be obtained before continuous IV therapy is instituted. Use in patients with underlying thrombocytopenia or other potential bleeding diathesis should be monitored especially closely. Use in the setting of epidural or spinal anesthesia must be carefully considered. Heparin is contraindicated in patients with active hemorrhaging and in those with allergies to porcine or bovine products. It should not be administered IM. Reversal of hemorrhagic complications may require protamine sulfate.

Supply
Bovine lung:

Vials, 1,000, 5,000, and 10,000 U/mL for SC injection.

Porcine intestine:

Vials, 10, 20, 25, 30, 50, 100, 300, 1,000, 2,500, 5,000, 7,500, 10,000, and 20,000 U/mL for SC injection.

In 5% dextrose, 40, 50, and 100 U/mL for IV administration.

In normal saline solution, 2, 50, and 100 U/mL for IV administration.

Dosage
General guidelines for deep venous thrombosis prophylaxis: 5,000 to 7,500 U injected SC twice daily. Adjustments may be necessary as clinically indicated.

General guidelines for full-dose continuous IV use: loading dose of 50 to 100 U/kg of body weight, followed by continuous infusion of 10 to 15 U/kg of body weight per hour.

Repeat bolus and/or readjust infusion rate to desired PTT initially every 6 hours and then daily after stable dose is achieved. Adjustments may be necessary as clinically indicated.

Warfarin Sodium (Coumadin)
Action
Warfarin indirectly alters the synthesis of functional coagulation factors by interfering with vitamin K activity, which is required for τ-carboxylation of factors II, VII, IX, and X.

Selected Indications
Prophylaxis and treatment of deep venous thrombosis, hypercoagulable states, and anti-phospholipid syndrome, and care after cerebrovascular accident.

Metabolism
Warfarin is generally well absorbed by the gastrointestinal tract, but the rate of absorption can be highly dependent on individual variability and the commercial source of the drug. Although peak levels of warfarin occur within hours after ingestion, its antithrombogenic activity does not depend on plasma levels but rather on levels of vitamin K-dependent factors, which may not be affected until at least 2 days after administration. IV administration of warfarin does not hasten the onset of activity. The effects of warfarin may be potentiated or diminished by innumerable foods and medications, all of which should be taken into careful consideration during treatment. Warfarin is inactivated in the liver, and the metabolites are excreted in urine.

Adverse Reactions
Hemorrhage is the most common adverse effect of warfarin. Potentially fatal necrosis of the skin or other tissue is a rare complication, most commonly seen in patients with defects or deficiencies in the antithrombotic factors protein C or protein S. This is usually seen early after initiation of therapy and is thought to be caused the rapid depletion of the vitamin K-dependent protein C, which results in a transient prothrombotic state. Another rare complication is cholesterol microembolization syndrome, which can result in systemic microvascular ischemia. Although the PT/INR is most sensitive to warfarin, the PTT can also be elevated at high doses.

Caution
Close monitoring of the PT/INR is required for appropriate dosing of warfarin, especially at the start of therapy or when changes in concurrent medications are made. Familiarity with drugs that may enhance or reduce the anticoagulant effects of warfarin is advised. Warfarin is contraindicated during pregnancy and in nursing women. IM injections should not be given to patients in an anticoagulated state. Patients with anti-phospholipid syndrome present an additional problem in that circulating antibodies may cause artifacts in the INR, which makes monitoring of anticoagulation difficult.

Supply
Tablets, 1, 2, 2.5, 4, 5, 7.5, and 10 mg.
Injectable solution, 5 mg.

Dosage
Daily dosing as dictated by desired INR. For most indications (e.g., treatment of deep venous thrombosis, atrial fibrillation), an INR of 2.0 to 3.0 is generally recommended. For patients with mechanical heart valves, an INR of 2.5 to 3.5 should be maintained. Patients with anti-phospholipid syndrome may require an INR of 3.0 to 4.0 or higher.

VASOACTIVE AGENTS
Vasoactive agents are useful in the management of systemic and pulmonary hypertension, Raynaud's phenomenon, and congestive heart failure. Vascular tone may be relaxed by (a) inhibition of sympathetic function (e.g., prazocin), (b) direct relaxation of smooth muscle (e.g., hydralazine), (c) calcium channel blockade (e.g., amlodipine,

diltiazem, nifedipine, verapamil), and (d) inhibition of ACE (e.g., captopril, enalapril). The use of ACE inhibitors, in particular, has drastically changed the outcome in diffuse systemic sclerosis. Included below is a small sampling of available agents.

Amlodipine (Norvasc)

Action

Calcium channel blocker that dilates coronary and peripheral arteries and arterioles.

Selected Indications

Hypertension, Raynaud's phenomenon.

Metabolism

Dose adjustment is not generally necessary in the setting of renal insufficiency. However, elimination can be reduced in the setting of hepatic impairment and in geriatric patients.

Adverse Reactions

Hypotension, bradycardia, dizziness, headache, congestive heart failure, pedal edema, nausea, and rash may occur. In Raynaud's phenomenon, all vasodilators may precipitate a vascular steal syndrome.

Caution

Avoid in patients with sick sinus syndrome, atrioventricular conduction disturbances, severe congestive heart failure, or hypotension (systolic blood pressure <90 mm Hg).

Supply

Tablets, 2.5, 5, and 10 mg.

Dosage

Initially, 2.5 mg daily.

Captopril (Capoten)

Action

ACE inhibitor that reduces peripheral vascular resistance and venous tone.

Selected Indications

Hypertension, treatment of scleroderma renal crisis, proteinuria.

Metabolism

Rapid oral absorption with peak blood levels at 1 hour. Captopril should be taken 1 hour before meals, as food reduces absorption. The drug is 25% to 30% protein-bound. Excretion is in urine.

Adverse Reactions

Rash occurs in 10%, dysgeusia in 7%, proteinuria in 2%, orthostatic hypotension in 2%, proteinuria in 1% to 2%, angioedema in 1%, cough in 0.5% to 2%, neutropenia in 0.3%, and renal failure in 0.1%. Gastric irritation and fever have been reported. Chronic cough may result in discontinuation of all ACE inhibitors.

Caution

Severe hypotension may be seen in salt-or volume-depleted patients, such as those on diuretics. Patients with congestive heart failure may have elevations in blood urea nitrogen and serum creatinine. Neutropenia with myeloid hypoplasia occurs mainly in patients with SLE or other autoimmune diseases. Complete blood cell count, urinalysis, and renal (especially serum potassium and creatinine) parameters should be checked frequently. Renal function and electrolyte abnormalities in patients with SLE in particular should be watched closely. The dosage should be decreased in patients with renal dysfunction.

Supply
Tablets, 12.5, 25, 50, and 100 mg.

Dosage
Initial dose is 12.5 mg three times daily, then 25 mg three times daily. After 1 to 2 weeks, the dosage may be increased to 50 mg three times daily, then at 1- to 2-week intervals to a maximum of 150 mg three times daily.

Diltiazem (Cardizem)
Action
Calcium channel blocker that dilates coronary and peripheral arteries and arterioles.

Selected Indications
Hypertension, Raynaud's phenomenon.

Metabolism
Diltiazem is absorbed with peak level in 3 hours and a half-life of 4 hours. It is 80% protein-bound. There is extensive hepatic metabolism.

Adverse Reactions
Hypotension, bradycardia, dizziness, headache, congestive heart failure, pedal edema, nausea, and rash may occur. In Raynaud's phenomenon, all vasodilators may precipitate a vascular steal syndrome.

Caution
Avoid in patients with sick sinus syndrome, atrioventricular conduction disturbances, severe congestive heart failure, or hypotension (systolic blood pressure <90 mm Hg). Diltiazem should not be used with cyclosporin A. There are data suggesting that extended-release forms may be safer than rapid-release preparations.

Supply
Tablets, 30, 60, 90, and 120 mg.
Extended-release capsules, 120 mg, 180 mg, 240 mg, and 300 mg.

Dosage
Initially 120 mg daily in single or divided doses. Can be increased as tolerated to 480 mg daily in single or divided doses.

Enalapril/Enalaprilat (Vasotec)
Action
ACE inhibitors that reduce peripheral vascular resistance and venous tone.

Selected Indications
Hypertension, treatment of scleroderma renal crisis, proteinuria.

Metabolism
Enalapril is the ethyl ester of enalaprilat. The gastrointestinal absorption of enalapril is good (about 55% to 75%) and does not appear to be affected by foods. In contrast, enalaprilat is poorly absorbed and is administered IV. Enalapril is a pro-drug that is activated by hepatic hydrolysis. Two-thirds of the drug and its metabolites are excreted in urine, and the remainder is eliminated in feces.

Adverse Reactions
Fewer than 5% of patients discontinue enalapril for adverse effects. These may include neurologic complaints (dizziness, vertigo), postural hypotension, deterioration of renal function, hypersensitivity reactions, leukopenia, dysgeusia, hyperkalemia, and chronic cough.

Caution
Severe hypotension may be seen in salt-or volume-depleted patients, such as those on diuretics. Patients with congestive heart failure may have elevations in blood urea nitrogen and serum creatinine. Complete blood cell count, urinalysis, and renal (especially serum potassium and creatinine) parameters should be checked frequently. Renal function and electrolyte abnormalities in patients with SLE in particular should be watched closely. Conversion between IV and oral dosing requires careful attention.

Supply
Enalapril tablets, 2.5, 5, 10, and 20 mg.
Enalaprilat injectable solution for IV use, 1.25 mg/mL.

Dosage
The initial dose of enalapril is 2.5 mg daily; the maximum is generally 40 mg daily in once- or twice-daily dosing. The initial dose of enalaprilat is 1.25 mg every 6 hours, which can be raised to 5 mg every 6 hours as indicated.

Nifedipine (Procardia, Adalat)
Action
Calcium channel blocker. Coronary and peripheral arterial vasodilation.

Selected Indications
Hypertension, Raynaud's phenomenon.

Metabolism
Well absorbed, with peak levels in 1 to 2 hours. Highly protein-bound. Completely metabolized in liver before excreted in urine.

Adverse Reactions
Hypotension, dizziness, headache, tachycardia, fatigue, edema, flushing, nausea, nasal congestion, and leg cramps have been noted. In Raynaud's phenomenon, all vasodilators may precipitate a vascular steal syndrome.

Caution
Close monitoring of blood pressure is recommended. There are data suggesting that extended-release forms of calcium channel blockers may be safer than rapid-release preparations.

Supply
Capsules, 10 and 20 mg.
Extended-release tablets, 30, 60, and 90 mg.

Dosage
Initially 30 mg daily in single or divided doses, which can be raised to 90 mg daily.

Prazocin (Minipress)
Action
Arterial and venous dilator that may act via α-adrenergic receptor blockade.

Selected Indications
Hypertension, Raynaud's phenomenon.

Metabolism
Peak plasma levels in 3 hours with half-life of 2 1/2 hours. It is highly protein-bound and extensively metabolized in the liver.

Adverse Reactions
Orthostatic hypotension, syncope, peripheral edema, fatigue, headache, dizziness, and nausea may occur. Rarely, urinary frequency, impotence, rash, and nasal congestion have been noted.

Caution
Symptomatic orthostatic hypotension with syncope may occur after the first dose. Therefore, the first dose should not exceed 1 mg and should be given at bedtime with instructions for the patient to remain in bed at least 3 hours. The dosage may be increased to 1 mg twice daily, then three times daily, with further gradual increments. Tolerance to hemodynamic effects may develop during long-term treatment.

Supply
Capsules, 1, 2, and 5 mg.

Dosage
The dosage is 1 mg three times daily, gradually increased to 20 mg/d in divided doses.

Verapamil (Calan, Covera, Isoptin, Verelan)
Action
Calcium channel blocker that reduces coronary and peripheral vascular resistance.

Selected Indications
Hypertension, Raynaud's phenomenon.

Metabolism
Excellent oral absorption with peak levels in 1 to 2 hours. It is 90% protein-bound. Half-life is 3 to 6 hours, with marked prolongation in patients with hepatic dysfunction. Extensive metabolism in the liver and excretion of active metabolites in urine.

Adverse Reactions
Hypotension, peripheral edema, bradycardia, heart block, congestive heart failure, headaches, dizziness, constipation, and abnormal serum liver chemistries may occur. In Raynaud's phenomenon, all vasodilators may precipitate a vascular steal syndrome.

Caution
Verapamil increases digoxin levels by 50% to 70%. It should be avoided in patients with sick sinus syndrome, severe congestive heart failure, or hepatic or renal impairment. There are data suggesting that extended-release forms of calcium channel blockers may be safer than rapid-release preparations.

Supply
Tablets, 40, 80, and 120 mg.
Extended-release tablets, 120, 180, and 240 mg.

Dosage
Initially 120 mg daily in single or divided dose; can be increased up to 480 mg daily.

SUPPLEMENTS AND MISCELLANEOUS

Chondroitin Sulfate/Glucosamine Sulfate
In the United States, chondroitin sulfate and glucosamine sulfate are regarded as nutritional supplements rather than as medicines and so have not been as rigorously studied for metabolism, efficacy, and toxicity.

Selected Indications
Osteoarthritis.

Action
Usually taken together, these agents are thought possibly to maintain synovial joint integrity by optimizing synthesis of collagen and glycosaminoglycans, stimulating hyaluronic acid secretion by chondrocytes, and inhibiting degradative enzymes.

Metabolism
Both agents are absorbed in the gastrointestinal tract. At least some of the compounds can then be traced to synovial joints.

Adverse Reactions
Mild gastrointestinal intolerances such as bloating and flatus are common but generally do not result in discontinuation.

Caution
No data are available on effects on fertility, pregnancy, or lactation.

Supply
Glucosamine sulfate, capsules and tablets, 500 mg.
Chondroitin sulfate, capsules and tablets, 400 mg.
Also available in combined forms.

Dosage
Glucosamine sulfate, 1,500 to 2,000 mg daily in divided doses.
Chondroitin sulfate, 1,200 to 1,600 mg daily in divided doses.

Cisapride (Propulsid)
Action
Cisapride is thought to enhance the release of acetylcholine at the myenteric plexus, thus promoting peristalsis.

Selected Indications
Gastrointestinal dysmotility, systemic sclerosis.

Metabolism
Cisapride is rapidly absorbed via the gastrointestinal tract, and peak plasma levels are reached within 2 hours. Gastrointestinal absorption is enhanced by concomitant administration of cimetidine and ranitidine. The mean half-life is between 6 and 12 hours. It is metabolized by the cytochrome P-450 3A4 enzyme. Its metabolites are excreted in both feces and urine. Although hepatic or renal impairment may cause accumulation of metabolites within plasma, no dose adjustments are generally necessary.

Adverse Reactions
Headache, sedation, nausea, and diarrhea are the most commonly reported adverse effects. These problems appear to be dose-dependent.

Caution
Rare cases of serious cardiac arrhythmias, including ventricular arrhythmias and *torsades de pointes,* have been reported; therefore, the use of cisapride in patients with conditions associated with QT prolongation should be avoided. Concomitant administration of drugs that inhibit cytochrome P-450 3A4 activity (e.g., ketoconazole, itraconazole, micronazole, erythromycin, and troleandomycin) may raise cisapride levels to cause prolongation of the QT interval and so is contraindicated. Cisapride may enhance the effects of sedatives.

Supply
Tablets, 10 and 20 mg.

Dosage
The dosage is 10 to 20 mg up to four times daily, taken orally 15 to 30 minutes before meals.

Hyaluronans (Hyalgan, Synvisc)
Action
Increases viscoelasticity of synovial fluid and possibly reduces cartilage degradation.

Selected Indications
Osteoarthritis.

Metabolism
High-molecular-weight fractions of sodium hyaluronate for sterile intraarticular injection are derived from chicken combs and are available in a buffered physiologic sodium chloride solution. The intraarticular half-life of sodium hyaluronate is less than 24 hours. Hylan G-F is a cross-linked derivative of sodium hyaluronate and appears to have a longer half-life. Hyaluronans are degraded by intraarticular enzymes, free radicals, and sheer forces. The degradation products are removed through lymphatics and undergo hepatic catabolism.

Adverse Reactions
Most adverse effects are related to symptoms associated with the site of injection, including pain, swelling, effusion, warmth, and redness. Some of these cases are exacerbations of gout or pseudogout. Self-limited allergic reactions have been reported.

Caution
At present, hyaluronans are approved only for osteoarthritis of the knee. Increases in knee inflammation after administration in the setting of inflammatory arthritides (e.g., RA and gout) have been noted. Because the source of the agent is rooster combs, precaution should be taken in patients with allergies to avian proteins, feathers, and egg products. Strict sterile technique is to be observed, and no injection should be attempted through skin that appears infected. Disinfectants containing quarternary ammonium salts should not be used for skin preparation.

Supply
Sodium hyaluronate (Hyalgan), sterile 2-mL vials.

Hylan G-F 20 (Synvisc), sterile 2-mL prefilled syringes.

Dosage
Sodium hyaluronate, 2 mL administered weekly by intraarticular injections during 5 weeks.

Hylan G-F 20, 2 mL administered weekly by intraarticular injections during 3 weeks.

Lansoprazole (Prevacid)

Action
Lansoprazole is a substituted benzimidazole that specifically inhibits the proton pump system on the secretory surface of the gastric parietal cell.

Selected Indications
Gastroesophageal reflux, gastroprotection against NSAIDs, systemic sclerosis.

Metabolism
Absorption of lansoprazole occurs after the drug leaves the stomach and is diminished when the drug is taken after eating. Lansoprazole is transformed into two active metabolites that act locally at the parietal cell, and so plasma levels do not reflect activity at the gastric mucosa. The drug is extensively metabolized by the liver, and its metabolites are excreted in both feces (67%) and urine (33%). Dose adjustment should be considered in patients with hepatic impairment.

Adverse Reactions
Lansoprazole is generally well tolerated. Minor reported adverse effects include gastrointestinal intolerance, diarrhea, nausea, vomiting, headache, dizziness, and rashes.

Caution
Lansoprazole may increase clearance of theophylline. It may also interfere with absorption of drugs (such as ketoconazole, ampicillin esters, and digoxin) for which gastric pH is an important determinant of bioavailability.

Supply
Delayed-release capsules, 15 and 30 mg.

Dosage
The dosage is 15 to 30 mg daily.

Lyme Disease Vaccine (LYMErix)
Action
Lyme disease vaccine is a recombinant form of the 257-amino acid outer surface protein A (Osp A) of *Borrelia burgdorferi,* the spirochete that causes Lyme disease. Immunoglobulins stimulated by the vaccine are thought to prevent infection via interaction with the bacterium, either within the human host or possibly within the tick vector after uptake of antibody into its midgut during a blood meal.

Selected Indications
Prevention of Lyme disease.

Metabolism
Optimal vaccination requires at least three doses during a 1-year period.

Adverse Reactions
Most adverse reactions usually occur within the first month after immunization. These include pain or local reaction at the injection site, myalgias, chills, rigors, fever, rash and influenza-like symptoms.

Caution
Patients with histories of hypersensitivity reactions to any components of the vaccine or to natural rubber should not receive the vaccine. Persons receiving immunosuppression therapy may not mount an optimal immune response. Only IM administration should be used, and so anticoagulation therapy is a relative contraindication. An association of unclear significance has been observed between antibiotic-resistant Lyme arthritis and immune reactivity to Osp A; accordingly, Lyme disease vaccination is not currently recommended in such patients.

Supply
Single-dose vials and prefilled syringes, 30 μg/0.5 mL.

Dosage
Three IM injections of 30 μg at 0, 1, and 12 months.

Metoclopramide (Reglan)
Action
Metoclopramide stimulates upper gastrointestinal peristalsis without stimulating gastric, biliary, or pancreatic secretions, possibly by sensitizing tissue to the effects of acetylcholine.

Selected Indications
Gastrointestinal dysmotility, systemic sclerosis.

Metabolism
Metoclopramide is rapidly absorbed via the gastrointestinal tract, and peak plasma levels are reached within 2 hours. The mean half-life is about 6 hours. It is partially metabolized by hepatic conjugation and is excreted primarily in urine. Patients with renal impairment may require dose adjustment.

Adverse Reactions
Central nervous system effects, including sedation, headache, restlessness, and cognitive or affective changes, may occur in more than 10% of patients. Extrapyramidal reactions, including acute dystonic reactions, akathisia, parkinsonian symptoms, and tardive dyskinesia, may occur.

Caution
Metoclopramide should not be used in patients with poorly controlled hypertension or in patients with pheochromocytoma. It is also contraindicated when acceleration of gastrointestinal motility is not desired, as in patients with acute hemorrhages. Patients at risk for extrapyramidal symptoms should not receive metoclopramide.

Supply
Tablets, 5 and 10 mg.
Syrup, 1 mg/mL.
Injectable, 5 mg/mL in 2-, 10-, and 30-mL vials.

Dosage
The dosage is 10 to 20 mg up to four times daily, taken orally 15 to 30 minutes before meals. A dose of 10 mg may be administered parenterally (either IM or IV) during 1 to 2 minutes.

Misoprostol (Cytotec)
Action
Misoprostol is a synthetic analog of prostaglandin E_1 with protective properties against gastric inflammation and ulceration induced by NSAIDs.

Selected Indications
Gastroprotection against NSAIDs.

Metabolism
Absorption of misoprostol is rapid but is diminished by food or antacids. It is converted into its active form via de-esterification. Most of the drug is excreted in urine, but dose adjustment is generally not necessary in the setting of renal impairment.

Adverse Reactions
Abdominal discomfort, flatulence, and diarrhea are commonly reported. Gynecologic symptoms, including spotting, cramps, hypermenorrhea, and dysmenorrhea, may also occur. Postmenopausal vaginal bleeding requires thorough evaluation.

Caution
Misoprostol has abortifacient properties and is contraindicated in pregnant women. Women of childbearing age must be warned of these properties and must comply with effective contraceptive methods before taking misoprostol.

Supply
Tablets, 100 and 200 μg.

Dosage
The dosage is 200 μg four times daily. It may be reduced to 100 μg four times daily if the higher dose is not tolerated.

Omeprazole (Prilosec)
Action
Omeprazole is a substituted benzimidazole that specifically inhibits the proton pump system on the secretory surface of the gastric parietal cell.

Selected Indications
Gastroesophageal reflux, gastroprotection against NSAIDs, systemic sclerosis.

Metabolism
Omeprazole is absorbed after leaving the stomach. Although the drug is easily absorbed after oral administration, extensive first-pass hepatic metabolism results in an absolute bioavailability of about 30% to 40% of that from an equivalent IV dose. Accordingly, bioavailability increases in persons with chronic liver disease. About three-fourths of the administered drug is excreted in urine, and the remainder is excreted in feces.

Adverse Reactions
Omeprazole is generally well tolerated. Minor reported adverse effects include gastrointestinal intolerance, diarrhea, nausea, vomiting, headache, dizziness, and rashes.

Caution
Omeprazole may interfere with the metabolism and increase plasma levels of warfarin, phenytoin, and diazepam. It may also interfere with absorption of drugs (such as ketoconazole, ampicillin esters, and digoxin) for which gastric pH is an important determinant of bioavailability.

Supply
Delayed-release capsules, 20 and 40 mg.

Dosage
The dosage is 20 to 40 mg daily.

Pilocarpine Hydrochloride (Salagen)
Action
Cholinergic parasympathomimetic agent that increases salivary gland secretions in Sjögren's syndrome.

Selected Indications
Xerostomia.

Metabolism
Peak levels are achieved within 1 hour after oral administration but are delayed with high-fat meals. Pilocarpine does not bind to serum proteins. It is thought to be inactivated at neuronal synapses and in plasma. Pilocarpine and its metabolites are excreted in urine.

Adverse Reactions
At dosages recommended for xerostomia, excessive sweating is the most commonly reported adverse effect, occurring in 40% of patients. Urinary frequency, flushing, and chills can also occur.

Caution
Pilocarpine is contraindicated and should be avoided in patients with underlying cardiovascular disease, in whom transient hemodynamic changes may not be tolerated, and in patients with uncontrolled asthma or chronic obstructive pulmonary disease. It should also not be used when miosis is undesirable. Concomitant use of β-adrenergic antagonists may result in conduction disturbances. Toxicity is caused by exaggeration of parasympathetic and cholinergic effects and may require treatment with atropine and hemodynamic support. Pregnant and nursing women should not be given pilocarpine. Pilocarpine should be avoided in patients with narrow-angle glaucoma.

Supply
Tablets, 5 mg.

Dosage
The dosage is 5 mg four times daily.

Sunscreens
Action
Absorption of ultraviolet (UV) light. Medium-wave (UVB, 280 to 320 nm) light is the major cause of sunburn and probably lupus-related skin reactions. Long-wave light (UVA, 320 to 400 nm) is the major cause of photosensitivity reactions.

Selected Indications
SLE, prevention of sun exposure while on medications.

Metabolism
Topical use only.

Adverse Reactions
Local hypersensitivity reactions to active compounds, vehicle, or both; contact dermatitis; photocontact dermatitis. Sunscreens may prevent cutaneous synthesis of vitamin D, especially in the elderly.

Caution
Patients allergic to thiazides, sulfa drugs, benzocaine, procaine, aniline dyes, and paraphenylenediamine may have allergic reactions to paraaminobenzoic acid (PABA), a common active ingredient. PABA-free preparations are available.

Dosage
Sunscreens are rated by sun protection factor (SPF, 0 to 50). Higher values reflect greater degrees of protection; preparations with an SPF of 30 or greater are recommended. Apply 1 to 2 hours before sun exposure and several times during exposure, especially after sweating or swimming. Reapplication does not extend the period of protection.

F. BASIC RHEUMATOLOGY LIBRARY

Stephen A. Paget and Allan Gibofsky

Textbooks

Canale ST. Campbell's operative orthopedics, 9th ed. St. Louis: Mosby, 1998.
Harris ED. *Rheumatoid arthritis.* Philadelphia: WB Saunders, 1997.
Kelley WN, et al. *Textbook of rheumatology,* 5th ed. Philadelphia: WB Saunders, 1997.
Klippel JH, Dieppe PA. *Rheumatology,* 2nd ed. London: Mosby, 1998.
Koopman WJ. *Arthritis and allied conditions,* 13th ed. Baltimore: Williams & Wilkins, 1997.
Lahita RG. *Systemic lupus erythematosus,* 3rd ed. San Diego: Academic Press, 1999.
Maddison PJ, et al. *Oxford textbook of rheumatology,* 2nd ed. Oxford, 1998.
Wallace DJ, Hahn BH. *Dubois' lupus erythematosus,* 5th ed. Philadelphia: Lea & Febiger, 1997.
Weisman MH, Weinblatt ME. *Treatment of rheumatic diseases.* Philadelphia: WB Saunders, 1995.

References

AHFS 99 Drug Information. Bethesda, MD: American Society of Health-System Pharmacists, 1999.
Physicians' Desk Reference, 53rd ed. Montvale, NJ: Medical Economics Company, 1999.

Journals

Annals of the Rheumatic Diseases. London: British Medical Association.
Arthritis and Rheumatism. Atlanta: American College of Rheumatology.
Bulletin on the Rheumatic Diseases. Atlanta: Arthritis Foundation.
Current Opinion in Rheumatology. Philadelphia: Lippincott Williams & Wilkins.
Journal of Rheumatology. Toronto: Journal of Rheumatology.
Lupus. London: Macmillan.
Rheumatic Disease Clinics of North America. Philadelphia: WB Saunders.
Rheumatology International. Heidelberg, Germany: Springer-Verlag.
Scandinavian Journal of Rheumatology and supplements. Oslo: Scandinavian University Press.
Seminars in Arthritis and Rheumatism. Philadelphia: WB Saunders.

Web Sites

American College of Rheumatology. www.rheumatology.org
Arthritis Foundation. www.arthritis.org

SUBJECT INDEX

Page numbers followed by the letter *f* indicate figures; numbers followed by the letter *t* indicate tables.

N

S